Pharmaceutical Practice

FOURTH EDITION

Edited by

A. J. Winfield BPharm PhD MRPharmS
Formerly Chairman, and Visiting Professor, Department of Pharmacy Practice,
Faculty of Pharmacy, Kuwait University, Kuwait

J. A. Rees BPharm MSc PhD Certificate in Health Promotion
Senior Lecturer, School of Pharmacy and Pharmaceutical Sciences, The University of
Manchester, Manchester, UK

I. Smith BSc(Hons) ClinDip FHEA MRPharmS
Boots Teacher Practitioner, The University of Manchester, Manchester, UK

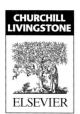

Edinburgh London New York Oxford Philadelphia St Louis Sydney Toronto 2009

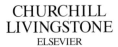

CHURCHILL
LIVINGSTONE
ELSEVIER

Fourth edition 2009
Third edition 2004
Second edition 1998
First edition 1990

ISBN 978-0-443-06906-2
  Reprinted 2010
International edition ISBN 978-0-443-06909-3
  Reprinted 2010

British Library Cataloguing in Publication Data
A catalogue record for this book is available from the British Library

Library of Congress Cataloging in Publication Data
A catalog record for this book is available from the Library of Congress

26179830

Notice
Knowledge and best practice in this field are constantly changing. As new research and experience broaden our knowledge, changes in practice, treatment and drug therapy may become necessary or appropriate. Readers are advised to check the most current information provided (i) on procedures featured or (ii) by the manufacturer of each product to be administered, to verify the recommended dose or formula, the method and duration of administration, and contraindications. It is the responsibility of the practitioner, relying on their own experience and knowledge of the patient, to make diagnoses, to determine dosages and the best treatment for each individual patient, and to take all appropriate safety precautions. To the fullest extent of the law, neither the Publisher nor the Editors assumes any liability for any injury and/or damage to persons or property arising out of or related to any use of the material contained in this book.

The Publisher

Printed in China

Contents

Arthur J. Winfield BPharm PhD MRPharmS
Academic and professional positions held: Senior Lecturer
and Head of Pharmacy Practice, Robert Gordon University,
Aberdeen; First Local Postgraduate Tutor for Scottish
Centre for Postqualification Pharmaceutical Education;
Academic Advisor and External Examiner for new Faculty of
Pharmacy, University of Kuwait and then became first
Chairman of Department of Pharmacy Practice, University
of Kuwait. Following retirement has been Visiting Professor,
Department of Pharmacy Practice, Faculty of Pharmacy,
Kuwait University, Kuwait
21 Routes of administration and dosage forms
26 Pharmaceutical calculations
30 Solutions
31 Suspensions
32 Emulsions
33 External preparations
34 Suppositories and pessaries
35 Powders and granules
36 Oral unit dosage forms
Appendix 2 Latin terms and abbreviations
Appendix 3 Systems of weights and measures

Judith A. Rees BPharm MSc PhD Certificate in Health
Promotion
Academic and professional positions held: Senior Lecturer,
School of Pharmacy and Pharmaceutical Sciences, The
University of Manchester, Manchester; External Examiner
for Pharmacy at University of Bath, Robert Gordon
University, DeMontfort University, Aston University, Kingston
University, University of Hertfordshire, School of Pharmacy,
London, UK
2 Models of pharmacy practice within healthcare systems
13 Communication skills for the pharmacist
25 Dispensing techniques (compounding and good
practice)
28 Labelling of dispensed medicines
43 Storage of medicines and waste disposal
44 Communication skills – role of the pharmacist in giving
advice and information

Ian Smith BSc(Hons) ClinDip FHEA MRPharmS
Academic and professional positions held: currently Boots
Teacher Practitioner, The University of Manchester,
Manchester, UK. Prior to this he held the same position in
Bradford University. He has also worked for Boots as a
Preregistration and Management Tutor in Nottingham and
as a store manager in Thirsk
24 The prescription

Darren Ashcroft BPharm MSc PhD MRPharmS
Reader in Medicines Usage & Safety and Director, Centre for
Innovation in Practice, School of Pharmacy and
Pharmaceutical Sciences, The University of Manchester,
Manchester, UK
9 Risk management

David R. Bethell BScPharm(Hons) MRPharmS MInstM
LPC Secretary, Wigan Branch Secretary, UK
43 Storage of medicines and waste disposal

Christine M. Bond BPharm MSc MEd PhD FRPharmS FPH
FHEA
Professor of Primary Care (Pharmacy), Head of Centre of
Academic Primary Care, University of Aberdeen; Consultant
in Pharmaceutical Public Health, NHS Grampian,
Aberdeen, UK
1 The role of pharmacy in healthcare

Derek G. Chapman BSc(Pharm) PhD MRPharmS
Lecturer, School of Pharmacy, Robert Gordon University,
Aberdeen, UK
27 Packaging
29 Production of sterile products
38 Parenteral products

Victoria Crabtree BPharm(Hons) MRPharmS
Teaching Fellow, School of Pharmacy and Pharmaceutical
Sciences, The University of Manchester, Manchester, UK
48 Services for vulnerable patients

Parastou Donyai BPharm(Hons) PhD MRPharmS PCTLHE
PGDPRM(Open)
Lecturer, School of Pharmacy, University of Reading,
Berkshire, UK
23 Information retrieval

Ivan O. Edafiogho BPharm MSc PhD PharmD
Associate Professor, Department of Pharmacy Practice,
Faculty of Pharmacy, Kuwait University, Kuwait
26 Pharmaceutical calculations

K. Hannes Enlund MSc(Pharm) DSc(Pharm)
Professor, Department of Pharmacy Practice, Faculty of
Pharmacy, Kuwait University, Kuwait
3 Socio-behavioural aspects of health and illness
4 Socio-behavioural aspects of treatment with medicines

Marthe M. Everard BSc(Pharm) MSc(Pharm) MSc(LSHTM) MRPharmS
Technical Officer, Department of Medicines Policy and Standards, World Health Organization, Geneva, Switzerland
7 WHO and the essential medicines concept

Isobel J. Featherstone MPharm MRPharmS
Locum pharmacist
13 Communication skills for the pharmacist

David Graham BSc MSc MRPharmS
Radiopharmacist, Department of Pharmacy, Aberdeen Royal Infirmary, Aberdeen, UK
42 Radiopharmacy

Felice S. Groundland BSc(Pharm) MRPharmS
Boots Teacher Practitioner, School of Pharmacy, University of Strathclyde, Glasgow, UK
14 Relationship with other members of the healthcare team

Jason Hall BSc MSc PhD MRPharmS PGCE MCPP
Senior Teaching Fellow, School of Pharmacy and Pharmaceutical Sciences, The University of Manchester, Manchester, UK
16 Access to medicines and prescribing – introduction
17 The prescribing process and evidence-based medicine

Lindsay Harper BSc(Hons) MRPharmS DipClin
Principal Clinical Pharmacist, Salford Royal NHS Foundation Trust, Salford Royal Hospital, Salford, UK
41 Parenteral nutrition and dialysis

Dyfrig A. Hughes BPharm MSc PhD MRPharmS
Reader in Pharmacoeconomics, Institute of Medical and Social Care Research, Bangor University, Bangor, UK
19 Drug evaluation and pharmacoeconomics

Janet Krska BSc PhD PGCert (Tertiary Level Teaching) PGCert (Health Economics) MRPharmS MCPP
Professor in Pharmacy Practice, School of Pharmacy and Biomolecular Sciences, Liverpool John Moores University, Liverpool, UK
11 Audit
18 Formularies
19 Drug evaluation and pharmacoeconomics

Liz Lamerton BSc(Hons) Pharmacy MRPharmS DipClin Pharm
Pharmacy Department, Salford Royal NHS Foundation Trust, Salford, UK
41 Parenteral nutrition and dialysis

Alison Littlewood MRPharmS MSc MCPP FHEA
Lead Pre-Registration Trainee Pharmacist Facilitator, NW Region, School of Pharmacy and Pharmaceutical Sciences, The University of Manchester, Manchester, UK
47 Monitoring the patient

G. Brian Lockwood BPharm PhD MRPharmS FHEA
Senior Lecturer, School of Pharmacy and Pharmaceutical Sciences, The University of Manchester, Manchester, UK
20 Complementary/alternative medicine

Richard C. O`Neill LLB LLM BPharm PhD MRPharmS
Associate Head, The School of Pharmacy, University of Hertfordshire, Hatfield, UK
12 Ethics

Karen Rice MPharm MRPharmS
Business Developement Manager, The Cohens Group, Lostock, Bolton, UK
45 Collection and delivery services

Peter M. Richards BPharm MRPharmS
Prescribing Adviser, Lincolnshire Teaching Primary Care Trust, Lincoln, UK
37 Inhaled route

R. Michael E. Richards OBE BPharm PhD DSc DPharmSci (Hons) DPharm(Hons) RPL(Thai)
Visiting Professor and Executive Consultant, Faculty of Pharmacy, University of Mahasarakham, Thailand
39 Ophthalmic products
Appendix 4 Presentation skills

Paul Rutter BPharm PhD MRPharmS
Principal Lecturer, School of Applied Sciences, University of Wolverhampton, Wolverhampton, UK
22 Prescribing for minor ailments

Ellen Schafheutle MSc PhD MRes MRPharmS
Research Fellow, School of Pharmacy and Pharmaceutical Sciences, The University of Manchester, Manchester, UK
6 Types of patient charges for medicines and their impact

Jenny Scott BSc(Pharm) PhD MRPharmS(IP) FHEA
Senior Lecturer, Department of Pharmacy and Pharmacology, University of Bath, Bath, UK
49 Substance use and misuse

Graham J. Sewell BPharm PhD MRPharmS MRSC CChem MIBiol CBiol
Professor of Clinical Pharmacy, School of Pharmacy, University of Kingston, Kingston upon Thames, UK
40 Specialized services

Raminder Sihota BSc(Hons) MRPharmS Dip Comm Pharm
Boots Teacher Practitioner, School of Pharmacy, University of Sunderland, Sunderland, UK
10 Continuing professional development and fitness to practise

Megan R. Thomas BSc(Med Sci) MB ChB DRCOG MRCP FRCPCH
Consultant Community Paediatrician, Blenheim House Child Development and Family Support Centre, Blackpool, UK
Appendix 1 Medical abbreviations
Appendix 4 Presentation skills

Simon J. Tweddell BPharm MRPharmS
Senior University Teacher, School of Pharmacy, University of Bradford, Bradford, UK
8 Clinical governance – an overview

Roger Walker BPharm PhD FRPharmS FFPH
Consultant in Pharmaceutical Public Health, National Public Health Service for Wales, Temple of Peace and Health, Cathays Park, Cardiff and Professor of Pharmacy Practice, Welsh School of Pharmacy, Cathays Park, Cardiff, UK
5 Pharmacy and public health

Marjorie C. Weiss BSc (Pharmacy) MSc (Clinical Pharmacy) MSc (Social Research Methods) DPhil MRPharmS
Professor of Pharmacy Practice and Medicine Use, Department of Pharmacy and Pharmacology, University of Bath, Bath, UK
46 Concordance

Mary Zargarani MPharm
Teaching Fellow, School of Pharmacy and Pharmaceutical Sciences, The University of Manchester, Manchester, UK
15 Record keeping

It is almost 5 years since the publication of the last edition of *Pharmaceutical Practice* and, as Bob Dylan wrote, 'The times they are a-changin'.' Indeed, many of the new ideas and concepts (fitness to practise and continuing professional development, governance, evidence-based practice, concordance, monitoring the patient) that were emerging 5 years ago are now fully embedded within pharmacy practice. Other more traditionally accepted areas of practice (record keeping, storage of medicines and waste disposal, collection and delivery services, services for vulnerable patients) have developed and their emphasis changed during this time period. Alongside these changes in pharmacy practice, society itself has changed (patient empowerment, patient choice, issues of consent and the development of a more ethically aware public, and the widespread availability of computers and the Internet), and many of these changes have had an impact on areas of pharmacy practice. Thus the content of this fourth edition of *Pharmaceutical Practice* has changed to take account of all these developments. Many new chapters have been included to cover all these new and/or developed areas of pharmacy practice and the original chapters have been updated or rewritten to include newer aspects of practice.

Besides the changing content of the book, one of the original editors (AJW) remains, acting as an anchor and guide to the two newer junior editors, and making sure the ethos of the previous editions is maintained – that is, the reader is provided with an up-to-date knowledge base for all aspects of good pharmacy practice, presented wherever possible, to encourage a professional attitude of always seeking to provide the highest standards of pharmaceutical care.

Many new authors have been recruited for this edition and they include full-time practising pharmacists, pharmacists with joint appointments with community or hospital pharmacies, and academic pharmacists. All these new authors have been chosen for their experience and expertise in the subject matter. Although this book is produced in the UK, many of the new and established authors do not hail from these shores and so international aspects of pharmacy practice are covered in this book.

Pharmaceutical Practice has been written to provide the reader with the traditional and pharmaceutically unique aspects of pharmacy practice, and in addition to offer the newer concepts and methods employed in the pursuit of quality pharmaceutical care for patients. Hopefully this book will provide the reader with a wide knowledge base of pharmacy practice and the skills required for the developing roles of a pharmacist in 2009 and beyond.

There are two companion volumes to *Pharmaceutical Practice*: *Aulton's Pharmaceutics: The Design and Manufacture of Medicines* third edition (2007) edited by M. E. Aulton, which provides greater detail on the scientific principles that underpin the design and manufacture of dosage forms and medicines; and *Clinical Pharmacy and Therapeutics* fourth edition (2007), edited by R. Walker and C. Whittlesea, which considers in greater detail aspects of treatment with drugs and clinical practice by pharmacists. These three books complement each other and readers should realize that information cannot be compartmentalized. It is detrimental to patients to ignore any aspect of the total knowledge base – all must be integrated if optimum pharmaceutical care is to be provided.

JAR
IS
AJW

Acknowledgements

The editors would like to take this opportunity to thank the many people who have helped to make this fourth edition possible. Since publication of the third edition, Professor Mike Richards has decided to 're-tire' as an editor. It is impossible to pay sufficient tribute to his input to previous editions. His decision has meant that new editors were required. It has been a pleasure working (as a new team) with both Judith Rees and Ian Smith. They have brought a different range of experience, which is reflected in the detailed content of this fourth edition.

New editors also bring new contacts, so we have been able to recruit many new authors for this edition. We are deeply grateful to all the authors for their willingness to contribute to this volume and for the time and effort they have spent researching their subjects and in preparing text – and for the way they have responded to e-mails!

Our special thanks are due to our families. Without their continued encouragement, support and assistance, an undertaking like this would not reach completion.

Those companies, organizations and individuals who have given permission to use or modify their materials or who have helpfully answered queries or provided information to our authors are thanked. Without this type of cooperation, any textbook cannot hope to present a worthwhile overview.

Thanks are also expressed to the publishers, in particular Ellen Green, Pauline Graham, Hannah Kenner and Carole McMurray, for their guidance and timely support throughout the preparation of this fourth edition. Professional guidance is always necessary. They have provided it as required and made our lives much easier.

Finally, we wish to thank you, our students, past and present, in the UK and Kuwait. We know that students do not appreciate how much their teachers learn from them, but we do! We hope that some of this is reflected in this book.

JAR
IS
AJW

In the initial stages of planning this fourth edition of *Pharmaceutical Practice* and considering what was needed to provide the reader with a rounded and full knowledge of pharmacy practice, we had to take cognizance of the fact that this subject has changed rapidly in the last few years. Thus, as indicated in the preface, this edition contains several new chapters by new authors and, in addition, the original chapters have been revamped and the content rewritten or brought up to date. Because of these changes, it was also necessary to rearrange the order of the chapters. In so doing, we have attempted to place the chapters into logical groupings or sections. These sections should make it easier for the reader to appreciate the new developments in pharmacy practice. We hope, however, that the use of these sections does not isolate and compartmentalize the subject matter, especially since many topics span the range of pharmacy practice activities; thus, where appropriate, we have indicated (cross-referenced) where the subject matter is referred to in another part of the book. In total there are five sections and appendices:

- Section 1 Pharmacy practice and society
- Section 2 Governance and good professional pharmaceutical practice
- Section 3 Pharmacy prescribing and selection of medicines
- Section 4 Dispensing and related pharmaceutical practice activities
- Section 5 Pharmacy services and monitoring the medicine-taking patient
- Appendices.

Section 1

In Section 1, the chapters address the wider aspects of pharmacy practice, the influence of society on pharmacy practice and vice versa, the organization of pharmacy practice within societies, and the impact of health or illness of patients and the supply of medicines within societies on pharmacy practice. These chapters also consider international features of pharmacy practice and medicines. The book opens with a detailed description of the development of pharmacy practice and the role it now plays within society. This chapter is followed by the way pharmacy practice is organized in different countries of the world, highlighting some of the similarities and differences. The next two chapters (3 and 4) cover the behavioural and sociological aspects of patients and their illnesses and treatment with drugs. An understanding of these two chapters should underpin many of the latter chapters, which consider self-care, patient empowerment and patient choice. The nature of public health and the role that pharmacy can play and should play in providing public health is the subject of Chapter 5. While Chapters 6 and 7 have a very international flavour, Chapter 6 considers the different methods by which patients are charged for their medicines and the impact it makes on the provider and patient, and Chapter 7 considers the essential medicines concept, which is important for many countries, including 'developed' countries.

Section 2

The chapters in this section all consider ways of providing good professional pharmacy practice, whether this involves evaluating and/or setting up 'ways of working' or developing the individual skills of the pharmacist. Chapter 8 sets the scene by describing what is meant by governance, all its component parts and how pharmacists can apply good governance to their daily working life. The nature of risk and how it can be managed to prevent accidents and provide a safer environment for patients receiving medicines is considered in Chapter 9. In Chapter 10, the need for pharmacists to demonstrate fitness to practise and provide evidence of continuing professional development is outlined as part of governance. Audit, as described in Chapter 11, is another aspect of governance and a way by which pharmacists can demonstrate that they meet standards and provide good services. Underpinning good professional practice is an appreciation and demonstration of an ethical stance by the pharmacist (Chapter 12), while

Chapter 13 outlines the ways in which pharmacists can develop good communication skills to develop their professional role. Pharmacists do not work in isolation and Chapter 14 considers the pharmacist's relationship with other members of the healthcare team as they provide good, effective and professional services. Chapter 15 describes the very necessary record keeping that pharmacists are required to maintain as evidence of professional practice.

Section 3

The emphasis in this section is on the development of non-medical prescribers, including pharmacists, and the safe and economic selection of effective medicines. Chapters 16 and 17 provide background and detailed information on prescribers, prescribing and the need for an evidence base. The development of formularies to reduce costs and help in the selection of medicines by prescribers is discussed in Chapter 18, while Chapter 19 develops the topic further by considering drug evaluations and pharmacoeconomics. The increasing use by the public of complementary and alternative medicines requires pharmacists to develop knowledge and skills to help with the selection of these products (Chapter 20). The increasingly varied routes of administering of medicines are dealt with in Chapter 21. Prescribing for minor ailments has always been a core role for pharmacists and Chapter 22 describes effective ways of assessing patients' symptoms and conditions to arrive at a differential diagnosis and hence become a more helpful and professional prescriber. In order to underpin the prescribing and selection of medicines, it is essential that the pharmacist can access good information, especially with the wealth of information available on the Internet: Chapter 23 addresses this important topic and skill.

Section 4

Dispensing and the preparation of extemporaneous products are at the core of traditional pharmacy practice. This section starts with Chapter 24 and the important task of checking the information on a prescription, and outlines a novel scheme for the clinical and legal checking of a prescription to ensure that it is appropriate for the patient. Chapter 25 describes dispensing techniques in general and Chapter 26

details how to perform pharmaceutical calculations. Packaging and labelling of dispensed products is considered in Chapters 27 and 28. Chapter 29 describes the set-up of sterile production areas and the sterility testing of pharmaceutical products. Then follows in Chapters 30–36 a systematic coverage of the different types of medicines, concentrating mainly on the extemporaneously prepared medicines that pharmacists may have to produce. From Chapter 37, the emphasis changes to more specialized medicines and the role of the pharmacist in ensuring their effective use. Chapter 37 discusses how medicines are given by inhalation, Chapter 38 by injection and Chapter 39 deals with ophthalmic products. Chapters 40–42 describe hospital-based services including specialized services, total parenteral nutrition, dialysis and radiopharmacy. Chapter 43 considers the storage of medicines in a pharmacy and their disposal as waste, when required. Chapter 44 completes the dispensing process by describing the communication skills required to provide advice to patients on their medicines.

Section 5

The chapters in this section consider the next stage after the patient has received their medicine(s), the pharmaceutical services provided to groups of patients and the monitoring of patients who take medicines. Chapter 45 outlines the provision of services to ensure that patients receive their prescribed medicines within the community setting. Chapter 46 considers concordance and the agreement between prescriber and patient on how, when and why to use medicines and whether the patient is fulfilling that agreement. Further monitoring of the patient's actual use of medicines and whether they understand how to take their medicines is followed up in Chapter 47. Chapters 48 and 49 consider how vulnerable patients and drug misusers can be helped by pharmacists and others to obtain and use correctly their medicines or drugs.

Appendices

The appendices supplement the chapters by providing information that either would not require a full chapter or is more appropriately situated outside of the chapters. Appendices 1 and 2 list medical and Latin abbreviations, both of which are useful to pharmacists as part of their job, but may need to be looked up because of their infrequent use. Appendix 3 provides reference to the various systems of weights and measures that may be encountered by pharmacists. Appendix 4 provides guidance on presentation skills; pharmacists throughout their professional careers require such skills. Key references and guidance to further reading for all the chapters are collated in Appendix 5.

For us as editors, it has been a daunting task to produce a textbook of a reasonable size that covers all the possible topics in pharmacy practice. We realize that it is possible only to provide an overview and supply key information. Any reader requiring more information on the topic should initially consult Appendix 5 for suggested additional reading, then use the information in Chapter 23 to practise their skills at information retrieval.

Finally, we acknowledge that changes will take place between writing and publishing that will mean that by the time this book appears in print some of it will almost certainly be out of date. This process of obsolescence will continue with time. Therefore it is suggested that readers keep up to date by reading current medical and pharmaceutical journals and literature.

Section One

Pharmacy Practice and Society

1

The role of pharmacy in health care

Christine M. Bond

STUDY POINTS

- The historical development of pharmacy
- The position of pharmacy within the National Health Service in the UK
- Recent developments in the services being provided by pharmacists
- The need for lifelong learning
- The public's attitudes to pharmacy

Introduction

Pharmacists are experts on the actions and uses of drugs, including their chemistry, their formulation into medicines and the ways in which they are used to manage diseases. The principal aim of the pharmacist is to use this expertise to improve patient care. Pharmacists are in close contact with patients and so have an important role both in assisting patients to make the best use of their prescribed medicines and in advising patients on the appropriate self-management of self-limiting and minor conditions. Increasingly this latter aspect includes over the counter (OTC) prescribing of effective and potent treatments. Pharmacists are also in close working relationships with other members of the healthcare team – doctors, nurses, dentists and others – where they are able to give advice on a wide range of issues surrounding the use of medicines.

Pharmacists are employed in many different areas of practice. These include the traditional ones of hospital and community practice as well as newer advisory roles at health authority/health board level and working directly with general practitioners as part of the core, practice-based primary healthcare team. Additionally, pharmacists are employed in the pharmaceutical industry and in academia.

Members of the general public are most likely to meet pharmacists in high street pharmacies or on a hospital ward. However, pharmacists also visit residential homes, make visits to patients' own homes and are now involved in running chronic disease clinics in primary and secondary care. In addition, pharmacists will also be contributing to the care of patients through their dealings with other members of the healthcare team in the hospital and community setting.

The changing role of pharmacy

Historically pharmacists and general practitioners have a common ancestry as apothecaries. Apothecaries both dispensed medicines prescribed by physicians and recommended medicines for those members of the public unable to afford physicians' fees. As the two professions of pharmacy and general practice emerged this remit split so that pharmacists became primarily responsible for the technical, dispensing aspects of this role. With the advent of the National Health Service (NHS) in the UK in 1948, and the philosophy of free medical care at the point of delivery, the advisory function of the pharmacist further decreased. As a result pharmacists spent more of their time in the dispensing of medicines – and derived an increased proportion of their income from it. At the same time, radical changes in the nature of dispensing itself, as described in the following paragraphs, occurred.

In the early years, many prescriptions were for extemporaneously prepared medicines, either following standard 'recipes' from formularies such as the

British Pharmacopoeia (BP) or *British Pharmaceutical Codex* (BPC), or following individual recipes written by the prescriber. The situation was similar in hospital pharmacy, where most prescriptions were prepared on an individual basis. There was some small-scale manufacture of a range of commonly used items. In both situations, pharmacists required manipulative and time-consuming skills to produce the medicines. Thus a wide range of preparations was made, including liquids for internal and external use, ointments, creams, poultices, plasters, eye drops and ointments, injections and solid dosage forms such as pills, capsules and moulded tablets.

Scientific advances have greatly increased the effectiveness of drugs but have also rendered them more complex, potentially more toxic and requiring more sophisticated use than their predecessors. The pharmaceutical industry developed in tandem with these drug developments, contributing to further scientific advances and producing manufactured medical products. This had a number of advantages. For one thing, there was an increased reliability in the product, which could be subjected to suitable quality assessment and assurance. This led to improved formulations, modifications to drug availability and increased use of tablets which have a greater convenience for the patient. Some doctors did not agree with the loss of flexibility in prescribing which resulted from having to use predetermined doses and combinations of materials. From the pharmacist's point of view there was a reduction in the time spent in the routine extemporaneous production of medicines, which many saw as an advantage. Others saw it as a reduction in the mystique associated with the professional role of the pharmacist (see Ch. 2 for a more detailed discussion on the professional roles of pharmacists). There was also an erosion of the technical skill base of the pharmacist. A look through copies of the BPC in the 1950s, 1960s and 1970s will show the reduction in the number and diversity of formulations included in the Formulary section. That section has been omitted from the most recent editions.

Some extemporaneous dispensing is still required and pharmacists remain the only professionals trained in these skills. For this reason, Section 4 of this book deals with the types of medicine used, the ingredients employed in them and describes some of the practical skills required to make products suitable for use by patients.

The changing patterns of work of the pharmacist, in community pharmacy in particular, led to an uncertainty about the future role of the pharmacist and a general consensus that pharmacists were no longer being utilized to their full potential. If the pharmacist was not required to compound medicines or to give general advice on diseases, what was the pharmacist to do?

The extended role

The need to review the future for pharmacy was first formally recognized in 1979 in a report on the NHS which had the remit to consider the best use and management of its financial and manpower resources. This was followed by a succession of key reports and papers which repeatedly identified the need to exploit the pharmacist's expertise and knowledge to better effect. Key among these reports was the Nuffield Report of 1986. This report, which included nearly 100 recommendations, led the way to many new initiatives, both by the profession and by the government, and laid the foundation for the recent developments in the practice of pharmacy, which are reflected in this book.

Radical change, as recommended in the Nuffield Report, does not necessarily happen quickly, particularly when regulations and statute are involved. In the 23 years since Nuffield was published there have been several different agendas which have come together and between them facilitated the paradigm shift for pharmacy envisaged in the Nuffield Report. These agendas will be briefly described below. They have finally resulted in extensive professional change, most recently articulated in the definitive statements about the role of pharmacy in the NHS plans for pharmacy in England (2000), Scotland (2001) and Wales (2002) and the subsequent new contractual frameworks for community pharmacy. In addition other regulatory changes have occurred as part of government policy to increase convenient public access to a wider range of medicines on the NHS. These changes reflect general societal trends to deregulate the professions while having in place a framework to ensure safe practice and a recognition that the public are increasingly well informed through widespread access to the Internet.

For pharmacy, therefore, two routes for the supply of prescription only medicines (POM) have opened up. Until recently POM medicines were only available on the prescription of a doctor or dentist, but as a result of the Crown Review in 1999, two significant changes emerged. First, patient group directions (PGDs) were introduced in 2000. A PGD is a written direction for the supply, or supply and administration, of a POM to persons generally by named groups of professionals. So, for example, under a PGD, community pharmacists could supply a specific POM antibiotic to people with a confirmed diagnostic infection, e.g. azithromycin for *Chlamydia*.

Second, prescribing rights for pharmacists, alongside nurses and some other healthcare professionals, have been introduced, initially as supplementary prescribers and more recently as independent prescribers. To carry out these prescribing roles, pharmacists must have undertaken additional postgraduate training and be accredited by the Royal Pharmaceutical Society of Great Britain (RPSGB). It is anticipated that the training will soon be routinely incorporated into undergraduate curricula.

The profession

The council of the RPSGB decided that it was necessary to allow all members to contribute to a radical appraisal of the profession, what it should be doing and how to achieve it. The 'Pharmacy in a New Age' consultation (familiarly referred to as PIANA) was launched in October 1995, with an invitation to all members to contribute their views to the council. These were combined into a subsequent document produced by the council in September 1996 called *Pharmacy in a New Age: The New Horizon*. This indicated that there was overwhelming agreement from pharmacists that the profession could not stand still. Four main areas in which pharmacy should make a major contribution to health outcomes were identified:

- *Management of prescribed medicines*. This covers drug development, provision of medicines, information and support, and ensuring patient needs are met safely, efficiently and conveniently so that they can get maximum benefit from their medicines.
- *Management of chronic conditions*. Here the need is to improve the quality of life and outcomes of treatment for the patient. Pharmacists may help by supplying medicines and advice, helping to develop local shared care protocols, ensuring that patients are taking or using their medicines properly and working as part of the healthcare team.
- *Management of common ailments*. Patients require reassurance and advice, with or without the use of non-prescription medicines, and referral to other professionals if necessary.

- *Promotion and support of healthy lifestyles*. Pharmacists can help people protect their own health through health screening, giving advice on healthy living and providing educational materials.

During the consultation process, pharmacists expressed their views on the way the profession should change. These, too, may be summarized under four main headings:

- *The strengths of pharmacy*. There was a high level of consensus that the knowledge base of pharmacy was very important. This is based on both the study of and experience with medicines and also in managing the medicines and handling relevant information. A second strength which was seen as important was pharmacists' availability and accessibility in a wide range of different locations in the heart of the community, such as conventional high street premises, health centres, supermarkets, hospitals and in people's homes. This accessibility is strengthened by easy communication with both patients and other professionals, giving pharmacists a pivotal position. The growth of information technology could be a potential threat to this, although pharmacists are noted for their adaptability.
- *Demonstrating the value of pharmacy*. Pharmacy must claim its rights as a profession and accept the responsibilities which come with this. Thus high standards must be set and achieved. Additionally, evidence must be produced which demonstrates clearly the value of pharmacy in health care. This will require research and professional audit (see Ch. 11). Further support for this development will come from increased continuing education and recognition achieved by effective promotion of the profession.
- *Changes in practice*. Three main areas where there could be an increase in services were identified. These are: the enhancement of services to patients (advice, counselling, domiciliary visits, health promotion and non-prescription medicine sales); improved relationships with other healthcare professionals (closer support for prescribers, medicine management, liaison between hospital and community pharmacy and different community pharmacists, training for other professionals and carers); and practice research and audit, continuing education and better use of information technology (all required to support the other developments). There was also a high

level of support for a reduction in the mechanical aspects of dispensing, sale of non-health-related products and routine paperwork associated with the NHS and business activities.

- *A sustainable future*. These elements could make up a sustainable future for the profession. In particular, pharmacy would be concerned with advice and counselling, dispensing, health promotion, the sale of non-prescription medicines, medicines management and as a first port of call for health care. Some of these may require changes in the setting of pharmaceutical provision and others may require different types of employment for pharmacists. Other changes which would be required included changes to the system of payment under the NHS, a rationalization of pharmacy distribution and at least two pharmacists being employed per community pharmacy.

The main output of this professional review was a commitment to take forward a more proactive, patient centred clinical role for pharmacy using pharmacists' skills and knowledge to best effect.

The NHS drugs budget

Health services are expensive to run. Governments try to reduce expenditure as far as possible through a range of methods. In the UK some medicines have been identified as being ineligible for prescribing on the NHS. The so-called Black List was introduced in 1984 to reduce the size of the NHS bill. Furthermore the introduction of computer technology into prescription pricing has enabled far more data to be produced than was previously possible. Doctors now receive a regular breakdown of the drugs they have prescribed and their prescribing costs. Chapter 18 considers the use of prescribing data (PACT or SPA) by pharmacists when advising doctors about reducing their prescribing costs.

However, despite these moves, and in common with other developed countries, UK drug costs are inexorably rising due to the greater availability of new effective treatments, patient demand and changes in patient demography (more older people). This has made many governments look at other ways of controlling this item of expenditure, and there are two ways in which pharmacists can have a role.

First, it is recognized that not all prescribing follows the current best evidence for cost-effective practice. Pharmacists are seen as a profession with the necessary knowledge to support quality in prescribing at a strategic and practice level. At a strategic level they can appraise the evidence and make recommendations for the inclusion of a drug in a formulary. At a general practice level pharmacists can advise prescribers on the best drugs to prescribe for individual patients, and community pharmacists are well placed to monitor and review repeat prescriptions, which account for 80% of all prescriptions in primary care.

Second, in a move to promote self-care, pharmacists can encourage patients to be responsible for their own health care and, by implication, remove the cost of treating what is known as 'minor illness' from the NHS. Many drugs previously only available on prescription (POM) are now available over the counter from pharmacies (P) or from any retail outlet general sales list (GSL). All drugs are classified into legal categories which restrict their supply in the interests of patient safety. The main categories are: prescription only medicines (POM); pharmacy medicines (sale only under the supervision of a pharmacist; P); and general sales list (sale from any retail outlet including pharmacies; GSL; see Ch. 2). These changes have resulted in many potent drugs now being available for sale from community pharmacies and the advisory role of the pharmacist has therefore been greatly enhanced. In 1983, ibuprofen and loperamide were the first of the many drugs to be deregulated in the following decades, and there is no obvious end to the process. Initially, deregulated drugs were for the management of conditions already diagnosed and treated by pharmacists, such as dyspepsia, but where the choice of effective remedy was limited. Then deregulations became more focused on extending the licensed indications for P sale, such as the inclusion of eczema as an allowable indication for topical hydrocortisone. Most recently, deregulations have increasingly been for new drugs for 'new' conditions, such as emergency hormonal contraception and statins. Conversely, the two non-sedating antihistamines terfenadine and astemizole are rare examples of the reclassification to POM because of the emergence of major safety concerns when these drugs were taken by increasing numbers of people. Terfenadine was subsequently removed totally from the UK market. Overall these moves have implications for the pharmacist's role as a first line provider of care for minor conditions, with a return to the traditional pre NHS advisory role including simple diagnosis and management.

The NHS workforce

As demand for health care grows, it is not only budgets that are stretched. Increasingly there are insufficient trained professionals to deliver services, and innovative ways of working need to be introduced to maximize the skills of the different professionals in the healthcare team. This has resulted in a recognition that many of the tasks previously undertaken by the medical profession, in both primary and secondary care, can be undertaken by other professions such as pharmacists and nurses. Thus, some of the professional roles originally identified by the profession, such as the management of chronic disease and a greater role in responding to symptoms, are now supported by the wider healthcare community because they can contribute to more effective health care for the population. As a result a team approach to managing health care has emerged.

The current and future roles of pharmacists

There are currently around 46 000 registered UK member pharmacists, including those who are working in different sectors of the profession as well as those who are in non-pharmacy-related posts or retired, both in Britain and overseas. The register is divided into practising and non-practising sections. There are 40 000 pharmacists on the 'practising' register, of whom approximately 70% work in community pharmacy, 20% in hospitals, 8% in primary care and 4% in the pharmaceutical industry. The next section will summarize the community, hospital and the other NHS roles as they are practised today, with indications of likely changes and challenges in the near future.

Community pharmacy

As a result of the final recognition of the pharmacist's role beyond solely dispensing, new community pharmacy contractual frameworks were agreed for England and Wales, and for Scotland, in the early part of this century. In England and Wales, the contract is based on a list of essential services to be delivered from all NHS contracted pharmacies, and then an advanced service specification for specially accredited pharmacists operating from enhanced premises with private consultation areas. At the time of writing the only advanced service is the medicines use review (MUR) and prescription intervention service. Enhanced services, which are negotiated locally with individual NHS primary care organizations, are also delivered. These are summarized in Box 1.1. In Scotland, the new contract is similar, but there is an emphasis on all pharmacists delivering all of the four core service areas: these are the acute medicines service (AMS), the chronic medicines service (CMS), the minor ailment service (MAS) and the public health service (PHS). More detail on these is provided in Box 1.2. In Northern Ireland, a new contract is proposed but is not yet delivered. However, whichever contractual framework pharmacists are operating under, the following generic services will be delivered.

Dispensing, repeat dispensing and medication review

Despite the recent contractual recognition of new clinical roles, which are described later, dispensing remains a core role of community pharmacy and would still account for the majority of a pharmacist's time. The preponderance of original pack dispensing means that, compared to even a decade ago, while the name may remain the same, the similarity ends there. The focus of dispensing now rests not only on accurate supply of medication but also on checking that the medication is appropriate for the patient and counselling the patient on its appropriate use. All community pharmacists maintain computerized patient medication records which are a record of previous prescriptions dispensed (see Chs 24 and 47). While not necessarily complete, since patients are not registered with an individual pharmacy, in practice the vast majority of patients, particularly those on regular prescribed medication, do use one pharmacy for the majority of their supplies. Thus pharmacists have a database of information which will allow them to check on issues such as accuracy of the new prescription, compliance and potential drug interactions.

In the future the dispensing role will be further enhanced as connection of community pharmacy into the NHS net becomes a reality. Electronic transmission of prescriptions is currently being universally implemented in England and Scotland. Under this scheme, GPs will send prescriptions to a central 'cyberstore' from which pharmacists can download the information using a unique identifier, and dispense the prescribed supplies or medications to the patient. Ultimately this electronic link should allow access by the pharmacist to

Box 1.1	

Community pharmacy contractual framework (England & Wales), introduced 2005

Essential services	Dispensing of prescribed medicine
	Repeat dispensing
	Disposal of unwanted medicines/waste management
Public health	Healthy lifestyle campaigns, prescription-linked healthy lifestyle interventions
Signposting	
Support for self-care	E.g. advise on treatment of minor illness including OTC medicine sale, maintain records of clinically significant products purchased
Clinical governance	E.g. in relation to public and patient involvement, monitoring by NHS, participation in clinical audit, undertaking risk management and supporting self and staff with education and professional development
	Appropriate use of information and compliance with statute such as the Data Protection Act 1998, the Human Right Act 1998, the NHS Code of Practice on Confidentiality, the Disability Discrimination Act 1995 and Health and Safety legislation
	Maintenance of patient medication records
Advanced services	Medicines use review
	A service initiated by either the pharmacist, the GP or the patient in which accredited pharmacists undertake structured concordance centred reviews with patients on multiple prescribed medicines. The aim is to help patients understand and comply with their treatment, identify problems if any, and provide a report to the patient and the GP
Enhanced services (locally negotiated)	A wide range of services such as alcohol screening, anticoagulation monitoring, asthma, care homes, care staff, controlled drugs, record cards, chronic obstructive pulmonary disease, databases, emergency hormonal contraception, gluten-free foods, *Helicobacter pylori* testing, minor ailments, needle and syringe exchange, needle collection, 'not dispensed scheme', out of hours, palliative care, Parkinson's disease, phlebotomy, point of care testing, prescription intervention, quality and outcomes framework, seasonal influenza, sexual health, smoking cessation, supervised administration (e.g. of methadone), vascular risk assessment, weight management and obesity

at least a selected portion of the patient's medical record, further enhancing the pharmacist's ability to assess the appropriateness of the prescription. It is hoped that there will also be a facility for pharmacists to write to the patient record, so that GPs will know whether or not prescriptions have been dispensed and what OTC drugs have been purchased.

A further enhanced dispensing role is in the management of repeat prescriptions, which until recently have been issued from GP surgeries with little clinical review. Following research projects which demonstrated that when given this responsibility, community pharmacists could identify previously unrecognized side-effects, adverse drug reactions and drug interactions, as well as saving almost a fifth of the costs of the drugs prescribed, this repeat dispensing service is

now part of the new community pharmacy contract (see Boxes 1.1 and 1.2).

This opportunistic clinical input at the point of dispensing is also being developed in a more systematic way, such that patients with targeted chronic conditions, such as coronary heart disease, have formal regular reviews with the community pharmacist about their medication and other disease-related behaviours. Again schemes like this, with research evidence of benefit in small studies, are currently undergoing national implementation through the new contractual frameworks. Such services, called medicines management (see Ch. 17), medicines use review (MUR) or chronic medicines services (CMS), are part of a more holistic approach often referred to as pharmaceutical care. Supplementary

New Scottish community pharmacy contract, introduced incrementally from 2006

There are four services delivered by all community pharmacies:

Minor ailment service (MAS) (from mid-2006)	The provision of a range of pharmacy and general sale list medicines (e.g. to treat skin problems, pain, coughs and colds) from the community pharmacy on the NHS to patients registered with that pharmacy and not normally paying an NHS prescription charge
Public health service (PHS) (from end 2006)	All interactions with patients should include provision of opportunistic healthy living advice, take part in four national campaigns a year, e.g. flu, vaccinations, meningitis by poster display and provision of health promotion messages, and offer smoking cessation service, emergency hormonal contraception supply and *Chlamydia* testing and treatment
Acute medication service (from July 2008)	Dispensing prescribed medicines, plus advice. Electronic transmission of prescriptions between GP and community pharmacy
Chronic medication service (anticipated mid-2009)	The management of long-term conditions by monitoring, medications review, adjustment of doses (by those with prescriber qualification), repeat dispensing

There are also optional services:

National funded optional services	E.g. palliative care, prescribing clinics
Locally negotiated services	These will also continue, e.g. services for drug misusers (needle exchange and supervised consumption), flu immunization and drugs as per the English contract (see Box 1.1)

and independent prescribing will greatly enhance this role for pharmacy.

Responding to symptoms

Provision of advice to customers presenting in the pharmacy for advice on self-care is now an accepted part of the work of a pharmacist which, as described earlier, has been enhanced by the increased armamentarium of pharmacy medicines. Advertising campaigns, particularly those by the National Pharmaceutical Association (NPA), have brought to public attention the advice which is available from the pharmacist, as have the commercial adverts from the pharmaceutical industry for their deregulated products. The increased emphasis on the provision of advice from community pharmacies has also extended to the counter staff, who require special training and must adhere to protocols. Some of the principles of responding to symptoms are dealt with in Chapter 22.

The full contribution of this advisory role to health care has been limited, to some extent, to the more advantaged sections of the population, particularly since the deregulation of many potent medicines referred to earlier. Many of these newer P medicines are relatively expensive, and those on lower incomes, and particularly those who are exempt from prescription charges, may in the past have attended their doctor only for the purpose of obtaining a free prescription for the drug. This has now been circumvented. Under the new contract in Scotland, all patients who would not normally pay for their prescription can access any medicine normally available without a prescription on the NHS from their local community pharmacist. Patients have to register with a community pharmacy to receive the service and all records are maintained centrally and electronically. Ultimately they will be able to be linked to other patient information through a unique patient identifier, known as the CHI (Community Health Index). In England, similar schemes also exist under the new contract but they are an enhanced, locally negotiated service rather than an essential service. At the time of writing, only about 25% of English community pharmacies provide this service.

Health promotion and health improvement

A large number of people pass through the nation's pharmacies in any one day; on the basis of prescription numbers this is frequently said to be 6 million people per day in the UK. Another way of looking at this is that over 90% of the population visit a community pharmacy in any single year. Thus the pharmacist is one of the best placed healthcare professionals to provide health promotion information and health ed-ucation material to the general public. This has now become part of the pharmacist's NHS contract and formalized as a core service to be delivered by all pharmacies in England and Wales, and Scotland. The service specification is generally limited to par-ticipation in healthy lifestyle campaigns and opportu-nistic intervention. More aspirational roles can also be delivered and there are extensive opportunities for proactive, targeted and specialist advice to be provid-ed from community pharmacies. The development of cancer and cardiovascular disease, major causes of morbidity and mortality, are both closely linked to lifestyle factors such as diet, exercise and smoking. Pharmacists can give out patient information leaflets on healthy nutrition, which may reduce the develop-ment of disease which would otherwise occur and lead to the need for expensive treatment. Smoking is considered to be the single biggest cause of prevent-able ill health. Pharmacists have a successful record in supporting smoking cessation though tailored face-to-face advice and the supply of smoking cessation products such as nicotine replacement therapies (see Ch. 5), and the vast majority of pharmacies are engaged in local smoking cessation schemes.

Services to specific patient groups

Certain groups of patients have particular needs which can be met by community pharmacists more cost effectively than by any other healthcare profes-sional. Such specific patient services often cause the remit of a profession to change almost overnight in response to an unexpected national issue. One such example is drug misuse and the spread of blood borne diseases such as hepatitis and AIDS. Drug misuse is an increasing problem in society today. It is now generally accepted that drug misusers have a right to treatment both to help them come off their addiction and to reduce the harm they may do, either to themselves or to society, until such time as they are ready to undergo detoxification. The vast majority of pharmacists will be involved to a greater or lesser extent in a number of ways, as discussed in

Chapter 49. In particular, pharmacists have become involved in needle exchange schemes and in instal-ment dispensing and supervised consumption of methadone. Because of the urgent need for these important services, and to some extent because of the unwillingness of some community pharmacists to become involved on the grounds of professional responsibility alone, these services have unusually been recognized by specific locally negotiated remu-neration packages. These local arrangements contin-ue within the new contracts.

Domiciliary visiting

Pharmacists have traditionally delivered oxygen to a patient's home, and many pharmacists will visit a small number of patients in their own home to deliver medicines and provide advice on their use. This will now be extended to include other situations where patients could benefit, such as on discharge from hos-pital, including highly specialized services (often called the 'hospital at home') where patients may be on palliative care, cytotoxic agents, intravenous antibiotics or artificial nutrition. These topics are dis-cussed in more detail in Chapters 40 and 41. As med-icines management services for people on chronic medication continue to evolve, and with more early hospital discharge, this could mean more domiciliary visits to housebound patients. There is also a separate but related need for services to be provided in care home settings, to include both advice on the storage and administration of medicines as well as clinical advice for individual patients (Ch. 48).

Personal control

One of the requirements of the current regulations is that a pharmacist has to be in personal control/super-vision of registered community pharmacy premises at all times. The principle is that the pharmacist should be aware of any transaction in which a medicine is provided to a member of the public and be able to intervene if deemed necessary. This requirement was intended to protect the public but it has been a barrier to innovative practice, and it has been interpreted as the pharmacist needing to be physically present in the pharmacy and aware of all transactions involving P and POM medicines. For single-handed pharmacists this has been difficult to combine with new roles under-taken outwith the pharmacy premises, such as domi-ciliary visits, or multi-professional meetings. A recent consultation reviewed this stringent requirement and recommended that the pharmacist can, under exceptional circumstances, leave their premises for professional reasons only, for short periods of time during the working day. The current Code of Ethics and Standards, released at the time of writing, promotes greater use of professional judgement, stating principles and removing detailed technical requirements. It remains to be seen exactly how it will be implemented.

A further challenge to established practice will also come from the increasing use of the Internet for personal shopping; and the acquisition of medicines, whether prescribed or purchased, will not be immune to such developments. Already mail order pharmacy and e-pharmacy are making small inroads into medicines distribution and supply, and challenge some of the principles of the Code of Ethics and professional practice points which encourage personal counselling wherever possible. Again, the new Code of Ethics and Standards has responded appropriately, with guidance to professionals on how they can still deliver the same standards of care as from face-to-face premises. Although online services are probably more developed in North America, such changes to practice are inevitable and need to be managed professionally, remembering that best care of the patient, rather than professional self-interest, must be the rationale of any decision making.

Out of hours services

The NHS call centres NHS Direct (England and Wales) and NHS 24 (Scotland) handle health-related telephone enquiries from the general public and triage them on to appropriate services. Referral to community pharmacy is one of the formal dispositions included in the algorithms used by the call handlers. It is intended, therefore, that the community pharmacist will not be bypassed by the new telephone help lines. It should also serve to educate the public about the role of the community pharmacist and to increase general awareness that the community pharmacy is just as much a part of the NHS as is the general practice. Audits of calls have revealed that a high proportion are linked to medicines and could have been handled directly by pharmacists. As a result pharmacists are now employed directly to provide online advice from NHS 24/ NHS Direct phone lines, and there is also a recognized need to divert the public back to the community pharmacist as the port of call during normal working hours. Finally there are moves to extend accessibility to face-to-face out of hours pharmaceutical advice through links between community pharmacies and out of hours centres.

Hospital pharmacy

Clinical pharmacy services have been established in the hospital setting for some time; indeed many of the innovations identified for community pharmacy come from earlier experience in hospitals. In general there is already a greater working together of the professions in the hospital setting compared to primary care, including pharmacists' involvement in medication history taking, active engagement in research, and for the provision of 24-hour services. In 1988, the NHS circular *Health Services Management: the Way Forward for Hospital Pharmaceutical Services* laid down the government policy aim as 'the achievement of better patient care and financial savings, through the more cost effective use of medicines, and improved use of pharmaceutical expertise obtained through the implementation of a clinical pharmacy service'. Two main components were identified. One is the overall management of medicines on the hospital ward. This is achieved through the provision of advice to medical and nursing staff, formulary management and ensuring the safe handling of medicines. The other component is the development of individual patient care plans. This is achieved through the provision of drug information and assisting patients with problems which may arise. In practice there are many stages and activities involved in these processes. A working group in Scotland published *Clinical Pharmacy in the Hospital Pharmaceutical Service: a Framework for Practice* in July 1996 (Clinical Resources Audit Group 1996). The framework advocates a systematic approach to enable the pharmacist to focus on the key areas and optimize the pharmaceutical input to patient care. Some of the thinking behind this document is discussed subsequently in Chapter 5.

There is a growing awareness of the problems which arise at the interface between community (primary) and hospital (secondary) care. Patients move in both directions. Their medical and pharmaceutical problems also move with them. Over the next few years it is hoped that a large proportion of these problems will have been resolved through the greater involvement of pharmacists at admission and discharge with effective (ultimately electronic) transfer of information, from hospital pharmacist to community pharmacist. As more patients are discharged early, and with more serious and specialized clinical conditions, there will need to be greater communication at this interface and possibly hospital pharmacists operating outwith their traditional secondary care base.

As in community pharmacy, technical skills for local manufacturing of individual products is also now greatly reduced and the skills of hospital pharmacists are more utilized in decisions about the cost-effective and clinically effective selection of drugs, and contributing to drug and therapeutic committees, formulary groups and quality assurance procedures. Issues of supply and efficient distribution of medicines are increasingly becoming automated.

Other NHS roles

Primary care pharmacy

During the 1990s there was increasing evidence of close working between pharmacists and the rest of the general practice based primary healthcare team. Doctors realized that pharmacists had many possible additional clinical roles in primary care, beyond their traditional community pharmacy premises. Many pharmacists now provide doctors with advice on GP formulary development (Ch. 18) and undertake patient medication reviews, either seeing patients face to face or through review of patient records, either globally or on an individual basis. They may also take responsibility for specific clinics following agreed protocols, such as anticoagulant and *Helicobacter pylori* assessment clinics. These pharmacists are known as primary care pharmacists. However, as community pharmacy develops along the lines described above, and IT links become the norm, it is envisaged that many of the tasks now done by primary care pharmacists will ultimately be carried out from the community pharmacy base.

Pharmaceutical advisers

As new NHS structures emerge in primary care, services are being delivered in an integrated way, involving the wider healthcare team as well as local authority managed services such as social work, and other community workers. In England these organizations are called primary care organizations, in Scotland community health partnerships, in Wales local health boards, and in Northern Ireland health and social services. Management teams for these organizations generally include a senior pharmacist who will coordinate pharmaceutical care for the organization, integrating community pharmacy into the delivery of core health care, and coordinating the primary care pharmacist workforce to achieve area wide goals in prescribing.

Pharmaceutical public health

Strategic health authorities in England and NHS boards in Scotland administer larger geographical areas. Most of these also have a senior pharmacist, operating at consultant level, as part of the public health team. They have a specific responsibility for local pharmacy strategy development, compliance with statutes and the managed entry of new drugs, as well as providing local professional leadership and advice on professional governance alongside their senior pharmacy colleagues in the trusts. Increasingly as professional boundaries begin to merge, they are also seen as public healthcare professionals and take their share of the generic public health workload. Many are now gaining formal recognition as public health practitioners through membership of the Faculty of Public Health or the UK Voluntary Register for Public Health Specialists.

The public's view

Increasingly patient satisfaction with new services is monitored in formal health services research projects, as part of innovative pilot schemes and for ongoing routine quality control. Indeed one of the requirements of the new contracts is that community pharmacists should 'have in place a system to enable patients to give feedback or evaluate services'. Large surveys of the public's opinion of community pharmacy services have also been conducted. In general such surveys find that the public are satisfied with the service they receive, and that pharmacy is a trusted profession. Research also tells us the public regard community pharmacy services as an important resource for them to access when managing symptoms of minor illness, and that they prefer to seek such advice from a pharmacist rather than a GP or one of the NHS online services. However, it is also shown that they are more wary of hypothetical situations in which pharmacists become involved in the delivery of new roles which have previously been delivered by GPs or nurses working with GPs. In particular older people are less open to new models of service, whereas younger people are much more positive. Once new services have been trialled, such as repeat dispensing, medicines management and prescribing, patient feedback is highly positive. Nonetheless, when asked whether or not they would prefer a doctor or pharmacist to provide the service, there is a status quo bias in favour of the GP. This is not really surprising, but the profession needs to be aware of this. New services have to earn their place in the public's esteem, building confidence in the quality of what they offer and the advantages of pharmacy delivered services. There is also a need for other healthcare professionals to value the pharmacist's new roles and to recognize their increasingly central place in the NHS team.

Quality assured NHS

Some high profile examples of substandard health care, most particularly the investigation into the standards of children's heart surgery at Bristol Royal Infirmary, have focused attention on the need to identify and learn from mistakes and to systematically assess and manage risk. There is now an increasing understanding of the components of a quality assured NHS, and the systems that need to be in place to support this.

Clinical effectiveness

Clinical effectiveness is a term often used to describe the extent to which clinical practice meets the highest known standards of care. Clinical governance is a term used to describe the accountability of an organizational grouping for ensuring that clinical effectiveness is practised by all functions for which it is responsible. Central to this is the use of evidence-based guidelines and protocols, which have increased dramatically in the past decade. (An overview is provided in Chapter 8.) These guidelines are a way of increasing the quality of service because they are developed after systematic searches of the research evidence and make recommendations for 'best practice' which are easily understood and widely accepted.

The extent to which guidelines are actually applied in particular situations should be measured by clinical audit. Chapter 11 aims to give the background to the need for audit and the different ways in which it may be carried out. Audit is also an important tool in the raising of standards of service delivery.

Training, research and development are also all important strands of clinical effectiveness, as are professional reflection and development. Structures established to deliver this agenda for pharmacy are described in more detail in the next section.

Continuing education and continuing professional development

In such a rapidly changing profession, there is a need for continual updating of knowledge. The RPSGB, through *The Pharmaceutical Journal*, has established a regular pattern of continuing education (CE) articles on a wide range of topics and has introduced a formal portfolio-based continuous professional development (CPD) initiative. The council of the RPSGB, through the Code of Ethics, requires that all pharmacists undertake at least 30 hours of continuing education each year. This is now monitored more closely through an online record which requires both details of activities undertaken and reflection on the values of the activities to practise. This approach is thus more about tailored personal and professional development.

Continuing education is further supported by the centres for postgraduate or post-qualification pharmaceutical education (CPPE). They are located in Manchester (England), Cardiff (Wales) and Belfast (Northern Ireland). The Scottish centre is amalgamated with sister organizations in medicine, dentistry, psychology and nursing as a special health board, the NHS Education for Scotland Board. This is an exciting development, once again reflecting new approaches to healthcare delivery and facilitating teamwork across professional boundaries. Courses from all four centres are provided free to pharmacists who are employed in the provision of pharmaceutical services to the NHS.

There is, therefore, good provision for continuing education, which pharmacists use to good effect. At the moment there is no requirement for a further assessment of competence once the pre-registration year is successfully completed but it is unlikely that this will remain the case for much longer.

The role of the RPSGB

The RPSGB has historically undertaken an unusual dual role as a professional body and a regulatory body. For the latter function it is responsible for the registration of pharmacists and premises, for the maintenance of standards though a network of inspectors, and for disciplining those who do not meet the required standard through the Statutory Committee. With increasing public concerns about standards of health care in general, the regulatory function is increasingly open to public scrutiny and the Council for the Regulation of Healthcare Professionals was established. As part of a recent review of the regulation of all healthcare professionals, arising from some high profile cases of suboptimal care, a recommendation has been made that the regulatory functions of the RPSGB will be delivered by an independent body, the General Pharmaceutical Council, and a new body for pharmacy should be created to deliver the complementary professional role. Again at the time of writing, the exact shape of this new body is unknown but it has been suggested it will be akin to that of a royal college, such as is established for the medical specialities. See Chapter 10 for further information on CPD and fitness to practice.

Pharmacy education

Undergraduate education

Teaching of pharmacy was traditionally under four subject headings: pharmaceutical chemistry, pharmaceutics, pharmacology and pharmacognosy. This was seen as a restraint on the development of new ideas of teaching to make the course more relevant to the profession. The course has to have a firm science base, building on knowledge acquired in secondary school, but be relevant to practice. Pharmacognosy is no longer a core part of the undergraduate curriculum. Pathology and therapeutics, law and ethics, and the teaching of dispensing practice all have their place alongside clinical pharmacy, which is now accepted as a subject in its own right and one of the most important parts of the course. The course also includes social and behavioural science – a broad subject area which covers many sociological and psychological aspects of disease and patients – and communication skills. Although communication cannot be learned solely by studying a book, it is still useful to have an understanding of the underpinning theoretical framework when learning to put good professional communication into practice. In this book, chapters have been included dealing with social and behavioural science (Chs 3 and 4), communication skills (Ch. 13) and counselling skills (Ch. 44).

Most schools of pharmacy involve both primary and secondary care pharmacy practitioners in undergraduate teaching. The aim of utilizing these teacher–practitioners is to ensure that the university course is relevant to current professional practice. This reflects the situation in other healthcare professions such as medicine. Other ways of learning from current practice as part of course provision are also used, such as visiting lecturers, making GP practice and hospital visits, using part-time teaching staff, staff secondment to practice and joint academic/practice research studies.

As a result of the need to harmonize the undergraduate courses across the EU as far as possible, all UK courses are now of 4 years, and at master level, with a further year of structured pre-registration training in a practice situation (see below).

Pre-registration training

The purpose of the pre-registration year is for the recent graduate to make the transition from student to a person who can practise effectively and independently as a member of the pharmacy profession. At the end of the year the pre-registration trainee has to pass a formal registration exam prior to entry to the register. Pre-registration training is carried out, in either hospital or community pharmacy practice, in a structured way with a competency-based assessment after 12 months. The recommendation to include both hospital and community practice in the pre-registration year has not yet been acted upon. Some of the differences between community and hospital practice are becoming less distinct as pharmacists in the community take on roles which in the past have been common in hospital practice, such as prescribing advice to doctors. In the future, it may be that a combined pre-registration year may be introduced and interchange between the two areas of practice will become easier to achieve than it is at present.

Higher degrees and research

As recently as the 1980s only a few taught MSc degrees were available. A wide range of such courses is now offered. Some are relatively short; others offer a postgraduate diploma or a master of science. Subject matter may be very specialized or more general. Study may be full time or part time. There are also distance learning courses for those who have limited opportunity to be away from their place of work. Additionally, taught PharmD courses are gaining in popularity and are provided from a small number of institutions across the UK. The programmes are intended to allow pharmacists to develop specialist skills in their chosen area, through formal learning, together with the conduct of either a substantive piece of research or work-based project.

Research has also developed, and research articles appear regularly in the *Pharmaceutical Journal* and the *International Journal of Pharmacy Practice* as well as other academic journals from medicine and primary care. There are practice research sessions at the British Pharmaceutical Conference each year, and there is an annual dedicated Health Service and Pharmacy Practice Research Conference. Many students are now graduating with a doctorate for studies undertaken in aspects of pharmacy practice, and, reflecting the integrated multidisciplinary delivery of care, many pharmacists are carrying out research in multidisciplinary research teams. The development of the discipline of pharmacy practice research has a lot to be proud of. The generation of research evidence of the clinical and cost-effective contribution which pharmacists can make to health care has had a key part to play in the innovations in professional practice we have seen in the past decade, and which have been summarized in this introductory chapter.

Conclusion

During the 20th century, pharmacy has undergone major changes. This process has accelerated since the introduction of the NHS in 1948, the Nuffield Report in 1986 and, most recently, the new plans for the NHS published at the turn of the century. As will be evident from reading this chapter, many changes are still ongoing, demonstrating the vibrant and dynamic nature of both the health service and of our profession. Pharmacists now deal with more potent and sophisticated medicines, requiring a different type of knowledge and a different skill set than was previously the case. At the same time, the public has become more aware of the services which are available from pharmacists. People are making increasing use of the pharmacist as a source of information and advice about minor conditions and non-prescription medicines. This is now

extending to the general public regarding pharmacists as a source of information and advice about their prescribed medicines and seeking help from pharmacists with any medication problems which they may encounter. This process is likely to develop further as society moves into the 21st century. We are also likely to see further changes reflecting the merging of professional boundaries and competency based delivery of health care. Thus generic healthcare professionals may emerge, and many may undertake tasks traditionally undertaken by one profession. In addition, in order to free up professional time, we can expect to see pharmacy technicians taking on greater responsibility for the technical aspects of the pharmacist's role while qualified pharmacists concentrate on cognitive functions and interact directly with the patient.

Pharmacists need to have the knowledge and adaptability to take a lead in these processes, so that they can have a key role in ensuring that the health care of the public can be delivered as efficiently as possible. The undergraduate pharmacy courses must reflect these changes to ensure that their graduates meet the demands of the future NHS workforce.

KEY POINTS

- The UK NHS came into being in 1948
- Early developments in the NHS were in hospital services, but this has gradually changed to focus on community practice
- Publication of the Nuffield Report in 1986 marked a watershed for pharmacy in the UK. It made nearly 100 radical recommendations for change, most of which have been implemented in community pharmacy; use of IT, links with GPs, responding to symptoms, health education, meeting patients' needs, re-regulation of POM to P medicines have all developed
- New community pharmacy contracts in the UK are delivering the vision together with regulatory changes such as patient group directions and supplementary and independent prescribing
- Education at undergraduate and postgraduate levels reflects these changes and pharmacy graduates are well trained for their new roles
- The public values the pharmacist but still has some reservations about too much care being delegated from doctors

2

Models of pharmacy practice within healthcare systems

Judith A. Rees

STUDY POINTS

- Some of the influences on pharmacy worldwide
- Private and public healthcare systems
- Classification of medicines, availability and advertising of medicines
- Different educational pathways for pharmacists
- Registration and regulation of pharmacists and pharmacies
- Types of community pharmacy organization
- Different types of hospital pharmacy

Introduction

The development and role of pharmacy practice in the UK was detailed in Chapter 1. It can be seen that the role of, and demands on, the pharmacist has come a long way from being an apothecary or simply a dispenser of medicines. Chapter 6 describes the types of patient charges for prescriptions and their impact. What becomes clear from these two chapters is that there are many methods used by healthcare systems in different countries to charge patients for their medicines. Also, lists of medicines have to be drawn up in less well developed or economically poorer countries to assist them provide basic essential medicines for their populations (see Ch. 7). Thus it becomes apparent that different countries, depending on their economic circumstances and their values (political or otherwise), have developed numerous different methods to provide and distribute medicines to their communities.

Most countries of the world have some system of healthcare provision and involve a range of healthcare

providers. The latter may range from very basically trained lay support or outreach workers to highly skilled, university-graduated, regulated and registered healthcare professionals. The skills and range of healthcare workers available in a country will depend mainly on the economic development of that country. Richer countries generally have more healthcare workers with more of them highly trained and skilled.

Healthcare provision throughout the world is not equitable. Although economically rich countries often help poorer countries with financial aid, medicines, medical equipment, advice and some healthcare professionals, etc., there is still inequality between countries. This can be demonstrated by comparing the average overall life expectancy between countries (Table 2.1).

Discussion of how equitable health care can be provided worldwide is outside the scope of this chapter. The chapter describes some of the actual healthcare systems to illustrate their diversity and, in particular, emphasizes the role of pharmacists, their education, regulation and registration, and the supply and distribution of medicines to a country's inhabitants. Rather than describing the healthcare provision and the role of pharmacists in every country in the world, the aim has been to look at trends, similarities and differences between countries.

Healthcare systems

No one healthcare system is perfect for all situations and equally no system will be totally static. Countries do look at other healthcare systems and often copy, emulate and subsume the perceived 'good ideas' into their own systems. Healthcare systems will change

Table 2.1 Life expectancy in years at birth for different countries

Country	Life expectancy at birth (years)
World average	67.2
Japan	82.6
Australia	81.2
Singapore	80.0
UK	79.4
USA	78.2
Lithuania	73.0
Saudi Arabia	72.8
India	64.7
Gambia	59.4
Kenya	54.1
Nigeria	46.9
Swaziland	39.6

depending on the economic stability, growth of the country and political or governmental changes. Other factors include changing demographics of the population, development of new medicines and medical technologies, the emergence of new diseases (e.g. HIV and AIDS) or the eradication of old diseases (e.g. smallpox). Most countries with the lowest life expectancies are those in which there are high incidence rates of HIV/AIDS, such as Swaziland, Botswana, Zimbabwe and Zambia. These countries also lack the finance to provide the population with antiretroviral drugs.

Pharmacists and/or pharmacy technicians (the names may vary in different countries) are present in most countries. Their roles may be widely different; for example in some countries the concept of pharmaceutical care or medicines management may not be accepted or well developed, so there will not be roles for pharmacists in those specialist areas. However, because of the increased availability of modern medicines of greater potency and cost, it becomes imperative that someone is responsible for their distribution and supply to the population, either via dispensed prescriptions or by sale over the counter. Due to their efficacy and side-effects, medicines are both potent and potentially dangerous. A rational dis-

tribution system safeguards the population by controlling the supply of medicines to the general public. In most countries pharmacists are normally given the authority to be the guardians of medicines. Thus they are the healthcare professionals with the responsibility for the safe, effective, rational and economic use of medicines. However, the extent of these responsibilities will be dependent on the healthcare system in the individual country and the legal controls placed on medicines, their supply and the healthcare professionals involved. Pharmacists will be employed in the pharmaceutical industry (if there is one in the country) as the developer and producer of manufactured medicines. Alternatively pharmacists will be engaged in controlling the importation of medicines, checking their authenticity and safety. Pharmacists or pharmacy technicians will be involved in the extemporaneous production or small-scale supply and distribution of medicines, whether in hospitals, in healthcare centres such as district clinics in remoter areas, or in pharmacies in the community.

Each country tends to develop its own system to accommodate its own particular needs and in line with its economic ability. Clearly the provision of pharmaceutical services and medicines will be different in a small economically rich country with good transportation and communication links when compared to that of a much poorer, geographically large country with remote areas and limited transportation and communication links.

The legal structure within a country will influence both the distribution of medicines and the place of the pharmacist in that distribution system. Laws may strictly regulate the production, distribution, marketing and supply of medicines, e.g. the UK Medicines Act 1968 and its subsequent amendments and subsuming of EU law. Other countries may have much less tight regulation of their medicines. The legislation in place will control, for example:

- Which medicines are available for purchase directly by the public
- Which medicines are only available on prescription
- Whether and which medicines can be advertised directly to the public
- Who can prescribe and who can dispense medicines.

Further legislation may regulate the education of potential pharmacists and whether they need to register with a state or professional body before being able to practise. For example, the Pharmacist and Pharmacy Technicians Order 2007 in the UK details the education, registration and fitness to practise of pharmacists and pharmacy technicians, as well as the procedure for disciplining or even removing a pharmacist or pharmacy technician from the register. Thus the legislation in place at any time in a country will have a direct effect on the ability of a person to become and remain a pharmacist and their opportunities for employment and career prospects. These will be explored in more detail.

UK healthcare systems

Pharmacists throughout the world have to operate within the particular healthcare system of their country. This will have a direct effect on their roles, responsibilities and employment opportunities. In most countries the aim is that all citizens have access to health care. This is called universality. However, how and whether this is achieved will differ between countries. Most countries have a private healthcare system running alongside a state or insurance-based system which will either fully or partially fund treatment. A system of claims and/or benefits may be in place for certain members of the country – for example the young, the old and the unemployed may receive free treatment.

In the UK, all the population (including visitors) are provided with a 'free' healthcare system provided by the National Health Service (NHS) which is funded through taxation. In the primary care sector, that is in the community, many healthcare professionals are independent but have contracts with the NHS to provide NHS services. For example doctors and dentists will have contracts with the NHS so that access to them is free, although in the case of dentists, while a dental check up is free, there is a co-payment scheme in operation for any treatment. In practice this means that patients can choose to be treated either as an NHS patient or as a private patient by their dentist, so the dentist operates in both the private sector and the NHS. Community pharmacists are similarly independent but most will have a contract with the NHS to provide dispensing and pharmaceutical services. This situation enables community pharmacists to dispense both private and NHS prescriptions and to provide private pharmaceutical services if they wish. The NHS also provides the secondary care structures such as hospitals, health centres/clinics, etc., and employs a wide range of healthcare professionals such as pharmacists, nurses, physiotherapists, nutritionists, social workers and doctors. Access to hospital treatment is free.

While most medicines are available on an NHS prescription, a few medicines, in particular some of the newer, more expensive drugs with limited long-term clinical evidence, may not be available. Thus if a person is financially able to afford these NHS-restricted medicines then a private prescription can be written alongside NHS prescriptions. Additionally community pharmacies, as independent retailers, can offer medicines as well as other goods for sale.

Alongside the NHS a private healthcare sector exists with a full range of hospitals and healthcare professionals and healthcare provision. Individuals choosing to be treated privately will have to cover all the associated costs. However, many individuals pay using insurance or private healthcare schemes which may be a benefit of their employment for themselves and their families.

For pharmacists the two systems mean that there are employment opportunities within both NHS and private hospitals. Likewise pharmacists employed in community pharmacy might find themselves dispensing both private and NHS prescriptions. Community pharmacists may find themselves providing medicines for minor ailments via a free NHS scheme to eligible patients, while other customers would have to buy the same medicine themselves because they are not eligible for the scheme. Thus pharmacists need to understand the healthcare systems in which they are working in order to be efficient and productive and provide a quality pharmaceutical service to their patients within the appropriate healthcare system.

Some other healthcare systems

In Australia the principle of universality aims to provide access to the same standard of care for all citizens based on a health insurance scheme called Medicare. All citizens contribute via the taxation system, depending on their ability to pay. However, unlike the UK NHS system, while access to public hospitals is free, cash benefits are paid from Medicare for the cost of access to general practitioners and other healthcare specialties, such as dentists and optometrists. Prescription medicines are provided from private pharmacies and a pharmaceutical benefits scheme exists which provides a co-payment scheme for prescriptions and lists of eligible medicines. The system is fairly complex with different levels of benefit depending on the status of the individual (welfare entitlement of the citizen) and the lists of eligible and non-authorized medicines. Patients may choose to pay extra for branded products rather than generically prescribed medicines. Australian pharmacists require a good understanding of the pharmaceutical benefits scheme and the medicines and brands of medicines available if they are to provide both a good pharmaceutical service for their patients and navigate the system.

In Ireland the emphasis of health care is on the individual arranging their own private medical and surgical services for themselves and their family. However, there is a free healthcare scheme in cases of hardship, called the General Medical Services (GMS). This scheme also covers all under 16-year-olds and those over 70 years of age. Community pharmacies are privately owned and have to enter into an agreement with the local health board to provide GMS services. GMS provides a system of health care in which many individuals are covered to a greater or lesser extent by a drug payment scheme and a long-term illness scheme. Both are very convoluted and provide a level of benefits for almost every group of patients. These benefits can include a range of subsidized or free medicines and appliances. While the aim is a private GMS, the work of pharmacists working within the system will be increased by the system.

These three healthcare schemes are a mixture of private and public. The public scheme either covers the majority of the population or picks up the poorer or more dependent sections of the population. In Saudi Arabia all nationals are provided with free health care and medicines. In that country, all community pharmacies are privately owned and are recompensed by the state for dispensing and the other pharmaceutical services that they provide.

The different healthcare systems described above, while not comprehensive, do indicate the variety of healthcare systems available. Clearly pharmacists have to work in the healthcare system of a particular country. This may impose different systems of working because of characteristics of the provisions for health care. It is essential that, whatever the situation, pharmacists provide the best pharmaceutical services for their patients within any limitations imposed on them by the national healthcare system.

Legal classification of medicines

The legal classification used for medicines in a country will have a direct impact on the practice of pharmacists. Most countries have laws to restrict access to

narcotic analgesics and other groups of potent medicines.

Some countries have a two-tier classification of drugs:
- 'Prescription only' with dispensing limited to pharmacists
- 'Non-prescription' medicines, also called 'general sales' or 'over the counter' (OTC) medicines. These medicines are available from pharmacies and also from other retail outlets such as grocers, supermarkets, newsagents and garage forecourts.

Some countries further divide non-prescription medicines into 'pharmacy medicines' and OTC medicines. 'Pharmacy medicines' are available for sale to the general public but only from a pharmacy and under the supervision of a pharmacist. Thus pharmacists have a direct input into the sale of these medicines. Germany, Ireland and the UK are examples of countries which have this three-tier classification. Australia also has a three-tier classification, but has further divided pharmacy medicines into those that can be sold:
- Only under the direct supervision of a pharmacist in a pharmacy and cannot be self-selected
- In a community pharmacy on a self-selection basis.

The USA, Estonia and Saudi Arabia are examples of countries with a two-tier system in which only pharmacists control access by the general public to prescription only medicines.

In recent years some medicines have been reclassified, usually from prescription only to pharmacy or general sales classifications. This allows more medicines to become available to the general public for purchase. It also gives the pharmacist more control over the sale of medicines classed as pharmacy medicines. Such a process has given pharmacists a more professional image and increased the professional content of their work. The reclassification process can go from general sales to prescription only, but this would only be expected if a drug was found to have major side-effects not suitable for a general sales medicine. This would be unusual.

Advertising and availability of medicines

Many countries have strict controls on the advertising of prescription only medicines. For example, advertising to anyone other than a healthcare professional is banned in the UK. These controls are to help protect the public from the potential misuse of medicines. However, in other countries, banning advertising is considered to be a constraint on trade and so advertising of prescription only medicines is allowed, as for example in China. With the advent of the Internet it is very difficult for any country to completely control the advertising of prescription only medicines, and the general public can now access both advertising and information about prescription only medicines via the Internet. Some of the information on these sites may contain inaccurate information. However, having acquired this knowledge some patients consider themselves (often incorrectly) to be knowledgeable about medicines. They may become very demanding of pharmacists and doctors in their quest to obtain a particular medicine.

The advertising of pharmacy medicines and general sales medicines is usually permitted. However, most countries will have, as a minimum, some guidelines to ensure that advertisements are truthful and do not make excessive claims for their products. Again, this advertising of pharmacy medicines may result in difficult patients who are not prepared for the pharmacist to advise against, or refuse to sanction, their purchase of a particular pharmacy medicine. Thus the laws governing the advertising of medicines in their country will influence the everyday work of community pharmacists.

The availability of medicines in a country is usually dependent on the general wealth of the country, with the richer countries usually having a full range of all the marketed medicines and the ability to import from other countries as required. Thus pharmacists in these countries will deal with many hundreds of different medicines, especially if there is a range of proprietary and generic medicines available for the same drug. Pharmacists will need to use their full range of knowledge and skill. This situation contrasts very sharply with poorer countries, in which even essential medicines (see Ch. 7) may not be available. In such countries the role of the pharmacist will be limited and some aspects of clinical pharmacy will not be possible.

Education of pharmacists

The education of pharmacists follows a similar pattern worldwide. This is not surprising since a few countries have exerted a wide influence through a history of domination. Europeans settled in many countries in their quest for discovery and wealth and thereby influenced the development of those countries. One example was the British, whose empire dominated many countries; the British Empire eventually evolved into the less dominant but still influential British Commonwealth.

More recently the creation of the European Community, later the European Union (EU), has resulted in the need to harmonize the education and recognition of professionals throughout member countries. This has resulted in a minimum of 4 years' undergraduate university education for the awarding of an accreditable pharmacy degree in the EU. An agreement to standardize the curricula between member countries within the EU has emerged. The 4-year degree is followed by a 1-year practical training (called pre-registration in the UK, internship in Germany) in a pharmaceutical setting and under the supervision of a pharmacist. In some countries the 1-year practical training may be incorporated into the degree structure, thereby lengthening the degree.

Countries as geographically widespread as New Zealand, Australia, Singapore, Brazil and Saudi Arabia have also developed this 4 plus 1 model of pharmaceutical education.

Registration as a pharmacist

The legislation in most countries requires registration as a pharmacist with a professional and/or regulatory body or the state. For example, Singapore has a Pharmacists Registration Act requiring pharmacists to register with Singapore's Pharmacy Board, while in the UK, the Pharmacy and Pharmacy Technicians Order is the legal basis setting out the registration requirements. Requirements usually include the prospective registrant to have achieved success in a professional examination, usually termed the registration examination, prior to applying for registration. Unless actually registered, a person cannot work as a pharmacist, even if they have completed all the educational and registration requirements. Pharmacists wishing to work in a country other than the one in which they were educated will usually have to complete further training. This is likely to include practical training and passing at least one examination. The latter may be equivalent to the registration examination, but may require more extensive knowledge before applying for registration in that country.

In the UK, prospective pharmacists have to successfully complete the pre-registration year and the registration examination before registering with the Royal Pharmaceutical Society of Great Britain (RPSGB).

The RPSGB is an example of a combined professional and regulatory body. Plans are in place to separate these two roles and establish a separate regulatory body which will register and monitor 'fitness to practice' of pharmacists (see Ch. 10). It will have disciplinary powers to deregister, if necessary. The other body will have a professional role. Similarly other countries, such as New Zealand, have recently and successfully separated these functions.

In South Africa, pharmacists must register with the South African Pharmacy Council, which is the statutory body. Its objectives include the control, promotion and maintenance of standards of pharmaceutical education and pharmacy practice. It also plays a role in the control and maintenance of the professional conduct of registered pharmacists. This system is an example of a separate registration body. Professional organizations exist in South Africa, including the Pharmaceutical Society of South Africa, to professionally represent pharmacists.

In Saudi Arabia, the Pharmacy Board of the Saudi Food and Drug Authority acts as the regulatory and registration body for pharmacy.

In very small countries such as Bermuda, which does not offer its own pharmacy degrees, overseas trained pharmacists are employed, usually with US, Canadian or UK degrees. They are required to undertake a 1-month pre-registration training to acquaint themselves with the Bermudan system before taking a pre-registration examination. Success in the examination will allow the individual to register as a pharmacist with the Pharmaceutical Council of Bermuda.

Most of the regulatory bodies place requirements on registered pharmacists including compliance with codes of practice or standards. For example, the South African Pharmacy Council publishes Rules for Good Pharmacy Practice and a list of products that should not be sold in a community pharmacy. Continuing professional development (CPD) is rapidly becoming a mandatory requirement for continuing registration as a pharmacist. Some countries require obligatory credits, for example Saudi Arabia requires 60 credits over 3 years. Other countries simply require the pharmacist to undertake CPD, while yet others, including the UK, require written records.

The requirement for registration and the concomitant application of 'rules of professional behaviour' and CPD places responsibilities and obligations on pharmacists in their practice of pharmacy. Ignorance of these 'rules' and CPD requirements may place a pharmacist in the position of being disciplined by the regulatory body and ultimately de-registered. Thus a knowledge of the continuing requirements for registration must influence how a pharmacist behaves professionally both at work and during leisure.

Community pharmacy

From the earlier description of healthcare systems, it is apparent that most community pharmacies are privately owned. State owned pharmacies were the norm in the former Soviet Bloc countries, but these have now been privatized. In some countries, for example Estonia and Switzerland, only pharmacists can own a pharmacy. Some countries limit the number of pharmacies which a pharmacist can own. In Germany, for example, pharmacists are limited to owning no more than four pharmacies, while in some Australian states the limit is no more than three pharmacies. In Finland, no pharmacist can own more than one pharmacy, but with permission, can own up to three 'subsidiaries' in the neighbourhood. In Finland, a 5–6-year masters degree in pharmacy is offered in addition to a 3-year bachelors degree, but a pharmacy can only be owned by a pharmacist with a masters degree.

In some countries the ownership of pharmacies is not restricted to pharmacists and the number of pharmacies owned is similarly not restricted. This arrangement gives rise to chains of pharmacies and pharmacies within supermarkets. The UK, Australia, USA, Lithuania and Saudi Arabia are examples of countries with this latter model. Some countries have regulations limiting the number of pharmacies within a geographical area or even the location of pharmacies.

In a similar way to the registration of a pharmacist, most countries will require a pharmacy to be registered and/or licensed with an appropriate body. This body may impose conditions on the pharmacy, such as required equipment, grades and numbers of staff, dispensary size, having counselling areas, places for health promotion leaflets, etc.

Some of these requirements mean that pharmacists in such pharmacies will be expected to use the counselling room for medication reviews. This is the case in the UK and Australia, for example. In some countries there may be an emphasis on the provision of health promotion advice, possibly accompanied by a leaflet. Other pharmacies will have testing equipment to provide, for example, cholesterol or *Chlamydia* testing. Yet other pharmacies may develop expertise in extemporaneous dispensing.

Thus, depending on the country in which they work, community pharmacists will find themselves able to own a pharmacy or be employed in an independent pharmacy or a chain or supermarket pharmacy. The registering or licensing body decides the conditions in which they work and the type of work that they are required to undertake. These different models will clearly affect the working conditions of a pharmacist.

Hospital pharmacy

Pharmacists may work in either private or public hospitals depending on the healthcare organization in the country. The role of hospital pharmacists in different countries will be dependent on the range of medicines available, the distribution systems in place and the extent of development of clinical pharmacy and other specialist areas.

Hospital pharmacy was originally concerned with the distribution and manufacturing of medicines. In many wealthier countries and those with an abundant supply of medicines this function has changed to one with more emphasis on clinical pharmacy and the rational and appropriate use of medicines. Thus pharmacists are not confined to the dispensary, but will conduct patient medication reviews, take part in ward rounds, provide therapeutic drug monitoring, deliver drug information services and advise on medicines management. Additionally, specialist pharmacists have evolved with the spread of clinical pharmacy in areas such as intensive care, HIV/AIDS and psychiatric pharmacy, for example. With a diminution of the manufacturing function, the distributive and manufacturing functions in hospital pharmacy are often delegated to others, for example pharmacy technicians, who develop their own areas of specialization.

In many countries, hospital pharmacists have developed their own organizations. An example is the Society of Hospital Pharmacists of Australia. These organizations unite hospital pharmacists, promote their role and provide routes for exchange of information and education and training.

Thus the practice of hospital pharmacy will depend on the country, the availability of medicines and the extent of development of clinical pharmacy.

Conclusion

While there are many similarities in the roles of pharmacists working in different countries, the dissimilarities are also evident. The role of pharmacists depends to a great extent on the healthcare systems in place. In most countries, there is a mix of private and public health care and most community pharmacists will be working in a private community pharmacy which will contract to provide pharmaceutical services to both private and state systems. Thus the pharmacist must have a wide understanding of the system of charging patients and the system for reimbursement from the public healthcare system. The role of hospital pharmacists is changing from distributive and manufacturing pharmacy to patient centred pharmacy. However, the role of all pharmacists will be dependent on the medicines available and their legal classifications.

KEY POINTS

- A wide spectrum of methods of healthcare provision is used around the world because no one system is ideal for all circumstances
- There is a lack of equity in healthcare provision with richer countries having more advanced systems, but often providing financial aid to poorer countries
- Healthcare systems must react to local needs
- The potency of modern medicines requires responsible distribution, usually by a pharmacist or technician, in order to protect the public
- Legal controls vary in classifying medicines, advertising, availability and dispensing of medicines
- Most countries provide health care to citizens, often alongside a private system, funded centrally or by insurance schemes
- Because of the diversity of schemes, pharmacists must be fully conversant with the scheme in the country in which they practise
- Most countries adopt a two-tier or three-tier classification of medicines and allow for reclassification
- Many countries allow advertising of pharmacy and general sales medicines but restrict or ban advertising of prescription medicines
- A 4-year plus 1 model for pharmacist education is normal, although 'registration' requirements vary
- Ownership of community pharmacies might be restricted in some countries by number, geography or pharmacist qualification

3

Socio-behavioural aspects of health and illness

K. Hannes Enlund

STUDY POINTS

- Why social and behavioural sciences are important in pharmacy
- The meaning of health and illness
- Factors incorporated into models of health
- How people behave when they are ill
- Behavioural aspects of health care
- Factors affecting the treatment process

Introduction

For a full understanding of the use of medicines and the role of pharmacy in health care it is necessary to consider sociological and psychological factors which often are tightly interwoven. These are still rather new areas within pharmacy education and research. Understanding and resolving medicine-related problems that result in suboptimal outcomes requires a scientific basis, and earlier attempts to solve these problems using 'common sense' approaches have been only partially successful. Therefore there is a need to broaden our perspectives by incorporating relevant social and behavioural theory and research.

The purpose of this and the next chapter is to give a broad overview of the health-related issues within a social and behavioural framework to show the importance of 'non-biological' factors in understanding health and illness with relevance to practising pharmacy. Illness can be seen either as a purely biophysical state or more comprehensively as a human societal state where behaviour varies with culture and other social factors. A common view is that the pure biomedical model underemphasizes the human aspects of patient care and neglects important psychosocial issues. The social sciences have a shared focus on understanding patterns and meaning of human behaviour, which distinguishes them from the physical and biological sciences.

Pharmacists have to deal with many social and behavioural issues in their daily work, either directly or indirectly. The contribution of social sciences to pharmacy and pharmacy practice can be summarized in the following three areas:

- Analysing pharmacy, i.e. helping in identifying important questions relating to the use of medicines, the practice of pharmacy and pharmacy as a profession
- Providing conceptual and explanatory frameworks for understanding human behaviour in a social context
- Providing tools to study the use of medicines and pharmacy.

The aim here is not to be all-inclusive, but rather to highlight important contributions from social and behavioural sciences. Many of the subjects presented could fill a book on their own, so it is evident that only a brief introduction to each subject is possible in this chapter. This chapter will focus on the definitions, dimensions and determinants of health and illness. For a pharmacist it is also very important to understand the different processes involved in illness behaviour and treatment. There is also an attempt to mention the major concepts and theories in each context. An overall framework is presented in Figure 3.1. The interested reader is referred to the specialized textbooks, other books and articles on the topic that are included in the further reading (Appendix 5).

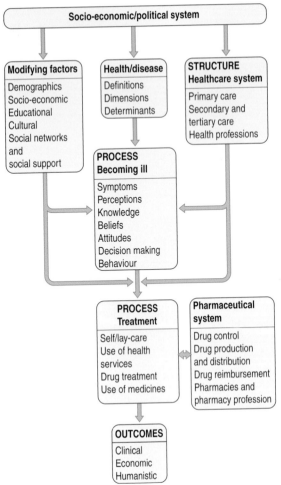

Figure 3.1 • A model of the social and behavioural factors involved in health and illness.

Defining health and illness

Health and illness mean different things to different people. Most young people take health for granted. We commonly think about health as the absence of signs that the body is not functioning properly or absence of symptoms of disease or injury. There is a tendency to dichotomize health; either you are healthy or not. However, health is not merely the absence of disease, but rather a continuum of different states. There are degrees of wellness and of illness. Disease, in contrast to illness, is something professionally defined and therefore also perceived to be more accurate. This has also become the essential framework for the organization we call health care. However, research shows that physicians and other experts vary greatly in their views on both physical and mental disorders and their connections. Therefore we can ask whether disease is well defined or even definable.

Illness is more a state defined by a layman or a reaction to a perceived biological alteration of the body or mind. It has both physical and social connotations. Illness is also highly individual. It is influenced by cultural, social and other factors. It is important to note that a person may have a disease and not be ill, might be ill but not have a disease or might have both an illness and a disease. Sickness is also a socially defined condition, a social status conferred on an individual by other members of the society. This will be further elaborated in the context of the sick role (p. 30).

The most widely used definition of health or wellness is that of the World Health Organization (WHO), which states that: 'Health is a state of complete physical, mental and social well-being and not merely the absence of diseases and infirmity'. This definition has been widely quoted, but is less used in daily practice in health care. The definition has to be seen more as a goal that is actively sought through positive actions and not merely as a passive way of avoiding disease-causing agents. Different definitions and models of health also have practical relevance, as they are needed to guide policymakers in their allocation of resources.

Dimensions of health

The WHO definition distinguishes physical, mental and social health. In some narrower definitions, only physical and mental health are included, thus implicitly excluding resource allocation for other areas. A broader definition may emphasize social and other dimensions as well. One of the dangers is that the broader the definition, the more we tend to medicalize our society as we include more and more everyday things as part of the responsibility of clinical medicine and public health (e.g. loneliness, attention deficit disorders, domestic violence). On the other hand, these broad definitions allow us to examine health issues more comprehensively. The definition used will also have economical and other consequences.

Most of us see physical health as being free from pain, physical disability, acute and chronic diseases and bodily discomfort, i.e. as the normal functioning of the body's cells, organs and systems. However, our prior experiences of disease, age, education and a variety of other personal and social factors will influence our perception of physical health.

Mental health is composed of the ability to deal constructively with reality and adapt to change without feeling threatened by it. A positive self-image and an ability to cope with stressors and develop intimate relationships are also part of mental health. Furthermore, enjoying the pleasures of ordinary life and making plans for the future are important aspects of mental health.

The role of spiritual health has raised less research interest. Some might consider this as merely part of the mental health dimension, while others argue that it is a separate dimension. It should not be confused with religion or religiousness. A sense of spiritual well-being is possible without belonging to an organized religion. Spiritual health has been characterized by Miller & Price (1998) as the ability to articulate and act on one's own basic purpose of life, giving and receiving love, trust, joy and peace, having a set of principles to live by, having a sense of selflessness, honour, integrity and sacrifice and being willing to help others achieve their full potential. By contrast, a negative spiritual health can be described by loss of meaning in one's life, self-centredness, lack of self-responsibility and a hopeless attitude.

The impact of social health on the well-being of the individual has been widely demonstrated. Social integration, social networks and social support have both direct and indirect influences on health. A low socio-economic status defined by educational level, income and occupation is closely related to higher morbidity and mortality.

Determinants and models of health

The history of medicine contains several theories, or frameworks, for the origins of disease. One of the earliest explanations was that mystical forces like evil spirits could cause physical and mental illness. The father of medicine, Hippocrates (460–370 BC), developed the humoral theory to explain why people get sick. According to this theory the body contains four fluids (blood, phlegm, yellow and black bile) called humours. When these are in balance we are in a state of health and, accordingly, when there is an imbalance we are sick.

In the Middle Ages illness was closely related to religious beliefs and sickness was often interpreted as God's punishment for doing evil things. Priests led most of the practice of medicine and became more involved in treating the ill, sometimes torturing the body to drive out evil spirits. After the Renaissance different scholars became more human-centred, one of the most influential in the 17th century being René Descartes. Descartes' impact on scientific thought has been extensive and lasted for centuries. His main health-related ideas can be summarized in three points: first he saw the body as a machine and described how action and sensation occur, second he proposed that body and mind, although separate, could communicate, and third that the soul in humans leaves the body at death.

In the following centuries scientists learned more and more how the body functions with the help of the microscope and other technical advances. New theories, like the germ theory, tried to explain disease by microbes, etc. All these advances led to the foundation of the current biomedical disease model, which proposes that all diseases or physical disorders can be explained by disturbances in physiological processes which result from injury, biochemical imbalances and bacterial or viral infections. The biomedical model assumes that disease is an affliction of the body and is separate from the psychological and social processes of the mind.

A more recent and comprehensive model is the biopsychosocial model that involves the interplay of biological, psychological and social aspects of a person's life.

Additionally, some ancient beliefs about ill health and disease, still prevalent among primitive tribes and in certain cultures, continue surprisingly strongly in industrialized countries alongside conventional medicine. Wrong behaviour, diet, dirty water, weather, accidents, black magic or witchcraft, spirits and God are all mentioned as causes of diseases. 'Don't wet your feet or you'll catch a cold' typifies certain superstitious thinking.

Genetic and biological determinants

In current medicine there is much interest in the genetic basis of disease. The origin of most health problems seems to lie in human genes. The newspapers have declared the finding of the alcoholism, antisocial behaviour and obesity genes among others. This leads to the lay impression that once the genetic code has been solved all health problems will also be solved without any need to pay attention to, for example, health habits. This is, of course, far too simplistic a way of thinking. The scientific interest in this field lies in interactions between genetic endowment and psychosocial factors in early childhood. Laboratory research with animals has shown that genetically predisposed spontaneously hypertensive rat pups cross-fostered by normotensive mothers did not develop hypertension as they matured. This study shows that poor genetic endowment can be overruled by favourable upbringing and environment.

Behavioural determinants

The leading causes of death today – heart disease, cancer, stroke and accidents – are all associated with behavioural risk factors. The origin of many chronic diseases such as diabetes and hypertension can be found in lifestyle factors. Sedentary lifestyle explains a lot of the causes of these diseases without the need to go to the gene level. Sometimes positive genetic endowment can explain why poor health habits are not leading to poor health. It is also remarkable that the remedy for most of these lifestyle diseases can be found in simple behavioural remedies like increased physical activity, reduced stress, balanced diet and quitting smoking.

Behaviour and mental processes are the focus of psychology and they involve cognition, emotion and motivation. Cognition involves perceiving, knowing, learning, remembering, thinking, interpreting, believing and problem solving. Emotion is a subjective feeling that affects and is affected by our thoughts, behaviour and physiology. Emotions can be positive/pleasant or negative/unpleasant. People whose emotions are more positive are less disease prone and more likely to recover quickly from an illness than those with more negative emotions. Motivation applies to explanations of why people behave the way they do, e.g. why they start a health-related activity or why they do not take their medicines as prescribed. Psychology is also interested in interpersonal relationships, which includes thinking, feeling and doing with someone else. Descriptions of cognition, affect, behaviour and interpersonal interactions overlap and it may be difficult to separate them; for example, in a situation causing anxiety the person may think he is not in control of the situation (cognitive component), he is afraid (affective) and his hands are sweating (behavioural) and he may ask somebody to help support him (interpersonal).

Stress is a condition that results when personal/environmental transactions lead the individual to perceive a discrepancy (real or not) between the demands of a situation and the resources of the person's biological, psychological or social system. The connection between body and mind is also reflected in how people react to stress. It can produce changes in the body's physiology and cause illness. Stress can release hormones, especially catecholamines and corticosteroids, by the endocrine system through arousal. Effects on the cardiovascular system can be important and stress-related emotions such as anxiety and depression can play a critical role in the balance of the immune system. Stress can be described as a stimulus. Events and circumstances that are perceived as threatening or harmful, and which produce feelings of tension, are called stressors. However, stress can also be seen as a response to stressors. The person's physiological and psychological response to a stressor is called strain. Stress can be seen as a process including stressors and strain and the relationship between the person and the environment as continuous interactions and adjustments.

Stress can also affect health through the person's behaviour. People who experience high levels of stress tend to behave in a way that increases their chances of becoming ill or injured. They consume more alcohol and drugs and smoke more than people who experience less stress. Accident rates are also higher among those with elevated stress.

Environmental determinants

The role of environmental factors (biological, chemical, physical, mechanical) in influencing human health is widely accepted. The main pathways into the human body are air (outdoor and indoor), water, food and soil. The role of these environmental factors in the pathogenesis of asthma, hay fever and others is clear. However, environmental factors have a much broader impact, starting in the prenatal phase (e.g. the use of drugs like thalidomide during pregnancy has led to severe birth defects).

The importance of the environment has been demonstrated in migrant and time-trend studies of disease. When people change environment their disease risk patterns change. One interesting demonstration is the case of Japanese migrants. The further they went across the Pacific the higher their incidence of coronary heart disease and the lower their rate of stroke. Japanese in Hawaii have rates of heart disease intermediate between those in Japan and those in California. Environment and lifestyle are the most probable explanations of these differences.

There is also a distinction between individual risk factors and environmental causes of disease. Differences in individual risk factors explain only a part of the variation in the occurrence of disease. While reducing high risk factors might be beneficial for the individual concerned, it makes a limited contribution to reducing disease rates in the whole population. Rose has suggested that the causes of individual differences in disease may be different from the causes of differences between populations. A risk factor does not necessarily cause the disease even if it is associated with it.

Socio-economic determinants

These factors are also 'environmental', but it can be debated as to whether they are genuine factors determining health or whether they only represent predisposing factors. Society establishes certain health values, which are often reflected in the media. These values can be both positive and negative. Being fit and healthy is 'good' and exemplifies a positive value, while celebrities smoking cigarettes or marijuana exemplify a negative value. The family is the closest and most continuous social relationship for most people. Therefore, many health-related habits, behaviours and attitudes are learned and modelled from this context. The degree of support or encouragement received from family members and friends for partaking in a health-related activity might be an important factor. This is dealt with in more detail later (p. 38).

In developing countries factors such as poverty, poor nutrition and poor resistance to pathogens are all interrelated with a poor health status of the population. Similarly, historical statistics from industrialized countries show that over the last two or three centuries there has been a strong positive correlation between improved health, life expectancy and improved economy. In most countries the relationship between socio-economic status and disease runs across the social hierarchy. This shows that the relationship between socio-economic status and health is a question of relative deprivation rather than absolute deprivation. This linear association can only be partially explained by lifestyle factors. Usually people with a higher socio-economic status have healthier habits than those from lower socio-economic groups. Similarly there are huge differences in life expectancy between western and eastern European countries that can be attributed to socio-economic factors.

Interaction of different factors

It is evident that no single factor can alone explain the health of a nation, demographic group or individual. It is difficult to capture all the relevant features and their relationships. Having good genes can prevent some people from getting a disease; on the other hand, somebody with poor genes can get ill regardless of a healthy lifestyle and other positive factors. Considering the impact of all aspects of a person's life as a total entity in understanding health and illness is called holism.

One comprehensive attempt to describe/model the interactions between different factors is the 'nested model of health'. This model consists of two levels of activity, the individual and the community level. The individual level is composed of five different categories:

- Psychosocial environment (e.g. personal housing)
- Microphysical environment (e.g. chemicals and noise)
- Work environment (e.g. work stress)
- Behavioural environment (e.g. smoking, alcohol use, exercise)
- Race/class/gender environment.

These environments are thought to affect each other and to affect and be affected by the individual. The individual level is nested/located in the centre of the community level. This community level, which is the main focus of health policy decision makers, is composed of four components, the political/economic climate (e.g. unemployment level), the macro physical environment (e.g. air quality), social justice/equity (e.g. social security system) and local control/cohesiveness (e.g. local planning efforts). These four components are interrelated and changes in them are expected to lead to changes in the health of individuals.

Process of illness

Becoming ill

Understanding illness behaviour can help pharmacists appreciate and accept why patients respond differently to seemingly similar pain or discomfort. The general criteria by which people view themselves as 'well' include a feeling of well-being, an absence of symptoms and an ability to perform normal functions. This is the baseline situation against which any changes are judged. When studying health-related behaviour it is important to consider how behaviour changes with the health status of the individual. Kasl & Cobb defined three types of behaviour that characterize three stages in the progress of disease:

- Health behaviour, which refers to any activity undertaken by people believing themselves to be healthy for the purpose of preventing disease or detecting it at an asymptomatic stage
- Illness behaviour, which involves any activity undertaken by people who feel ill, to define the state of their health and to discover a suitable remedy
- Sick-role behaviour, which refers to the activity undertaken for the purpose of getting well by those who consider themselves ill.

Ways of identifying and reacting to symptoms

Symptoms can be classified into three broad groups: those symptoms noted by the patient, symptoms noted by behavioural changes and patient complaints. A behaviour which in some situations is regarded as normal can in other situations be regarded as a sign of illness. Not all symptoms can be regarded as medical, as they may have a natural explanation, like tiredness. Different symptoms may be perceived very differently, depending on the person, setting and situation. Differences in illness behaviour occur as a function of the immediate experience, past experiences and the patient's information processing, organizing and recall. The significance of symptoms is judged according to the degree of interference with normal activities, the clarity of symptoms, the person's tolerance threshold, familiarity of symptoms, assumptions about cause and prognoses, interpersonal influence from the lay-referral system and other life crises making the symptoms appear more severe. The subjective and psychosocial aspects of an incident can be more important in determining decision and action than the symptoms themselves.

The experience of illness involves affective and cognitive reactions to illness, in which the patient undergoes emotional changes and attempts to understand the illness. Bernstein & Bernstein have described these emotional reactions to illness and treatment in the following ways:

- Emotional reactions directly related to illness or treatment, including fear, anxiety and a feeling of

damage and frustration caused by loss of habitual gratification and pleasure

- Reactions determined primarily by life experience before or during illness, such as anger, dependency and guilt
- Complications such as depression and loss of self-esteem.

Women are more likely than men to interpret discomfort as a medical symptom; they also recall and report more symptoms. These differences may partly be explained by a higher interest in and concern with health issues among women than men. The family often plays an active role in the symptom identification process. Other family members may recognize some symptoms before the person does. The family also takes part in the interpretation process of symptoms. The culture is also an important factor influencing the process of symptom identification and evaluation. Some cultures describe more readily common symptoms as medical, while others tend to suppress signs of medical symptoms. There might also be differences between generations in this respect. What was earlier considered as normal may today be seen as something requiring medical attention. The individual's feeling of anxiety may also explain the symptom levels, since high anxiety has been associated with the identification of many symptoms.

Sick-role behaviour

When people perceive themselves to be sick they adopt the so-called 'sick-role behaviour'. According to Parsons this includes the following components:

- The patient is not blamed for being sick
- The patient is exempt from work and other responsibilities
- The illness is seen as legitimate as long as the patient accepts the undesirability of it
- The patient is expected to seek competent help to get well again.

It has been found that not all people follow these patterns of the sick role and it should be seen more as a general framework for understanding illness behaviour. However, this framework is not able to explain variations within illness behaviour; it is not applicable to chronic disease and often not to mental illness. There are also certain diseases where there might be some unwillingness to grant the exemptions from blame. These include certain conditions related to smoking, overuse of alcohol and AIDS. But even epilepsy has been stigmatized in many cultures.

The role of personality in illness

Personality has been shown to be associated with illness. People who have high levels of anxiety, depression and anger/hostility traits seem to be more disease prone than others. These emotions are part of reactions to different types of stress. People handle stressful situations in different ways. People who approach stressful situations more positively and hopefully are less disease prone and also tend to recover more quickly if they get ill. People who are ill need to overcome their negative thoughts and feelings in order to recover more quickly.

The cardiologists Friedman and Rosenman were the first ones to describe differences in behavioural and emotional style, when studying the behaviour of heart patients. These patterns have been named Type A and Type B behaviour. The Type A behaviour pattern is characterized by:

- A competitive achievement orientation, including a high level of self-criticism and striving towards goals without feeling a sense of joy in achievements
- Time urgency, e.g. tight scheduling of commitments, impatience with time delays and unproductive time
- Anger/hostility which is easily aroused. This component, especially, seems to be detrimental to good health. Type A individuals respond more quickly and strongly to stress, often seeing stressors as threats to their personal control.

The Type A pattern may also increase the person's probability of getting into stressful situations. The relationships between Type A behaviour and psychosocial factors are very complex, involving multiple levels of human experience.

Type B behaviour is opposite to Type A, with individuals taking life more easily with little competitiveness, time urgency and hostility. Interestingly the overall evidence for an association between Type A and B behaviour and general illnesses is weak and inconsistent. However, many studies, but not all, have shown a clear association between Type A behaviour and coronary heart disease.

Health knowledge, beliefs and attitudes

There are different definitions of what this knowledge is. Sometimes it may include a variety of things such as beliefs, expectations, norms and cognitive perceptions. If this is the case, knowledge has to be considered in a wider framework than merely having some factual knowledge about diseases and treatment. One of the goals in current health care is to improve the patient's problem solving capacity. The starting point is providing the necessary information and improving the factual knowledge of the patient. It has been shown several times that knowledge alone is not sufficient to ensure change in behaviour, which is often the goal. Preventive behaviours, the treatment process and taking medications all require a certain amount of knowledge. The current trend emphasizing guided self-care in chronic diseases such as asthma, diabetes and hypertension requires a well-informed patient. The aim is to produce patients who actively participate in their own treatment. In research settings, the narrow approach towards knowledge usually involves using a knowledge index (set of questions) that the patient has to answer before and after an educational intervention.

Attitudes have been defined as states of readiness or predisposition, feeling for or against something, which predisposes to particular responses. They involve emotions (feelings) and knowledge (or beliefs) about the object and emanate in behaviour. Attitudes are not inherited but learned and, though relatively stable, are modifiable by education.

The health belief model

The health belief model, which was originally developed by Rosenstock and his colleagues to predict the use of preventive health services, has been extensively used during the last two decades to try to explain various health behaviours. The model was further developed for predicting health behaviour in chronic diseases and reformulated for predicting compliance with healthcare regimens.

The elements of the model are subjective perceptions which can be modified, at least in theory. According to the model, the probability that a person will take a preventive health action – that is, perform some health, illness or sick-role behaviour – is a function of:

- The perceived susceptibility to the health problem or disease
- The perceived severity of medical and social consequences of the disease
- The perceived benefits and barriers (costs) related to the recommended behaviour.

According to the model, the more vulnerable the person feels and the more serious the disease the more likely it is the person will act. Furthermore, various factors that result from the perceptions are expected to modify this motivating force. These factors include demographic, socio-economic and therapy-related factors as well as the illness itself and the prescribed regimen. Prior contact with the disease or knowledge about the disease may modify the behaviour. Some incidents, so-called 'cues to action', are also expected to trigger the behaviour. These include, for example, a mass media campaign, magazine article, advice from significant others or illness of a family member or friend.

The concept of perception is important in the health belief model. It is the patient's and not the pharmacist's perceptions that drive the decisions and behaviours of the patient. In studies of compliance with prescribed medications the concept of personal susceptibility has been modified because the illness has already been diagnosed. One approach includes examining the individual's estimate of or belief in the accuracy of the diagnosis. This concept has also been extended to estimating resusceptibility or measuring the individual's subjective feelings of vulnerability to various other diseases or to illness in general. Studies show that in hypertension, for example, the threat posed by hypertension and the perceived effectiveness of treatment in reducing this threat seem to be important predictors of compliance. Likewise the perceived control over one's own health is important. There is some controversy about the chronology of these beliefs and whether they precede or develop simultaneously with health behaviour.

The health belief model and common sense might tell us that the patient's decision to seek health care, accept a diagnosis and engage in health-related behaviours would be related to the seriousness of the disease. Research indicates this may not always be the case. Patients' health behaviours are a function of many psychosocial variables. Reasons why humans may behave illogically are dealt with in more detail in the section 'The conflict theory', below, and also in the section 'Decision analysis and behavioural decision theory' (p. 34).

The theory of reasoned action

According to the theory of reasoned action by Ajzen & Fishbein, a person's intention is the best predictor of what he will do. The person's intention is determined by his attitude regarding the behaviour and whether he thinks it is a good or bad thing to do. This assess-

ment is based on behavioural beliefs about possible outcomes of the behaviour and evaluations of whether these outcomes would be rewarding. The other attitude represents the impact of social pressure or influence. These are based on normative beliefs regarding others' opinions about the behaviour and the person's motivation to follow those opinions, i.e. what do other people think I should do? The theory proposes that the subjective norm and the attitude regarding the behaviour combine to produce an intention, which leads to the behaviour.

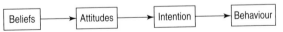

Beliefs → Attitudes → Intention → Behaviour

If behaviour is determined by beliefs, this raises the question of what factors determine beliefs? These factors would include things like age, sex, education, social class, culture and personality traits. These variables influence behaviour indirectly rather than directly. One of the problems with the theory is that people do not always do what they plan, i.e. intentions and behaviour are only moderately related. Another problem is that people do not always act rationally. Irrational decisions such as delaying medical treatment when symptoms exist cannot be explained by the model. Neither does the model include prior experiences with the behaviour, which might be an important factor to consider, since past behaviour is a strong predictor of future practice of that behaviour.

The conflict theory

The conflict theory has been used to explain rational and irrational decision making. According to the model the process a person is using in arriving at a health-related decision involves five stages. It starts when something challenges the person's current course of action. It can be a threat (e.g. symptom) or a mass media alert about, for example, the danger of narcotics or an opportunity (e.g. free membership to a health club). The different stages of the conflict theory model are:

- Assessing the challenge, i.e. whether the risk is serious enough. The assessment may involve thoughts such as the risk is not real, it is irrelevant or inapplicable. If the risk is not considered serious enough, the behaviour continues as before and the decision-making process stops.
- Assessing alternatives, i.e. the search for alternatives for dealing with the risk starts when the risk is acknowledged. This stage ends when the

suitability of available alternatives has been surveyed.

- Weighing alternatives, i.e. the pros and cons of each alternative are weighed to find the best option.
- Making a final choice and committing to it.
- Adhering despite negative feedback, i.e. after starting a new behaviour people may have second thoughts about it if the environment is not supportive or it gives negative feedback.

The decision process can be aborted at any point. Errors in decision making are often caused by stress, information overload, group pressure and other factors. The way people cope with stress has an important role in health, illness and sick-role behaviour. According to the conflict theory, a person's coping with a conflict is dependent on the presence and absence of risks, hope and adequate time. Different combinations of these may result in different types of behavioural response. For example, when there are perceptions of high risk in changing the behaviour and no hope in finding a better alternative, a high level of stress is experienced. Denial and shifting responsibility to someone else are typical responses, with delays in seeking care when needed. The perception of serious risk, and belief in a better alternative, but also a perception of running out of time, also create high levels of stress. People search desperately for solutions and may choose an alternative hastily if promised immediate relief. Different untested cancer quacks are good examples where unscrupulous people try to make use of this kind of situation. The perception of serious risk, with a belief that a better alternative will become available and there is time to search for it, results in low levels of stress and rational choices.

Locus of control

It has been claimed that how individuals perceive their ability to influence disease and the treatment is an important determinant of health behaviour. People have been categorized into two groups: those with an internal locus of control and those with an external locus of control. The former tend to perceive that they are in control of their own health by their actions and behaviour, while the latter consider that health is externally determined and their actions have little or no effect. Therefore those with a strongly internal locus of control should tend to practise behaviours that prevent illness and promote health. Research has shown that this is the case, but the relationship

is not very strong. This shows that the locus of control is just one factor among many others that determine health behaviour. Belief in internal control is likely to have a greater impact among people who place a higher value on their health than among those who do not.

Self-efficacy and social learning

Sometimes performing a health action is hard to do because it is technically difficult or it may involve several steps. Therefore the belief in the success in doing something – called self-efficacy – may be an important determinant in choosing or not choosing to change behaviour. People develop a sense of efficacy through their successes and failures, observations of others' experiences and assessments of their abilities by others. People assess their efficacy based on the effort that is required, complexity of the task and situational factors, e.g. the possibility of receiving help if needed. People who think they are not able to quit smoking will not even try, while people who believe they can succeed will try and eventually some may even succeed.

Those with a strong sense of self-efficacy show less psychological strain in response to stressors than those with a weak sense of efficacy. People differ in the degree to which they believe they have control over the things that happen in their lives. Those who experience prolonged, high levels of stress and lack a sense of personal control tend to feel helpless. Having a strong sense of control seems to benefit health and adjustment to sickness.

As environmental factors and expectations directed towards the individuals change, they must either intensify their activities or change their environment. Individuals have different capabilities of coping and different coping strategies. According to the social learning theory, people change their environment with the help of symbols they choose in accordance with their values, norms and goals. On the other hand, the environment changes the individual's behaviour by rewarding beneficial activities and punishing or not rewarding activities that harm the environment. Through the socialization process the individual adopts the values and norms of the community, is socialized as its member and gains identity. Through this process the individual has learned to act efficiently in social systems.

Antonowsky has used the 'sense of coherence' concept, which is an extensive and constant feeling of an individual's internal and external environment being in harmony with each other. Every individual has characteristic psychosocial potentials that include material resources, intelligence, knowledge, coping strategies, social support, arts, religion, philosophy and health behaviour. Antonowsky calls a sense of coherence 'salutogenic' or health generating. Disease–health is a continuum, at one end of which is a high degree of coherence and health (ease) and at the other end a low degree of coherence and illness (disease). External factors that the individual considers threatening mobilize the defence mechanisms and cause stress conditions in the individual. Prolonged stress is disease generating and causes the condition dis-ease.

Coping

Because of the emotional and physical strain that accompanies it, stress is uncomfortable and people are motivated to do things that reduce their stress. The concept of coping is used to describe how people adjust to stressful situations in their life. Coping is the process by which people try to manage the perceived discrepancy between the demands and resources they appraise in stressful situations. Coping means the ability to meet the demands of new situations and solve the problems with which one is confronted. Coping is determined by situational and personal determinants. At the individual level, external factors turn into stress factors if previous experiences together with personality traits, consciously or unconsciously, are considered as threatening or diminish self-esteem. Coping efforts can be quite varied and do not necessarily lead to a solution of the problem. It can help the person to alter his perception of a discrepancy, tolerate or accept the harm or threat and escape or avoid the situation. The coping process is not a single event.

Coping mechanisms

Coping can alter the problem or it can regulate the emotional response causing the stress reaction to the problem. Behavioural approaches include using alcohol or drugs, seeking social support from friends or simply watching TV. Cognitive approaches involve how people think about the stressful situation, e.g. changing the meaning of the situation. Emotion-focused approaches are used when people think they cannot do anything to change the stressful situation. Problem-focused coping is used to reduce the demands of the stressful situation or to expand the

capacity and resources to deal with it. The two types of coping can also be used together. Sarafino (2005) has summarized commonly used methods of coping as follows:

- The direct method, i.e. doing something specifically and directly to cope with a stressor, for example negotiating, consulting, arguing, running away
- Seeking information and acquiring knowledge about the stressful situation
- Turning to others, i.e. seeking help, reassurance and comfort from family and friends
- Resigned acceptance, i.e. the person comes to terms with the situation and accepts it as it is
- Emotional discharge, i.e. expressing feelings or reducing tension by taking, for example, alcohol or drugs, smoking cigarettes
- Intrapsychic processes, i.e. cognitive redefinition, for example the 'things could be worse' attitude.

Decision analysis and behavioural decision theory

Decision analysis is a systematic way of studying the process of decision making among patients, pharmacists and physicians. This is a widely used tool in pharmacoeconomics today (see Ch. 19). It usually involves assigning numbers to perceived values of the therapeutic outcomes and the probability that the outcome will occur. This gives a utility of each outcome and the one with the highest utility would be chosen. One problem is that humans do not always make decisions logically or treat information as value free.

Why don't humans behave logically? One explanation that has been offered is that humans are biased when making decisions under uncertainty because we fail to appreciate randomness. We believe that there are known causes and effects for all phenomena and we have a need to be able to explain outcomes. It is easier to explain, even incorrectly, than to have to deal with uncertain situations. People also tend to be inconsistent in judgment, often because of difficulties in remembering how a judgment was made. Another reason is that we seldom receive feedback from negative decisions, for example if we decide *not* to take the medicine we do not know how effective it would have been.

Behaviour decision theory has been used to understand how patients make decisions about their medicine and health-related behaviour. These include acquisition of information, information processing, making decisions under uncertainty and interpreting outcomes of that decision. It has been found that patients are more likely to take a health risk to avoid an aversive situation than to gain a positive health outcome. Patients are also more likely to choose a certain outcome than an outcome with a high probability of occurrence, even if the certain outcome is less valued than that one with a high probability of occurrence. When a person has already invested time and money on a product or activity they are likely to continue it, even if it does not appear to be effective.

Hogarth has described different biases that people tend to have in decision making which may be helpful in understanding patient choices about health behaviour. We tend to believe more in well-publicized events than in those that are less publicized. This has direct links with the consumer's choice of well-advertised over the counter (OTC) medicines. There is a tendency to believe what matches our existing beliefs. This selective perception has direct implications for health education in pharmacies. We also tend to believe real incidents more than abstract statistics. Positive experiences from a family member quitting smoking is more likely to be effective than showing statistics about future (uncertain) consequences of smoking. Two incidents occurring close in time and place tend to be regarded as causal. Becoming ill after having taken a medicine (regardless of cause and effect) would usually trigger a response of aversion next time seeing the same medicine. We are reluctant to change our beliefs, even when given new data, and tend to discount the new information rather than discount our belief. Very few instances of an occurrence are needed for us to form a new belief if it has a strong effect upon us. This has direct implications to the experience of side-effects of drugs. We also believe something is more likely to happen if we want it to happen. A decision that was successful is more likely to be considered to be due to the knowledge and wisdom of the decision maker. On the other hand, a decision resulting in bad outcomes is likely to be blamed on others.

Theory into practice – the process of behaviour change

A lot of pharmacists' activities will focus on changing the behaviour of patients. Without going into the ethical aspects of behaviour change, we will concentrate on the process of change. It has been proved several times that merely using common sense is not enough to reach permanent behaviour change. Using a common-sense approach would assume that, given the facts, people will be able to change their behaviour in a direction anticipated by the healthcare professional. A simple example illustrates the limits of this approach – why do so many people still smoke cigarettes despite knowing all the negative consequences of smoking?

Even if many of the behavioural theories are far from complete or comprehensive, they may guide us in improving the outcome of behavioural interventions. Behaviour change includes a long list of steps that need to be taken before it is finalized:

- The process starts with *attention*. The person needs to be exposed to the message; this might be a counselling session by the pharmacist or a health campaign in the mass media. If the same message is repeated from different sources and these sources are regarded as credible, the likelihood of change grows. Therefore it is important that the information received from physicians and pharmacists is congruent. If patients receive mixed messages they are more likely to ignore them.
- Attention is followed by *motivation*. The person must feel motivated to change their behaviour. It is well known that immediate rewards are more motivating than anticipated rewards after several years.
- Next the person has to *comprehend* the message to be able to act upon it, but they also need to learn some facts, i.e. improve their knowledge base. These facts need to be simple and match the local culture.
- The following step is *persuasion*, i.e. the person needs to 'change their attitude'.
- Furthermore they might need to learn some new techniques and skills in how to take or handle the medication. Demonstration and guided practice are the best ways of handling this step.
- The person must also be able to perform the skills and maintain the learned skills, which include self-efficacy training and feedback of success. Many experiments with a long enough follow-up show that positive results can be achieved with pharmacists' interventions, but when the experiment is over, the results soon deteriorate to pre-experiment levels.
- Continuous reinforcement is necessary to maintain good results in any intervention, be it changing medicine-taking behaviour or modification of preventive health behaviour.

The treatment process

Self- and lay care

During the 1970s and 1980s a new trend emphasizing the role of the individual and patient emerged as a part of a more general trend called consumerism. People have become more committed to getting and taking control of their own lives and assessing the impact of their behaviour on their health. Different self-care and self-help movements were a direct result of this trend. The same trend has been obvious in most countries although the starting time and speed of it has varied. At the same time the dominant role of health-care personnel has diminished. With new information sources, and especially the Internet, the trend continues to grow and spread to countries where physicians and other healthcare personnel still dominate. This new trend has included a much more critical attitude towards what is being done in health care and the quality of care given. Patients are asking more questions, seeking more information and taking a more active role in their health care. They have a better basic education and greater knowledge, especially about their own disease and treatment of that disease.

The new trend has also put increasing demands on pharmacists regarding their knowledge base, especially in therapeutics but also in communication. The priorities in treatment goals may differ between the patient and the treating physician and this calls for negotiation. One aspect is that patients' views have to be taken seriously.

According to the self-care philosophy, people should be given more responsibility for their own health. One way this can be achieved is to emphasize the role of self-care in treating minor ailments using home remedies and an increased number of self-medication products. Especially in the 1980s and early 1990s this trend was obvious in many countries. The most common 'action' in response to a perceived health problem has been to ignore the problem or wait for a few days. It is estimated that some 30–40% of health problems are dealt with in this way. Of those who take some action, 75–80% self-diagnose and use self-treatment, while only 20–25% seek professional care. Therefore a seemingly small change in this ratio (towards using more professional care) has a substantial impact and burden on the official healthcare system. Of those who use self-treatment, some 70–90% are self-medicating, and of those self-medicating, some 80% are using OTC drugs. Home remedies such as onion, garlic and warm drinks, as well as different herbal products, vitamins and minerals, are widely used all over the world. Some of the newly emerging preparations are marketed with high promises of eternal youth and health, the evidence base for which is nonexistent or weak.

Before people decide to seek medical care for their symptoms they get and seek advice from friends, relatives and co-workers. These advisors form a lay referral network that provides its own information and interpretation regarding the symptoms, recommending home remedies, self-medication, professional help or consulting another 'lay expert' who may have had a similar problem.

The pharmacy is often the first place where people come to seek help within the healthcare system. Increased self-care includes also potential risks in that lay people may not be able to distinguish between serious and non-serious symptoms. Certain situations may demand professional care without further delay caused by inappropriate self-medication practices. The lay referral network can in some cases be guilty of causing delay in seeking care. This treatment delay has been divided into three stages: appraisal delay, illness delay and utilization delay. Appraisal delay is the time it takes to interpret a symptom as a part of an illness. Illness delay is the time between recognizing the illness and the decision to seek care. Finally, utilization delay is the time between the decision to seek care and actually using a health service.

There has also been concern about misuse of OTC drugs such as laxatives, codeine-containing cough medicines, etc. The other side of the coin is saved resources in health care when there is less reliance on professionals. This seems to be an important aspect as healthcare budgets tend to increase more rapidly than the general inflation rate.

Primary care

Simultaneously with emerging self-care, the concept of primary health care was introduced. In 1977 the World Health Assembly of the World Health Organization adopted the concept of Health for All by the Year 2000. The following year this concept was translated into the so-called Alma Ata Declaration at the Alma Ata conference on primary health care. The focus was on making health care more accessible and lowering the healthcare costs and thus improving the quality of life for the whole population. According to the declaration, primary health care should include:

- Education about prevailing health problems
- Methods of identifying, preventing and controlling them
- Promotion of food supply and proper nutrition
- Adequate water supply and basic sanitation
- Maternal and child health care including family planning
- Immunization against the major infectious diseases
- Prevention and control of locally endemic diseases
- Appropriate treatment of common diseases and injuries
- Promotion of mental health
- Provision of essential drugs.

Primary health care focuses on principal health problems and must be part of national health policy and planning. The conference recommended a re-evaluation of health priorities, putting less emphasis on curative facilities, especially in third world countries. The conference also called for cooperation and commitment in striving for an acceptable level of health for all people by the year 2000.

The scope of public health is population based rather than individually based. Public health problems are not a series of individuals presenting diseases to a healthcare provider for cure, alleviation or prevention, but are considered in the context of the community. It is a public health problem to determine the prevalence of a disease in the community, compare that with figures from previous years and plan health services to reduce the prevalence. Public health includes enumeration, analysing and planning, but also specific actions to be taken. Public health exists on two levels: the micro level, for example performing some public health function such as immunization or preventing inappropriate use of illicit drugs, and the macro level, with activities like planning or policy formulation.

Factors influencing the use of health services

The structures of the healthcare systems in different countries have a lot of similarities but also a lot of differences. The system is the sum of historical development, culture and economic factors. In some countries there are actually several different systems in place within the healthcare system. It is not within the scope of this chapter to describe these different systems, rather to highlight some of the current issues in organizing the health care of the citizens and to highlight some socio-behavioural factors influencing the provision of care. It may seem obvious that when having bad angina you will need hospital care and you will be provided with all the technical know-how and help in dealing with the problem. However, the country you happen to live in, the insurance policy you have, the services available, quality of care, etc. will all influence the outcome of the disease. The organization and financing of health care, the environment of medical care, social and cultural factors all influence the care that you will receive.

Demographic factors

Several important differences have been reported between different age groups and between genders. However, few reports have been able to validate the reasons for these differences. As mentioned before, it is well known that women report more symptoms and that they have a lower threshold of pain and discomfort and are more likely to seek care. Men are more hesitant than women to admit to having symptoms and to seek medical care for these symptoms. This can be a result of perceived sex-role stereotypes – men should be tough and independent and ignore or endure pain. Women use physician services more than men in all age groups except for the first few years of life. Regardless of this, men have a higher mortality and shorter life expectancy at all ages.

In general, young children and the elderly use physician services more often than adolescents and young adults. Age differences in health behaviour cannot be explained by biological ageing alone. Elderly people have different views on health and illness, symptoms, healthcare use and drugs. There is a danger in labelling all elderly people as having similar attitudes concerning health issues, but, as with younger persons, among the elderly there are also a wide variety of views on health and treatment. Certain ideas are more prevalent among the elderly than the young. The differences can partly be explained by so-called cohort effects, meaning people of the same age have been exposed to the same kind of experiences and attitudes in society and therefore are also likely to share certain behavioural characteristics.

Cultural and socio-economic factors

Ethnic and cultural background may explain some differences in symptom experience, how people seek medical care and how they take their medicines. In the 1950s a classic study about how people deal with pain found big differences between Italian, Jewish, Irish and Yankee (Old American) hospitalized patients. Italian and Jewish patients were more likely to respond emotionally and expressively to pain than Irish or Yankee patients, who tended to deny pain. Italian and Jewish patients showed their pain by crying, complaining and demanding, while the Irish and Yankee patients preferred to hide their pain and withdraw from others. More recent studies among immigrants in the USA found that the differences in willingness to tolerate pain diminish in succeeding generations. Other similar studies have shown cultural differences among European countries and the USA, e.g. in perception of fever and the need to medicate children's fever.

There are also differences in seeking care according to social class, education and income. These factors all point in the same direction – those who are better off also use more health services. Different models of why people seek or do not seek health services have been proposed. The health belief model has also been used in this context.

Social support

Social environments and networks are important in the growth, development and health of people. Social support is an important factor in all phases of the process of illness and the treatment process. Social support relates directly to the general and universal needs of people. The best known theory is that by Maslow. According to his theory, human needs are hierarchical, starting with basic physiological needs, followed by safety needs, belongingness and love needs, esteem needs, and finishing with the highest – self-actualization needs. A slightly modified and simplified model is that by Allardt; according to Allardt, people's needs include standard of living (having), social relations (loving) and forms of self-actualization (being). Social relations include social networks and belonging to them is the basis of one's identity and social existence. Social support is the term used for different forms of emotional and material support. The nature of social support is reciprocal. It can be support provided directly by one person to another or indirectly through the system or community.

Forms and levels of social support

- *Material or instrumental support* includes money, goods, auxiliary appliances and medicine
- *Operational support* includes service, transportation and rehabilitation
- *Informational support* includes advice, directions, feedback, education and training
- *Emotional support* involves the expression of caring, empathy, love and encouragement
- *Mental support* involves a common ideology, belief and philosophy.

Social support has two dimensions, a qualitative and a quantitative dimension. It can also be subjective and objective in nature. The quality of social support can be measured only by subjective assessments. When providing material support the quantitative aspect is more prominent (medicines an exception); in the other support forms the qualitative aspect (including timing) is more important than the quantitative aspect. Thus a small functioning support network is better than a broad but passive one.

Social support has been divided into primary, secondary and tertiary levels based on the intimacy of the social relationships. The primary level includes family and close friends, the secondary level includes friends, colleagues and neighbours and the tertiary level acquaintances, authorities, public and private services. Social support can be provided by a lay person (usually on the primary and secondary level) or a professional (usually on the tertiary level). Recently different organizations have started training courses for lay providers of support aiming at strengthening the second level of support. Social support has both direct effects on health and well-being and indirect stress-buffering effects on coping in stressful situations.

The research on the effects of social support on health goes back to the late 1940s and early 1950s. The first studies in this area showed that lack of social support exposes people to recurrent accidents, suicide and risk of catching tuberculosis. In the 1970s the emphasis was on relationships between social support structures and health in communities. It was shown that the lack of social support increases the incidence of coronary heart disease, mortality due to myocardial infarction and total mortality in the population. It has also been shown that social support is important in perceived health and in reducing hypertension. Social support also has a positive effect on physical, social and emotional recovery. It reduces the need for medication and speeds up symptom amelioration. The positive effects of social support in different stages of illness can be summarized as follows:

- In the prevention of illness it can reduce insecurity and anxiety
- In the acute stage of illness it has a calming effect giving a sense of security
- In the rehabilitation phase it can improve adherence to medical regimens.

The side-effects to the patient of excessive social support or poor quality support may include increasing the passiveness of the patient, creating dependence, reducing self-confidence and self-esteem and causing feelings of shame and guilt.

KEY POINTS

- Social and behavioural issues can help explain non-biological aspects of health
- Illness is a person's reaction to a perceived alteration of body or mind, while disease is something which is professionally defined
- Health has been defined by the WHO as a 'state of complete physical, mental and social well-being and not merely the absence of disease and infirmity'
- Apart from biophysical factors, health is also affected by behavioural, environmental and socio-economic determinants
- People react differently to symptoms as a consequence of many factors
- Family, culture, gender and age influence response to symptoms
- Type A behaviour is more closely associated with illness than Type B behaviour
- The knowledge which a person has will affect his response to illness
- According to the health belief model, the patient's perception is most important in determining patient behaviour and decisions
- The theory of reasoned action suggests that beliefs give rise to attitudes, which form intentions which lead to behaviour
- The conflict theory can be used to explain rational and irrational decision making
- People use a wide range of coping mechanisms when under stress
- Humans may not reach decisions logically for many reasons, with biases being particularly important
- Behaviour is seldom changed as a result of providing facts, but results from a long series of stages
- Through the self-care philosophy, patients are increasingly encouraged to be responsible for their own health, placing increasing demands on pharmacists
- The 1978 Alma Ata Declaration defines the content of primary care which should be available to all
- Demographic, cultural and socio-economic factors influence the use of health services
- Social support networks may be primary, secondary or tertiary and are important for the health of individuals

4

Socio-behavioural aspects of treatment with medicines

K. Hannes Enlund

STUDY POINTS

- Functions of medicines
- Societal perspectives on rational use of medicines
- Factors affecting the treatment process with medicines
- Sociological and behavioural aspects of use and prescribing of medicines
- A sociological perspective of pharmacy and the pharmacy profession
- Measuring outcomes

Introduction

In attempting to understand the treatment process with medicines we can partially apply the same theoretical models as for illness behaviour presented in the previous chapter (see also Fig. 3.1). It is also feasible to regard the treatment process from a macro and a micro perspective. The macro perspective includes an analysis of the different systems and structural components in place to ensure a rational use of medicines, which is one of the primary goals of the system. The micro perspective includes the patient level and the interaction between patient and practitioner.

When explaining patient behaviour in taking or not taking medicines and the interaction with the environment we can, for example, use the social learning theory and the concept of self-efficacy (see p. 33). The health belief model (see p. 31) has been used to explain patients' adherence in taking medicines. In addition, we need to understand the behaviour of the physician when prescribing the medicines and dealing with the patient. Likewise our interest is to understand the behaviour of the pharmacist and the patient–physician–pharmacist interactions. Different models and theories provide a slightly different perspective on the use of medicines, and the adequacy of the theory often depends on the question being addressed. Because this is a relatively new research area there are still many gaps in our understanding of the different processes involved and their interactions.

Functions of medicines

Social and behavioural scientists have proposed that medicines and use of medicines also serve important latent functions for the individual and society. In this context it is important to have a wide definition of the word 'medicines'. The functions may be the same as the approved medical uses or may be hidden functions. Barber and later Svarstad have identified a long list of these functions:

- Therapeutic function – the conventional use of medicines to prevent, treat and cure disease
- Placebo function – to show concern and satisfy patient
- Coping function – to relieve feelings of failure, stress, grief, sadness, loneliness
- Self-regulatory function – to exercise control over disorder or life
- Social control function – to manage behaviour of demanding or disruptive patients, hyperactive children
- Recreational function – to relax, enjoy company of others, experience pleasurable feelings

- Religious function – to seek religious meaning or experience
- Cosmetic function – to beautify skin, hair and body image
- Appetitive function – to allay hunger or control the desire for food
- Instrumental function – to improve academic, athletic or work performance
- Sexual function – to increase sexual ability
- Fertility function – to control fertility
- Research function – to gain knowledge and understanding of human behaviour
- Diagnostic function – to help make diagnosis
- Status-conferring function – to gain social status, prestige, income.

A societal perspective on rational use of medicines

Defining rational use

Rational use of medicines has been defined as the safe, effective, appropriate and economic use of medicines. The definition as such seems to be clear and straightforward, but how do we define 'safe' and the other components of the definition? Safety relates to aspects like relative and absolute safety. It is well known that all medicines have side-effects, some less and some more. The safety aspect has to be assessed from many different angles, e.g. the severity of the disease, the available treatment options including medicines and non-medicines options, long-term or short-term treatment, whether the medicine is to cure or control symptoms, any risks of overdoses and other possible factors.

Effectiveness relates to the question of how well the medicine works in daily practice when used by unselected populations and patients having co-morbidities and other medications. Efficacy relates to a clinical trial type of situation, where we want to know the maximum effect of the medicine in a particular disease and when it is optimally used in selected patients with as few confounding factors as possible, such as co-morbidities and other medicines used simultaneously.

Appropriateness refers to how a medicine is being prescribed and used in and by patients, including aspects such as appropriate indication, with no contraindications, appropriate dosage and administration. Duration of treatment should be optimal and the medicine should be correctly dispensed with appropriate and sufficient information and counselling. To achieve the intended effects, the medicine also needs to be correctly used by the patient.

The economic aspect does not refer merely to price; rather, a cost-effectiveness approach needs to be applied, where all factors are assessed. A somewhat more expensive medicine may be preferable to a less expensive medicine, for example because it has better treatment outcomes or fewer side-effects. We should also be aware of hidden costs, such as a need for more extensive laboratory tests, which may increase the total cost of a particular treatment (see Ch. 19).

National medicines policy

Ensuring rational use of medicines requires that there are appropriate structures in place and that the processes involved are functioning well. The starting point and frame of reference is the national medicines policy (NMP). The role of an NMP is usually discussed in the context of medicine-related issues in developing countries. In industrialized countries it has received much less attention, because many key issues and policies regarding medicines and their rational use are already in place. However, the global crisis in healthcare financing, especially the medicines budget, has created a momentum to look more closely at medicine policies in industrialized countries too. When trying to understand the general principles that can be applied to all countries it is helpful to use the guidelines that have been proposed for developing countries, and from there try to understand how the system works and what might be the strong and weak points in each particular country.

The NMP can be seen as a guide for action, including the goals and priorities set by the government, the main strategies and approaches. It also serves as a framework in the coordination of different activities. Depending on cultural, historical and socio-economic factors there are differences in objectives, strategies and approaches between countries, but some common components can be distinguished. The goals for an NMP can be divided into:

- Health-related goals, which entail making essential medicines available, ensuring the safety, efficacy and quality of medicines, and promoting rational prescribing, dispensing and use of medicines
- Economic goals, which may include lowering the cost of medicines and providing jobs in the pharmaceutical sector
- National development goals, which may include increasing the skills of personnel in pharmacy,

medicine, etc. and encouraging industrial activities in the manufacturing of medicines.

There is further discussion of these issues in Chapter 7.

Ensuring safety of medicines

Why is it important to regulate and control the medicine sector with special laws and regulations? The medicine sector is of concern to the whole population. Most citizens will use medicines and related services on a regular basis and therefore the functioning of the sector is of common interest. There are also many parties involved – patients, healthcare providers, manufacturers and sales people – requiring detailed rules for interaction and functioning. The consequences from the lack of medicines or their misuse might be serious. History has shown that informal controls are not sufficient or respected. Generally there is little disagreement about the need to regulate the medicine sector; the disagreement lies rather in the extent to which it should be regulated.

Legislation and regulation include different health-related laws, pharmacy law, trademark and patent laws, criminal law, international treaties (e.g. on narcotic and psychotropic drugs) and governmental decrees. Sometimes there may be a lack of political will or a weak infrastructure to enforce the laws. When looking at the legal situation in the medicine sector in different countries, the problems seem to be more often in the enforcement of legislation than in the lack of legislation.

Registration of medicines is a key tool in assuring the safety, quality and efficacy of a new medicine being introduced on the market. In this connection the new medicine will also be scheduled to a certain category such as prescription or over the counter (OTC) medicine. The infrastructure that will assure quality, safety and efficacy can be ascertained by licensing and inspection of manufacturers, distributors and the premises, but also by setting some standards on the professionals working there. There is wide international cooperation in this field among the different competent authorities. Nevertheless every now and then the media have reports about counterfeit products and toxic products sold to the public, sometimes with disastrous consequences. News such as somebody having replaced glycerin with diethyleneglycol in paracetamol syrups intended for small children should not be possible with all the controls in place today.

Pharmaco-epidemiological studies are used to assure the safety of new medicines after they have been accepted on the market. This kind of information can supplement that available from pre-marketing studies; it can also give a better quantification of the incidence of known adverse drug reactions (ADRs), and also of the beneficial effects. For ethical and other reasons it is not always suitable to perform clinical trials on certain patient groups such as children, elderly people and pregnant women in the early phase of a new product. It is also important to establish how other medicines and diseases may alter the positive effects. New types of information not available from pre-marketing studies, such as rare undetected ADRs, long-term effects that manifest only after long use or after long latency periods, and effects with low frequency are also the concern of pharmaco-epidemiological studies. Further aspects on the safety and evaluation of medicines are dealt with in Chapters 19 and 47.

Ensuring the availability of medicines

Availability of medicines is one of the key requirements in a well functioning pharmaceutical system. This includes a functioning manufacturing and importation system of medicines, good procurement and distribution practices. These functions are often taken for granted in industrialized countries, while in developing countries they are key issues for a functioning system. In developing countries the maintenance of a constant supply of medicines, keeping them in good condition and minimizing losses due to spoilage and expiry are issues that need to be solved to assure the availability of medicines to the population.

With more and more sophisticated new medicines, the prices of new products are beyond reach for a large part of the population if no mechanisms like price control or reimbursement/insurance systems are in place. Economic availability of medicines will be a major policy issue in all countries during the next few years. With national medicine budgets increasing annually by more than 10%, there is a doubling of the budget every 5–6 years.

Use of medicines

Medicine (drug) use or utilization studies and pharmaco-epidemiological studies during the last 25 years have basically tried to describe who are using the medicines and how much are being used. On a macro level, factors influencing medicine consumption include among others: size of population, age and gender distributions, occupational structure, income levels (gross national product), availability of health services, number and type of health facilities, number and type of personnel, social insurance and reimbursement mechanisms.

Medicine use studies have also been used to identify different types of 'irrational use', e.g. overuse of psychotropics and antibiotics in the 1970s and 1980s (such as people using them, when not indicated, for too long periods and habitual use of analgesics every morning without a medical reason). There has also been a lot of interest in the 'underuse' of medicines for major chronic diseases such as hypertension, diabetes and elevated lipids (not starting or stopping treatment, 'drug holidays', taking only half of what is prescribed). Underuse, together with misuse or erratic use (wrong way of administration, taking with contraindicated medicines/food, etc.), has been one of the main focuses of patient adherence studies. From these studies we know something about the use of medicines and its clinical, social and economic consequences (see also Ch. 46).

Attempts to understand the medicine use behaviours of patients have been less common. However, more recently, a new research line has emerged using qualitative research methods such as in-depth interviews. These studies have focused more on what people think about their medicines, on their motives when taking or not taking them, their attitudes and beliefs about medicines and their experiences and expectations.

Some general consumer behaviour models have been used to explain non-prescription and prescription purchases. In one American study the medicine attributes that consumers rated as important included possible side-effects, physician recommendation, strength, prior use, price and the availability of generic versions. Medicines are not ordinary goods and consumers acknowledge this. According to one purchase theory, purchase motivations can also be characterized as being either transformational (positive) or informational (negative). Positive purchases are made to enhance or generate a positive situation or state of mind (e.g. clothes, music) and negative purchases to minimize or prevent negative situations (e.g. car service). Negative purchases are based on (rational) choices like perceived benefits and convenience (and therefore require more information), while positive purchases are more emotional and based on subjective appeal

and positive shopping experience. Research has shown that OTC medicines and vitamins are neutral on the positive–negative dimension and oral contraceptives highly negative. This type of research is still not very well developed within the pharmaceutical field.

Like general illness behaviour, medicine use occurs in a social context. Choosing self-medication or consulting a physician to obtain prescription medicines is not based solely on symptoms or clinical aspects. The concept of social knowledge has been used to describe collective understanding, which is based on available information and nature of prior experiences. Family members, friends, work colleagues and their experiences, books and the media in addition to our own experiences, form the basis of social knowledge of medicines. Montagne has described some interesting social conceptions or fundamental principles about medicines in peoples' minds, which he calls 'pharmacomythologies'. It is a common belief among lay people that a specific medicine produces only one 'main' effect, which is positive. Other effects are considered as negative or 'side'-effects. Likewise it is believed that a medicine produces the same main effect every time it is taken and in each person who takes it. This means that medicine effects are caused by the taken medicine and the effect of the medicine is a property residing inside the chemical compound and not a function of some change in a living organism. This easily leads to the belief that medicines cure the diseases.

The general health behaviour models and theories previously presented – such as the health belief model, theory of reasoned action, social learning theory, conflict theory and behavioural decision theory – can all be used to explain certain types of behaviour related to taking medicines. Basic decision-making and problem-solving skills are important components of patients' seemingly rational and irrational behaviours. As presented earlier, the choices do not always follow the criteria of medical rationality, but may seem quite rational to the patient. It may be useful to consider rationality as a continuum rather than either/or. The degree of rationality is also influenced by social knowledge and the micro and macro environment, as described earlier, as well as the actual health problem.

Improving public understanding of medicines

During the last few years there have been different attempts both in developed and developing countries to improve knowledge and understanding about medicines among the general public. This can be seen as an attempt to influence and improve (from a medical point of view) social knowledge related to medicines and health in general. Campaigns such as 'Ask about your medicines' are good examples of this kind of activity. A more balanced partnership between consumer-patients and healthcare providers is one of the goals in such activities. A better appreciation of the limits of medicines and a lessening of the belief that there is a 'pill for every ill' are examples of the goals of such efforts.

The general public also needs to develop a more critical attitude towards advertising and other commercial information, which may often fail to give objective information about medicines. The use of medicines should be seen within the context of a society, community, family and individual, recognizing cultural diversity in concepts of health and illness or how medicines work. Improvement of the public's knowledge about medicines should start at school. To facilitate informed choices on use of medicines, public education should be accompanied by supportive legislation and controls on availability of medicines. Non-governmental organizations, community groups and consumer and professional organizations should be involved in the planning and implementation of such programmes. Effective public education requires a commitment to and understanding of the need for improved communication between healthcare providers and patients. This should also be reflected in the basic and continuing education of healthcare personnel.

Prescribing

The process of prescribing has gained a lot of interest lately because of ever increasing medicine costs and the concern for rational prescribing from a clinical point of view (see also Ch. 17). Before this, social scientists had studied aspects such as the decision-making process in prescribing and the adoption of new medicines, using the 'diffusion of innovations' theory. Concern about prescribing habits is not new. In 1752 the famous Swedish physician and botanist Carl von Linne mentioned in a paper 21 different reasons for irrational prescribing, including factors like outdated knowledge, wrong diagnosis and chemical incompatibility, which are still relevant aspects when assessing rationality of prescribing. It is noteworthy that he used pharmacy records as his source of information.

Functions of prescriptions

Besides the pharmacological-therapeutic use, physicians may sometimes use medicine knowingly or unknowingly for other reasons too. According to Smith (2002), these can be either patient or physician centred. He has also presented a long list of latent functions of prescriptions in addition to their intended and recognized functions (method of therapy, legal document, record source and means of communication). Medicines may be used to stimulate the patient's expectations for recovery and to meet patients' expectations, e.g. the use of antibiotics for viral infections or boosting a patient's morale in intractable diseases. The physician may also want to gain some time to diagnose the condition more precisely. The medicine also legitimizes the physician–patient relationship. The prescription is a sign of the physician's power to heal and his efforts to try to heal and care for the patient. For the patient the prescription is a sign and symbol that they really are ill. Thus it also legitimizes their sick role and confirms that they have fulfilled one of the obligations of the sick role, to try to become well again (p. 30). Finally the physician uses the prescription to communicate to the patient that the office visit is over. Sometimes it may be difficult to distinguish between rational/pharmacological and non-pharmacological use of medicines. It can also raise ethical dilemmas, for example when purposely using placebos. Is the physician in this case cheating and/or behaving in a paternalistic way, when he should have an honest and trustful physician–patient relationship?

Choosing the right medicine

Therapeutic effect is the most important criterion when the physician decides which medicine to prescribe. When treating severe cases this aspect is even more important. A second consideration is the incidence and severity of side-effects. It has been shown that physicians tend to concentrate on a few serious side-effects. The medical situation often determines the acceptable level of side-effects. Economic aspects have a lower priority than the first two dimensions. Low cost or actual amount paid by the patient has a minor role due to reimbursement systems in place in most industrialized countries. If patients pay, the physician gives more attention to cost. Patient convenience and compliance may be decision criteria in

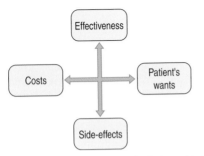

Figure 4.1 ● The factors which must be balanced in treating patients (after Barber).

situations when medically similar preparations are available, e.g. suppositories not being recommended when oral preparations are feasible. When prescribing for children, taste may be an important factor to consider (see Ch. 30).

In studies concerning the adoption of new medicines, it was shown that those physicians at the centre of a professional network tended to be innovators and started prescribing the new medicine at an early point. An early adopter in one therapeutic area might not necessarily be an early adopter in another therapeutic area. The opinion of colleagues is important; two physicians in close contact with each other tend to start a new medicine at the same time. Also the type of practice is an important factor. Physicians working alone adopt a new preparation more slowly than those working in group practices.

Barber has shown the dilemma the physician faces when choosing the right medicine. The problem is summarized in the question of how to find the right balance between the areas shown in Figure 4.1:

- Maximizing the effectiveness of treatment
- Minimizing the side-effects
- Minimizing costs
- Taking into account patient's wants and wishes.

Models to study prescribing

Several studies have tried to find typical characteristics of prescribing physicians and their work settings that would explain both irrational prescribing and prescribing in general. Basically three types of models and approaches have been used:

- Models focusing on demographic and practice variables which give descriptive information about what and how physicians tend to prescribe. These variables are often difficult or impossible to change, but these types of study point to where the focus should be put and indicate possible points for intervention
- Models focusing on psychosocial issues related to physician–patient interaction
- Models focusing on cognitive theories behind prescribing decisions. These studies focus on how physicians evaluate the available information and their decision-making process.

There seems to be no general competency to prescribe rationally, since a physician may prescribe rationally in one area and irrationally in another. This could be expected if, for example, an ophthalmologist prescribed for cardiac conditions. Younger and more recently graduated physicians usually seem to prescribe more rationally than older physicians. It has been found that physicians with a negative attitude towards the use of medicines for social problems tend to prescribe fewer psychotropic medicines. The availability of non-medicine alternatives (e.g. cognitive therapy) reduces benzodiazepine prescribing. Also the social environment may be important in prescribing, for example during the Gulf War, benzodiazepine prescribing doubled in Israel compared with the period before and after the conflict. A more cosmopolitan attitude and a more critical attitude towards commercial information were associated with more careful prescribing of risky medicines in one study. Another study showed that 'less rational prescribers', defined as those with a high rate of benzodiazepine prescriptions, rely more on commercial information from the pharmaceutical industry than others. Professional satisfaction and reading professional material seem to translate into better prescribing.

Many physicians base their selection of medicines on their own experience, which may not be an accurate base for rational selection. The probability of observing rare but important side-effects is very small for an individual physician. The same biases that were mentioned earlier affecting patients' decision making also affect physicians' decision making. If they have high initial positive expectations before starting a new treatment, the outcomes will be interpreted in a way that meets these expectations. Negative aspects will not be accounted for. Only positive aspects transform into writing more new prescriptions. Irrational prescribing is also often legitimized by positive personal experiences from prescribing or using that medicine. High medical uncertainty may also contribute to irrational prescribing. On the other hand it may also result in seeking information from many sources to reduce this uncertainty.

Certain patient factors also influence the probability of receiving a prescription for psychotropic medicines. The most widely studied factors have been age and gender. The elderly are usually prescribed more than younger people, which may be a reflection of a higher rate of symptoms and psychological distress. There is also a tendency to write more repeat prescriptions for the elderly, partly reflecting the type of medication being prescribed. Women are prescribed psychotropic medicines more often, which is partly explained by a higher consultation rate. The sex of the physician does not seem to influence this tendency to prescribe more for women. Physicians' expectations that women have more psychological–emotional disorders that can be treated successfully with benzodiazepines may also partly explain the difference.

Influencing prescribing

Providing information and employing educational programmes to change physicians' prescribing behaviour has become an integral part of the pharmacist's new role. Pharmacists participate in this kind of activity as part of their daily work, but also in formal trials or programmes in community and institutional settings. Several experimental studies have shown that pharmacists providing information and educating physicians produce positive effects on knowledge and attitudes, but the effects on prescribing behaviour have usually been modest. Providing physicians with printed material alone will not influence prescribing habits.

Individual feedback coupled with one-to-one education is the method most likely to be successful. Educational outreach or academic detailing has been studied and practised for the last 20 years. It follows the same principles as do medical representatives for pharmaceutical companies in their promotional activities. The basic principles are that physicians need to be interviewed in their own office where they are most receptive, the facilitators (often pharmacists) should be well presented and briefed, and the messages should be concise, clear and relevant to the prescriber. The programme should also be ongoing with repeat visits on a regular basis to maintain the contact and keep the messages up to date. The second major strategy includes managerial and regulatory activities such as use of limited lists (e.g. for reimbursement purposes), hospital or regional drug and therapeutic committees and formularies, structured medicine order forms (e.g. special forms for narcotics), drug utilization review (DUR) and treatment guidelines.

Pharmacies and the pharmacy profession

Historically a pharmacy has been the place for preparing and dispensing medicines. The first known pharmacy was established in the year 766 in Baghdad. In Europe the first pharmacies date back to the 11th century. In ancient times the same person acted as both doctor and pharmacist, i.e. diagnosed, prescribed and prepared the medicines for the patient. But in 1231 the German emperor and king of Sicily, Frederick II of Hohenstaufen in the edict of Palermo, legally separated the professions of medicine and pharmacy. Physicians were to diagnose and prescribe medicines, while pharmacists were to be responsible for preparing the medicines and providing these to the patients. Pharmacies were also designated to certain areas, where they had the monopoly of selling medicines. Certain physicians were also to oversee the work of pharmacists. Frederick also laid down rules about the education of healthcare professionals. These and other provisions given by him were the basis of legislation and practice of pharmacy in many European countries until the 20th century.

Elsewhere the distinction between the medical and pharmaceutical professions has not always been so clear and we can still find dispensing doctors today. However, in most countries, through the last centuries, pharmacists have acted as the 'poor man's doctor', diagnosing and prescribing. It should be remembered that the classification of medicines into prescription and OTC medicines has happened only fairly recently. Some other countries have similar legislation in place, but it is not enforced. The system of dispensing doctors has been defended based on availability and grounds of patient convenience. The problems related to the system are an apparent conflict of interest, which is present when the income of the physician depends on the volume and price of medicines prescribed. This problem has been highlighted in Japan, which also has one of the highest costs of medicines per capita in the world and where prescription medicines are mainly distributed by physicians. The same conflict of interest is often mentioned in the context of the professional and business roles of the pharmacist, especially concerning sales of non-prescription medicines.

There has been much discussion about the occupational status of pharmacists. Is pharmacy a true profession or not? Two major approaches have been used by academics in trying to answer the question.

One approach is to look at the functions pharmacists perform for society, asking if they are vital for the society. The second approach is to look at certain characteristic traits of the occupation and determine whether they fulfil typical traits of a profession. During the last 50 years, different traits have been mentioned by different academics, but there are some common ones. In the 1950s, Lewis & Maude mentioned the following traits that characterize a profession:

- Registration or state certification embodying standards of training and practice in some statutory form
- A fiduciary practitioner–client relationship
- An ethical code
- A ban on the advertising of services
- Independence from external control.

Most authors agree that the basic traits of a learned profession are advanced and lengthy training in a highly specialized body of knowledge. This knowledge is to be used in the service of society and mankind. Research and abstract reasoning are the ways of expanding this unique body of knowledge. The services provided by a profession are also related to the degree of impact or danger they may have on individuals or society. Besides the expert knowledge the professional possesses, he must also exert his professional judgement to the benefit of the client. Co-workers in the same or related occupations acknowledge the level of expertise of the profession, which is also important in legitimating the practice. There is also a certain level of trust that the public must place in the work performance of the professional. Professionals themselves define which kind of activities are allowed and what privileges members may claim. They also define, through ethical codes and legislation, which they have often themselves had an opportunity to draw up, the type of controls that guarantee the social privileges given to them (like autonomy of action, monopoly of practice, remuneration) are not abused.

Role of pharmacists

The origin of the pharmacy profession was in the unique knowledge base and skills needed to compound a drug product. With the growth of the pharmaceutical industry, this function decreased throughout the 20th century, especially in the 1950s and 1960s. Today it is impossible for the individual pharmacist in the pharmacy to compound similar products to those of the pharmaceutical industry. Also the pharmacist's traditional role of procuring and storing crude drugs has vanished. As the pharmacist's knowledge about the proper preparation, storage and handling of medicines is still greater than any other professional group, the quality assurance aspects of medicines are still their responsibility. Both the society and the profession have defined that the duty of the profession is to ensure that the medicines provided to patients are safely and accurately dispensed. The question raised in the 1960s was whether the status of pharmacy as a profession could be maintained if it were based solely on storing and distributing medicines. The discussion was referred to as 'the profession in search of a role'. This discussion was one contributory factor in the rise of the clinical pharmacy movement in the USA starting in the 1960s. The debate about the pharmacist's role has continued ever since, with new developments like the pharmaceutical care movement and the 'extended role' of the pharmacist in the 1990s. Today there seems to be some kind of consensus among pharmacy spokespersons that the future of pharmacy as a profession lies in pharmaceutical care. In different countries, however, there seem to be different interpretations about what pharmaceutical care is all about. Another question is to what extent the profession at the grassroot level has embraced this philosophy and to what extent it is being practised in everyday pharmacy practice.

International guidelines for good pharmacy practice by the FIP

The International Pharmacy Federation (FIP) has issued its guidelines for good pharmacy practice (GPP), stating that the mission of pharmacy practice is to provide medications and other healthcare products and services and to help people and society to make the best use of them. The concept of GPP is based mainly on the concept of pharmaceutical care. The patient and community are the primary beneficiaries of the pharmacist's actions and the pharmacist's first concern must be the welfare of the patient in all settings. The core of pharmacy activity is the supply of medication and other healthcare products of assured quality, appropriate information and advice to the patient and monitoring the effects of their use. From an international perspective, a rather new aspect is the quest for the pharmacist's contribution to the promotion of rational and economic prescribing and appropriate medicine use. According to GPP the objective of each element of pharmacy service should be relevant to the individual, clearly defined and effectively communicated to all those involved.

In satisfying GPP requirements, professional factors should be the main philosophy underlying practice. Economic factors are also important, but they should not be the driving force. Pharmacists should give their input to decisions on medicine use, and a therapeutic partnership with physicians and good relationships with other pharmacists are important. Pharmacists are also responsible for the evaluation and improvement of the quality of services given. There is a need for keeping patient profiles and to record pharmacists' interventions (see also Ch. 15). Pharmacists need independent, comprehensive, objective and current information about medicines. They should also accept personal responsibility for lifelong learning and educational programmes should address changes in practice. National standards of GPP need to be put in place and adhered to.

According to the guidelines there are four main elements of GPP: promotion of good health, supply and use of medicines, self-care and influencing prescribing and medicine use. It also encompasses cooperation with other healthcare professionals in health promotion activities, including the minimization of abuse and misuse of medicines. Professional assessment of promotional materials for medicines should also be carried out and evaluated as well as information about medicines and health care disseminated to the public. The involvement in all stages of clinical trials is also recommended. The guidelines include further areas within the four main elements that need to be addressed, such as national standards for facilities for confidential conversation, provision of general advice on health matters, involvement in health campaigns and the quality assurance of equipment used and advice given in diagnostic testing. In the supply and use of prescribed medicines, standards are needed for facilities, procedures and use of personnel. Assessment of the prescription by the pharmacist should include therapeutic aspects (pharmaceutical and pharmacological), appropriateness for the individual and social, legal and economic aspects.

Furthermore, national standards are needed for information sources, competence of pharmacists and medication records. Advice should be given to ensure that the patient receives and understands sufficient oral and written information. It is also important to have standards on how to follow up the effect of prescribed treatments and the recording of professional activities. When trying to influence prescribing and medicine use, general rational prescribing policies and national standards are needed. In research and practice documentation, pharmacists have a professional responsibility to document professional practice experience and activities and to conduct and/or participate in pharmacy practice research and therapy research. These guidelines form an international consensus on current practice of pharmacy and point to the direction for national guidelines and efforts to improve it.

Outcomes of medical treatment

Evaluation and outcomes research

Evaluation and outcomes research are fairly new topics within pharmacy. They are integral elements of pharmaceutical care and much more effort needs to be put into these aspects of pharmacy practice and research in the future. Evaluation has been defined as making a comparative assessment of the value of the intervention, using systematically collected and analysed data, in order to make informed decisions about how to act or to understand causal mechanisms and general principles. One important aspect from society's point of view is the question 'What are we getting for our money?' According to the model originally proposed by Donabedian, evaluation of health care can focus on:

- Structure – e.g. facilities, equipment, money, number and qualification of personnel
- Process – e.g. activities by staff and patients, prescribing, counselling
- Outcomes – e.g. intermediate outcomes such as patients' knowledge and behaviour, and final outcomes such as cure of the disease.

Traditionally evaluation has focused on structure and process and to a lesser extent on outcomes. More recently a whole new research field has emerged within health care called 'outcomes research'.

One difficulty in health-related outcomes research is to demonstrate the linkages between the three elements of the model: structure–process–outcome. For example, will a new computer-based patient medication record system in the pharmacy (structure) improve the follow-up of a patient (process), so that the pharmacist is able to detect more efficiently a medicine-related problem in the use of the antihypertensive medicine with the outcome of lowered blood pressure and the patient feeling better and living a healthier, longer and happier life (outcome)? Even if there is little empirical evidence, it is the general view that good structure leads to a more appropriate process resulting in better outcomes.

A general observation in the healthcare field is that we still lack evidence of many widely used procedures and interventions. Since the mid 1960s new medicines have undergone clinical trials and an official evaluation through the registration process. This does not mean that all medicines currently on the market or being marketed are safe, effective, economic or appropriate. Furthermore, even if we have only high-quality medicines on the market, the outcome of medical treatment is ultimately dependent on how the medicines are being prescribed by physicians and used by patients.

Within the pharmaceutical field a more comprehensive framework has been proposed by Kozma and his colleagues. This model, named ECHO, classifies outcomes in three categories: *e*conomic, *cl*inical and *h*umanistic *o*utcomes. Clinical outcomes have been defined as medical events that occur as a result of the condition or its treatment. Economic outcomes are the direct, indirect and intangible costs compared with consequences of medical treatment alternatives. Humanistic outcomes include well-being, health-related quality of life and patient satisfaction.

Health-related quality of life

The primary objective of health care is to improve patients' quality of life. To what extent this objective is achieved often remains unanswered. This may be due to lack of proper measures, the knowledge and attitudes of healthcare providers or some other factor. The central feature and objective of pharmaceutical care is to achieve outcomes by identifying, solving and preventing medicine-related problems that will improve a patient's quality of life. In experimental settings this has been shown to be the case. To what extent it is achieved in ordinary everyday practice is still an open question.

A classic list of outcomes in medical care has been crystallized in the 'five Ds' – death, disease, disability, discomfort and dissatisfaction. These include a wide range of different aspects, but are all negative terms. They will give partial answers to the questions about

the quality of life of the patient, but are not sufficient to cover all aspects of quality of life. The term 'health-related quality of life' has been used quite differently in the literature and daily practice. Explicit definitions are quite rare because of the multidimensionality of the concept. The domains of health-related quality of life usually include functional health (physical activity, mobility and self-care), emotional health (anxiety, stress, depression, spiritual well-being) social and role functioning (personal and community interactions, work and household activities), cognitive functioning (memory), perceptions of general well-being and life satisfaction, and perceived symptoms.

Health-related quality of life has been measured with disease-specific instruments and general or generic instruments, e.g. health profiles and measures based on utilities. Disease-specific instruments provide a greater detail concerning functioning and well-being in that particular disease. The disease-specific measures (e.g. those used in hypertension and asthma) can also be further categorized as population specific (e.g. elderly), function specific (e.g. sexual) and condition specific (e.g. pain). Examples of these instruments include the Asthma Quality of Life Questionnaire and the Diabetes Quality of Life Questionnaire.

The generic measures include health profiles, which constitute a number of questions covering the different aspects giving separate scores for each domain of life mentioned earlier. Examples include the Nottingham Health Profile, Sickness Impact Profile, McMaster Index and SF-36. The advantage of health profiles is that they provide a comprehensive array of scores that is multidimensional. If the measure used is sensitive enough, through the profile we may be able to distinguish, for example, when a medicine influences the emotional domain while having no effect on the functional health domain.

The utility-based measures incorporate specific patient health states while adjusting for the preferences (utilities) for the health state. The outcome scores range from 0 to 1, where 0 represent quality of life associated with death and 1 represents perfect health. The preferences have been empirically tested in different populations and been through a validation process. These utility-based measures have been extensively used in pharmacoeconomics research and more specifically in cost–utility analysis (see Ch. 19).

The most accurate and comprehensive end result may be achieved by using both a generic and a disease-specific measure when possible. The focus in current medicine is more on patient-perceived impact on long-term morbidity than on limiting mortality. It is good to remember that medicines can both increase and decrease the quality of life. The goal of medical therapy is to improve health and make patients feel better. Physiological measures may change without people feeling any better. Treatment of mildly elevated blood pressure is a good example of this. Nevertheless, treatment may improve subjective health without any measurable changes in clinical parameters. There may also be a trade-off between positive treatment outcomes and adverse events.

Client and patient satisfaction

An important aspect when measuring the outcomes of pharmacy practice and pharmaceutical interventions is the satisfaction of clients and patients. Measurement of client satisfaction can be an important tool in quality assurance of pharmacy practice (see also Ch. 11). There are difficulties in defining the quality of pharmacy services. One approach is to divide the quality into a technical dimension (i.e. what is offered) and a functional dimension (i.e. how it is offered). Different proposals have been made to cover different aspects of service provision in general. One comprehensive model is that by Parasuram. He distinguishes between 10 different dimensions: reliability, responsiveness, competence, access, courtesy, communication, credibility, security, understanding/knowing the customer and tangibles. Hedvall has presented a somewhat simplified model. She has proposed four dimensions: professionalism, commitment, confidentiality and milieu, which also contain the essence of what Parasuram has proposed. Customers may have difficulties in distinguishing between all 10 dimensions and some of them tend to overlap. The proposed dimensions represent important aspects to both prescription and self-care clients visiting the pharmacy. These aspects also have a direct linkage to communication skills and pharmaceutical care.

Measurement of patient satisfaction has usually focused more specifically on aspects in providing care. Cleary & McNeil have listed the following dimensions that are typically covered in the measurements of patient satisfaction: accessibility and availability of care, convenience, technical quality, physical setting, efficacy, personal aspects of care, continuity and economic aspects. In these dimensions we can distinguish a technical or cognitively based evaluation of the services offered and also an emotional or affective aspect – how well they are offered. The significance of client satisfaction can be correlated to patronage, patient adherence, and ultimately to the survival of the pharmacy profession.

KEY POINTS

- Medicines have a wider function than merely treating disease
- Rational use of medicines is defined in terms of safety, effectiveness, appropriateness and economics
- Society expects medicines used to be safe and attempts to achieve this by employing legislation and regulation supported by pharmaco-epidemiological studies
- Patients' medicine use behaviour is influenced by complex social and behavioural factors
- Prescribing is a complex process in which the prescriber has to balance cost, effectiveness, side-effects and the patient's wants
- The professional status of pharmacy can be determined from its role in society and the service characteristics of pharmacists in society
- Pharmacy is changing from a 'storage and supply' function only to include an advisory and monitoring role in the context of pharmaceutical care
- Evaluation of health care is achieved by measuring structure, process and outcomes
- Outcomes may be economic, clinical or humanistic
- Health-related quality of life can be assessed using disease-specific questionnaires or general health profiles

5

Pharmacy and public health

Roger Walker

STUDY POINTS

- The principles of public health
- The determinants of health and lifestyle determinants of health
- Different measures of deprivation
- What is public health pharmacy?
- Opportunities for pharmacists to be involved in public health pharmacy

Introduction

Over the past 30 years, pharmacists have received wide recognition for their considerable knowledge, skills and expertise in dealing with medicine-related issues at the level of the individual patient. In contrast, they appear to have struggled with the concept of contributing to the wider public health agenda. Perhaps this has arisen because pharmacists are most comfortable operating in situations where they determine the agenda and their work is focused on tackling medicine-related issues. Working with other agencies as part of a multidisciplinary team to address population-wide public health issues is a relatively new challenge that requires additional knowledge and skills.

There is an irony to the current situation because for many years pharmacists have addressed a range of public health issues by giving lifestyle advice on issues such as smoking cessation, diet, substance misuse, sexual health, alcohol and exercise to the population they serve. Pharmacists have, however, generally failed to recognize these as public health interventions. Perhaps only in recent years has pharmacy started to recognize its public health contribution following the publication

of key government strategies to develop public health pharmacy (Department of Health 2005). This chapter will help the reader better understand the principles of public health and the partnerships required to deliver the public health agenda and identify what the pharmacist can contribute.

What is public health pharmacy?

There are many definitions of public health in common use but perhaps the one most widely used in the UK is: 'The science and art of preventing disease, prolonging life and promoting health through the organized efforts and informed choices of society' (Acheson 1998).

Central to this definition is the concept that promoting public health is not solely an evidence-based science. For those working within public health there is also a need to understand different sociological groupings within society and work with others to support and persuade the population or sectors within society to make changes that may bring health benefit. This can also be interpreted as promoting a 'health service' in which resources are expended on both encouraging people to adopt a healthy lifestyle and protecting them from communicable diseases. This is in contrast to an 'ill health service' that many feel the current health-care system resembles and which primarily targets resources at those who are ill.

Typically, those employed in public health work across organizations such as local health service bodies, local authorities and local communities in settings ranging from acute hospital trusts and local health organizations through to local authorities, social services and the voluntary sector. Much of the work is long term and will take several years before any outcomes materialize that will have a lasting impact on health.

As a corollary to the definition of public health presented above, public health pharmacy can be defined as: 'The informed application of pharmaceutical knowledge, skills and resources to promote public health'. This definition (Walker 2000) reflects a pragmatic approach to public health pharmacy and can be applied to whatever the preferred definition of public health is. This approach has proved useful to help understand what pharmacy can contribute but it has misled some to believe that public health pharmacy is a discipline in its own right. This is incorrect. Public health requires a multidisciplinary team approach and pharmacy is but one of the contributors, and often with a strong focus on medicine-related issues.

If pharmacy restricts its public health contribution to medicine-related issues, and given that taking a medicine is the most common intervention in health care, it will always be in a position to have some impact on public health. However, to influence the wider determinants of health is more challenging and requires an appreciation that more than 70% of what determines an individual's health lies outside the domain of the health services and within demographic, social, economic and environmental conditions. To neglect these wider determinants will result in pharmacy failing to make its optimal contribution to public health. For example, there is limited opportunity to improve the health of a patient with asthma by counselling them on the correct use of their inhaler when wider public health issues are influencing treatment outcome. The individual may live in poorly heated, damp, infested accommodation, have a low paid job that involves working in a dusty or dirty environment, be poorly educated, have few or no friends or family to support them and have poor mental health. In addition, they may continue to smoke cigarettes, take little exercise and eat too many cheap, high fat content foods. It is clear that these factors will impact on good disease management, but the influential factors are often much less obvious than described above. To be aware of the wider determinants of health is important as each carries a significant health burden. Moreover, many health burdens have a significant link with deprivation. A number of these are summarized in Table 5.1.

Wider determinants of health

Most measures of population health show that it has improved markedly over the past 150 years. For example, life expectancy in England and Wales has improved in every decade since the 1840s. In 1841 life

Table 5.1 Examples of indicators that have been shown to have a significant association with deprivation

Domain	Indicator	Increased deprivation significantly associated with indicator
Lifestyle health determinant	Smoking	Yes
	Excess alcohol consumption	No
	Healthy diet	Yes
	Physical inactivity	Yes
Health status	Obesity	Yes
	Physical functioning	Yes
	Bodily pain	Yes
	General health	Yes
	Vitality	Yes
	Social functioning	Yes
	Role – emotional	Yes
	Mental health	Yes
	Low birth weight	Yes

Continued over

Table 5.1 *(Continued)*

Illness and injury	Depression and/or anxiety	Yes
	Hearing	Yes
	Eyesight	Yes
	Limiting long-term illness	Yes
	Arthritis	Yes
	Back pain	Yes
	Respiratory disease	Yes
	Asthma	Yes
	Diabetes	Yes
	High blood pressure	Yes
	Heart disease	Yes
	Angina	Yes
	Heart failure	No
	Cancer registrations	Yes
	Pedestrian injury 4–16 years reported to police	Yes
	Pedestrian injury 65+ years reported to police	Yes
	Pedestrian injury 5–14 years hospital inpatient	Yes
Use of health service	Dentist	Yes
	Family doctor	Yes
	Hospital inpatient (persons)	Yes
	Coronary heart disease admission	Yes
	Angiography	Yes
	Revascularization	Yes
	Hip replacement	Yes
	Knee replacement	No
	Lens replacement	No
	Infant mortality	Yes
Deaths	All-cause persons	Yes
	All-cause females	Yes
	All-cause males	Yes
	All cancer	Yes
	Colorectal cancer	Yes
	Lung cancer	Yes
	Breast cancer	Yes
	Coronary heart disease	No
	Stroke	Yes
	Respiratory disease	Yes
	Unintentional injury	Yes
	Road traffic injury	Yes
	Unintentional fall	Yes
	Suicide	Yes

expectancy for males was 41 and this had increased to 75 years by 1998. The equivalent improvement for females was from 43 to 80 years of age. Much of the improvement seen has been the result of environmental and social changes rather than developments in medicine and health care. Despite these overall improvements, social inequalities have widened, with improvements in the health of the most disadvan-taged groups being relatively small. To illustrate these inequalities we can look at the life expectancy of those who live in the most and least deprived areas of our big cities. In Scotland, for example, people living in the most deprived districts of Glasgow have a life expectancy 12 year shorter than those in the most affluent areas (NHS Health Scotland 2004). In London, boroughs a few miles apart have markedly

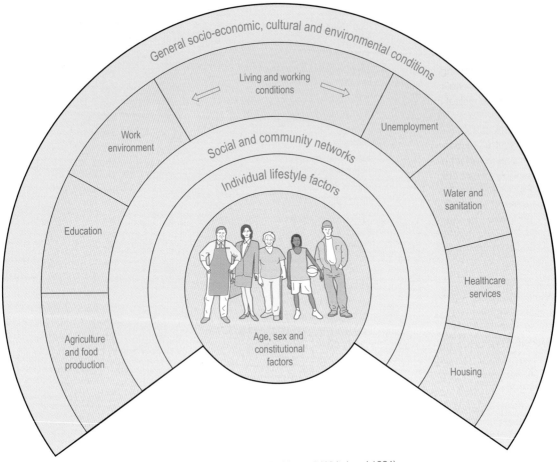

Figure 5.1 • Schematic model of the determinants of health (Dahlgren & Whitehead 1991).

different life expectancies. Each of the eight tube stations on the Jubilee line from Westminster to Canning Town represents a decline of one further additional year in life expectancy for the resident population (Department of Health 2004).

The landmark work of Dahlgren & Whitehead (1991) highlighted the main factors that determine the health of a given population (Fig. 5.1). The age, gender and genetic make-up of an individual clearly influence the health potential of that individual although each is fixed and non-modifiable. Other factors that influence health and which can be modified to have a favourable impact include addressing individual lifestyle factors such as smoking, diet and physical activity. Improving interactions with friends and relatives, and developing mutual support within a community can help sustain health. Other wider influences on health include living and working conditions, food provision, access to essential goods and services, and the

overall socio-economic, cultural and environmental conditions. There are too many factors to discuss in detail here, but a number of the relevant, key determinants are outlined below. However, the simple message is that, whether attempting to evaluate mortality, morbidity or self-reported health, and regardless of whether it is income, class, house ownership, deprivation, social exclusion or similar indicator or combination of indicators that is used as the socio-economic indicator, those who are worse off in society have poorer health.

Employment and unemployment

Both employment and unemployment can be associated with adverse effects on health. Job security has also been recognized as important for well-being. The trend towards less secure, short-term employment

Box 5.1

Examples of the health burden on individuals who may be unemployed

- Increased smoking
- Increased alcohol consumption
- Reduced physical activity and exercise
- Increased use of illicit drugs
- Increased sexual risk-taking and sexually transmitted diseases
- Increased weight gain
- Reduced psychological well-being, e.g. self-harm, depression, anxiety
- Increased morbidity
- Increased premature mortality from diseases such as coronary heart disease
- Social exclusion and isolation

affects everyone but is a particular problem for less skilled manual workers. Unemployment imposes a number of health burdens on the unemployed and some of these are summarized in Box 5.1.

In addition to job security there is considerable evidence that greater control over work is associated with positive health such as lower coronary heart disease, fewer musculoskeletal disorders, reduced mental illness and less sickness absence. The relationship between status in the workforce and health has been demonstrated across the gradient from the top jobs to those at the bottom. The landmark studies with civil servants in Whitehall, London (Marmot et al 1984, 1991) demonstrated that even those in the next grade down from the top had worse health than those in the top posts. Despite being in well paid and relatively secure posts, a health gradient was observed across a range of disorders when compared to those in the top posts.

A confounding issue when trying to interpret the effect of unemployment on health is that people with poorer health are more likely to be unemployed. This is particularly true for people with long-term conditions although this does not fully explain why the unemployed have poorer health.

Environment air quality

One of the most enduring images of poor air quality are the photographs taken in the 1950s of London in a dense smog. Pollution arising from the burning of domestic coal accounted for a significant number of premature deaths among Londoners. In the London smog of 1952 there was almost a threefold increase in death in the over 65s, while deaths from bronchitis and emphysema rose 9.5-fold, pneumonia and influenza increased 4.1-fold and myocardial degeneration increased almost threefold, along with associated increases in hospital admissions. Although the sulphur dioxide and black smoke from domestic coal is now a thing of the past, other pollutants have taken their place, notably from burning petrol and diesel in cars and other forms of transport. Ambient levels of air pollution continue to be associated with raised morbidity and mortality and are particularly hazardous to the elderly, children and those with pre-existing disease.

Crime

Crime affects not only the health of the victim but also that of the community involved. Fear of crime is a real phenomenon that impacts on both health and well-being. As a consequence of crime or the perception of crime, people make adjustments to their lifestyle and behaviour such as not going out after dark, not going out alone, avoiding certain areas, not using public transport and avoiding young people. Because crime is often concentrated in particular neighbourhoods and the avoidance measures outlined above are adopted, this can weaken social ties and undermine social cohesion in these neighbourhoods.

Energy and housing

It is recognized that energy obtained from fossil fuels must be reduced to meet international commitments on global warming and reduce their associated adverse impact on health. In many UK cities the trend is for falling use by industry but increased use by transport.

Heating of houses must also become more energy efficient. Typically housing for low income families is the most inefficient with the use of electric fires at standard tariff prices costing three times more than gas central heating. There is a fuel poverty strategy in the UK which seeks to provide heating and insulation improvement for those who spend 10% or more of their income on heating their home. Cold homes exacerbate many existing illnesses such as asthma and make the individual prone to respiratory infections (Box 5.2). In addition, fuel poverty brings opportunity loss. Poor families spend a disproportionate amount of their income in keeping warm and this has an adverse effect on their social well-being, ability to adopt a healthy lifestyle and overall quality of life.

Examples of the health burden of poor housing

- Increased respiratory infections
- Increased cardiovascular morbidity (cold housing)
- Increased risk of infection due to overcrowding
- Increased risk of accidents due to faulty wiring, dangerous appliances, lack of smoke alarms, cluttered conditions
- Increased risk of infestation with rats and cockroaches and the associated health risks
- Increased risk of indoor pollutants, e.g. carbon monoxide, radon, lead

Lifestyle determinants of health

The individual lifestyle determinants of health represent the areas in which pharmacy has traditionally made its most significant contribution to public health. It is therefore important to appreciate that poverty is associated with a number of behaviours that may have an adverse impact on health. For example, poor people are less likely to eat a good diet and more likely to have a sedentary lifestyle, be obese and abuse alcohol. Cigarette smoking has one of the strongest associations with social disadvantage, with higher levels recorded in more deprived sectors of the population, and this in turn has the greatest cost in terms of premature death.

Smoking

In 2006 tobacco smoking was the main avoidable cause of premature death in the UK, responsible for more than 120 000 deaths. Smoking causes a wide range of serious illnesses including cancer of the lung, respiratory tract, oesophagus, bladder, kidney, stomach and pancreas, respiratory disease including chronic obstructive lung disease and pneumonia, circulatory disease such as heart disease, strokes and aneurysms, and digestive disorders such as ulcers of the stomach and duodenum. Second-hand smoke also puts others at risk and has been linked to lung cancer, strokes, respiratory disorders and infections, particularly in children.

In 2007, before the introduction of the ban on smoking in public in England, Wales and Northern Ireland (smoking in public was banned in 2006 in Scotland), approximately 28% of men and 23% of women were smokers, accounting for up to 10 million people in England alone. This remains a significant problem despite the decline in smoking seen over the past 30 years from the 53% of men and 42% of women who smoked in the mid 1970s. Factors that continue to predict the likelihood of smoking include challenging material circumstances, cultural deprivation and stressful marital, personal and household circumstances.

To reduce the health burden of smoking, a number of public health strategies have been put in place and these include reducing the public's exposure to second-hand smoke, providing more support for smokers to stop, raising public awareness of the health effects of smoking and the benefits of stopping smoking and reducing tobacco advertising and the impact of tobacco promotion, and regulating the sales and design of cigarette packets.

With respect to the no smoking agenda the major contribution of pharmacy is in raising awareness of the harm caused by smoking, supporting strategies to reduce the adverse impact of smoking on health, identifying smokers who want to stop and providing these individuals with behavioural support or referring them to alternative sources of smoking cessation support.

Pharmacists are often in a unique position to discuss smoking cessation and opportunities to raise the topic with individuals who visit them and who may be unhappy with their health, have respiratory problems or dental problems, be proactively seeking other lifestyle advice such as cholesterol or blood pressure testing, requesting health-related products such as cough medicines or alternative/complementary therapies such as St John's wort, purchasing smoking cessation-related products or presenting a prescription for nicotine replacement therapy, bupropion or varenicline – all are potential windows of opportunity for pharmaceutical intervention.

Weight management

The UK is experiencing one of the world's fastest growing rates of obesity. In 2006 obesity was considered to be at epidemic proportions with almost 24% of men and women classified as obese and 25% of children aged 11–15 years of age being overweight or obese. Such classification is often based on determining the body mass index (BMI: defined as weight in kilograms divided by the square of height in metres) of an individual. A BMI in the range of $25 \, \text{kg/m}^2$ to $30 \, \text{kg/m}^2$ indicates the individual is overweight while a BMI of greater than $30 \, \text{kg/m}^2$ indicates obesity.

Being overweight can seriously affect an individual's health and may lead to high blood pressure, type II diabetes, cardiovascular disease, many cancers including colorectal and prostate cancers in men and breast or endometrial cancer in women, osteoarthritis, poor self-image and decreased life expectancy.

Increasingly the measurement of waist circumference is being undertaken as it presents a simple way of assessing someone's risk rather than measuring BMI. Men are at an increased health risk if their waist measurement is ≥ 94 cm and at substantially increased health risk if the measurement is ≥ 102 cm. Equivalent waist measurements for women are ≥ 80 cm and ≥ 88 cm.

Raising issues of weight management can be difficult but opportunities for the pharmacist to intervene may arise when a person complains of being unhappy with their weight, short of breath or having mobility problems associated with back or hip pain. Alternatively, opportunities may arise when individuals request products such as slimming aids, blood pressure monitors, cholesterol monitoring kits, alternative or complementary therapies for use in weight loss or receive prescribed or purchased medicines for arthritis, diabetes, cardiovascular or respiratory disease. Key advice to be offered will need to address healthy eating and exercise.

Alcohol

Excessive alcohol intake is associated with a range of health problems including serious liver disease, disorders of the stomach and pancreas, anxiety and depression, sexual problems, high blood pressure and cardiac disease, involvement in accidents, particularly car crashes, a range of cancers, including those of the mouth, throat, liver, colon and breast, and becoming overweight or obese.

Alcohol misuse currently accounts for approximately 22 000 deaths each year, with consumption above the recommended limits of 3 units per day for men and 2 units per day for women being exceeded by 22% of adult females and 39% of adult males. Of equal concern is the fact that 20% of the population in England drink to get drunk (binge drink). This is defined as consuming more than 8 units for men and more than 6 units for women and is strongly associated with involvement in accidents and with cardiovascular disease.

Most people are sensitive about revealing the details of their drinking habits; however, opportunities for pharmacists to raise awareness of sensible drinking may arise when individuals present with a hangover, headache, indigestion, or complain of

insomnia, excessive tiredness, depression, stress, being overweight or report having been involved in a minor accident. Individuals seeking advice about testing blood pressure or dietary information, requesting products for hangovers, painkillers or antacids, and requesting kits to test drinks for contaminants also present opportunities for intervention. Requests for alternative medicines/complementary therapies that may be used to treat alcohol-related problems, or supplying a prescribed or over the counter medicine known to interact with alcohol are further opportunities that may allow discussion with the individual.

Exercise

Regular exercise for adults that is equivalent to at least 30 minutes a day of moderate physical activity on 5 or more days of the week, can help prevent or manage a range of disorders including cardiovascular disease, type II diabetes, musculoskeletal disorders, mental illness and a range of cancers. Children are required to undertake at least 60 minutes of moderate activity each day to promote healthy growth, development and psychological well-being. Recent surveys have shown less than 37% of adult men and 24% of women undertake sufficient exercise to gain any health benefit. Older people need to maintain their mobility and undertake regular daily activity, and attempts to improve strength, coordination and balance may be particularly beneficial.

Clearly the amount of physical activity an individual needs to undertake will be influenced by their daily routine and the nature of their job. Opportunities for the pharmacist to raise issues relating to physical activity may arise when people are unhappy with their weight, complain of being short of breath or tired, have mobility problems, suffer from depression or stress, or have difficulty sleeping. Again, when an individual seeks advice about monitoring blood pressure or cholesterol levels or requests dietary information on how to lose weight, it may be opportune to discuss exercise-related issues. Likewise the purchase of support equipment, for example for knees, requesting alternative or complementary medicines to provide energy, or obtaining prescribed or purchased medicines for blood pressure may be additional opportunities.

Measuring deprivation

Although a number of different approaches have been developed to measure the deprivation of a given population, most have significant limitations.

Over recent years new tools have emerged to give more robust estimates of deprivation. One of the most widely used measures of deprivation has been the Townsend index, which produces a composite score for relative deprivation based on four variables obtained from the national census undertaken every 10 years in the UK. These variables include proportion of:

- Households with no car
- Households not owner occupied
- Unemployed economically active persons aged 16–59 years (females) and 16–64 years (males)
- Households overcrowded.

The Townsend index has a number of limitations, including a lack of validity in rural areas where, unlike urban areas, ownership of a car may be a necessity at all levels of deprivation. The Townsend index continues to be widely used because its construction is independent of health-related variables and the component data are captured in the national census. However, over recent years each of the constituent countries in the UK has developed its own approach to measuring deprivation. As a consequence it is increasingly difficult to compare deprivation across, for example, England and Wales. In England a new index was introduced in 2004 to measure multiple deprivation based on seven distinct domains:

- Income: captures the proportion of the population in an area living on low income
- Employment: measures unemployment assessed as the involuntary exclusion of those of working age from work
- Health deprivation and disability: identifies areas with high rates of premature deaths or whose quality of life is impaired by poor health or who are disabled
- Education, skills and training: captures education deprivation for children and young people and the level of skills and qualifications among the working age adult population
- Barriers to housing and services: measures wider barriers such as household overcrowding, homelessness, difficulty of becoming an owner occupier and geographical barriers such as distance to GP premises, convenience store, primary school and Post Office
- Crime: measures the incidence of recorded crime in an area for burglary, theft, criminal damage and violence

- Living environment: measures the quality of the indoor living environment and the outdoor living environment including air quality and road traffic accidents involving injury to pedestrians and cyclists.

From the above it can be seen that the Index of Multiple Deprivation 2004 is based on the principle of distinct dimensions of deprivation that can be recognized and measured separately. Individuals may be counted in one or more domains depending on the type of deprivation they experience. The final deprivation score is a composite, weighted score of each of the seven domains. In 2007 there were 354 local authorities in England and each could be given a score and a rank on the index of multiple deprivation. The lower the rank the more deprived the district.

In comparison to the English index, the Welsh Index of Multiple Deprivation 2005 is compiled from seven similar indicators of deprivation: income, employment, health, education, housing, access to services and environment. However, the data sources utilized in the domains vary between the two countries and therefore the scores obtained cannot be used to compare deprivation in England and Wales. Even within a single country small differences in deprivation scores mean little and the scores do not really allow you to determine how much more deprived one area is compared to another. Likewise, where two areas have markedly different deprivation scores, one area may be considered less deprived than the other, but not more affluent, i.e. the indices are a measure of deprivation and not affluence.

Changing habits and lifestyle

To assist people in making changes to their habits and lifestyle there is a need to recognize the part played by socio-cultural influences and the environment. There are many models that are used to help understand the change process. One that has found use within public health is the 'three Es model for lifestyle change'. In this model three stages are identified:

- Encouragement
- Empowerment
- Environment.

Encouragement involves raising awareness that may include the use of adverts, leaflets, one-to-one advice and targeted campaigns. This stage of the change process is used to act as a trigger for people to make healthy choices, or at least consider the healthy options. By itself, encouragement is unlikely to bring about sustained change in the population without empowerment and changes to environmental factors.

Empowerment involves the education and development of the individual and the community. Central to empowerment is the development of knowledge, life skills and confidence that will enable individuals, groups or populations to make the healthy choice. This process will be enhanced by the pharmacist, who can instil confidence in patients rather than undermining them, and by making changes to environmental factors.

Environment changes are targeted at the social, cultural, economic and physical surroundings in which people live and work. These changes aim to make the healthy choice the easy option.

A good example that can be used to illustrate this process is the need for the wider population to reduce their intake of salt to less than 6 g per day. *Encouragement* could involve a campaign to raise awareness of the daily intake of salt and the harmful effect of excessive intake; *empowerment* might target the labels on food and ensure they are easy for everyone to understand and to know what they are consuming; changes to the *environment* could involve a reduction in the salt content of prepared foods by manufacturers and the availability of low salt options in supermarkets and restaurants, thereby making it easier for consumers to reduce dietary salt intake.

Conclusion

This chapter has highlighted the key determinants of health and focused on areas of lifestyle advice where the pharmacist has traditionally contributed to the public health agenda. Hopefully it is apparent to the reader that to make a substantive contribution to public health, pharmacy will need to build on its current roles. Some public health pharmacy roles, such as assessing the health and social needs of communities through involvement in surveillance, surveys and information gathering exercises, acting as an advocate for local communities on health issues, and building sustainable communities or working in partnership with relevant statutory and voluntary services to promote and protect the health of the public, may be seen as roles best undertaken by individuals who choose to specialize in public health. Nevertheless, a large number of public health activities can be undertaken from a pharmacy, whether it is located in the community or hospital sector. Some of these are identified in Box 5.3.

Box 5.3

Examples of public health roles that could be undertaken by most pharmacies

- Develop closer working relationships with local authorities and other non-pharmacy bodies to influence the wider determinants of health
- Develop community leaders and health champions from within pharmacy
- Develop pharmacy services in deprived areas to provide additional pharmaceutical support and tackle health inequalities
- Provide information and advice to the public on health improvement and health protection
- Improve medicines and health literacy of patients, public and carers
- Provide access to, or signpost, health information resources and services
- Provide lifestyle advice for individuals with disease risk factors
- Provide services to promote self-care
- Promote health literacy and participate in national campaigns
- Provide stop smoking services
- Provide sexual health services, e.g. emergency hormonal contraception (EHC), *Chlamydia* screening, free condoms
- Provide healthy weight programmes
- Provide safe use of alcohol services
- Provide health screening services
- Encourage immunization uptake and provide immunization services
- Monitor and track safe use of medicines including reporting of adverse reactions
- Promote safe, efficient and effective use of prescribed and purchased medicines
- Develop medicines management programmes for those with chronic conditions
- Make pharmacies more accessible for difficult to reach groups, e.g. men, teenagers

KEY POINTS

- Pharmacist have many opportunities to promote health
- Public health pharmacy can be defined in many ways
- More than 70% of the factors affecting an individual's health are outside the domain of the health services
- Public health has improved markedly during the past 150 years
- During this time, social inequalities have widened, with disadvantaged groups showing little improvement
- A wide range of factors affect the health of an individual, some of which are fixed, while others can be modified

- Both employment and unemployment are associated with adverse health effects
- Air pollution is associated with raised morbidity and mortality
- It is with individual lifestyle determinants that pharmacists have had a traditional role
- Community pharmacists may offer support with smoking cessation, weight management, exercise and problems with alcohol
- Measures of deprivation vary from one country to another
- While these details vary, the main factors are income, employment, health, education, housing, crime and the environment
- To help people change lifestyle or habit, think – encouragement, empowerment, environment

Chapter Six

Types of patient charges for medicines and their impact

Ellen Schafheutle

STUDY POINTS

- Know the reasons for charging patients for (part of) their prescribed medicines
- Define the different types of co-payments for medicines
- Understand the effect of patient charges on uptake of medicines
- Differentiate between essential and less essential medicines, and the differing effect of charges on them
- Define patient groups that are likely to be most susceptible/vulnerable to the impact of medication cost
- Describe strategies patients use to manage or reduce medication cost
- Describe strategies healthcare professionals, especially pharmacists, can use to help patients cope with medication cost sharing issues

Introduction

Healthcare expenditure has been rising steadily over the past decades, and with the ever evolving advent of new technologies and treatments this trend is likely to continue. In the developed world payment for health care is usually covered by third-party payment systems to which the population (or members) contribute in the form of regular insurance premiums or taxes. However, paying for health care and medicines through such third-party providers removes the price barrier to consumption, as healthcare services become – or rather appear – free to the patient on access. Getting patients to contribute something when accessing health care is thus seen as the reintroduction of such a price barrier, with the aim of deterring unnecessary access and medicines use, and thus reducing potential waste. Such contributions or payments borne by patients are commonly referred to as cost sharing, as they make a contribution to the actual cost of treatment. Besides creating a cost barrier to (unnecessary) demand, cost sharing also creates another form of revenue to the healthcare provider.

Cost sharing can be levied on some or all types of health care. In some countries patients have to pay when visiting a doctor. In the UK, for example, patients have to contribute considerably towards dental and optical care, but visits to family doctors and hospitals are free. One particular form of cost sharing that is relatively easily defined, identified and implemented is on prescribed medicines. The impact of this cost has been widely studied and is of particular interest to pharmacists, which is why it is the focus of this chapter.

Types of cost sharing arrangements

Essentially, there are three types of cost sharing for medicines, i.e. the cost the patient has to pay themselves, out-of-pocket, in order to obtain prescribed medication. These are a:

- Flat rate fixed charge, usually called a prescription charge
- Percentage co-payment system
- Deductible system.

A *prescription charge* is a fixed fee that is payable per item on a prescription, or per prescription (containing one or more items). Flat rate prescription charges are independent of actual drug cost and exist in Austria and the UK. They are used in combination with other forms of cost sharing in Finland and Germany.

Percentage co-payment (also termed 'co-insurance') is probably the most common form of cost sharing and is based on a percentage payment of actual drug cost. The percentage amount that is payable by the patient can vary depending on the type of medicine and the seriousness of the underlying pathology. In France, for example, patients have to pay 35% of actual cost towards medicines that are classed as being of major therapeutic value, but have to contribute 65% for those where therapeutic value is judged as moderate or low. Certain drugs, treating conditions that are considered as 'not usually of a serious nature', may need to be paid in full, and many drugs that are available to buy over the counter (OTC) from pharmacies fall into this category.

In a *deductible system* a patient has to pay 100% of the cost of their prescribed medication up to a set amount (the deductible), after which the cost is subsidized. This system is often combined with a percentage co-payment or prescription charge once the deductible has been reached.

Protection mechanisms and exemptions

In many countries cost sharing arrangements are accompanied by mechanisms to protect vulnerable groups against undue or excessive expenses for drugs. Such protection mechanisms can take the form of reduced (i.e. subsidized) payments, exemptions, caps on expenditure, or complementary insurance to cover all or part of out-of-pocket cost sharing. These protection mechanisms may be available to all (e.g. complementary insurance), or apply to particular types of drugs, e.g. essential drugs treating chronic or life-threatening conditions. They may also apply to particular groups in the population, who can access prescribed drugs at a reduced or no cost (i.e. exempt). Criteria that usually define vulnerable groups and qualify for exemption or subsidy are:

- *Clinical conditions* – commonly those defined as chronic or life-threatening and requiring essential medication, usually implemented as a list of qualifying conditions or drugs. (In the UK, for example, patients requiring medication for type I or type II diabetes are exempt.)

- *Level of income* – where people on low incomes are protected against undue expense.
- *Age* – children are exempt in Austria, Germany, Ireland, New Zealand, Sweden and the UK; older people are exempt or have reduced cost sharing arrangements in Australia, Austria, Belgium, Canada, Denmark, Ireland, New Zealand, Portugal, Spain, the UK and the US. (NB: definitions for 'children' and 'older people' differ in the different countries, the latter being linked to retirement in some.)

Caps on co-payments

Only a few countries (e.g. New Zealand and Sweden) have reduced medication co-payments for high users, but many have some form of cap. Caps are sometimes also referred to as out-of-pocket maximums and define the maximum amount a patient should be asked to cost share. Caps can either apply per prescription or be annual caps. Caps per prescription exist, for example in Taiwan. Annual caps are probably more common and can either apply to the whole of the population (e.g. Sweden and Norway) or only to certain groups, such as the chronically ill (e.g. Denmark, Finland and Germany). Some countries also have systems where medication co-payments are tax deductible (e.g. Ireland and Portugal).

Complementary insurance

Complementary insurance covering the cost of prescription co-payments is another form of protection mechanism; patients who have bought this type of insurance do not have to cost share or, if they are asked to pay an amount out-of-pocket, are subsequently reimbursed. Complementary insurance is widespread in France (*mutuelle*) but can also be found in a number of other countries. In England, Scotland and Northern Ireland a so-called prepayment certificate (PPC) exists, which can be bought to cover the cost of any prescription charges over a 3- or 12-month period, thus providing a cap through advance payment. The problem with complementary insurance and PPCs is that they only alleviate the financial burden for those that can afford to purchase this cover, which raises equity concerns.

Impact of cost sharing on drug use and health outcomes

Impact on drug consumption

A large body of international literature exists showing that cost sharing reduces access to health services in general (where cost sharing applies), and use of prescribed medication in particular. This is, of course, one of the aims of having such a policy in place, whereby patients respond to cost sharing by assessing whether a visit to their doctor, and the use of prescribed medication in particular, are seen as important enough to warrant the relevant out-of-pocket payment. For unnecessary visits or self-limiting conditions that patients may be able to treat themselves (either through self-care or the use of self-medication remedies, for example), avoiding the use of formal health care may be the most appropriate action. This will save cost to the patient, as no cost sharing is incurred, or possibly a reduced amount is paid if OTC remedies are purchased. It further reduces resource use by the health service itself (third party payment), which is the aim of a cost sharing policy.

Differential effect on essential and less essential medication

Cost sharing should therefore only affect patient demand that may not be entirely clinically necessary. It should thus also only affect the use of less essential medication. The latter is defined as medication that provides symptomatic relief without having an effect on any underlying disease process (see Table 6.1 for a more detailed definition). Indeed, the negative effect of cost sharing on drug utilization has been found to be more pronounced for non-essential drugs, but it does also reduce the use of essential medication (Soumerai et al 1987; Stuart & Grana 1998). As the terminology suggests (see Table 6.1), essential drugs are those whose withdrawal would have important effects on morbidity and mortality, and thus a cost-related reduction in essential medication is likely to have a negative effect on health outcomes.

Effect on health outcomes

Even though there are not as many studies that show that a cost-related reduction in the use of essential medicines impacts negatively on health outcomes, convincing large-scale evidence does exist. Tamblyn et al (2001) used interrupted time series analysis to examine the effect of the Quebec drug policy reform, where a 25% co-payment and income linked caps were introduced. Using a random sample of 93 950 elderly persons and 55 333 adult welfare recipients, the authors showed that the use of essential drugs decreased by 9.12% and 14.42% in the two groups; and the use of less essential drugs decreased by 15.14% and 22.39% respectively. The authors further demonstrated an increase in emergency department visits and serious adverse events (defined as hospitalization, nursing home admission or mortality) in association with the decrease of essential drugs use, but not in association with the reduction in less essential drugs. They thus established a causal link between the reduction in drug use in response to cost sharing and a negative effect on health outcomes.

Table 6.1 Definitions of essential and non-essential medications (Tamblyn et al 2001)

Drug category	Definition	Drugs included in categories
Essential drugs	'Medications that prevent deterioration in health or prolong life and would not likely be prescribed in the absence of a definitive diagnosis'	Insulin, anticoagulants, angiotensin converting enzyme inhibitors, lipid-reducing medication, antihypertensives, furosemide, β-blockers, antiarrhythmics, aspirin, antivirals, thyroid medication, neuroleptics, antidepressants, anticonvulsants, antiparkinson drugs, prednisone, β-agonists, inhaled steroids, ciclosporin
Less essential drugs	'Medications that may provide relief of symptoms but will likely have no effect on the underlying disease process'	

Furthermore, Rice & Matsuoka (2004) and Lexchin & Grootendorst (2004) provide two independently published reviews of the literature on the impact of prescription medicine fees on drug and health service use, as well as health status. They both conclude that cost sharing leads to a decrease in essential drug use and a decline in health status in vulnerable populations.

Negative effect on healthcare use and resources

If cost-related reduction in the use of essential medication leads to worse health outcomes, this will invariably lead to an increased use of healthcare services (such as increased numbers of visits, increased hospital admission and additional treatment and medication). This, in turn, will have an effect on resource use, as all such increased health service use will need to be funded. It is thus important to note that any savings in drug spend (due to a reduction in drug use because of cost sharing) may be offset by cost increases in other healthcare areas. However, very few studies exist that have demonstrated such a link. Soumerai et al (1994) assessed the effect of a Medicaid imposed cap, allowing a maximum of three prescriptions a month, on 268 permanently disabled, non-institutionalized patients with schizophrenia. They demonstrated a decrease in the use of essential mental health drugs and a concomitant increase in the use of acute mental health services among low-income patients. They estimated that the average increase in mental healthcare costs per patient during the cap exceeded the savings in drug costs to Medicaid by a factor of 17. From a societal perspective this runs counter to the aim of any cost sharing policy.

Effect of cost sharing on different population groups

Besides having differing effects on essential versus less essential drugs, cost sharing can also affect different groups in the population to differing extents. The elderly, people with disabilities (including mental health problems), those taking medication for chronic conditions and people on low incomes are particularly vulnerable and susceptible (Lundberg et al 1998; Safran et al 2005; Stuart & Grana 1998). Essentially, these are the groups that are most likely to have high morbidity and high use of essential medication, while

being least likely to be able to afford cost sharing. To protect them, many countries have exemptions and other protection mechanisms in place, which have already been mentioned.

Impact of cost sharing on patients and healthcare professionals

The preceding sections have provided insight into the fact that medication cost sharing reduces drug utilization, and that certain groups of patients are more vulnerable or susceptible to this effect, particularly those on low incomes or regular medicine users. However, these studies provide little detail on how drug utilization is reduced, i.e. how individual patients cope with the cost of their medication. Rather than relying on the analysis of large insurance reimbursement or claims databases that provided much of the above evidence, studies that employed methodologies involving direct contact with patients have explored this. In-depth interviews and focus groups have provided some of the depth and detail on how patients cope with medication cost, and questionnaire surveys have allowed quantification of this information (Cox et al 2001; Cox & Henderson 2002; Safran et al 2005; Schafheutle et al 2002, 2004).

Effect of cost sharing on patients – coping strategies

From these studies we know that patients respond to cost sharing in complex ways. Furthermore, there are many factors that can impact on whether patients decide to adhere to their medication, and cost is just one of them. Indeed, medication cost is often not an overriding factor when patients decide whether to adhere to their prescribed medication regimen or not, but it can be at least a mediator. If patients perceive their condition as serious and the prescribed treatment as one providing an important health benefit, cost is less likely to have an effect. On the other hand, if a condition is judged to be less serious, and where treatment may be mainly symptomatic rather than curative, cost is more likely to impact. The evidence presented in the previous section, where cost sharing was shown to have a greater effect on less essential than essential medication, supports this.

The actual amount of cost sharing is also important, and the higher it is the more likely it is to impact on patients' management behaviour (called 'price elasticity'). Patients' 'affordability factors' are also important, where patients on lower incomes and with competing demands on the resources they have available are more likely to be affected by cost sharing than patients on higher incomes, without affordability issues.

When cost sharing does affect patients' management behaviour, patients respond by using a variety and combination of strategies, which all aim to either make the cost manageable or reduce it. Their use is strongly influenced by patients' income and affordability, where people on below average incomes are significantly more likely to use these cost reduction strategies than those on above average incomes (Schafheutle et al 2004).

In order to cope with cost sharing, patients may decide to:

- Not have their medication dispensed at all
- Take less of their medication to make it last longer
- Delay having their prescription dispensed until they have money available
- Borrow money to pay for their prescription
- Prioritize, i.e. get only some items dispensed if more than one has been prescribed.

In some cases patients may also decide not to go to the doctor to avoid getting a prescription that would then need to be paid for, a strategy that will be particularly prominent in systems where cost sharing also exists for physician visits.

Patients in all types of cost sharing systems use many of the above strategies, as they reduce patients' out-of-pocket expense for prescription medicines regardless of the type of cost sharing that is in place. However, some strategies are only used in certain systems, as their effectiveness in terms of cost reduction depends on the particular type of cost sharing system. A UK specific strategy, for example, would be to buy a pre-payment certificate, while the specific French strategy is to buy the complementary insurance 'mutuelle'. Strategies that are specific to patients who pay a proportional co-payment are to:

- Shop around at different pharmacies which may offer different discounts
- Purchase their prescribed medication cheaper in another country (e.g. Mexico if from USA)
- Apply to a pharmaceutical company's Prescription Drug Patient Assistance Program (USA).

Asking for cheaper generic drugs instead of more expensive brands is also a strategy likely to be used in countries with proportional co-payments.

Self-medication strategies

Patients may also respond to high medication cost sharing for prescribed medicines by opting to access cheaper OTC remedies, if they are available. This approach is only likely to work in systems with a flat prescription charge, where the cost of the charge is generally higher than the cost of many OTC products (such as in the UK). Buying OTC products will also be a strategy in countries where (some or all) OTC products are not prescribable (blacklisted), or are not covered (i.e. paid for) by the healthcare system (such as France, Germany and the Netherlands).

It is further interesting to note that patients are price sensitive when making self-medication choices (Schafheutle et al 2004). Especially if they experience affordability issues, patients consider the price of different OTC products and may choose a cheaper alternative. Conversely, in some cases paying a prescription charge works out cheaper than buying one of the more expensive OTC products, which may make some patients more likely to visit the doctor rather than self-medicate. (This may be different in countries where patients have to pay out-of-pocket when they visit a doctor.)

Involving the prescriber

Prescribers also have a number of options available to them which allow them to, in effect, prescribe in a way that gives patients best 'value for money'. The types of strategies they can use, again, depend on the cost sharing system within which they operate. In a flat fee charge system (e.g. Austria, Germany or the UK), they can, for example, issue a prescription for a longer supply or a larger pack size, as this allows patients to obtain a larger supply for the same fixed charge. UK and German doctors may issue a private prescription (in the UK alongside an NHS one) for low cost drugs whose actual price is less than the flat fee prescription charge. In a proportional co-payment system, physicians can issue prescriptions for cheaper generic rather than branded items.

Physicians may try to prescribe more 'effectively' by issuing fewer items, provided this does not compromise the clinical effectiveness of their treatment. They may also prescribe a drug that may be more likely to be effective straight off and not require several attempts at finding a suitable drug, each requiring a further charge (one example being a prescription for a proton pump inhibitor for those that pay, rather than an H_2 antagonist, in the management of dyspepsia). UK doctors have further mentioned issuing samples that have been left by pharmaceutical industry representatives (thus avoiding any patient charge) or packs that were returned unused by patients (the latter, however, is not usually a legal strategy; Weiss et al 2001). Doctors also have a role to play in recommending money-saving options, such as the availability of pre-payment certificates (UK) or complementary insurance, or suggesting cheaper OTC alternatives.

For prescribing doctors to be likely to use strategies that will help patients to afford their medication, doctors need to be aware that patients pay and that they do, in fact, experience affordability issues. However, patients are generally reluctant or embarrassed to raise issues of cost and affordability with their doctor, as they consider this to be their own problem rather than that of their doctor, whose role they see as choosing the clinically most appropriate treatment. Nevertheless, if cost sharing impacts negatively on patients' adherence to prescribed regimens, this can undermine their effectiveness, particularly if the medicines in questions are essential. In order for doctors to be able to find the best treatment for their patients, they need to know whether their patients adhere to their medication, and if not, why not.

The role of community pharmacies

In most countries, community pharmacies are the places where patients go to have their prescriptions dispensed. This is therefore also the place where patients have to pay the amount that is due for medication cost sharing, which makes it likely that patients will raise issues of cost and affordability there. Pharmacists and their staff thus have an important role to play in response to patients' cost and affordability issues, and the impact this may have on their decisions not to adhere to their prescribed medication regimen as intended. Pharmacists can support patients to make appropriate decisions, using some of the above mentioned patient strategies. They can, for example, raise awareness of complementary insurance programmes (or the pre-payment certificates in the UK), recommend generic substitution or the purchase of a cheaper OTC product where available.

However, pharmacists will also be faced by patients delaying prescriptions, prioritizing certain items, i.e. getting only some dispensed, or choosing not to have any of their medication dispensed, because they cannot afford (or do not want) to pay the medication cost sharing amount that is due. In some cases these requests will relate to essential medication where adherence is crucial to achieving full health benefit. In other words, cost-related non-adherence may lead to worse health outcomes for these patients. An example might be that a patient only wants to get his β-agonist inhaler dispensed when he also requires a steroid inhaler. Or patients may choose not to take medication for hypertension, as the effect of this medication is not immediately evident to them and any long-term benefits are intangible.

Pharmacists have an important role in advising patients about the action and benefits of their medication and the importance of adherence in order to fully achieve this benefit. If understanding is increased, patients who can afford to pay may choose to do so. Nevertheless, this advice is unlikely to work for those patients who simply cannot afford to pay the cost sharing. In these cases pharmacists may want to liaise with doctors and other members of the healthcare team to discuss options to support this patient's treatment. Pharmacists and their staff may also be able to inform patients about the availability of income-related systems for exemptions or subsidy and how to go about applying for them (pharmacies may even have the relevant forms available).

To ensure that issues of cost and affordability are raised where necessary, pharmacists could incorporate appropriate questioning into pharmaceutical care plans, or when conducting medication use reviews. They should also ensure that they communicate any relevant information to the prescribing doctor and any other relevant healthcare professionals, so that a therapeutic plan can be discussed and agreed which meets the patient's clinical and other needs in the best (and most affordable) way.

Conclusion

Cost sharing for medicines is a mechanism used in many healthcare systems with the aim of deterring unnecessary demand and thus containing healthcare and drug expenditure. Drug use is indeed reduced when cost sharing is implemented, but essential as well as less essential medicines are affected. This can have a negative impact on health outcomes, requiring additional healthcare services and treatment, leading to increased resource use.

Certain groups of patients are particularly susceptible or vulnerable to the negative impact of cost sharing, namely the elderly, people who take regular medication for chronic conditions and people on low incomes. These are, in effect, people who may experience problems affording prescribed medication, either due to regular and thus relatively large expenses for (sometimes multiple) chronic conditions or simply because they only have a limited income and thus limited resources available for payment. Many countries therefore have protective mechanisms in place which provide exemption or reduced payments. Caps and complementary insurance may also be available. The criteria that are used for such protection are usually based on clinical condition and/or need, income and age, thus aiming to protect those identified as most vulnerable.

Patients use many strategies to keep medication cost to a minimum. Some are appropriate but others jeopardize treatment with essential medicines where adherence is crucial to achieve the desired health benefit. Patients commonly do not communicate issues of cost and affordability, or the strategies they use to cope with cost sharing, to their doctors. They are, however, more likely to raise these issues in community pharmacies as the places where money is exchanged when getting prescribed medication dispensed. This provides pharmacists and their staff with the important opportunity to explore cost issues and inform patients about the importance of adherence to essential medicines. They can also advise patients about options for managing cost sharing, such as exemptions and complementary insurance or PPCs. Pharmacists can also liaise with physicians and other healthcare professionals to inform and thus facilitate a jointly agreed treatment plan that takes account of cost sharing and affordability as much as possible.

KEY POINTS

- There are different types of cost sharing systems: flat fee prescription charges; proportional co-payments (co-insurance); and deductibles
- These systems are in place to deter unnecessary demand and thus avoid waste
- Many cost sharing programmes have protection mechanisms in place for vulnerable groups (elderly, chronically ill, low incomes)
- Medication cost sharing reduces drug consumption
- The reduction in drug use in response to cost sharing is more pronounced for less essential medicines than essential ones
- Patients use a variety of strategies to cope with medication costs, and these depend on the types of cost sharing within their country
- Healthcare professionals, including physicians and pharmacists, can advise on the importance of adherence and help with medication cost

7

WHO and the essential medicines concept

Marthe M. Everard

STUDY POINTS

- Core functions of WHO
- Model List of Essential Medicines based on the essential medicines concept
- Description of essential medicines
- Need for essential medicines for children

Introduction

The 20th century witnessed revolutionary progress in improving human health, leading to dramatic declines in mortality and equally dramatic increases in life expectancy. Income growth, higher educational levels, improved sanitation and better food all contributed to this progress. The development of pharmaceuticals, particularly essential medicines, also played an important role (WHO 1999).

The work of the world's leading international public health agency, the World Health Organization (WHO), covers numerous health-related technical areas, supporting its overall objective of 'the attainment by all peoples of the highest level of health'. Much has been achieved in the pharmaceutical sector since the essential medicines concept was introduced in 1975 and the first Model List of Essential Medicines was launched in 1977. Today, three out of four countries in the world have national essential medicines lists as the basis for public procurement, reimbursement schemes, training, supervision and patient information (WHO 2004a). More importantly, in 1977 less than half the world's population had regular access to essential medicines. Today, through a combination of public and private health systems, nearly two-thirds of the world's population is estimated to

have access to effective treatments essential for their health needs (WHO 2004a). Essential medicines are one of the most cost-effective elements in modern health care.

The World Health Organization

Established in 1948, WHO is a specialized agency of the United Nations system. It is the technical and professional body concerned with international public health issues. When WHO was endorsed on 7 April 1948 by the United Nations it had fewer than 60 member states; in 2007, it had 193 (WHO 2007a). Its definition of health and its overall objective are provided in Box 7.1 (WHO 2007b).

WHO can offer a range of opportunities for cooperating with its member states, with its headquarters in Geneva, Switzerland, dealing with global issues, and its six regional offices focusing on technical support and national capacity building. The organization's presence in 147 countries allows a close relationship with ministries of health (WHO 2007a). WHO was in official relations with almost 190 non-governmental and voluntary organizations involved in health promotion and healthcare provision in 2006 (WHO 2007a). It also collaborates closely with the other agencies of the United Nations system in health-related activities (WHO 2007a). Increasingly, WHO plays a leading role in various public health-related initiatives, the so-called public–private partnerships, which should be seen as public sector programmes with private or commercial sector participation (WHO 2008).

WHO continues to promote the efforts of international health cooperation that was initiated by the first

Box 7.1

The WHO definition of health

WHO's constitution describes health as: 'a state of complete physical, mental and social well-being and not merely the absence of disease or infirmity'. Its overall objective is: 'the attainment by all peoples of the highest possible level of health'.

International Sanitary Conference in Paris in 1851, when nations joined forces to combat common health threats such as plague, yellow fever, cholera, leprosy, tuberculosis, smallpox and typhus. Some of these diseases still exist today, though smallpox has been eradicated and other diseases are in the process of being eliminated, for example polio, measles and leprosy (WHO 2007c).

In 1897, aspirin was introduced as the first synthetic pharmaceutical product. The 20th century saw the discovery and further development of pharmaceutical products, such as the introduction of penicillin (1928), the measles vaccine (1943), streptomycin, the first antitubercular drug (1945) and chloroquine, the first antimalarial drug (1946). In the 1950s the first clinical uses of oral contraceptives and of medicines for diabetes and mental illness were introduced, and later medicines for other infectious and cardiovascular diseases (WHO 2007c).

Also in the 20th century, there were significant gains in life expectancy of 20–40 years worldwide. This was mainly due to declining infant and child mortality rates, maternal mortality rates and fertility rates, a drastic reduction in the disease burden of infectious diseases caused by effective preventive actions and improved treatment. In addition, general sanitation measures and immunization programmes were implemented. These achievements were the results of dedicated international health efforts (WHO 1999, 2007c).

Despite these successes, the current situation indicates that not all people have benefited equally from improvements in health status and access to healthcare services. It is estimated that more than 1 billion people are still excluded from adequate health care (WHO 1999). Low income countries face ill health, mainly through communicable diseases, due to poverty-related conditions such as inadequate food, water and sanitation, housing, education and health services. The emergence of the HIV epidemic, the resurgence of tuberculosis and malaria, and tobacco-related diseases are also

factors. In high income countries ill health, mainly through non-communicable diseases, results mainly from excessive eating, drinking and smoking, using and abusing narcotic medicines, and from environmental pollution and urbanization (WHO 1999).

Based on the experience of containing severe acute respiratory syndrome (SARS) and the threat of an avian flu outbreak worldwide, WHO is reinforcing its lead role in limiting the international spread of epidemics and other public health emergencies. The organization has to consider this diversity of health challenges in order to develop strategies and programmes to meet the health needs of its member states (WHO 2007c).

WHO fulfils its objectives through its core functions which underpin the global health agenda set out in a framework for an organization-wide programme of work, and is linked to the achievement of the millennium development goals. WHO's six core functions can be divided into normative work and technical cooperation and are listed below (WHO 2007d):

- Providing leadership on matters critical to health and engaging in partnerships where joint action is needed
- Shaping the research agenda and stimulating the generation, translation and dissemination of valuable knowledge
- Setting norms and standards and promoting and monitoring their implementation
- Articulating ethical and evidence-based policy options
- Providing technical support, catalysing change and building sustainable institutional capacity
- Monitoring the health situation and assessing health trends.

The global health agenda is a guide for all stakeholders, not for WHO alone, and it outlines seven priority areas. The first three areas are closely related to health: investing in health to reduce poverty; building individual and global health security; and promoting universal coverage, gender equality and health-related human rights. The other four areas focus on specific tasks such as: tackling the determinants of health; strengthening health systems and equitable access; harnessing knowledge, science and technology; and strengthening governance, leadership and accountability (WHO 2007d).

Many countries rely on WHO norms and standards, including quality assurance, especially for biological, pharmaceutical and diagnostic products. WHO will continue to encourage efforts, including those of industry, to develop new and affordable biological, pharmaceutical and diagnostic products. WHO has expanded its global normative work after the adoption by its member states of the WHO Framework Convention for Tobacco Control and the revised International Health Regulations in 2005 and through the establishment of its commissions on macroeconomics and health (2002), intellectual property rights, innovation and public health (2003), and the social determinants of health (2005) (WHO 2007d).

WHO's work in essential medicines

The departments of Medicines Policy and Standards (PSM) and Technical Cooperation for Essential Drugs and Traditional Medicine (TCM) are central to WHO's goal in medicines to help save lives and improve health by ensuring the quality, efficacy, safety and rational use of medicines, including traditional medicines, and by promoting equitable and sustainable access to essential medicines, particularly for the poor and disadvantaged (WHO 2004a). Essential medicines are one of the most cost-effective elements in modern health care and their potential health and economic impact is considerable in terms of saving lives, reducing suffering, and protecting, maintaining and restoring health.

Besides norm and standard setting for essential medicines, WHO provides guidance on regulatory standards, defines international non-proprietary names, provides therapeutic advice, such as standard treatment guidelines, and produces a Model List of Essential Medicines and a Model Formulary. Technical assistance to member states is also provided on the development and implementation of their national medicines policies. A national medicines policy is a commitment to a goal and a guide for action, providing a framework in which the national goals, objectives and priorities are formulated for both the public and private pharmaceutical sectors. It identifies strategies needed to achieve these objectives (WHO 2004a).

The essential medicines concept

During the 1970s a growing number of low-income countries had more than 20 000 different brands of pharmaceutical products circulating in their markets. This situation was similar to that in high-income countries, despite the differences in their prevailing common diseases and their socio-economic positions. Also, pharmaceutical products were promoted and marketed with little concern for the different health needs and priorities of individual countries (WHO 2006a).

In the mid 1970s some governments of low-income countries (Costa Rica, Cuba and Sri Lanka) started to realize that if medicines were to meet the real health needs of the majority of their populations and be equally available to all, then criteria had to be set, especially for selection of medicines. The concept of essential medicines was born. This concept proved to have a positive impact on drug procurement, distribution, use and prices as well (WHO 2006a).

The concept of essential medicines is forward looking (Quick 1997). It incorporates the need to:

- Regularly update medicines selections to reflect new therapeutic options and changing therapeutic needs
- Ensure drug quality
- Continue to develop better medicines, medicines for emerging diseases and medicines to meet changing resistance patterns.

The concept of essential medicines encourages health systems to focus on access to those medicines that represent the best balance of quality, safety, efficacy and cost to meet the priority health needs within a given healthcare setting. The implementation of the concept of essential medicines is intended to be flexible and adaptable to many different situations; exactly which medicines are regarded as essential remains a national responsibility (Quick 1997).

The Model List of Essential Medicines

In 1977, inspired by the essential medicines concept, a WHO expert committee discussed the question of how many medicines were really needed to treat common health problems. It concluded that approximately 208 individual medicines and vaccines could be considered essential and together could provide safe, effective treatment for the majority of communicable and non-communicable diseases. Moreover, the majority of drug products were off patent and could be produced at relatively low cost (WHO 2006b). In the same year, the first Model List of Essential Drugs was published by WHO and has since been updated every

2 years. It was met with a mixture of surprise, opposition and enthusiasm by the medical and pharmaceutical establishment and created a revolution in international public health (Quick 1997).

Essential medicines are defined as those medicines that satisfy the priority healthcare needs of the population. Essential medicines are selected with due regard to disease prevalence, evidence on efficacy and safety, and comparative cost-effectiveness. Essential medicines are intended to be available within the context of functioning health systems at all times in adequate amounts, in the appropriate dosage forms, with assured quality, and at a price the individual and the community can afford.

The WHO Model List is a guide for the development of national and institutional essential medicine lists. It was not designed as a global attempt to establish a uniform medicines list, as this is neither feasible nor realistic. However, for the past 30 years the Model List has led to a global acceptance of the concept of essential medicines as a powerful means to promote health equity. By the end of 2003, 156 member states had official essential medicines lists, of which 99 had been updated in the previous 5 years. Most countries have national lists and some have provincial or state lists as well. National lists of essential medicines usually relate closely to national guidelines for clinical healthcare practice. Therefore, they can be used as decision-making tools for drug procurement in the public sector, for schemes that reimburse medicine costs, for medicine donations and local medicine production. Moreover, they can be used as educational tools for the training and supervision of health workers and used as informational tools for consumers (Quick 1997; Fig. 7.1). National lists should reflect the national priorities in medication needs. This does not imply that no other medicines are useful, but simply that in a given context those medicines selected are the ones most needed for the national health services. They should, therefore, be available at all times in adequate amounts and in the proper dosage forms (Quick 1997). Access to essential medicines of assured quality is fundamental for the optimal performance of a healthcare system. Uninterrupted supplies of essential medicines to a great extent determine the credibility of health services (Quick 1997).

Many international organizations, including UNICEF, UNHCR and UNFPA as well as non-governmental organizations and international non-profit medicine supply agencies, have adopted the essential medicines concept and base their medicine supply lists largely on the WHO Model List (Quick 1997).

In 1999, the WHO Expert Committee on the Use of Essential Medicines reviewed the procedures for updating the Model List. They recommended to WHO that the process of developing the list should be seen as an example of a model drug evaluation procedure for national drug and therapeutics committees (Quick 1997). It should be a systematic and transparent process. In addition, the methods for updating the Model List should be revised because selection of medicines should be evidence based rather than consensus based, should have a clearer link between essential medicines and guidelines for clinical health care, and should consider the high cost of many new and effective medicines. At the beginning of 2002, the Model List was revised by the expert committee, applying the new procedure (Quick 1997).

Updated selection criteria

The updated criteria for the selection of essential medicines are based on several factors, including public health relevance and the availability of data on the efficacy, safety and comparative cost-effectiveness of available treatments. Most essential medicines should be formulated as single compounds. Fixed-dose combination products are selected only when the combination has a proven advantage in therapeutic effect, safety or compliance over single compounds administered separately. When making cost comparisons between medicines, the cost of the total treatment, not only the unit cost of the medicine, is considered. Factors such as stability in various climatic conditions, the need for special diagnostic or treatment facilities and pharmacokinetic properties are also considered if appropriate.

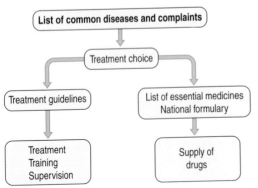

Figure 7.1 • Relationship between treatment guidelines and a list of essential medicines (WHO 2002).

When adequate scientific evidence is not available on current treatment of a priority disease, the expert committee may either defer the issue until more evidence becomes available, or choose to make recommendations based on expert opinion and experience. Cost and cost-effectiveness comparisons may be made among alternative treatments within the same therapeutic group (Quick 1997; see also Ch. 19).

In adapting the Model List to their own needs, countries often consider factors such as local demography and the pattern of prevalent diseases; treatment facilities; training and experience of available personnel; local availability of individual pharmaceutical products; financial resources; and environmental factors.

In March 2007, the 15th Model List of Essential Medicines was prepared by the WHO expert committee. This Model List contains 346 individual medicines for the treatment of infectious and chronic diseases which affect populations worldwide (WHO 2007e). Over the last 30 years, 199 (2005) new medicines were added to and 99 (2005) medicines deleted from the Model List.

The Model List has a 'core' list indicating the minimum drug needs for a basic healthcare system and a 'complementary' list including mainly essential medicines for priority diseases which may be cost-effective but not necessarily affordable (Quick 1997). The Model List reflects a model product, developed through a model process, and both models can be used for advocacy purposes (Quick 1997).

The WHO Model Formulary

In 1995, the WHO expert committee recommended that WHO should develop a Model Formulary which would complement the WHO Model List. It would provide independent information on essential medicines for pharmaceutical policy makers and prescribers worldwide. A Model Formulary would be a useful resource for countries wishing to develop their own national formulary.

The first edition of the Model Formulary was launched in 2002 based on the 12th Model List. The electronic version of the Model Formulary is intended as a starting point for developing national or institutional formularies by adapting the text of the Model Formulary for their own national list of essential medicines. A third edition of the Model Formulary will be based on the 15th Model List (2007) and will be available in 2008 (WHO 2004b).

The need for essential medicines for children

Over thirty years ago, in 1977, the first Model List of Essential Drugs was launched. This list defined medicines that satisfy the priority healthcare needs of the population, but until now the Model List has not included many medicines specifically for children. Every year there are over 40 million deaths in developing countries and over 10 million among children under 5 years of age (WHO 2005). The six main causes of death are pneumonia, diarrhoea, malaria, preterm birth, asphyxia and pneumonia/sepsis in newborn babies and these account for 73% of all deaths in the under fives. In addition, AIDS claims over 300 000 deaths in children under 15 years annually. Under-nutrition is a contributing cause of death in over 60% of diarrhoea cases, 57% of malaria cases and 52% of pneumonia cases (WHO 2005).

For all these conditions, essential medicines are available and are life saving. However, access to safe, effective and affordable essential medicines for children ('paediatric formulations') remains a problem. In particular, the HIV pandemic has highlighted the urgent need for adequate formulations for children as well as for acute infectious diseases, where medicines are either not available on the market or not financially or geographically accessible (WHO 2007f).

Studies of current practice worldwide revealed that healthcare workers estimate the dose of medicines by assuming that children are small adults, which is physiologically incorrect. They often dispense medicines to small children by using fractions of adult dosage forms such as half or quarter tablets, or by crushing tablets or opening capsules – both meant for adults. These strategies are not recommended and can result in either under- or overdosing, with potential efficacy and safety problems. Even if formulations for children are available, many healthcare workers may not know how to prescribe these medicines appropriately (WHO 2007f).

In May 2007, the World Health Assembly endorsed the WHO resolution on 'Better Medicines for Children', including the development of a Model List of Essential Medicines for Children (WHO 2007f). Therefore, WHO updated their Model List of Essential Medicines to include essential medicines for children, based on their clinical needs and the burden of disease. This resulted in the publication of the first Essential Medicines List for Children in July 2007. Based on this list, WHO will identify the appropriate dosage forms and strengths of medicines for children, develop and promote quality standards and support mechanisms for licensing of children's essential medicines by drug regulatory authorities. WHO will, in partnership with UNICEF, encourage manufacturers to develop appropriate medicines at affordable prices.

In view of the need to achieve the millennium development goals on the reduction of malnutrition and child and maternal mortality, and the focus of the director-general of WHO on improving health in Africa (WHO 2007a), developing a Model List of Essential Medicines for Children will become a powerful tool for reducing infant and child mortality.

Given that in 2007 it was 30 years since the first essential medicines list was published, this was also an opportunity for WHO to promote the essential medicines concept and WHO is looking to the future by creating a Model List of Essential Medicines for Children.

Conclusion

Over the years, the essential medicines concept has become a global concept and is a powerful tool to promote health equity. Although originally intended for low-income countries, an increasing number of high-income countries also use its key components. Health systems, from basic health systems in the poorest countries to highly developed national health insurance schemes in the industrialized countries, have recognized both its therapeutic and its economic benefits. This recognition has been triggered by the introduction of many new and often expensive drug therapies, increasing drug costs and by observed quality variations in healthcare provision (Quick 1997).

The essential medicines concept is now widely accepted as a highly pragmatic approach to providing the best of modern evidence-based and cost-effective health services. It is as valid today as it was when first introduced in 1975. The concept does not exclude all other medicines but focuses on those medicines that have the best balance of quality, safety, efficacy and cost for a given health service (Quick 1997). Moreover, the concept is forward looking. It stimulates research and development for better pharmaceutical formulations and for more efficient responses to new or re-emerging diseases. It has also been adopted by international and bilateral aid agencies and by non-governmental

organizations that include strategies on rational drug selection, supply and use in their programmes of work (Quick 1997).

In its present form, the Model List aims to identify cost-effective medicines for priority conditions, together with the reasons for their inclusion, linked to evidence-based clinical guidelines and with special emphasis on public health aspects and considerations of value for money. Information that supports the selection of essential medicines, such as relevant WHO clinical guidelines, systematic reviews, key references and indicative cost information, is being made available via the WHO website. The Model List's primary function is to facilitate the work of national and institutional committees in developing national and institutional lists of essential medicines.

Moreover, the list has also resulted in greater international coordination in healthcare development and in health emergency situations (Quick 1997). Linked to the Model List, the WHO Model Formulary provides independent information on essential medicines for pharmaceutical policy makers and prescribers worldwide. It is also a useful resource for countries wishing to develop their own national formulary (WHO 2004b).

Millions of children die each year because they do not have access to medicines that are child-specific. Access to safe, effective and affordable essential medicines for children is a global problem (WHO 2007f). There is an urgent need for adequate formulations in acute and chronic care and treatment of children. Medicines for children do not exist or are not available on the local market, or are unaffordable.

The WHO World Health Assembly resolution on 'Better Medicines for Children' supports the development of a Model List of Essential Medicines for Children which will identify the gaps in the range of medicines and formulations specifically for children (WHO 2007f).

KEY POINTS

- WHO was founded in 1948 and has 193 member states (2007)
- Health is described as 'a state of complete physical, mental and social well-being and not merely the absence of disease or infirmity'
- The essential medicines concept was launched in 1975, and encourages health systems to focus on access to those medicines that represent the best balance of quality, safety, efficacy and cost to meet the priority health needs within a given healthcare setting

- The first Model List of Essential Medicines was published by WHO in 1977 and included 208 individual medicines
- The 15th Model List, updated in 2007, consists of 346 essential medicines divided into a 'core' and 'complementary' list
- The Model List reflects a model product and a model process, which can both be used for advocacy
- A new Model List of Essential Medicines for Children will guide the need for new and improved formulations for children

Section Two

Governance and Good Professional Pharmaceutical Practice

Clinical governance – an overview

Simon J. Tweddell

STUDY POINTS

- Clinical governance, what it is and why it is necessary
- The use of standards for delivering quality services
- The role of clinical governance in modern day pharmacy
- Regulation of pharmacists
- How to deal with errors made by pharmacists

Introduction

Clinical governance is defined by the Department of Health as 'the system through which NHS organisations are accountable for continuously improving the quality of their services and safeguarding high standards of care, by creating an environment in which clinical excellence will flourish'.

Clinical governance

Why is clinical governance necessary?

Clinical governance was introduced following a series of well publicized lapses in patient quality in the 1990s as part of a broader government agenda to improve the quality of care delivered to patients by the NHS. It is a set of processes that healthcare professionals are expected to work with in order to learn from the successes and failures of both their own practice and those of others and to promote an open culture where experiences are shared to promote best practice for their patients.

When was clinical governance introduced?

The NHS document *A First Class Service: Quality in the New NHS* (Department of Health 1998) introduced the term 'clinical governance' stating that 'for the first time, the NHS will be required to adopt a structured and coherent approach to clinical quality, placing duties and expectations on local healthcare organisations as well as individuals. Effective clinical governance will make it clear that quality is everybody's business'.

What is clinical governance?

The NHS publication *Clinical Governance: Quality in the NHS* (1999) outlines four main components of clinical governance. These are:

- Clear lines of responsibility and accountability for the overall quality of clinical care
- A comprehensive programme of quality improvement activities
- Clear policies aimed at managing risks
- Procedures for all professional groups to identify and remedy poor performance.

The publication also provides examples of quality improvement activities, including:

- Audit programmes (see Ch. 11)
- Ensuring evidence-based practice (see Ch. 17)

- Implementation of clinical standards
- Continuing professional development
- Monitoring of clinical care and high-quality record keeping (see Chs 15 and 47)
- Research and development to promote 'an evaluation culture'.

Clinical governance should underpin the practice of all healthcare professionals as they strive for the best quality of care for their patients and continually seek improvement in their practice. Practising good clinical governance ensures a consistent approach to decision making, minimizes risk and ensures that patients are the priority and focus of the professional practice of pharmacists and all other healthcare professionals.

Quality

Standards for quality

Standards are set by clinical guidelines such as the National Service Frameworks (NSFs). These are documents that aim to guide decisions in a specific area of health care, as defined by an authoritative examination of current evidence. Decisions to prescribe medicines should be evidence based. Evidence-based medicine is defined as the use of clinical methods and decision making that have been thoroughly tested by properly controlled, peer-reviewed medical research.

Delivering quality

Quality health care should be delivered by well trained and motivated healthcare professionals who are well managed and are committed to self-development through continuing professional development (CPD; see Ch. 10). NHS staff should communicate openly with other healthcare professionals and should be encouraged to share best practice. Errors, service failures or 'near misses' should be recorded, reflected upon and shared among others so they are not repeated and a 'no-blame' culture should be adopted for mistakes. NHS staff should be regularly appraised on their performance and poor performance identified and remedied. The NHS document *Organisation with a Memory* (Department of Health 2000) requires that mechanisms are introduced for ensuring that, where lessons are identified, the necessary changes are put into practice and a wider appreciation of the value of preventing, analysing and learning from errors becomes the norm.

Monitoring quality

Quality of care should be monitored through a process of clinical audits, clear policies aimed at managing risks and involvement of patients and the public in an open and transparent health service.

The audit cycle could include the following:

- Decide criteria for ideal/best practice
- Measure current practice
- Feedback findings and set locally agreed targets
- Implement change to move from current practice to ideal
- Re-audit practice after changes in place and provide feedback to those involved
- Repeat audit cycle until practice meets agreed targets.

Clinical governance and pharmacy

The NHS document *Clinical Governance in Community Pharmacy* (Department of Health 2001) first introduced clinical governance into community pharmacy, although it was not part of the contract at that time. Clinical governance facilitators were introduced at a local level, whose role was to inform and educate community pharmacists on the primary care organizations' policies for good clinical governance. The new contract for community pharmacists was launched in April 2005 with the inclusion of clinical governance as an essential component of the terms of service. The new contract requirements on clinical governance include the following areas:

- Patient and public involvement
- Clinical audit
- Risk management including the implementation of standard operating procedures (SOPs)
- Clinical effectiveness programmes, e.g. practising evidence-based pharmaceutical care
- Staffing and staff management
- Education, training and CPD
- Use of information, for example storing patient information confidentially.

Professional governance

Professional governance in the pharmacy profession forms part of clinical governance, the aim of which is to:

- Ensure that pharmacists work to accepted standards of personal and professional conduct, put their patients' needs before their own and behave with integrity and probity.

Professional governance in pharmacy could be defined as:

- The process by which the pharmacy profession works with its members to ensure that patients receive an optimal standard of pharmaceutical care and maintains confidence in the profession.

Duty of care

Pharmacists have a duty of care to the public and their patients imposed by law to ensure that the public is protected. The law would expect that pharmacists practise pharmacy to a level of competence expected by the profession and indeed practised by the average pharmacist. Pharmacists are expected to exercise reasonable care when supplying the public and patients with medicines and pharmaceutical and other professional advice. In their practice, pharmacists are subject to criminal law (e.g. Medicines Act, Misuse of Drugs Act), administrative law (e.g. contractual agreements with the primary care organizations), civil law and the Code of Ethics of the Royal Pharmaceutical Society of Great Britain (RPSGB).

Mistakes or errors do happen. However, the vast majority of these are relatively minor and are usually quickly and easily rectified without concern. Unless a pharmacist causes deliberate harm to a patient it is unlikely that he or she would be subject to criminal charges; however, this is a possibility. In fact, a pharmacist and pre-registration trainee were initially charged with manslaughter following the incorrect dispensing of a supply of peppermint water that caused the death of a 3-week-old baby in 1998. The charge of manslaughter was later dropped in favour of prosecution under the Medicines Act instead.

Negligence

If the mistake by a pharmacist does lead to resulting damages then a more likely charge of negligence may be pursued in a civil court. For a breach in a duty of care to be proven then the prosecution must prove that a duty of care exists, that this duty of care has been breached and that the patient has suffered damages resulting from the breach. Often an expert witness from the pharmacy profession would be called to explain how a 'standard' or 'normal' member of the profession would have acted in this case.

The Code of Ethics

Pharmacists are also subject to the RPSGB Code of Ethics (see later) and should a pharmacist act in a manner that falls below the standards expected of members of the profession, then he or she may be subject to internal investigations conducted by the RPSGB.

Professional governance and regulation procedures in pharmacy

You may remember that one of the key components of clinical governance is that there must be 'Procedures for all professional groups to identify and remedy poor performance'. This role in the governance of the professional is vital to ensure that patients are protected and confidence in the profession is maintained. This role currently falls within the remit of the RPSGB; however, by 2010, parliamentary time permitting, this role will be undertaken by a new regulatory body for pharmacists and pharmacy technicians. The new independent General Pharmaceutical Council (GPhC) was proposed in the government White Paper entitled Trust, Assurance and Safety and will be approved in 2009 ready to take on the substantive functions of the GPhC in 2010. It is proposed that the GPhC will:

- Set standards for pre-registration and post-registration education and training
- Set standards for the conduct and ethics expected of registrants
- Set standards for practice and performance
- Set standards for the content and frequency of monitoring of CPD
- Approve courses, institutions and qualifications
- Maintain registers of pharmacists, pharmacy technicians and premises

- Determine initial fitness to practise of potential registrants
- Investigate impaired fitness to practise and adjudicate fitness to practise cases.

To complicate matters in the meantime, the RPSGB has had to implement new fitness to practise committees in 2007 following the publication of the Pharmacists and Pharmacy Technicians Order 2007. The order came into force on 7 February 2007 and new fitness to practise rules came into force on 30 March 2007 (see later). The order established three new statutory committees:

- Investigating Committee (replaces Infringements Committee)
- Health Committee (new committee)
- Disciplinary Committee (replaces Statutory Committee).

Under the old rules the RPSGB was only able to consider allegations of misconduct and had limited sanctions available to it. Under the new scheme the RPSGB is able to consider a wider range of allegations including those relating to a registrant's health, and has a number of new sanctions including imposing conditions on registration and suspensions from the registers of up to 1 year, as well as the power to direct removal of the registrant's name from the appropriate registers.

Investigating Committee

The Investigating Committee receives an 'allegation' and determines in the first instance whether that allegation should be referred to either the Disciplinary Committee or the Health Committee. If referral is unnecessary then it may issue:

- A warning or advice to the person concerned in connection with any matter arising out of or related to the allegation
- Advice to any other person or other body involved in its investigation of the allegation on any matter arising out of or related to the allegation.

Health Committee

The Health Committee determines whether or not the fitness to practise of the person of whom the allegation is made is impaired based on the health of the person. If the committee finds that fitness to practise is impaired it may:

- Issue a warning to the person concerned and advice to any other person or other body involved in its investigation of the allegation
- Give a direction that the person's registration shall be suspended for a period not exceeding 12 months
- Give a direction that the person's registration shall be conditional upon compliance with specified requirements that the committee thinks fit to impose for the protection of the public or in the person's own interests.

Disciplinary Committee

The Disciplinary Committee determines whether or not the fitness to practise of the person of whom the allegation is made is impaired based on allegations that are not normally health related. If the committee finds that fitness to practise is impaired it may:

- Issue a warning to the person concerned and advice to any other person or other body involved in its investigation of the allegation
- Give a direction that the person concerned be removed from the register
- Give a direction that the person's registration shall be suspended for a period not exceeding 12 months
- Give a direction that the person's registration shall be conditional upon compliance with specified requirements that the committee thinks fit to impose for the protection of the public or in the person's own interests.

When things go wrong

Pharmacists are only human and, despite best intentions and safeguards, mistakes do happen. It is how mistakes are dealt with and whether or not lessons are learned from them that will normally determine whether incidents are referred for further investigation.

When a dispensing error occurs the pharmacist is ideally placed to determine the potential risk to the patient. When dealing with dispensing or prescribing mistakes it is vital that pharmacists place the welfare of the patient first and seek immediate medical attention if necessary. An investigating committee would take a very dim view of pharmacists covering up a mistake, not assessing the risk of a mistake to the health of a patient or repeated mistakes where they have clearly not taken remedial action in preventing errors from recurring.

Dealing with errors

While this is not a comprehensive checklist it may be helpful to consider the following when an error occurs:

- Is there any risk to the welfare of the patient? If yes refer to GP/Accident and Emergency, phoning ahead if necessary
- Who do I need to inform? e.g. patient's GP, superintendent pharmacist, family member of patient, RPSGB inspector, primary care trust (PCT) personnel. It is better for you to proactively raise the error with these stakeholders rather than them to hear of it from the patient, patient's solicitor, etc.
- How did the mistake happen?
- Could I have prevented it from occurring?
- Document what happened in your medication error log and describe all steps taken to remedy the error
- Review procedures in light of your own internal investigation/self-reflection.

Preventing mistakes

- Ensure SOPs for the supply of medicines are in place and regularly used, evaluated and reviewed
- Ensure that one person is not the sole dispenser and checker of the supply of medicines
- Ensure that medicines with similar sounding names or with similar company livery are not placed next to each other
- Separate different strengths of medicines from one another by placing another medicine between the two different strengths.

Medication error logs

When a medication error does occur it is seen as good practice to record the error in a medication error log. Pharmacists should maintain such a log as part of practising good clinical governance and its use should form part of the SOP for dispensing. In March 2007 the council of the RPSGB agreed the criteria for which single dispensing errors are likely to amount to misconduct and would warrant referral to the Investigating Committee (Box 8.1). The criteria for referral include both the lack of systems to record errors in the pharmacy and the failure to make an error log if the pharmacist was aware that

one had occurred. The RPSGB inspectorate may, as part of the routine visits to a pharmacy, ask to see evidence that a system is in place to deal with dispensing errors, including the maintenance and use of medication error logs. Inspectors will not normally ask to view the actual logs unless investigating a specific complaint relating to a dispensing error, and may then request to see that specific medication error log. The RPSGB has also stated that it may be

Box 8.1

Criteria for consideration of single dispensing errors

Single dispensing errors are not likely to be referred to the Investigating Committee unless one or more of the following statements is true:

- There is potential for, or evidence that, the dispensing error caused moderate or severe harm or death (the definitions of these are from the National Patient Safety Agency (NPSA) definitions for grading patient safety incidents – see Box 8.2)
- There is evidence that the dispensing error was a deliberate attempt to cause harm to patients or the public
- There is evidence of ill health or substance abuse by the pharmacist
- There is evidence that the individual departed from agreed safe protocols or SOPs and in doing so took an unacceptable risk
- There are no systems to record errors in the pharmacy (this should result in the superintendent/pharmacy owner being referred)
- There has been a failure to make an error log (if aware of the error)
- There are no systems to learn from errors in the pharmacy (this should result in the superintendent/pharmacy owner being referred)
- No attempt has been made to learn from the specific error
- The society's inspector has previously given advice that would have prevented the error if it had been implemented
- There has been an attempt to cover up the alleged dispensing error
- There has been a failure to cooperate with an investigation carried out by the society's inspector or other investigatory body
- There is evidence of other misconduct that would form the basis of a complaint
- Failure to apologize/provide an explanation to the patient/representative (if aware of the error)
- There is relevant history within the past 3 years

particularly helpful if the error log describes any review of systems carried out at the pharmacy in light of the incident. If there are concerns regarding a pharmacist's fitness to practise then it may be that the entire medication error log may be examined, particularly if there was a concern for public safety.

NPSA definitions for grading patient safety incidents are shown in Box 8.2. See also Examples 8.1 and 8.2.

Box 8.2

NPSA definitions for grading patient safety incidents

- No harm
  Incident prevented – any patient safety incident that had the potential to cause harm but was prevented, and no harm was caused to patients receiving NHS-funded care. Incident not prevented – any patient safety incident that occurred but no harm was caused to patients receiving NHS-funded care
- Low harm
  Any patient safety incident that required extra observation or minor treatment and caused minimal harm to one or more patients receiving NHS-funded care. (Minor treatment is defined as first aid, additional therapy or additional medication. It does not include any extra stay in hospital or any extra time as an outpatient, or continued treatment over and above the treatment already planned; nor does it include a return to surgery or readmission)
- Moderate harm
  Any patient safety incident that resulted in a moderate increase in treatment and that caused significant but not permanent harm to one or more patients receiving NHS-funded care. (Moderate increase in treatment is defined as a return to surgery, an unplanned readmission, a prolonged episode of care, extra time in hospital or as an outpatient, cancelling of treatment or transfer to another area such as intensive care as a result of the incident)

- Severe harm
  Any patient safety incident that appears to have resulted in permanent harm to one or more patients receiving NHS-funded care. (Permanent harm directly related to the incident and not related to the natural course of the patient's illness or underlying condition is defined as permanent lessening of bodily functions, sensory, motor, physiological or intellectual, including removal of the wrong limb or organ, or brain damage)
- Death
  Any patient safety incident that directly resulted in the death of one or more patients receiving NHS-funded care. (The death must be related to the incident rather than to the natural course of the patient's illness or underlying condition)

KEY POINTS

- Clinical governance was introduced to improve the quality of care to patients
- The four main components are: lines of responsibility, programme of quality improvement, risk management policies and remedying poor performance
- Standards are set by national service frameworks
- Errors or near misses should be recorded, reflected upon and shared with others
- Quality of care should be subject to clinical audit
- The 2005 contract for community pharmacists included clinical governance as a requirement
- During practice, pharmacists are subject to both criminal and administrative law
- Currently the RPSGB has three committees with responsibility in these areas – Investigating Committee, Health Committee and Disciplinary Committee
- A new General Pharmaceutical Council will take on the RPSGB role of governance
- Mistakes will happen – how they are dealt with and learned from is most important
- When an error is made, the welfare of the patient is paramount
- A medication error log should be used to record all lapses – and this should be part of a SOP

Example 8.1

You are a community pharmacist manager and you are asked to deal with a complaint from Mrs A.B. who claims she was supplied with the wrong medication for her mother yesterday. You establish that she was supplied with 28 amiodarone 100 mg tablets instead of 28 atenolol 100 mg tablets. What action should you take?

It is important to first of all establish whether or not the patient has taken any of the incorrect medication. If so, then you are best placed to use your knowledge of medicines to determine the risk to the patient. If there is any risk to the health of the patient then you must advise the patient to seek urgent medical attention. It may be necessary to telephone the A&E department in advance of the patient arriving to provide as many details as you can. It would also be good practice to telephone the patient's GP to inform them of the risk to the patient.

Mrs A.B. informs you that her mother did take one of the amiodarone tablets this morning.

You should advise her not to take any more and ask her to seek medical attention. You should then phone the

patient's GP to discuss the incident. The Code of Ethics for Pharmacists and Pharmacy Technicians requires you to 'make the care of patients your first concern'. Once you have taken all reasonable steps to assure the patient's health and safety have been considered then it is important to document the incident in the medication error log while it is fresh in your mind. If you are working for a company then you should inform the superintendent pharmacist and if appropriate you could also seek advice from the RPSGB inspectorate.

How should you reflect on this incident and prevent it or similar errors from reoccurring?

Pharmacists and other healthcare professionals are only human and accordingly dispensing and prescribing errors do happen. What is important is to learn from them and take action to prevent this or other similar errors from occurring. Good clinical governance involves auditing and reflecting on our own professional practice and when something goes wrong taking action to improve systems and minimize risk.

Example 8.2

You receive a letter from the PCT indicating that there is a member of the public purporting to be a medical practitioner who is contacting pharmacies in the area with a view to obtaining illegal supplies of prescription only medicines (POMs) and controlled drugs. What action should you take now and what should you do if you find that you have supplied him with a medicine illegally?

Practising good clinical governance is not just about preventing mistakes from recurring, it is about auditing our policies and SOPs to ensure they protect the public and are robust enough to allow for all eventualities, including preventing medicines getting on to the black market.
In this case you should ensure that your SOP requires that all personal requests for prescription only medicines and controlled drugs by persons purporting to be medical practitioners, whether in person or by telephone, are dealt with personally by the responsible pharmacist and all early warning letters such as these are made available to all pharmacists practising from your pharmacy. It is essential that all unknown doctors are authenticated and if necessary confirmation verified by a phone call to the

medical practice and if necessary the General Medical Council.

While reviewing your procedures with the pharmacy assistants, a member of staff indicates that a doctor visited the pharmacy last Saturday requesting the purchase of a number of medicines. She informs you that the relief pharmacist dealt with the requests. You check the POM register but find no record of the sale of POM medicines to a GP last Saturday. What should you do now?

You must act on this information and assure yourself that POMs were not supplied illegally from the pharmacy. Although you were not the responsible pharmacist last Saturday you would be as culpable as the pharmacist who was if you later found out that the public was put at risk and you did nothing about it.
You should contact the pharmacist in charge on that day to ascertain the facts. If POMs or controlled drugs (CDs) were sold to a member of the public who was purporting to be a doctor then you must inform the police, the PCT, the superintendent pharmacist and the RPSGB inspector. You should make a full record of the events that occurred and ask the relief pharmacist to do likewise.

9

Risk management

Darren M. Ashcroft

STUDY POINTS

- The use of human error models to understand the causes of patient safety incidents
- Risk management techniques that can be used to understand the 'root causes' of an incident
- Some of the common risks in the pharmacy setting
- The National Patient Safety Agency's 'Seven Steps to Patient Safety'
- A structured approach to undertaking risk assessment in the pharmacy

Introduction

Risk – the probability that an adverse event will occur – is a normal part of daily life. We all continuously face risks and make decisions about them. Each day we decide when it is safe to cross the road and when it is more sensible to wait; we may choose to travel by car rather than walk. In these everyday choices, we assess the potential risks and benefits, and select a plan of action. Risk management is all about this process of anticipating potential hazards and reducing the likelihood of a problem occurring. However, before thinking about how to minimize or eliminate the possibility of errors, it is important to first consider how errors occur.

Human error models

Human error can be considered in two ways: the person approach and the systems approach. Traditionally, the person approach has been the dominant approach used in health care. This focuses on the errors of individuals, blaming them for forgetfulness, inattention, carelessness, negligence or recklessness. It has been widely acknowledged that blaming individuals does not encourage reporting and learning from errors, and the development of an effective risk management culture within healthcare settings depends critically on establishing an open reporting culture.

During the past decade, there has been increased interest to understand how management practices and other workplace factors impact on patient safety. The systems approach acknowledges that humans are imperfect and errors are to be expected, even in the best organizations. Rather than focusing on the individual, the systems approach concentrates on the conditions under which individuals work, trying to build defences to avoid errors or to mitigate their effects. James Reason (2000) classified medical errors into two types, *active* and *latent* failures, where active failures are unsafe acts (for example dispensing the wrong drug) committed by individuals who are at the 'sharp end' of health care, while latent failures are more distant from the actual incident and reflect failures in management or other organizational factors.

Active failures

Active failures take a variety of forms, such as slips, lapses, mistakes and procedural violations, as shown in Figure 9.1.

Slips occur when there has been a lack of attention, despite the fact that the individual has all the necessary skills to complete the task successfully. Lapses involve memory failures, such as forgetting your

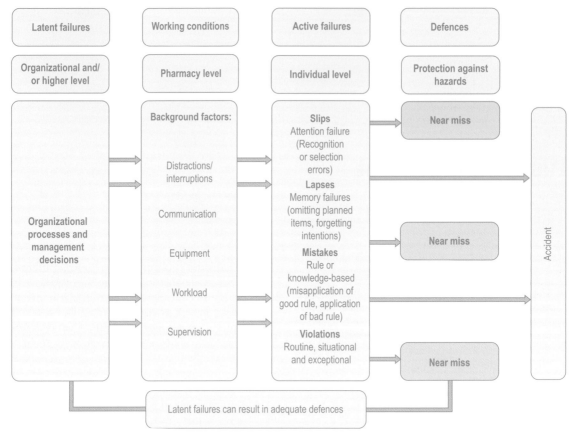

Figure 9.1 • Reason's (2000) four-stage model of human error theory.

intentions or omitting planned actions. In contrast, mistakes happen when we are in conscious control of the situation, but successfully execute the wrong plan of action. For instance, selecting the wrong plan can come about because of an incorrect assessment of the situation, such as arriving at the wrong diagnosis for an individual asking for an effective treatment for an 'upset stomach'.

Violations, on the other hand, involve deliberate deviations from the procedures or best way of performing a task, such as not following standard operating procedures (see Chs 7, 24 and 43) within the pharmacy. Several types of violations have been described; these are outlined in Box 9.1.

Each of these error types (slips, lapses, mistakes, violations) requires different strategies to be implemented to avoid similar events occurring in the future. Better system defences, such as redesigning the workplace, can help to minimize slips and lapses. Improved training and rigorous checking procedures can prevent some mistakes. Developing relevant procedures and protocols, ensuring effec-

tive implementation with the provision of the necessary resources and support are all important in promoting compliance and therefore avoiding procedural violations.

 Box 9.1

Types of procedural violations

Optimizing violations occur when skill and experience lead the individual to think that the rules do not apply to them

Routine violations occur when it becomes accepted practice to break a rule within the organization

Situational violations occur when the situation necessitates rule breaking, for example there are not enough staff or there is not enough time to carry out all the required checks

Exceptional violations arise when the rules that are in place are not able to deal with a novel situation

Latent failures

Latent failures are those whose adverse consequences may lie dormant, only becoming evident when they combine with other factors. These usually stem from poor decisions, made at a different time and place, by more senior members of the organization or people operating at a different level, such as the headquarters of a pharmacy chain. Latent failures have two kinds of adverse effect: they can lead to error and violation provoking conditions in the workplace (e.g. time pressures, understaffing, inadequate equipment, inexperience) or they can create weaknesses in the defences (e.g. unworkable procedures or design problems).

The investigation of many threats to patient safety has shown that there are usually multiple causes and they tend to occur when there is an unfortunate combination of active and latent failures. Reason (2000) proposed the 'Swiss cheese model'

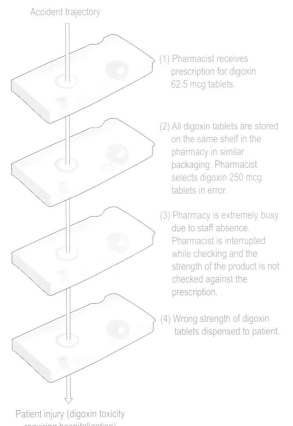

Accident trajectory

(1) Pharmacist receives prescription for digoxin 62.5 mcg tablets.

(2) All digoxin tablets are stored on the same shelf in the pharmacy in similar packaging. Pharmacist selects digoxin 250 mcg tablets in error.

(3) Pharmacy is extremely busy due to staff absence. Pharmacist is interrupted while checking and the strength of the product is not checked against the prescription.

(4) Wrong strength of digoxin tablets dispensed to patient.

Patient injury (digoxin toxicity requiring hospitalization)

Figure 9.2 • 'Swiss cheese' model showing how failures in the pharmacy can lead to patient harm.

to illustrate how accidents can occur within systems. This analogy compares the defensive layers of the system to layers of Swiss cheese, each having holes that represent safety failures. The presence of holes in one slice may not result in an accident because the other slices act as safeguards. However, the holes in the layers may temporarily line up, creating an opportunity for an accident. Figure 9.2 shows how multiple failures in the pharmacy setting can result in patient harm.

Risk management tools

There are a number of useful techniques that can be used to help understand the underlying causes of adverse events and help identify actions that can be put in place to avoid similar events occurring in the future. For instance, root cause analysis (RCA) provides a framework to reflect on an actual or potential error, working back across the sequence of events. RCA aims to uncover the underlying, contributory and causal factors that resulted in an error, and also understand better the protective factors that may have prevented harm from occurring. It is important to include all those involved in the incident in order clearly to map out the chronology of events. The analysis is then used to identify areas for change and possible solutions, to help minimize the reoccurrence of the event in the future. Various methods can be used for RCA including the use of a 'fishbone diagram' in which each of the 'bones' reflect different system failures, or the use of timelines where a chronological chain of events is mapped and tracked.

Failure modes and effects analysis (FMEA) is a systematic tool for evaluating a process and identifying where and how it might fail. It also assesses the relative impact of different types of failure and so prioritizes which areas need attention first. In addition, it can be used to assess the likelihood of the event reoccurring following changes to the system. The FMEA process involves:

- Mapping out the steps of the process through group discussion
- Identification of possible failure modes (what could go wrong?) by brainstorming
- For each error type or failure mode identified, a cause (why should failure happen?) and effect (what would be the consequences of each failure?) are attributed, together with scores for likelihood of occurrence, likelihood of detection and severity.

Multiplication of these three scores generates a risk priority number (RPN) which can be used to prioritize changes within the pharmacy.

Risk to patients in the pharmacy setting

It is increasingly recognized that risks within healthcare organizations, including pharmacies, are diverse and complex, and not just confined to specific activities. An accurate estimate of the extent and causes of adverse events that originate from the pharmacy is difficult to obtain since different methods have been used to collect the data.

Research has, however, suggested that in the UK, for every 10 000 prescription items dispensed in community pharmacies, there are likely to be at least 26 dispensing incidents. Most threats do not result in actual patient harm, but have the potential to do so. The most common types of events include incorrect product selection (60%) and labelling errors (33%). Organizational factors are associated with the majority of these errors including issues concerning distractions while assembling and checking prescriptions, poor communication, excessive workload and inadequate staffing.

Studies have also reported on practice variation in the way in which non-prescription medicines are sold and advice is communicated to patients in community pharmacies, suggesting that in some cases pharmacy services may be deficient or sub-optimal. Over the last decade, the Consumers' Association in the UK has repeatedly criticized deficiencies in the level of advice, questioning and referral of consumers to other healthcare professionals from community pharmacies.

It is also important to consider risks to pharmacy staff and customers through failures to comply with health and safety legislation. The Health and Safety at Work Act 1974 is the guiding piece of legislation placing responsibilities on employers and employees to carry out risk assessments. Pharmacies should have a health and safety policy in place with responsibilities allocated to specific members of staff. Key areas of concern that are relevant to the pharmacy setting include having an effective procedures manual dealing with control of substances hazardous to health, fire precautions, workplace equipment, the pharmacy environment (such as unsafe furniture and fittings) and first aid.

Developments in health policy

In 2000, the Chief Medical Officer (CMO) for England published *An Organisation With A Memory* (OWAM; Department of Health 2000). This was a report of an expert group on learning from adverse events in the NHS, drawing on insights from human error and risk management as applied in other high-risk industries, such as aviation and nuclear power. The report presented international evidence on the scale and impact of adverse events and made reference to the lack of systems in the NHS that allowed there to be learning from adverse events. The expert group concluded that the NHS could benefit greatly by applying these risk management principles to health care.

The report also recommended as one of its four key targets that there should be a 40% reduction in the number of serious errors involving prescribed drugs. In 2004, the Chief Pharmaceutical Officer for England published *Building a Safer NHS for Patients: Improving Medication Safety* (Department of Health 2004), which outlined strategies aimed at reducing the occurrence of prescribing, dispensing and administration errors drawing on experience and models of good practice within the NHS and worldwide.

More recent requirements, forming part of the essential services of the contractual framework for community pharmacy in England and Wales, has meant that standard operating procedures (SOPs) covering the dispensing process need to be in place in pharmacies. In addition, all pharmacies should be able to demonstrate evidence of recording, reporting, monitoring, analysing and learning from patient safety incidents. Furthermore, pharmacists are now expected to be competent in risk management, including the application of root cause analysis (RCA).

National Patient Safety Agency (NPSA)

Following the publication of the highly influential OWAM report, the National Patient Safety Agency (NPSA) was established in June 2001 to coordinate efforts to report and learn from patient safety incidents. The NPSA has published guidance for NHS organizations on the seven steps that they should take in order to improve patient safety (as described in Box 9.2). It is clear that risk management is firmly incorporated into this guidance.

Box 9.2

Seven steps to patient safety

Build a safety culture – create a culture that is open and fair

Lead and support staff – establish a clear and strong focus on patient safety throughout the organization

Integrate risk management activity – develop systems and processes to manage the risks and identify and assess things that could go wrong

Promote reporting – ensure that staff can easily report incidents locally and nationally

Involve and communicate with patients and the public – develop ways to communicate openly with and listen to patients

Learn and share safety lessons – use root cause analysis to learn how and why incidents happen

Implement solutions to prevent harm – embed lessons through practices, processes or systems

Of particular interest, the NPSA has also published recommendations on the labelling and presentation of a dispensed medicine as well as suggestions on how to promote the safe use of medicines. In addition, it has also published recommendations on changes in the general dispensing environment that can improve patient safety (http://www.npsa.nhs.uk).

The risk management process

The risk management process is about the planning, organization and development of a strategy that will identify, assess and ultimately minimize risk. The process can be represented by a sequence of steps but there is much overlap and often there is integration between all the steps.

Step 1: Establish the context

It is essential to identify all the legal and professional requirements for the pharmacy and to respond appropriately, since most of these will be needed for accreditation purposes or to satisfy a risk insurer or commissioner of pharmaceutical services. In the UK, pharmacies are routinely inspected by the Royal Pharmaceutical Society. Community pharmacies in England and Wales are also required to take part in

Box 9.3

Approaches that can be used to identify risks

Direct observation of working practices within the pharmacy

Incident reports of adverse events and near misses

Interviews and questionnaires of patients and staff

Complaints from patients, or other healthcare professionals

Litigation and compensation claims

an annual monitoring visit from representatives of their primary care trust (PCT) to check compliance with the community pharmacy controls assurance framework.

Step 2: Identification of risk

It is important to take into account things that have gone wrong in the past or near miss incidents that have previously occurred. Box 9.3 lists a variety of methods that can be used to identify risks in the pharmacy, and different approaches can be used in combination. Each method will identify different aspects about the frequency and nature of risks in the pharmacy.

Step 3: Analysis of risk

Once a risk has been identified, it should be analysed to determine what action needs to be taken. Ideally, the risk should be eliminated, but often this may not be possible and efforts need to be taken to minimize its potential impact. The use of rigorous risk management techniques such as RCA and FMEA can play an important role at this stage.

The following factors should be considered:
- The likelihood that an adverse event will occur
- Its potential impact (seriousness)
- The availability of methods to reduce the chance of the event happening
- The costs (financial and other) of solutions to minimize the occurrence of similar events in the future.

This will involve making decisions about risks that are rare but potentially very serious compared with risks that are very common but have a low probability of causing harm.

Step 4: Manage the risk

A range of choices is often available to manage the identified risks. The decision is largely determined by the financial cost of implementation balanced against the potential benefits (such as the cost of compensation if an adverse event occurred). The cost of preventing one major, but very rare, adverse event may be very great when compared with preventing hundreds of more minor adverse events.

Risk control

It may not be possible to eliminate all the identified risks, but preventative steps can be introduced that minimize the likelihood of an adverse event occurring.

Risk acceptance

This involves the recognition that the risk cannot be entirely removed, but at least it can be known and anticipated.

Risk avoidance

It may be possible to avoid the risk by understanding the causes of the risk and taking appropriate actions. An example is the recognition that company branding may result in different medications, such as digoxin tablets (see Fig. 9.2), being packaged in similar ways. This risk can be reduced by using different manufacturers so that different medications are clearly distinguishable.

Step 5: Auditing and reviewing performance

Finally, the effectiveness of the approaches used to identify, analyse and treat risks should be reviewed.

The role of audit is essential, in which risk management standards are set and monitored to see if the standards have been met. Following audit, the cycle of organizing, planning, measurement and review should reoccur to support continuous improvement within the pharmacy.

Conclusion

Risk management is an essential role for pharmacists to protect patients from harm. An understanding of human error models and risk management techniques can be used to analyse the possible risks in a working pharmacy environment and thus manage the risks.

KEY POINTS

- Risk is a normal part of daily life, but risk management attempts to minimize or eliminate risk
- Errors can be classified as active or latent
- Active failures are things like slips, lapses, mistakes and procedural violations by a pharmacist
- Latent failures often arise as a result of poor decisions by other, more senior people
- Techniques such as root cause analysis (RCA) are useful risk management tools
- A systematic tool such as failure modes and effects analysis (FMEA) has three main steps – mapping, identification and specifying cause and effect. Together they produce a risk priority number (RPN)
- Adoption of standard operating procedures (SOPs) is a contractual requirement for community pharmacies
- The National Patient Safety Agency (NPSA) coordinates efforts to learn from incidents
- Risk management processes have five essential stages: establish a context; identify the risks; analyse the risks; manage the risks; audit and review performance

10

Continuing professional development and fitness to practise

Raminder Sihota

STUDY POINTS

- Continuing professional development (CPD) and why it concerns pharmacists
- The CPD cycle
- Recording evidence of CPD
- Fitness to practise and its regulation

Introduction

The term continuing professional development (CPD) is familiar to most people and yet is frequently misunderstood. This chapter is designed to develop an understanding of CPD and to consider the importance to pharmacists of individual active engagement in an ongoing programme of CPD.

A search of the World Wide Web for the phrase 'continuing professional development' recently returned more than 30 million hits. The web search showed the phrase is not specific to pharmacy and pharmacists. The results included reference to CPD for teachers, psychotherapists, lawyers, architects, healthcare professionals and many more. Thus, a wide range of people in varying professions all over the world are involved in CPD. These professionals all recognize the value of planned CPD. In most professions CPD is not optional but mandatory. In the UK and many other countries (see Ch. 2) CPD is mandatory for pharmacists. It is relevant to all practising pharmacists, whether experienced and full time or newly qualified and just starting their career. CPD for pharmacists is part of being a professional with an obligation on all to continue to enhance their own knowledge and skills throughout their career and working life.

CPD is related to, and indeed part of, clinical governance (see Ch. 8). Clinical governance is about both continuous quality improvement and being accountable for quality improvement. As such, CPD is an integral part of clinical governance and it involves all healthcare professionals. Those healthcare professionals working in the UK NHS will find there are specific requirements for clinical governance and CPD which are mandatory. The Community Pharmacy Contract (England and Wales) with the NHS states a clear need for community pharmacists to be undertaking and maintaining CPD records within the clinical governance requirements (essential service number eight). In addition to this, the Code of Ethics of the Royal Pharmaceutical Society of Great Britain (RPSGB) places further obligations on pharmacists. Before any service is offered, whether to prescribers, patients or others, a pharmacist must ensure that whoever is delivering the service has a relevant level of competence, skill or knowledge in that area. CPD allows the pharmacist to provide evidence and demonstrate competence.

What is continuing professional development?

CPD means many things to many people. The NHS defines it as 'a process of lifelong learning for all individuals and teams which meets the needs of patients and delivers the health outcomes and healthcare priorities of the NHS and which enables professionals to expand and fulfill their potential' (Department of Health 1998). While this definition is accurate, it is somewhat lengthy. An easier option is to consider the three words individually:

- Continuing – this is about lifelong learning, an ongoing (or continuing) process regardless of age of the pharmacist or the stage of their career
- Professional – this is focused on individual competence in a professional role, i.e. it is to do with the work of the pharmacist
- Development – this is about identifying and undertaking learning that improves the personal skills of the pharmacist to enhance patient care and career development, i.e. it changes for the better the work of the pharmacist.

CPD can be defined as the process of reflection, planning, action and evaluation through which pharmacists continuously develop their knowledge, skills, attitudes and behaviours throughout their professional careers. CPD in the UK applies to both pharmacists and registered pharmacy technicians.

The RPSGB began introducing a framework for CPD for pharmacists in 2002. CPD was developed in pharmacy as a response to the profession's wishes, expressed in a consultation exercise for the Pharmacy in a New Age (PIANA) project in the 1990s, and in response to the requirements of the Health Act 1999.

Today, the concept of CPD remains a relatively new idea and process for pharmacists. Prior to the introduction of the CPD framework, pharmacists had to engage in 30 hours of continuing education each year in line with the professional obligation stated in their code of ethics. This requirement has been replaced with a formal need for CPD records to be completed and retained for the duration of a pharmacist's career in order to demonstrate the pharmacist is competent to be undertaking the role they are working in at the time.

CPD gives a pharmacist the opportunity to demonstrate to their employer, the NHS, and to patients that they are maintaining and building their own professional capabilities.

Background to CPD

The requirement for formal CPD arose from an increasing pressure on the government to ensure healthcare professions operate in a 'professional' manner. Professional accountability has been highlighted by many well documented high-profile reports and incidents. For instance, the Kennedy Report, published in 2001, highlighted gaps in the way the medical profession and the professions allied to medicine kept abreast

of changing techniques, knowledge, methods and processes, etc. The report made recommendations for ongoing professional development and suggested CPD should not focus solely on clinical skills but should encompass both attitudes and communication skills.

The Pharmacists and Pharmacy Technicians Order 2007 in the UK initiated the final steps for mandatory CPD for practising pharmacists registered with the RPSGB. This means that pharmacists must keep a record of their development which shows they are 'actively' keeping up to date with the knowledge they use day to day. By keeping up to date they are able to demonstrate ongoing competence in their current role, or roles that they wish to pursue in the future.

The RPSGB format for recording CPD involves keeping a written record of an activity or event, demonstrating that the pharmacist has learned from a situation relevant to their professional role.

Pharmacists gain from taking ownership of their CPD, since CPD is a personal activity: it is specific to each pharmacist. No two pharmacists will have the same CPD records. CPD is designed to help pharmacists structure and plan ways to ensure that their skills are constantly being updated and renewed. CPD puts pharmacists in control of their learning.

CPD cycle

CPD is defined as a systematic, ongoing, cyclical process of self-directed learning. It should enable pharmacists to do their job more effectively and involves employers as well as individuals.

CPD is a four-stage process which helps the pharmacist plan their learning and track, record and reflect on learning and development. The learning may be clinical or related to a skill, attitude or behaviour

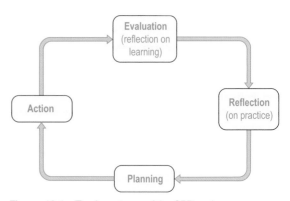

Figure 10.1 • The four stages of the CPD cycle.

associated with the pharmacist's role. The four stages are often depicted as a cyclical process. The RPSGB recording system is based on the four stages of the CPD cycle.

The four stages of the cycle are shown in Figure 10.1 and involve:

- Reflection on practice
- Planning
- Action
- Evaluation (reflection on learning).

Reflection on practice

Reflection involves the pharmacist spending time reflecting on current performance and how work is undertaken. The reflection time aids in the pharmacist identifying personal learning and development needs. The pharmacist is the best person to identify their own personal learning needs. Reflection involves the pharmacist thinking about how daily tasks are carried out, the areas in which the pharmacist feels knowledge or skills are weak or events have happened which indicate a pharmacist needs to improve knowledge or skills in that area.

Sometimes a particular situation or event will draw the attention of the pharmacist to a weakness in knowledge, ability or systems of work which, if not addressed, could cause further problems. This is called a critical incident (see Ch. 9).

When reflecting, there are several questions the pharmacist may ask:

- What knowledge gaps do I have when undertaking my current role?
- What areas do I need to develop to further progress my career?
- What have I done recently which I could improve next time?
- What do I want to be able to do?
- What extra skills can I offer my patients that would be of benefit to them?
- What skills could I develop that would help deliver my organization goals more effectively?

Other ways of identifying learning needs or knowledge, skill, attitude or behaviour gaps is for the pharmacist to consider the following activities:

- Asking colleagues for feedback on one's own practice – how do they think you are doing? What do they think you could do differently?
- Participating in new activities

- Formulating a development plan to structure future development
- Questions from customers
- Learning from a past event, sometimes referred to as critical incident analysis
- Appraisals
- Professional audit, measuring one's own standard against current competencies for the role of a pharmacist in a similar role.

When identifying learning needs, the pharmacist must remember to keep the learning need simple. A learning need broken down into bite-size pieces is easier to address. The process of reflecting on what a pharmacist does not know or is unable to do results in identification of training needs.

Planning

Having identified learning needs, the pharmacist next needs to plan what can be done to meet these learning needs and how it can be achieved. At this stage, if several learning needs have been identified the pharmacist will have to prioritize learning. When prioritizing, the pharmacist needs to consider the impact of the learning on one's self, on colleagues, on the organization worked for and on the patient.

If the pharmacist has identified more than one learning need then it may be that more than one CPD cycle needs to be started. When planning actions to meet learning objectives, the pharmacist needs to consider:

- What level of competence needs to be reached?
- When does the learning objective need to be met by?
- What will be the impact of the learning on customers, colleagues, the organization and the pharmacist?
- What activities can be undertaken to best meet needs?
- What activities lead to the best learning? (This will differ for each pharmacist.)

Additionally, at this stage the pharmacist needs to consider what the consequence of not undertaking the learning would be. If the pharmacist realizes that the learning need is no longer urgent or important, then it is appropriate not to take it any further.

When considering how to meet learning needs, there are a number of ways that learning can be undertaken. The RPSGB suggests pharmacists be creative and not limit themselves to formal or certificated courses. Pharmacists may wish to consider the following methods (this list is not exhaustive):

- Talking to a colleague
- Attending a course
- Reading a book, article or journal
- Research
- Work shadowing
- Coaching another individual
- Everyday experience (learning on the job)
- Talking to patients
- Computer assisted learning
- Deputizing for someone
- Audit.

It is important to recognize pharmacists all learn in different ways and all have preferences. It may be worthwhile considering options which may have not been considered before.

Action

At this stage of the cycle, once the plan is complete for what needs to happen, it is time for the pharmacist to put the plan into action and commence learning. Action is simply carrying out the plan. While this sounds simple, the time taken to undertake the learning needs to be built into the plan and the timetable adhered to.

While undertaking the actions, the pharmacist should throughout be asking:

- What have I gained from this action?
- How might this action benefit my practice?

As these questions are answered, a record should be made of what has been learned.

Evaluation (reflection on learning)

As with all development, evaluating what learning has been undertaken and how it has been undertaken is important. During the evaluation process, pharmacists should consider a series of questions:

- Has the activity achieved what the original learning objective was?
- Has any learning occurred?
- Have any further learning needs been identified?
- Has an opportunity to apply the learning occurred? If so, was there any feedback?

In some cases pharmacists may find that what has been learned is not what they set out to learn. In this case the pharmacist needs to revisit the original learning need and consider if the requirement to undertake further actions is still necessary for their practice. If the pharmacist decides the learning need is still valid, then this will lead the pharmacist into a new CPD cycle or alternatively the pharmacist can go back a couple of steps in the cycle and add in different actions.

If the pharmacist does not have the learning need any longer because it is no longer relevant or it has been overtaken by other priorities or events, then the pharmacist may exit the CPD cycle there.

Assessing whether the learning undertaken has been effective

A further question that the pharmacist needs to ask is: 'Can my practice now be shown to have improved as a result of the learning experience or is further learning required?' Realistically, true evaluation may not occur for some weeks or months, since an opportunity to apply learning may not occur sooner.

Scheduled learning vs unscheduled learning

The CPD cycle is a circle – each stage flows into the next. There are three entry points into the cycle – 'Reflection on practice', 'Planning' and 'Action'. The exit (end point) is always 'Evaluation', when the impact of the learning undertaken is reviewed.

Scheduled learning is another term given to CPD which enters the process at 'Reflection on practice'. This is when someone or something leads the pharmacist to identify a learning need or knowledge gap and plan ways that the pharmacist can meet this need or gap. This can be as simple as someone asking the pharmacist a question that the pharmacist does not know the answer to.

Unscheduled learning is learning that starts from 'Action'. This is learning that happens unexpectedly through someone or something. It is learning that was not planned and has not happened consciously.

All entry points into the CPD cycle are valid. Ordinarily a pharmacist would have a mixture of cycles, some starting at 'Reflection' or 'Planning', which indicates the pharmacist is thinking about his practice and planning appropriate actions, and some entries starting at 'Action', which indicates the pharmacist is receptive to new ideas and concepts as they arise.

Recording CPD

The CPD four-stage cyclical process should be documented to demonstrate learning is being undertaken which meets the needs of the individuals and the organizations in which the pharmacist works. The RPSGB has issued guidance stating the requirement to record CPD in a specially designed format. The RPSGB gives additional guidance stating how much CPD a pharmacist records is dependent on personal development needs. It is advised that a pharmacist focus on the quality of the process and recording rather than the quantity.

Generally a pharmacist needs to aim to record at least one CPD entry each month, although ordinarily most pharmacists will undertake greater CPD daily in the course of professional work.

The time taken to undertake a CPD cycle may be hours, days, weeks, months or, for some learning needs, years. The length of time taken to record a CPD cycle is about 30 minutes. This time includes the pharmacist recording the cycle and the thinking during the process. It is worth acknowledging that initially it may take longer than 30 minutes but as a pharmacist becomes more familiar and experienced in the process this time should reduce.

The CPD framework described is designed specifically for use by both pharmacists and technicians registered with the RPSGB. The framework was piloted with 500 pharmacists in all branches of the profession. Many of these pharmacists found that CPD was not an onerous burden and in fact it increased their personal satisfaction from work.

The RPSGB is of the view that pharmacists will need to submit their CPD records periodically for review to the RPSGB or equivalent regulatory body. This periodic review is likely to be every 3–5 years. The method of review will involve evaluating the records against a set of evaluation criteria.

In summary, CPD describes any activity – whether formal course, informal query from a patient or personal study – that helps a pharmacist do their job better, resulting in a more competent service to cus-tomers, line manager, colleagues and the organization, and helps the pharmacist progress faster in their career. CPD is a cyclical process. For everyone, the need for the updating of knowledge and skills is a continuous one. Pharmacists moving from one post to another may need new skills. Pharmacists may find job descriptions change over time and new developments in practice need to be implemented, which may also require new skills and knowledge. Learning does not stop after the first degree course, or after the pre-registration year or after completing a postgraduate qualification. Learning continues throughout life. What CPD does is to focus that learning on the needs of the individuals and the organizations which employ them.

Fitness to practise

Pharmacy in the UK is in a period of regulatory change. Regulations regarding fitness to practise in pharmacy have recently been implemented. It is well recognized throughout the pharmacy profession that this form of regulation is necessary in order to maintain and develop public confidence in pharmacists and other healthcare professions. In the past there has been a concern over disparity between regulation of different professions. Some professions being 'over-regulated' and others 'under-regulated' has impaired public confidence.

The UK Government in 2007 published a document entitled *Trust, Assurance and Safety – The Regulation of Health Professionals in the 21st Century*. This outlined proposals to ensure patient, public and professional confidence in the healthcare professionals' watchdogs to improve patient safety and ensure the fair treatment of healthcare professionals. Further proposals also suggested healthcare professionals will be required to prove their fitness to practise every 5 years. How this will impact on pharmacists and what role CPD has to play in proving fitness to practise and revalidation is very much in its embryonic stages.

Within the pharmacy profession, moves for additional broader regulation have commenced through the Pharmacists and Pharmacy Technicians Order 2007 which aims to bring pharmacist regulation into line with other professions. The main provisions in the order are as follows:

- Pharmacists to undergo CPD so that registrants keep their knowledge, skills and aptitudes up to date as long as they continue practising

- A wider range of powers and sanctions relating to investigating and dealing with allegations of impaired fitness to practise. These include impairment through ill health as well as performance and conduct, and impairment related to criminal convictions
- Introduction of sanctions, including the ability to suspend registrants when necessary to protect the public while their fitness to practise is being investigated and adjudicated
- The ability to restrict the practice of those unfit practitioners to areas in which they are safe to practise by attaching conditions to their registration
- New powers enabling the RPSGB to disclose fitness to practise information where that is in the public interest
- The requirement for others to disclose information to the RPSGB about fitness to practise matters
- A new duty to cooperate with other public authorities and bodies with an interest in pharmacy matters
- New powers to require practising registrants to be covered by an adequate and appropriate indemnity arrangement.

Declaration of fitness to practise

Pharmacists are required to make an annual fitness to practise declaration to the RPSGB. The declaration signed by practising pharmacists confirms their commitment to the Code of Ethics, to work under the standards and guidance published by the RPSGB and to undertake CPD. The declaration also confirms that the signatory has not been or is not the subject of any regulatory, civil or criminal proceedings or investigations relevant to their fitness to practise. Non-practising pharmacists sign a declaration to confirm they will not practise.

Pharmacists who fail to make an annual declaration are sent a letter by the RPSGB advising them that a note will be made on their file, and that until a declaration is received they will not be eligible for a letter of good standing or a certificate of current professional statement; this includes a complete fitness to practise check for inclusion in NHS pharmaceutical provider lists. Following the receipt of the letter the pharmacist has 2 months to provide a declaration; failure to do so will lead to an automatic removal of name from the Pharmaceutical Register.

In addition to the annual declaration pharmacists have a responsibility under the Code of Ethics to promptly declare to relevant parties, including the RPSGB, their employer and other relevant authority, any circumstances following completion of a declaration that may call into question their fitness to practise. The RPSGB states that pharmacists have a responsibility to notify their profession to the police should they be charged with any offence.

Roles of the statutory committees in fitness to practise

The Pharmacists and Pharmacy Technicians Order 2007 for fitness to practise has established three new statutory committees: the Investigating Committee, the Health Committee and the Disciplinary Committee (see Ch. 8).

In the past, the RPSGB had powers to consider allegations of misconduct and to make decisions and recommendations based on the misconduct. Under the changes introduced by the Pharmacists and Pharmacy Technicians Order 2007, the RPSGB is able to consider a wider range of allegations, including those relating to a registrant's physical and mental health. The Pharmacists and Pharmacy Technicians Order 2007 provides the RPSGB's new statutory committees with a wider range of sanctions and options for disposal. The new Investigating Committee has the power, in certain circumstances and where the allegation is admitted, to accept written undertakings. The Disciplinary and Health Committees have the power to impose conditions on registration and to suspend a person's name from the register for a period of up to 1 year, as well as the power to direct removal from the register.

Conclusion

In summary, the Pharmacists and Pharmacy Technicians Order 2007 states the fitness to practise guidance for pharmacists and pharmacy technicians in respect of standards of conduct, practice and performance, and the need to disclose information will change from time to time. It is important for all practising pharmacists to be engaged in regular CPD regarding updating their knowledge of practice, regulation and legislative changes within their field of work.

KEY POINTS

- CPD is a feature of most professions
- CPD is part of clinical governance, is required as part of NHS contracts, and is an obligation in the Code of Ethics for pharmacists
- The CPD cycle involves reflection, planning, action, evaluation
- Entry into the cycle can be at any of the first three stages; exit is always at evaluation, but may lead into further cycles
- The RPSGB requires pharmacists to record all CPD activity, which will be reviewed periodically
- Recent changes have introduced the concept of fitness to practise
- In renewing their annual membership of the RPSGB, pharmacists make a declaration about their fitness to practise

11

Audit

Janet Krska

STUDY POINTS

- Audit as part of clinical governance
- The relationship between practice research, service evaluation and audit
- Types of audit
- Structures, processes and outcomes which may be audited
- The stages in the audit cycle: standard setting, data collection, comparison with standards, identifying problems, implementing change, re-audit
- Learning from audit

Introduction: what is audit?

Audit concerns the quality of professional activities and services. Audit is carried out to determine whether best practice is being delivered and, equally importantly, to improve practice. Audit is part of clinical governance (see Ch. 8) – probably the key part – therefore it forms part of the quality improvement work which takes place within all NHS organizations. It can be described as 'improving the care of patients by looking at what you do, learning from it and if necessary, changing practice'.

Audit is based around standards of practice. The hallmark of a professional is that they maintain standards of professional practice, which exist to protect the public from poor-quality services. Audit provides a method of accountability, both to the public and to government, which demonstrates that standards are being met or, if not, that action is being taken to remedy the situation. It also provides managers with information about the quality of the services

their staff deliver. Although this may seem somewhat threatening, ultimately the aim of audit is to improve the efficiency and effectiveness of services, to promote higher standards and to improve the outcome for patients. It also allows changes in practice to be evaluated. Therefore it is an essential component of any professional's work and an integral part of day-to-day practice.

Most healthcare professionals' activities have an impact on patients, either directly or indirectly, so can be described as a clinical service. Audit of these services is therefore clinical audit. Clinical audit is defined by the National Institute for Health and Clinical Excellence (NICE) as 'a quality improvement process that seeks to improve patient care and outcomes through systematic review of care against explicit criteria and the implementation of change'. All NHS trusts in the UK must support audit, so should have a central audit office which provides training and help in designing audits and collates the results of clinical audits. All NHS staff are expected to participate in clinical audit. Community pharmacists are required to participate in two clinical audits each year, one based on their own practice and one multidisciplinary audit organized by their local primary care organization.

There are actually few instances where pharmacists provide a clinical service to patients in isolation from other healthcare professionals. The provision of advice and sale of non-prescription medicines may be one such area, but most services will impact on or be affected by service provision by other professionals, so can be regarded as multidisciplinary. The audit of these clinical services should ideally also be multidisciplinary. The users of services should also be involved in audit whenever possible, perhaps by asking patient representatives to join the audit team. They can provide important insight into what aspects of a service would benefit from audit and can help to set the criteria against which performance will be audited.

Relationship between practice research, service evaluation and audit

It is important to understand the relationship between practice research, service evaluation and audit. Practice research is designed to establish what is best practice. An example of this would be a randomized controlled trial of pharmacists undertaking a new service compared to normal care. In a controlled trial, patients are often carefully selected, using inclusion and exclusion criteria, special documentation and outcome measures are used which may differ from those used in routine practice and all aspects of the service being studied must be standardized.

To implement a new service into routine practice further development will be required. Many aspects of a new service are likely to differ from those used in a research situation and may differ between practice settings. All new services will then need to be evaluated, which may involve determining the views of service providers and users, collecting data on the outcomes for patients who use the service and finding out if publicity is adequate. Changes may be necessary if problems are identified in service evaluation.

Once a service is running smoothly it should then be subject to audit. This will involve setting standards for the service and measuring actual practice against these standards. Findings from research and service evaluations can contribute to standard setting in audit.

Although there are many similarities in the methods used to obtain data for research and for audit, there are important differences. In research, it is important to have controlled studies, to be able to extrapolate the results and to have large enough samples to demonstrate statistical significance of any differences between groups. None of these applies to audit. Audit compares actual practice to a predetermined level of best practice, not to a control. The results of audit apply to a particular situation and should not be

extrapolated. Audit can be even applied to a single case; large numbers are not required.

Types of audit

Audit may be of three types, depending on who undertakes it. These are:

- Self-audit
- Peer or group audit
- External audit.

Self-audit is undertaken by individuals and is part of a professional work attitude in which critical appraisal of actions taken and of their results is constantly being made. While anyone can do self-audit, it is most likely to be used by pharmacists who work in isolation, such as in single-handed community pharmacies. There are many examples of self-audits, such as those on availability of leaflets, facilities within the pharmacy, owing items and patient counselling, which fulfil the requirements of the pharmacy contract. See the Royal Pharmaceutical Society of Great Britain (RPSGB) website for audit packs on these topics.

Peer audit is undertaken by people within the same peer group, which usually means the same profession. Peer audit involves joint setting of standards by an audit team. For example, pharmacists from several hospitals which provide similar services could get together and audit each other's service. In primary care, pharmacists within or between primary care trusts (PCTs) could compare their practices. Another way of doing this is benchmarking – a process of defining a level of care set as a goal to be attained. Here standards are set against those identified by a leading centre, such as a teaching hospital.

External audit is carried out by people other than those actually providing the service and so is perceived as threatening by those whose services are being audited. It may be more objective in its criticisms than self or peer audit, but there may be less enthusiasm for corrective action to improve services. If standards are imposed, there is a perceived threat if an individual's performance is not of the standard required. It is possible to involve those whose services are to be audited in deciding what best practice should be and in making improvements to make external audit more acceptable. NHS services are subject to external audit carried out by the Healthcare Commission, which conducts national audits in England and Wales. The data produced enable comparisons to be made between different NHS trusts and enable sharing of good practice.

Multidisciplinary audit is the most common type of group audit and is usually preferred for clinical audit, but it is essential to ensure that one subgroup is not auditing the activities of another subgroup. This would lead to tensions and be counterproductive. For example, in an audit of doctors' prescribing errors detected by pharmacists, pharmacists cannot set the standard for an acceptable level of errors without the involvement of the doctors. If they are not part of the audit team, there is little chance of improvement. Pharmacists are often involved in carrying out audits of clinical practice, for example audit of prescribing against NICE clinical guidelines. In this situation, it is also important that the prescribers are involved in setting the standards.

What is measured in audit?

There are three aspects of any services and activities which can be audited. These are:

- The structures or resources involved
- The processes used
- The outcomes of the activity.

Structures are the resources available to help deliver services or carry out activities. Examples are staff, their expertise and knowledge, books, learning materials or training courses, drug stocks, equipment, layout of premises.

Processes are the systems and procedures which take place when carrying out an activity and may include quality assurance procedures and policies and protocols of all types. Examples are: procedures for dealing with patients' own medicines in hospital, prescribing policies and disease management protocols.

Outcomes are the results of the activity and are arguably the most important aspect of any activity. In pharmaceutical audits such as drug procurement or distribution or standards of premises, outcomes should be easily identified and measurable. In many clinical audits, some outcomes are relatively easily measured, for example changes in parameters such as blood pressure, INR (international normalized ratio) control and serum biochemistry. Surrogate outcomes can also be used, such as the drugs or doses prescribed. However, outcomes which involve a change in health status, attitude or behaviour may be very difficult to measure.

Any individual audit can examine structures, processes and outcomes individually or together.

The audit cycle

Audit is a continuous process, which follows a cycle of measurement, evaluation and improvement. The basic cycle is shown in Figure 11.1, but audit can also be seen as a spiral in which standards are continuously raised as practice improves.

Before starting an audit, first identify its purpose. This will derive from the desire to improve the quality of the service. For example, the purpose may be 'to improve the dispensing turnaround time' or 'to increase the proportion of patients counselled about their new medicines'. It may be appropriate to conduct a 'baseline audit' to find out if indeed there is a need to improve service quality. A baseline audit is a small study in which data are collected before standards are set. Once it is known that there is a need to improve services, the audit cycle incorporates:

- The setting of standards for practice
- Measuring actual practice
- Comparing the two
- Finding out any reasons why best practice is not being achieved
- Changing aspects of practice to improve this.

Although the process is continuous, it is not practicable to audit all activities or services all the time. A baseline audit may help to decide whether improvements are possible and routine monitoring may be instituted instead of repeat audits to ensure that best practice, once attained, is maintained.

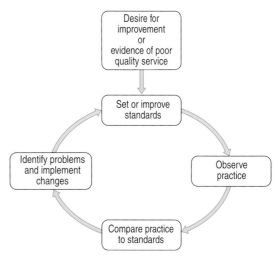

Figure 11.1 • The audit cycle.

Setting standards

All audits should be based on standards which are widely accepted (i.e. best practice). The Medicines, Ethics and Practice guide may help to set standards for many aspects of pharmacy services. Other documents can also be used to develop standards, such as national service frameworks, practice guidelines or clinical guidelines for individual medical conditions. Several standards are usually set for any individual audit, relating to resources, processes or outcomes.

Because audit is about comparing actual practice to standards of best practice, numerical values need to be added which will allow this. A guideline may suggest a criterion, for example that patients receiving warfarin should be counselled about avoiding aspirin. For this to form a useful standard for audit, it needs to be clarified whether this applies to all patients, i.e. 100%. This numerical value is the target, which, together with the criterion, forms the standard or 'level of performance'. It is then easy to measure whether this occurs in practice. Many clinical guidelines suggest audit standards and criteria.

A target level of 100% is termed an ideal standard but this may not be achievable. The level set may need to be a compromise between what is desirable and what is possible, since resources may be limited. This would be an optimal standard. Using the previous example, it may be considered at the outset that there are insufficient staff to ensure that 100% of patients receiving warfarin could be counselled about avoiding aspirin. A compromise could be that 100% of patients prescribed warfarin for the first time receive this advice. Another type of standard is the minimal standard, which, as its name implies, is the minimum acceptable level of service and is often used in external audits.

If there are no published guidelines or standards, they will need to be devised. This may involve searching the literature, for example recent journals, textbooks or educational material. Whether devising standards from scratch or making guidelines into standards, it is important that the whole audit team is involved in devising them. This may include doctors, nurses, health visitors, technical staff and non-medical staff, such as receptionists or porters, and patients or their carers. Inclusion avoids the potential feeling of threat which may be created by audit. Anyone excluded at this stage would perceive the audit as external, and refuse to help improve performance, which could mean the whole exercise is a waste of time.

Once standards have been set, the next stage of audit involves collecting data on actual practice.

Observing practice

Many audits require a simple form onto which data from other sources are transferred. In audits involving structures, checklists are often most useful; those involving processes may use checklists or may need space for other types of data, while auditing clinical outcomes may require additional methods such as questionnaires. As with any data collection, it is important that the information obtained is able to answer the questions asked. In the case of an audit, the question(s) may be relatively simple, such as 'What percentage of patients receiving warfarin are counselled?'

It is often useful to incorporate some measure of potential factors which may influence practice within the data collection. So, in addition to finding out whether local clinical guidelines are being used by examining medical records, it is worth issuing a questionnaire to those expected to use the guidelines to find out their views on whether the guidelines are readily available, are in an acceptable format and meet their needs. In an audit of warfarin counselling, it is useful to collect data on how busy the pharmacy is when each patient presents their prescription and how many staff trained to provide advice were available. This may mean that the data collection procedures may need to anticipate some potential causes of failing to provide best practice.

Before setting out to devise a data collection form, it is always worth finding out whether a similar audit has been done before, so you can adapt or modify the data collection procedures used. Some useful data collection sheets for a wide range of audits are available from the RPSGB website. These include audits of pharmacy processes such as prescription waiting times, responding to symptoms and referrals to GPs. If you do need to design a new procedure, the data collection must fulfil some basic requirements (Box 11.1). First the data collected must be able to address the purpose of the audit. The method of data collection must be valid and reliable. If sampling procedures are used, they too must be appropriate, avoiding bias and, equally importantly, it must be feasible to carry them out.

Validity is the extent to which what is measured is actually what is supposed to be measured. To use the warfarin counselling example again, the standard was

Box 11.1

Requirements for data collection procedures

- Provide information required
- Validity
- Reliability
- Controlled for bias
- Adequate sampling technique
- Feasible
- Quantitative or qualitative
- Retrospective or prospective
- Routinely or specially collected
- Pilot study

about advice concerning aspirin. If the only data collected involved the number of patients who were counselled and not what advice they were given about aspirin, these data would be invalid, since they did not measure what they set out to measure.

Reliability is a measure of the consistency or reproducibility of the data collection procedure. Good reliability can be difficult to achieve when trying to measure outcomes in health care. It is therefore important to use recognized measures wherever possible. Reliability may also vary among individuals collecting data, despite their using the same data collection tool. It is important to check this and ensure that they are doing the same thing before they start to collect data.

Sampling is important in collecting data for audit, because the data should be unbiased and representative of actual practice. It may be that the numbers and time involved are small enough that all examples of the activity are included in data collection procedures. In the case of large numbers, it may be easier to include just a proportion in the audit. If so, a plan is needed which ensures that those selected are representative. Many different sampling methods could be used, including random (using number tables or computer) or systematic (such as every tenth patient presenting a prescription for warfarin). Another way is to decide in advance that a certain percentage of the total population (a quota) will be sampled, usually ensuring that they will be typical of the population in important characteristics. These techniques require that the total population size within the audit period is known. A large population may also need to be stratified into subgroups first before sampling, for example patients with new prescriptions and patients with repeats.

Sampling, or even large numbers, may not always be necessary. Since audit is about a particular service or activity, carried out by one or more particular individual professionals, an audit can be carried out on a service provided to one patient. It is still the determination of whether actual practice equates to best practice.

Feasibility of data collection is very important. It must be possible to collect the data required to answer the question. It is often necessary to incorporate data collection for audit into routine work, so the time taken is an important consideration. Some data may already be collected on a routine basis, which can be used to answer audit questions. Data kept on patient medication records or on medicine use review (MUR) records may be useful for some audits. Some pharmacies routinely log the time when prescriptions are handed in and given out, so an audit of turnaround time could easily be carried out using these data. Hospitals routinely collect data on length of stay and number of admissions, discharges and deaths, which may be useful outcome measures. Often data have to be specially collected for the audit, which is where the data collection tools come in.

Data for audit can be either quantitative or qualitative in nature. Qualitative data are often useful in obtaining opinions about services or for measuring outcomes in patients. Large numbers are not required for producing qualitative data. It may be useful to undertake qualitative work which can then be used to help design a good data collection tool to be used in a quantitative way, using larger numbers. Quantitative audit may generate large amounts of data, which require subsequent analysis, usually using statistics. These may be purely descriptive or simple comparative statistics.

Whether the data collected are retrospective or prospective depends to a large extent on the topic of the audit and the data available. Retrospective audit can only be undertaken if good records of activities have been kept. Prospective audits should ensure that the data required are recorded, even if only for the audit period. There is a possibility of practice changing during the audit period simply because the audit is being undertaken. This may not always be a problem if practice is better than usual and if audit is continuous, since the ultimate aim is to improve services. It is more important to be aware of this effect if practice is measured periodically, although it is very difficult to control for.

In large audits, piloting the data collection tool using a sample similar to those to be included in the audit is a valuable way of finding out if it is suitable. This should avoid the discovery that there were difficulties in interpretation or that vital information has not been recorded after acquiring large amounts of data.

Comparing practice to standards

This is the evaluation stage of audit, in which actual practice is compared to best practice. First the data obtained must be analysed and presented. Most audit data require only descriptive analysis, such as percentages, means or medians, along with ranges and standard deviations to show the spread of the data. Comparative statistical tests are useful for looking at one or more subgroups of quantitative data. This could be for different data collection periods (audit cycles) or for subgroups within one audit. Examples where comparison may be useful are three different pharmacies' prescription turnaround times or the counselling frequencies for patients presenting prescriptions for warfarin for the first time compared to those who have taken it before. The statistical test must be appropriate for the type of data. Chi-square is used for nonparametric data, such as frequencies. For parametric data which are normally distributed, t-tests can be used. When statistics are used in an audit, it is important to consider the practical significance of the data. An improvement which is statistically significant may not always be of practical significance and vice versa. In presenting data, graphics can be particularly useful, as tables can be discouraging to many people. This is particularly important in a group audit, where everyone needs to see the results. Simple graphics, such as pie charts or bar charts, should be adequate.

Data collected for audit purposes relate to the activities of individual professionals and to their effects on patients. It is therefore essential to maintain confidentiality. Permission is required before any information about one individual's practice is given to other members of the audit team. Managers who may need this sort of information should be part of the audit team anyway. The general results of an audit should, however, be made available to others, after ensuring that no individual practitioner or patient can be identified. This is essential if the audit is to improve services, as it will help others to learn and allow comparisons to be made.

When comparing the results of audits between centres, there will most probably be differences – perhaps in staffing levels, population served, case mix and so on – which could account for differences in apparent performance. Any unusual situations which occurred during the audit and which may have affected performance should be highlighted. Also any errors in data collection must be identified, which may mean data have to be excluded from analysis as they could be unrepresentative of what should have happened. It is most important to remember that the results of any audit should not be extrapolated beyond the sample audited. Audit applies to a particular activity, carried out by particular individuals and involving particular patients.

Providing the standards for the audit have been set appropriately, it should be relatively easy to determine whether they have been achieved. Often the most difficult part of audit is finding out why best practice is not being delivered and ensuring that improvement occurs.

Identifying problems

It is little use simply finding out that a service fails to meet a given standard. The underlying causes of failure need to be established and the data collection procedures should have attempted to identify some of these. Suboptimal practice can arise for a variety of reasons, such as inadequate skills or knowledge, poor systems of work or the behaviour of individuals within a team. Each should be examined as a possible contributory factor to disappointing results of an audit. Simple lack of awareness, for example, about local clinical guidelines can contribute to their lack of use. Lack of skill may be related to infrequency of carrying out a particular activity. Both are relatively easily remedied. Both behaviour and the way in which work is organized are more difficult to change. The strategies adopted for effecting change will need to differ depending on which of these underlying causes is present.

Implementing changes

Achieving improvement in practice requires a change in behaviour. Change can be threatening simply because of its novelty. It may also involve increased work and is often resisted. This is why everyone whose work pattern may need to change should be active members of the audit team from the start. Change must be seen as leading to improvement in performance and ultimately patient benefit.

The changes proposed to improve practice must be closely tailored to the underlying cause of the sub-optimal audit results. They should be specific to the situation which has been audited, rather than general. They should be non-threatening and may need to be introduced gradually. Change may require resources, including time. It may also have other knock-on effects which need to be anticipated. The effect of changes must be monitored, to see whether they have been successful. This can be done by re-audit or by continuous monitoring if routinely collected data can be used.

Re-audit

Sometimes it may be appropriate to reconsider the standards before undertaking a further period of data collection.

Standards which were set too high may always be unattainable, although this may not have been apparent before practice was measured. It is equally possible to have used low standards and to have found they were surpassed. In this case it may be appropriate to raise them, which is a good way of improving practice. Whether or not the standards remain the same, a second period of measuring practice is needed if changes have been implemented, so that the effectiveness of these changes can be determined.

It is always difficult to change behaviour and improvements in practice may be short-lived. It may therefore be necessary to repeat audits at regular intervals to reinforce the desired practice and maintain the improvement in service.

Learning through audit

If the prevailing view of an audit which shows performance to be less than the standard set is that there are lots of reasons which could excuse this result, then little has been learned from undertaking the audit. Evaluating your service may be difficult, but it may also teach you a lot about yourself and the staff with whom you work. For example, it is of little use to suggest that the reason there were so many dispensing errors during the audit was that there was a new locum employed for part of the time. It is much more valuable to consider what information you have available for locums about your dispensing procedures and indeed whether your dispensing procedures are adequate.

If the results of an audit were suboptimal, but much as expected, is this because staff have been accepting of poor practices in the past? Have staff been aware of the need for improvements in systems but felt unable to suggest changes? Have staff been wanting more training but known that there is no money available to pay for it? All these are hypothetical situations, but you can see how conducting audit may have more learning than just what needs to be done to improve services. In this way, carrying out audit can contribute to continuous professional development and so has benefits both for you and, ultimately, for the patient.

KEY POINTS

- Pharmacists need to audit their practice to show that they meet appropriate standards
- The main aim of audit must be to improve standards of service and outcomes for patients
- There are similarities and differences between audit, service evaluation and practice research
- The three main types of audit are self-, peer and external audit
- An audit may examine structures, processes or outcomes
- Criteria should be formulated into standards for audit which may be ideal, optimal or minimal
- Standard setting should involve at least all those involved in delivering the service being audited
- Data collection must address the purpose of the audit and have the potential to identify reasons for failure to meet the standard
- Sampling must ensure that the data collected in an audit are representative of the total activity
- Piloting the data collection tool ensures that it is suitable and comprehensive
- Comparison with standards will normally involve very simple descriptive or statistical analysis
- Confidentiality must be respected, but outcomes should be shared with all the audit team
- Implementing change is a key part of audit
- Re-audit tests whether changes have led to improved achievement of standards

Chapter Twelve

Ethics

Richard C. O'Neill

STUDY POINTS

- The major ethical theories and principles applied to decision making in health care
- The key limitations of each ethical theory
- The distinction between morals, ethics and law
- Ethical decision-making frameworks
- Ethics relating to pharmacy

Introduction

The aim of this chapter is to introduce the concept of ethics, briefly explain ethical theories and principles and relate these to issues of relevance in pharmacy and healthcare practice.

Morals, values and ethics

The terms 'ethics' and 'morals', 'ethical' and 'moral' are often used interchangeably. They are almost synonymous in that an ethical action is one that is morally acceptable. However, they are not identical. Morals usually refers to practices; ethics is concerned with evaluating such practices. Morality is concerned with the standards of right or wrong behaviour, the values and duties adopted by individuals, groups and society. Personal morals arise from religious beliefs, political views, prejudices, cultural and family backgrounds.

Values are those ideals, beliefs, attitudes and characteristics considered to be valuable and worthwhile by an individual, a group or society in general. Personal values are acquired over a long period of time through interaction with family, friends, school, work, colleagues and role models, and develop and change throughout life. The way in which a person makes personal and professional judgments and choices is influenced by the way they organize, rank and prioritize values in a personal value system.

Ethics is the branch of philosophy that deals with the moral dimension of human life. Ethics deals with what is right and wrong, good and bad, what ought and ought not to be done. It is concerned with actions and judging whether an action is right or wrong and justifying this. The study of ethics is commonly grouped into three areas:

- Descriptive ethics simply describes the way things are – how people in different societies actually behave
- Meta-ethics is concerned with analysis of the language people use when they discuss a moral issue, for example the meaning of the words 'right' and 'wrong'
- Normative ethics is concerned with how things ought to be, how people should behave and how people justify decisions when faced with situations of moral choice. It attempts to generate the norms or standards of the right action.

Descriptive ethics is about facts while normative ethics is about values. One cannot argue from the one to the other. The way things are is not necessarily a guide to how they should be.

Ethical theories

Ethical theories provide a framework within which the acceptability of actions and the morality of judgments can be assessed. Absolutist theories rest on the assumption that there is an absolute right or wrong.

Relativistic or reason-based theories rest on the assumption that right or wrong can depend purely on what any society, group or individual believes.

Normative theories of ethics

Normative theories are distinguished by the way in which they provide ethical guidance:

- Virtue ethics locate the highest moral value in the development of persons
- Consequentialist (or utilitarian) theories evaluate actions by reference to their outcomes
- Deontological theories hold that actions are intrinsically right or wrong.

These are summarized in Table 12.1.

Virtue ethics

The word ethics is derived from the Greek *ethos*, meaning a person's character, nature or disposition. Virtue ethics has its roots in the work of Socrates, Plato and Aristotle, and places emphasis on the character of the person performing the action rather than on the action itself.

Virtue ethicists stress the importance of inner character traits such as honesty, courage, faithfulness, trustworthiness and integrity. Healthcare professionals are expected to demonstrate such characteristics (or virtues), having been inculcated in them throughout education and training.

Socrates (470–399 BC) taught the priority of personal integrity in terms of a person's duty to himself.

Plato (427–347 BC) emphasized four cardinal virtues: wisdom, courage, temperance and justice. Others virtues were fortitude, generosity, self-respect, good temper and sincerity. Hierarchies of virtues have changed over time.

Aristotle (384–322 BC) was concerned with what makes a good person rather than what makes a good action. He believed that being moral involved rationally applying good sense to find the middle way between one extreme or another, for example courage is the mean between cowardice and rashness (Box 12.1).

Table 12.1 Comparison of main ethical theories

Ethical theory	Virtue based	Duty based (deontology)	Consequentialism (utilitarianism)
Perspective	Actor based	Action based	Action based
Features	Emphasis placed on character and motivation	Emphasis on the manner of the action; act out of a sense of duty; moral rules are those that pass the categorical imperative test; means count; never right to treat people as just means to an end	Emphasis on the outcome or outcome of the action; no action in itself is good or bad; ends count
Morally correct action	Right action is that which a virtuous person would do	Right action is that following duty	Right action is that with the greatest usefulness; greatest good for the greatest number
Strengths	More personal; supports actions done for virtuous reasons; not bound by rules	Sets clear rules/moral boundaries; follow duty not inclination; based on reason–no subjectivity; consistent	Practical; flexible; results orientated; no conflicting rules; moral form of democracy
Weaknesses	No universally agreed list of virtues; concerned with good character rather than the specific problem; difficulties in resolving moral conflicts or competing claims in practice; may do harm despite virtue	Questions about where rules originate; can be inflexible; not as simple as consequentialism; difficulties when rules conflict; follow duty regardless of results; ends cannot justify means even if outcome is good	Relies on single criterion when many factors need to be considered; difficulties in identifying who and what should be considered; difficulties quantifying utility; uncertainties in consequences of actions/speculative; can lack justice; does not consider individual rights; ends can justify means; bad or unjust acts permissible

Box 12.1

Examples of Aristotle's moral virtues and the golden mean

Excess	Mean	Deficiency
Rashness	Courage	Cowardice
Boastfulness	Truthfulness	Understatement
Irascibility	Patience	Lack of spirit
Vulgarity	Magnificence	Pettiness

Modern Aristotelians believe that ethics should be concentrating more on how people should live their lives, advising which ethical characteristics people should try to develop and habituating people into having good dispositions so that moral behaviour becomes almost instinctive.

Consequentialism and utilitarianism

For consequentialists, whether an action is morally right or wrong depends on the action's 'ethos' or usefulness.

Utilitarians consider that an action should be judged according to the results it achieves. Bentham argued that actions are right if they maximize pleasure (good) and minimize pain (evil) for the majority of people. Since he believed everyone had an equal right to pleasure, everyone counted in the assessment of benefits of an action.

Later it was argued that not all forms of pleasure and happiness were equal and other values such as duty, love and respect should be considered. The goal of ethics is not only the pleasure (happiness) of the individual, but also the greatest pleasure (happiness) for the greatest number.

Recent utilitarian theorists have advocated taking into account the preferences of persons concerned. This approach has become widely used in areas of applied and professional ethics and assumes that there should be equal consideration of interests. While accepting that not all have equal interests (animals compared with humans for example), all should be treated in a way that is appropriate.

The simplicity and practical usefulness of utilitarianism is one of its main benefits. If an act is likely to produce the greatest good for the greatest number then it is right – if it does not, it is wrong.

Deontology

Deontology refers to a group of normative ethical theories that emphasize moral duties and rules. They are referred to as non-consequentialist since some actions are inherently right or wrong, regardless of their consequences. There are acts we have the duty to perform because these acts are good in themselves (i.e. intrinsically good); and we have a duty to refrain from acts that are intrinsically bad or wrong.

Kantianism

Kantianism is the most comprehensive deontological ethical theory named after Immanuel Kant (1724–1804). He believed that people, not God, imposed morality because they were rational beings. Kant suggested that moral duty could be determined by the use of reason about the act in question. This categorical imperative exists as several versions, the two best known being:

- First version: 'Act only on that maxim through which you can at the same time will that it should become a universal law.'

This means that 'unless you are able to say that everyone must act like this, then you should not act like it'. Something is morally right, or wrong, only if it applies for everyone. It would be inconsistent and irrational to decide, for example, that you could steal from others, but they could not steal from you. Thus, reason demands that we do not steal unless everyone is allowed to steal.

- Second version: 'Act in such a way that you always treat humanity, whether in your own person or in the person of any other, never simply as a means, but always at the same time as an end.'

People must be treated as ends in themselves and not as a means to an end. This means that all people are equal and deserve equal respect. There are certain ways we must not treat people, no matter how much usefulness might be produced by treating them in those ways (for example not lying to a patient). A consequentialist, by contrast, does not believe it is wrong to use people as means – if the ends justify the means, lying is permissible.

This second version has been very influential in medical ethics as it can be translated as saying it is necessary to treat people as autonomous agents capable of making their own decisions. The concept of autonomy and respecting an autonomous decision demonstrates respect for the person as an 'end in itself'.

Ross's prima facie duties

Ross recognized that a number of obligations present themselves in practical situations and that we must weigh up the various options available when deciding which course of action is morally correct (Hawley 2007). Ross distinguished duties as 'prima facie' or 'actual' duties. A prima facie duty is one that is always to be performed unless it conflicts with an equal or stronger duty. The stronger duty becomes an actual duty that must be carried out for the action to be morally correct. The prima facie duty to keep a promise (fidelity), for example, could be over-ridden if it was not in a person's best interests. Ross identified seven prima facie duties:

- Fidelity – duty to keep promises, honour contracts and agreements, tell the truth, be faithful
- Reparation – duty to rectify a wrong done to another
- Gratitude – duty to repay acts of kindness
- Beneficence – duty to make things better for other persons
- Non-maleficence – duty not to make other persons worse off
- Justice – duty to distribute pleasure or happiness, goods and benefits in accordance with the merit of persons concerned
- Self-improvement – duty to improve one's own condition.

Conflict of duties can only be resolved by considered judgment in a particular situation: there is no general ranking of the duties. The morally correct action is the one that produces the greatest balance of prima facie rightness to prima facie wrongness. However, the principle of non-maleficence is considered to take precedence over the principle of beneficence when they come into conflict. Ross's theory has greatly influenced the 'four-principles' approach to medical ethics (see later) as it introduced the idea of sorting and weighing principles.

Deontology and rights

The rights of persons are closely associated with duty. Using someone as a means to an end infringes that person's 'rights', such as rights to freedom and choice. This 'right' could be derived from the capacity to reason or to make choices, so that healthcare professionals, for example, are obliged to respect rational wishes of patients.

In every case the deontological norm has boundaries. What lies outside those boundaries is not forbidden. Thus lying is wrong while withholding a truth may be perfectly permissible. This is because withholding a truth is not lying. If more than one option is morally acceptable, the individual can choose which

to carry out. By contrast, a consequentialist must always select the best option.

Principlism and the four ethical principles

Principlism, introduced in the late 1970s, is now a widely applied bioethical framework for identifying key moral issues and as a starting point for looking at ethical dilemmas. It identifies four prima facie moral commitments relevant in health care and compatible with the major ethical theories. These enable a simple, accessible approach when the ethical theories themselves can be considered to be too general to guide particular decisions. Being conditional, the principles allow a stronger case to overrule a weaker one in a particular circumstance.

The four 'principles' are:

- Autonomy – self governance and respect for persons
- Non-maleficence – avoiding harm
- Beneficence – providing good
- Justice – fairness.

These are supplemented with four 'rules':

- Veracity
- Privacy
- Confidentiality
- Fidelity.

Autonomy

Autonomy encompasses the capacity to think, decide and act freely and independently. Respect for autonomy flows from the recognition that all rational beings have unconditional worth, and each has the capacity to determine his or her own destiny. People should be seen as ends in themselves and not treated simply as means to the ends of others.

Autonomy generally brings about the best outcome. Individuals should be allowed to develop their potential according to their own personal convictions provided these do not interfere with a like expression of freedom by others. A person's autonomy should be respected unless it causes harm to others. Liberty should not be limited on the sole grounds that a person's choice would harm them – competent adults should be free to risk their own health and well-being without interference. Respectfulness can be considered a characteristic of a virtuous person.

Three types of autonomy have been suggested:
- Autonomy of thought – thinking for oneself, making decisions, believing things, making moral assessments
- Autonomy of will (intention) – freedom to do things on the basis of one's deliberations
- Autonomy of action – ability to act.

Autonomy is perhaps the dominant principle of medical ethics. Autonomy is the basis of informed consent and truthfulness, privacy and confidentiality. Other proposed 'principles' such as fidelity (faithfulness) and veracity (truthfulness) can be considered to come under the umbrella of autonomy. Autonomy means that patients can choose what type of treatment they would prefer given a choice, and even choose not to be treated. Autonomy also involves helping the patient to come to his or her own decision. Where a patient is able to make an informed decision, this should be respected even when it appears to be detrimental, illogical or immoral. However, healthcare providers must also be able to recognize situations where a patient is unable to act autonomously. Of course, a person may even make an autonomous decision to leave decision making to someone else.

Autonomy and patient preferences or wishes are not absolute and must be weighed against competing liberties and interests. The opposite of autonomy is paternalism. Paternalism over-rides the principle of respect for autonomy and involves making decisions on behalf of another, usually justified by appealing to the principle of beneficence (the duty to do good) or non-maleficence (the duty not to harm). In the past paternalistic practice was common, but in modern society it is less acceptable, although weak (soft) paternalism can be justified in some cases, such as when acting in the best interests of an incompetent patient. However, strong (hard) paternalism, ignoring or over-riding a competent person's wishes, is difficult to justify.

Non-maleficence

Non-maleficence means not doing harm, often expressed as 'First, do no harm' – a simplification from the Greek 4th century BC Hippocratic oath.

Non-maleficence requires healthcare providers to do everything in their ability to avoid causing, and where possible actively avoid causing, either intentional or unintentional harm. This would include maintenance of competence through continuing education, always acting within the scope of practice and individual ability and doing everything to avoid making mistakes that can harm the patient. Healthcare providers have an ethical (if not legal) obligation to report behaviours by others that adversely (or could adversely) affect the health, safety or welfare of patients – an obligation to report others who are incompetent, impaired (such as from fatigue, alcohol, drugs or mental illness) or are unethical.

Beneficence

Beneficence is an obligation to do good. To benefit the patient is a fundamental goal of health care. Most people enter a healthcare profession because of the opportunity to help others and each profession will have its own definition of what 'good' means.

Beneficence and non-maleficence are often seen as two sides of the same coin. However, while there is a general positive obligation not to do harm, providing benefit (typically to a specific individual) is not always possible.

Desire to help others can come into conflict with the principle of autonomy, as when a patient chooses a course of action that does not appear to coincide with his or her best interest. Beneficence also frequently comes into conflict with non-maleficence. Most medical and therapeutic interventions are associated with some harm (for example, the pain associated with immunization) and benefits have to be balanced against risks. In such instances, we rely on beneficence to ensure that any harm is performed for a greater good.

Beneficence involves doing what is best for the patient. This does raise the question of who should judge what is best. Conflicts between beneficence and autonomy can occur when a competent patient chooses a course of action that the healthcare professional does not consider is in his or her best interests.

Justice

Justice is often synonymous with fairness and equity: a moral obligation to act on the basis of fair adjudication between competing claims. All people of equal need are entitled to be treated equally in the distribution of benefits and burdens regardless of race, gender, religion and socio-economic status, etc. Justice requires that only morally defensible differences among people be used to decide who gets what. Decisions should not be based on capricious or illogical reasons. The logical opposite of justice is discrimination.

Various factors can be used as criteria for the distribution of various resources, for example to each (after Beauchamp & Childress 2001):

- According to their need
- According to their merit
- According to their worth/contribution to society
- An equal share
- According to their effort.

Justice is about equal access to health care. Not all patients have an equal need and it is not always possible to provide the same level of care to all patients at all times. Consequently, a system has to be established to provide care as fairly as possible. For example, in emergency departments, a system of triage is applied in which the most critical patients are treated first on the basis of clinical need.

The four rules

Beauchamp & Childress (2001) analysed veracity, privacy, confidentiality and fidelity in the context of the professional–patient relationship.

Veracity

Veracity is the obligation to tell the truth and is an essential component of informed consent and hence respect for autonomy. It is also closely linked to obligations of fidelity, trust and promise keeping. Veracity is not limited to cases of informed consent. Veracity provides for open and meaningful communication that is an absolute necessity in any moral relationship between two persons. The relationship between healthcare professional and patient needs to be based on mutual trust and honesty.

To Beauchamp & Childress, veracity is prima facie binding. It is not absolute, and non-disclosure, deceiving and lying could be justified when veracity conflicts with other principles such as non-maleficence. Non-disclosure or benevolent deception, but not involving lying, would be more easily justified, as it is less likely to threaten the relationship of trust.

With the complexity and uncertainties of modern medicine, complete honesty and 'whole truth' can be an oversimplification. Just what the truth is can be a matter of clinical judgment. Issues concerning how much information should be given, to whom and in what circumstances create continuing difficulties for healthcare professionals. The obligation of veracity often conflicts with obligations of confidentiality and privacy.

Whistle blowing, calling the attention of authorities to unethical, illegal or incompetent actions of others, is based on the ethical principles of non-maleficence and veracity.

Privacy

An obligation to respect privacy can be seen to come under the ethical principle of respect for a person's autonomy. Privacy relates to a right to restrict access to what a person regards as private and personal and not to be invaded. Beauchamp & Childress consider privacy to include decisions about sharing or withholding information about one's body or mind, one's thoughts, beliefs and feelings.

Confidentiality

Confidentiality relates to the duty to maintain confidence and thereby respect privacy. Beauchamp & Childress define privacy as allowing individuals to limit access to information about themselves and confidentiality as allowing individuals to control access to information they have shared.

Fidelity

Fidelity is the obligation of faithfulness and is concerned with acting in good faith, keeping promises, fulfilling agreements, integrity and honesty. Among the duties of fidelity is the duty of loyalty and an obligation to put the patient's interest first. Issues can arise when there are conflicts of interest or divided loyalties.

Principlist ethics and research

Principlist ethics have dominated the field of health research. The National Commission for the Protection of Human Subjects of Biomedical and Behavioural Research, in the Belmont Report of 1979, identified three basic ethical principles (the so-called Belmont principles):

- Respect for persons
- Beneficence
- Justice.

Respect for persons incorporated two ethical convictions: that individuals should be treated as autonomous agents; and that persons with diminished autonomy are entitled to protection.

Beneficence required that persons be treated in an ethical manner and their decisions respected and protected from harm. It incorporated the concept of non-maleficence by maximizing possible benefits and minimizing possible harms.

Justice required fairness in distribution of benefits and burdens associated with research and subject selection.

Morals and law

Both laws and morals can be considered to be guidelines for conduct. Laws establish minimum standards of behaviour that everyone must meet. The law is influenced by moral and ethical principles but they do not necessarily match. Laws may not necessarily be ethical and many things that are not illegal may still be wrong. Morality is a system of right and wrong enforced through societal pressure. Morals tend to be simple and general rather than precisely defined. They provide general rules that should be applied in particular instances according to circumstances and an individual's conscience. In general, morals correspond to what is done in a society and accord with customs and traditions. Personal morals relate to the values and beliefs that provide the framework for an individual's decisions and actions. Ethics lies somewhat between law and morality. Ethical standards need to be precisely defined but are subject to individual interpretation. Ethics seeks ideal or maximal standards of behaviour.

All law has some moral basis, and in medicine, law, morality and ethics are inextricably linked. Many acts of parliament associated with health care are far from ethically neutral. There are many areas – research on embryos and embryonic stem cells for example – that are a source of deep moral divisions. Sometimes the law acts almost in a knee-jerk fashion, responding to society's moral disquiet, for example the Surrogacy Arrangements Act 1990 prohibiting commercialization of surrogacy and the Human Reproductive Cloning Act 2001 prohibiting the planting of cloned embryos in a womb were both rushed through parliament. Medical science and technology are continuously advancing and at a pace. Situations are having to be addressed before society has had time to thoroughly think them through.

Applied and professional ethics

Applied ethics is the branch of ethics that is concerned with the analysis of specific, controversial issues, arising in specific cases. It uses ethical theories and principles to form judgments. Applied ethics covers a number of areas including business ethics, environmental ethics and bioethics. Bioethics, a contraction of biomedical ethics, is concerned with the interface between the life sciences and ethics. It encompasses medical or healthcare ethics and focuses on issues that arise in healthcare or clinical settings. Professional ethics includes group standards and norms as well as individual ethics.

Ethical issues in health care

Advances and changes in health care and medical technology, the changing relationship between professional and patient and the changing interprofessional roles and their relationships all require an increased ethical awareness in healthcare professionals. Healthcare professionals need to be able to answer ethical questions, work out solutions to ethical problems and resolve ethical dilemmas. Some current issues such as medical research and resource allocation (rationing) appear to reflect a more utilitarian approach to ethics. Issues surrounding the beginning and end of life, cloning and reproductive technologies, and genetic testing clearly do not evoke utilitarian principles alone. In a pluralistic society, there are many different and strongly held moral viewpoints (moral pluralism) which apply to medicine, as is clearly demonstrated with issues such as abortion and euthanasia.

One area, for example, where significant challenges in ethics are likely to occur is in relation to death and dying. The issue of euthanasia encompasses a number of concepts used in moral discussion, such as autonomy, the sanctity of life, quality of life, medical futility, best interests, acts and omissions, double effect and slippery slopes.

The doctrine of double effect embraces two effects, an intended good effect and an unintended secondary bad effect. This justifies giving pain-relief treatment to terminally ill patients provided it is given with the primary intention of relieving pain, and excuses any unavoidable, but unwanted, life-shortening effect of doing so. The central core of the doctrine is the moral distinction between intention and foresight.

The moral distinction between passive and active euthanasia rests largely on the distinction between acts and omissions. To actively end life is both morally and legally wrong, whereas to withhold life-saving treatment could, in some circumstances, be seen as the right thing.

The slippery slope argument is one used against the practice of voluntary euthanasia. The sanctioning of some mildly objectionable practice inevitably leads to some highly objectionable practice. Thus by permitting voluntary euthanasia this will lead down a slippery slope to involuntary active euthanasia.

Ethics and pharmacy

There are legal, ethical and professional implications to every decision and action taken by a pharmacist. While dramatic ethical dilemmas may not be the norm of everyday practice, each encounter with a patient raises ethical issues. Most do not present a dilemma. A dilemma arises from fundamental conflicts among beliefs, duties and principles. An expanded role and increased patient contact increases the opportunity for ethical issues to arise. Pharmacists need to become more comfortable with decision making in conditions of uncertainty. Ethics in practice involves such varied issues as pharmacist–patient relationships, empathy, responsibility and accountability, privacy and confidentiality issues, compliance and adherence, responding to errors, maintaining competence, supply of emergency contraception, abuse of over the counter medicines, supply of homoeopathic medicines, supply of unlicensed medicines, etc. (see Chs 6, 10, 13, 14, 20, 44, 46, 47, 48 and 49).

Ethical dilemmas are not restricted to clinical issues. Studies have reported a willingness of students to engage in some sort of academic dishonesty (Aggarwal et al 2002; Rennie & Crosby 2001). This demonstrates the importance of nurturing and enhancing ethical behaviour in students and helping them to find their 'moral compasses'. Dilemmas may also arise in areas of practice, for example areas of possible conflict of interest, areas concerning NHS fees and remuneration (e.g. dispensing a prescription item at a loss; Thimbleby 2003), as well as personal behaviour, whistle blowing and research, etc.

Professional ethics and law

Laws can be considered an empowering force in healthcare ethics. They define the legal aspects of practice, rights of patients and duties of healthcare professionals. Negligence involves a failure to meet obligations to others and, by attributing fault or blame, clearly has a moral dimension. Standards of care have a moral as well as legal and professional dimension.

However, the law is seen as setting minimum standards, while the others aim for the maximum.

Professional ethics are concerned with the principles of professional conduct concerning the rights and duties of the profession and the professional person himself or herself.

Professional codes and oaths

Professional ethics are concerned with professional values and philosophies. Health professions articulate their profession's values and standards of conduct, and the rights and responsibilities of their members in an ethical code. Codes exist to encourage optimal behaviour and promote a sense of community between members. While codes tend to emphasize duties and responsibilities (deontologically based), a feature of many is their aspirational nature – they strive for upper ideals. They make explicit, to both members and the public, the expectations and ideals central to the profession and so help ensure public trust and confidence in professional practice. Law and professional guidelines alone are unlikely to be an effective way of maintaining professional competence and behaviour. Standards of care are as much about ethics as they are about skills.

Various oaths and codes exist in health care (e.g. the Hippocratic oath), their content having evolved (Box 12.2). Reference to autonomy and justice, as well as the obligation and virtue or veracity, has traditionally been ignored in medical codes (Gillon 1985) and also in pharmacy codes (Rogers & John 2006).

Both law and ethics influence the formulation of the code of ethics and, more recently, so do the ethical principles: respect for people is related to autonomy, competence to non-maleficence and integrity to fidelity. The Code of Ethics for Pharmacists and Pharmacy Technicians 2007 now adopts a principled approach, identifying ethical principles and including inherent value attitudes and behaviours that characterize a

Box 12.2

Origins of codes of ethics

Traditional	**Contemporary**
Duty based	Principles based
Stress beneficence, non-maleficence and professional etiquette	Stress autonomy and justice

good pharmacist (Wingfield 2007a, b, c). The code is intended to promote professional judgment and support professional discretion.

Health care requires a multidisciplinary approach and healthcare professionals can be expected to share some common ethical rules. A shared code of ethics has been advocated and principles identified based on the Tavistock principles (Berwick et al 2001; Smith et al 1999a, b):

- Rights – people have a right to health and health care
- Balance – care of individual patients is central, but the health of populations is also our concern
- Comprehensiveness – in addition to treating illness, we have an obligation to ease suffering, minimize disability, prevent disease and promote health
- Cooperation – health care succeeds only if we cooperate with those we serve, each other and those in other sectors
- Improvement – improving health care is a serious and continuing responsibility
- Safety – do no harm
- Openness – being open, honest and trustworthy is vital in health care.

There has been a resurgence of interest in medical oaths in recent years (Hurwitz & Richardson 1997; Sritharan et al 2001) and such a personal professional pledge has been advocated in pharmacy (Hawksworth 2003, 2004). This could take the form of a personal affirmation encompassing the four ethical principles, some of the virtues such as integrity, honesty, compassion and other key obligations concerned with working practice such as confidentiality and consent.

Ethical decision making

In making ethical decisions, healthcare professionals can refer to law, professional codes and guidelines and to the principles and theories of ethics. Common sense, beliefs and values, intuition and experience also all play a role in influencing the decision. The first step in the process is to recognize that an ethical issue is involved and it is not purely a matter of law or professional etiquette. Ethical issues arise when there is confusion about competing alternatives for action, when interests compete and when none of the alternatives is entirely satisfactory. It typically prompts the question: 'What should I do?' or 'What ought I to do?' This requires a moral awareness or sensitivity. The next stage requires critical thinking and an ability to

make ethical judgments. Typically this benefits from following a structured approach such as:

- Obtaining knowledge of all the pertinent facts
- Identifying the specific ethical issue(s)
- Framing these issues in the context of ethical theories and principles
- Considering – weighing up all available information in order to identify options
- Choosing an option
- Justifying the reasoning behind the decisions
- Reviewing and reflecting.

Wingfield & Badcott (2007) have set out in detail a methodology for ethical decision making, based on a four-stage approach:

- Gather relevant facts
- Prioritize and ascribe values
- Generate options
- Choose an option.

Gathering relevant facts includes ascertaining what law (criminal, civil, NHS) applies and what guidance (codes and guidelines) is available. The second stage is identifying all the individual parties involved and attempting to balance their disparate interests. The third stage involves asking the question 'What COULD I do in this situation?' and the final stage, asking the question 'What SHOULD I do in this situation?' – recognizing that decisions may have to be justified. Finally, so as to develop decision-making skills, professional judgment and practice experience, once the decision has been made and any consequences realized, reflection is required (Wingfield & Badcott 2007).

When applying ethical principles, the principles involved should be identified, asking whether any of these are in competition, and whether one principle should take priority over another. The ethically correct option is typically one that fulfils the most principles. There may not always be right and wrong answers to situations, but there are better and worse ways of dealing with them. The better way would be to analyse an ethical problem by following a structured framework that enables the theories and principles to be critically reviewed and applied.

The importance of reflection cannot be emphasized enough. Most people make decisions at great speed and with little reflection. Experienced pharmacists often do not recognize the processes they use when making difficult choices. By slowing down the process, and breaking it up into stages and steps, it is possible to analyse how decisions were reached. An analysis of what was done, and why, can prove helpful the next time a situation presents with a difficult decision to make.

The virtuous pharmacist

Ethical principles do not in themselves solve ethical dilemmas but merely act as starting points to help identify the issues and concerns. Principles need to be supplemented with compassion, empathy and common sense.

At its simplest, the ethical principles become merely a checklist. Beauchamp & Childress (2001) were keen to assert that the principles-based approach was not designed to provide simple solutions to complex ethical dilemmas:

> Principles do not provide precise or specific guidelines for every conceivable set of circumstances. Principles require judgement, which in turn depends on the character, moral discernment, and a person's sense of responsibility and accountability... Often what counts most in the moral life is not consistent adherence to principles and rules, but reliable character, moral good sense, and emotional responsiveness.
>
> (Beauchamp & Childress 2001, p. 462)

The four focal virtues

One or two virtuous traits do not amount to a virtuous person. A virtuous professional requires a virtuous character, according to Beauchamp & Childress. To that end, they identified four focal virtues:

- Compassion – 'regard for the welfare of others. It combines an attitude of active regard for another's welfare with an imaginative awareness and emotional response of deep sympathy and discomfort at the other person's misfortune or suffering'
- Discernment – 'includes the ability to make judgements and reach decisions without being unduly influenced by extraneous considerations, fears, or personal attachments'
- Trustworthiness – 'Trust is a confident belief in and reliance upon the ability and moral character of another person'
- Integrity – 'means soundness, reliability, wholeness, and integration of moral character ...[it] means fidelity in adherence to moral norms'.

Mapping of values associated with pharmacy (Benson 2006, Benson et al 2007, BMA 1995) have been undertaken in recent years and have identified some of the basic and ancient virtues.

Being a professional is concerned with personal development and striving for professional and moral excellence. In response to the question 'What is a good doctor?', Tonks (2002) identified the following qualities:

- Compassion
- Understanding
- Empathy
- Honesty
- Competence
- Commitment
- Humanity.

The education of a healthcare professional is more than the acquisition of knowledge and skills. There is the need to learn professional behaviour and to acquire a new identity – a professional identity. From entering a professional programme, professionalism, the development of character traits and behaviours associated with professionalism, and the development of a commitment to ethical principles must be nurtured. This process continues throughout professional life.

Conclusion

Why is ethics important and why do healthcare professionals need to study ethics? Because it helps us to consider different perspectives, to respect others and the different needs of others. It helps us to take note of a patient's wishes. It helps personal and professional development. Autonomous professionals are required to make judgments and take decisions and it helps us to analyse these actions and their consequences.

Healthcare professionals have a responsibility to work ethically and personal standards, competence and high ethical standards are essential. Individual reflection on personal standards and ethics is vital. Excellence is not a state but a journey. It requires constant effort and never quite reaching the final destination. Aristotle recognized that it was not easy to be virtuous – otherwise we would not praise it.

KEY POINTS

- Ethics is associated with choices, judgments and decisions, encompassing concepts such as right and wrong, values, duty and obligation. Importantly, ethics is critically reflective and analytical

- Three main ethical theories inform biomedical ethics: utilitarianism, deontology and virtue theory
- Utilitarianism is the most prominent consequentialist theory and actions are judged by their usefulness
- Deontology emphasizes duty and motives

- Virtue theory stresses the importance of the actor's character
- The four key ethical principles in medical ethics are autonomy, non-maleficence, beneficence and justice
- Ethical principles serve as a stimulus to identify ethical conflicts and aid decision making
- A coherent and consistent approach to ethical decision making is needed and requires critical analysis and reflective thinking

13

Communication skills for the pharmacist

Judith A. Rees and Isobel J. Featherstone

STUDY POINTS

- Elements of communication
- Assumptions and expectations
- What is communication?
- Listening skills
- Questioning skills
- The Calgary–Cambridge model
- Patterns of behaviour in communication
- Empathy and its facilitation
- Barriers to communication in the pharmacy
- Confidentiality
- Communicating with those with special needs
- Handling difficult situations

Introduction

Joan is a community pharmacist. At the end of the working day she thinks back to what has happened that day. She has discussed with customers their choice of over the counter (OTC) medicines, advised patients how to use their prescription medicines, conducted a medicines use review, phoned the local GP about a potential drug interaction, supervised a methadone addict, spoken briefly to the district nurse, who popped in to pick up some dressings for a patient, explained to a patient who needed to fill in a prescription exempt payment form, negotiated with her boss about a day off, interviewed a potential sales assistant, disciplined a sales assistant, exchanged pleasantries with the delivery person and had been introduced to the new chairman of the local pharmaceutical committee at lunchtime.

Ravi, a hospital pharmacist, similarly looked back at his working day. He had spent time on the wards discussing drug-related matters with junior doctors and nurses, as well as undertaking medication histories with a couple of patients and talking to a patient about their discharge medication. The latter task involved him phoning the patient's GP and local pharmacist to arrange a continuity of medicine supply. He had helped run an induction course for pre-registration students and given a seminar at the lunchtime journal club for fellow pharmacists. Later in the day he had attended a committee meeting on developing policies for the safe use of medicines in the hospital. Representatives of other healthcare professionals and administrators in the hospital attended this meeting. He had finished off his day with a brief spell supervising the dispensary, when he had to deal with a complaint from a prescriber about an alleged aggressive phone call from pharmacy earlier in the day.

From the above descriptions of two pharmacists' very different working days, it can be seen that while each is performing pharmaceutical tasks, all of these tasks required the use of communication skills. In fact, almost everything we do in life depends on communication. Pharmacists spend a large proportion of each working day communicating with other people – patients, doctors, other healthcare professionals, staff and others. Poor communication has the potential to cause a range of problems, from misunderstandings with healthcare professionals and others caused by incomplete/poor communication to inappropriate or incomplete advice on the use of medication causing potential harm to a patient/customer.

Thus there is a need for effective communication skills for pharmacists. But how effective is our communication? Many are able to talk at length, but do our listeners benefit from our words? Others may find talking to strangers difficult. Good communication demands effort, thought, time and a willingness to learn how to make the process effective. Some people find that good communication is difficult to achieve and an awareness of this fact is an important first step to improvement.

This chapter considers some of the elements of successful communication, looking first at the ways in which we assume things about other people and how this can influence our attitudes and then at the processes involved in communication, listening and questioning skills. A total model for an effective pharmacist–patient consultation is outlined, followed by the barriers to effective communication in pharmacy. The importance of confidentiality and the needs of special groups are considered. Finally there are some difficult situations to consider and practise.

Assumptions and expectations

It is said that you never get a second chance to make a first impression. When we meet somebody for the first time we make assumptions about that person. We often put people into categories and the assumptions lead to expectations of their behaviour, jobs and character.

This initial judgment of a person is often based purely on what we see and hear and includes appearance, dress, age, gender, race and physical disabilities. It is important that we are aware of these assumptions in order to avoid stereotyping people. For example, the impression we have of a person wearing a hooded jacket, baseball cap and jeans may be very different from that of the same person wearing a designer shirt and smart trousers. Conversely, people will make assumptions about us based on initial impressions; e.g. a pharmacist wearing a smart suit in a clean, clinical environment may inspire more confidence than a pharmacist wearing a scruffy jumper and working in a cluttered, untidy environment.

It is well documented that age and gender may affect how we communicate with people because of assumptions and expectations. We should not assume that people in wheelchairs cannot communicate effectively. Likewise, we must ensure that we direct our communication at an appropriate physical level and to the appropriate person (that is, to the patient in the wheelchair, not the person pushing it!).

Demeanour

The way in which people present themselves will lead to certain judgments being made. For example, people who stride aggressively towards someone else may make the person being approached feel defensive because the assumption may be made that they have come to make a complaint. However, people who approach hesitantly may lead to the assumption that this person needs help and advice, perhaps on a potentially embarrassing matter. Both assumptions may be wrong but will affect our behaviour and attitude in subsequent communication with this person.

Tone of speech, accents and common expressions

All of these have an impact on communication. Our response to a person speaking with a whining, complaining tone will differ from our response to someone who greets us in a friendly welcoming manner. Similarly, a cultured, 'BBC' English accent may invoke a different response from that to someone with a strong local accent.

No one experiences the same situation in the same way. While people may appear to be doing similar things, they will have different feelings about them. We can only guess what people are thinking or feeling from how they look and from their behaviour. For example, we may think that people are nervous if they move restlessly or twitch, but that may not be the case. It is also useful for us to consider how aware we are of our own behaviour and appearance and what message this may give to other people.

What is communication?

Communication is more than just talking. It is generally agreed that in any communication the actual words (the talking) convey only about 10% of the message. This is called verbal communication. The other 90% is transmitted by non-verbal communication which consists of how it is said (about 40%) and body language (about 50%). Non-verbal communication is well described in Chapters 22 and 44 and so is not discussed here, but see Example 13.1.

Example 13.1

To test your awareness of communication and assumptions there is a simple exercise. To be effective, you must not read the questions which follow just yet. Spend about 5 minutes talking to a person who you do not know very well – there is no particular topic, just let the conversation flow. After this time, turn away from each other and each write down your answers to the following questions:

1. What did you notice about your partner? What type of facial expression did he/she have? What was his/her posture (or gestures) like? How did he/she speak – tone, speed, volume? What does this tell you about him/her?
2. How aware were you of your own non-verbal communication? What was your facial expression? How were you sitting (posture, position in relation to your partner), gesturing and speaking?

3. What assumptions did you make about your partner? For example, what is his/her taste in food, political persuasion, favourite TV programmes, family background?
4. How accurate were the assumptions that you made? Ask your partner.
5. Do these assumptions say anything about you and the initial judgments you make of people based on sex, age, class, dress, etc.?

Now come back together and share your answers about each other – do they surprise you? If you complete this exercise without 'cheating' you will realize just how many assumptions we make about other people with no evidence for them – and how wrong some of them are!

The communication process

Argyle (1983) describes the message process as a sender encoding a message which is then decoded by the receiver:

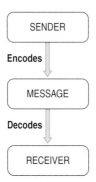

Mistakes can be made by both sender and receiver. The sender may not send the message they wished to send or they may sometimes intentionally seek to deceive. At the receiving end the message may not be decoded correctly. Poor communication skills contribute to these mistakes in encoding and decoding. Messages are not normally one way and if we send a message then we generally expect a reply, and so in replying the receiver becomes the sender and the sender becomes the receiver. While the messages may be going backwards and forwards between two people, effective communication becomes a helical model. In other words, what one person says influences how the other person responds in a spiral fash-

ion with reiteration and repetition, coming back around the spiral at a different level each time.

Pharmacists tend to see contact with patients/customers as either getting information out of, or imparting advice to them. However this ignores the vital purpose of communication, which is to initiate and enhance the relationship with their patients/customers. If this can be achieved, then pharmacists will be perceived as more 'patient friendly' and more supportive of patients. Indeed good communication skills will make it easier for a pharmacist to seek information and advise patients.

Listening skills

Communication is not just about saying the right words; it involves listening correctly. If we do not listen properly, then it means we are not decoding the message that is being sent to us. In other words, however good the patient is at telling the pharmacist their symptoms, if the pharmacist does not listen correctly then the patient may be given the wrong diagnosis or the wrong medicine or the wrong advice. Listening and hearing are different. Hearing is a physical ability while listening is a skill. Listening skills enable a person to make sense of and understand what another person is saying. The listening process is an active one that consists of three basic steps, namely hearing, understanding and judging. The hearing stage means listening enough to catch what the person is saying. The understanding stage takes the listener from hearing to understanding the message in his or her own way (this may not be what was intended by the speaker). The judging stage takes the understanding stage and questions whether it makes sense. Do I believe what I have heard? Is it credible? Have I really understood what I have been told or have I misinterpreted the meaning?

How to be a good listener

Listening, like other skills, takes practice. Tips for developing good listening skills are shown in Box 13.1.

Box 13.1

Tips for being a good listener

- Always look attentive to the person who is speaking. Maintain eye contact and stand/sit facing them. Try not to fidget or move around too much. Do not stare at the floor or look at some other object in the room
- Focus your mind on what is being said. Do not let your mind wander, even if you think you know what is going to be said or you think you have heard it all before
- Always let the speaker finish what they are saying. Do not interrupt – speakers prefer to finish what they were trying to say. In addition, interruption tends to imply that you were not listening
- Let yourself finish listening before you start to talk. Listening is an active process and you cannot really listen if you are busy thinking how to reply
- Listen for the main ideas of the message. The main ideas may be repeated several times by the speaker
- Ask appropriate questions or repeat what has been said in your own words if you are not sure that your understanding is correct
- Give feedback to the speaker by nodding to show you understand (but only if you do). It may be helpful to smile, laugh, grimace or just be silent to let the speaker know that you are listening. Leaning towards the speaker may show you are interested in what the speaker has to say and give them encouragement
- Do not forget the non-verbal side of communication. The speaker may be demonstrating many non-verbal clues and gestures, which may indicate their true feelings. So in the listening process use your eyes as well as your ears

In a pharmacy, avoid listening across a barrier such as a counter or desk, or getting too close and invading a patient's 'intimate zone'

Questioning skills

Pharmacists need effective questioning skills to obtain information from patients/customers. Examples of situations in which questioning skills are used include:

- Drug history taking
- Requests for treatment of minor ailments
- Probing a patient's knowledge of how they take/use their medicines
- Determining the need for an emergency supply.

Effective questioning skills involve the use of different types of questions, namely open and closed questions. These are explained fully in Chapter 44 and their use is discussed in the questioning of patients in the treatment of minor ailments (Ch. 22).

Effective questioning can also be used in symptom analysis, which is another approach to assessing a patient's presenting symptoms. The mnemonic PQRST provides key questions which will help pharmacists to obtain an overview of symptoms, although additional questions can be added, for example 'Is the patient taking any concurrent medication?' The PQRST approach to symptom analysis is shown in Box 13.2.

However, questioning skills do not apply only to pharmacist–patient/customer situations. Good questioning skills are required in staff training, implementing procedures and other management tasks, as well as

Box 13.2

PQRST symptom analysis

- P = Precipitating/palliative factors
  Ask: What were you doing when the problem started? Does anything make it better/worse, such as medicine or change in position?
- Q = Quality/quantity
  Ask: Can you describe the symptom? How often are you experiencing it? What does it feel/look like or sound like?
- R = Region/radiation/related symptoms
  Ask: Can you point to where the problem is? Does it occur or spread anywhere else? Do you have any other symptoms? (These symptoms may be related to the presenting symptoms)
- S = Severity
  Ask: Is the symptom mild, moderate or severe? Asking the patient to grade on a scale 0–10 may help
- T = Timing
  Ask: When did the symptom start? How often does it occur? How long does it last?

dealing with other healthcare professionals and administrative staff.

On many occasions questioning skills may not be in a face-to-face situation. Often a pharmacist has to communicate by telephone with, for example, a GP, a dentist, a district nurse, nursing home staff, hospital staff or patients' relatives. The major drawback of this type of communication is that reliance is put solely on good verbal communication skills and not on the non-verbal aspect of communication. In these circumstances, it is vital to obtain the information as quickly and efficiently as possible. At the same time, the pharmacist must remain professional, give out accurate advice and offer reassurance if necessary. For example, when a GP phones to order a prescription medicine for a patient, the pharmacist is required to ask specific questions to ensure that all information is accurate. As another example, a patient phones to ask about a prescription item that may have been incorrectly dispensed, and, using good questioning skills, the pharmacist would check the prescription information, identify the patient's concerns and be able to take appropriate action.

A model for guiding the pharmacist–patient interview

The Calgary–Cambridge model was developed in 1996 to aid the teaching of communication training programmes for medical students. Since that time it has been adopted widely by medical schools and has been used in other related disciplines (see Ch. 46 in which its use is described for the development of a concordance model for pharmacy, involving patients in decisions about their medicines). The Calgary–Cambridge model is designed to specifically integrate communication skills with the content skills of traditional medical history and thus the approach can be used by pharmacists for their core tasks, such as drug history taking and the interviewing of patients to determine the best treatment of presenting minor ailments.

The Calgary–Cambridge model has five main stages, namely:

- Initiating the session
- Gathering information
- Physical examination
- Explanation and planning
- Closing the session.

Concomitantly and alongside these stages, the model provides for two further ongoing stages:

- Providing structure to the interview
- Building the relationship.

Providing the structure to the interview involves:

- *Summarizing* at the end of a line of enquiry to make sure there is mutual understanding between the pharmacist/prescriber and the patient/customer, before continuing
- *Signposting* – in other words indicating to the patient when moving from one section to the next, e.g. gathering information and explaining
- *Sequencing* – this means developing a logical sequence which is apparent to the patient, in other words do not interrupt information gathering to explain and then go back to information gathering
- *Timing* – this means keeping to time and not being able to close the session or closing abruptly because the time has run out.

Building the relationship during the interview involves:

- *Developing rapport* – being aware of non-verbal behaviour clues and involving the patient in the interview process. Developing rapport has four areas:
  o Acceptance of the patient, their views and feelings and being non-judgmental
  o Empathy with the patient by showing an understanding and appreciation of the patient's feelings or predicament (see later in this chapter, p. 131)
  o Support which expresses itself as concern for the patient, a willingness to help, an acknowledgement of their coping efforts and self-care, e.g. use of OTC medicines, and offering a partnership approach (see Chs 44 and 46)
  o Sensitivity, which includes dealing sensitively with embarrassing and disturbing topics.

Some sensitive areas can be seen in Table 13.1.

An awareness of non-verbal behaviour is the next step in building the relationship. The awareness relates to the interviewers themselves – are they demonstrating good eye contact and other features of positive non-verbal behaviour? Are they picking up on any cues displayed by the patient's non-verbal behaviour? Any note taking or reading (or use of computers these days) should not interrupt or affect the dialogue.

In building the relationship it is important to involve the patient and to share thoughts with them (e.g. 'I think we are looking for a medicine that doesn't cause drowsiness'), to provide a rationale

Table 13.1 Types of patients' problems and the communication difficulties which they present

Problem type	Examples	Communication difficulties
Embarrassing problems	Contraception; disorders of the reproductive system; hyperhydrosis; skin conditions	Obtaining privacy in the pharmacy. Establishing a common language of understanding. Demonstrating empathy and understanding. Establishing trust and confidentiality. Not exhibiting negative non-verbal behaviour
Emotional/ psychological	Anxiety; depression; marital problems; drug abuse and dependence; stress	Demonstrating empathy and understanding. Insufficient time for counselling. Evaluating patient's immediate needs. Establishing the nature and amount of advice to be given. Establishing two-way listening

Problems of handicap
  Sensory
  Physical
  Communicative
  Mental
  Psychological
  Social
	
	Blindness, deafness
	Paralysis, congenital deformity
	Speech impairment
	Educationally subnormal
	Personality disorders
	Introversion
		Making inaccurate judgments regarding personality, intellect, etc. Providing effective explanations. Listening and taking sufficient time with patient. Overcoming social barriers

Terminal illness		Knowing what to say and how to say it. Establishing patient's feelings
Financial problems		Interpreting cues given off by patient. Not embarrassing the patient regarding cost of medicines

for questions (e.g. explain why you need to know about concurrent prescribed medicines when recommending an OTC cough medicine), and to explain and ask permission if a physical examination is necessary.

We will now consider in more detail the stages of the interview process relevant to current pharmacy practice according to the Calgary–Cambridge model in order.

Initiating the session

Preparation involves the interviewer (the pharmacist) preparing him- or herself and focusing on the session. For example, in community pharmacy, a customer may request to see the pharmacist. The pharmacist will need to finish off at an appropriate point whatever task they were doing, probably take a few breaths and then focus on meeting the patient. At this moment it is important to establish initial rapport by greeting the patient, introducing yourself, the role and nature of the interview (e.g. a pharmacist conducting a drug medication history) and obtain consent, if necessary. The next step is to identify the reasons for the consultation by an opening question such as, for a patient requesting to see the pharmacist, 'I understand that you would

like to speak to me – how can I help?' The patient's answer must be listened to attentively and then the pharmacist needs to check and confirm the list of problems/queries/issues with the patient. During this stage the pharmacist should pick up on any verbal and non-verbal behaviour cues and help facilitate the patient's responses. To complete this stage an agenda for the interview is negotiated (e.g. 'so you would like me to recommend a medicine to help relieve your cough that doesn't make you drowsy? Is that right?').

Gathering information

An initial exploration of the patient's problems, either disease or illness, is necessary and the patient should be encouraged to 'tell their tale' in their own words. Clearly the pharmacist needs to listen attentively and question appropriately using different types of question (open and closed) and suitable use of language (e.g. avoiding jargon and very technical language but not in a patronizing way). The pharmacist needs to be aware of verbal and non-verbal cues and the possible need to facilitate responses. It may be necessary to clarify what the person is saying (e.g. 'What do you exactly mean by a stomach cold?'). Certainly it will be necessary to periodically summarize to check your own understanding of what the patient has said. This summarizing also allows the patient to correct any misinterpretation. A further exploration of the disease framework may be necessary and this may include symptoms analysis (see, for example, the PQRST symptoms analysis in Box 13.2) and more focused closed questions. The patient's perspective is taken into account by the Calgary–Cambridge model at this stage in the interview, when a further exploration of the illness from the patient's perspective is undertaken. This further exploration investigates the following:

- The patient's ideas and concerns, i.e. the patient's beliefs on the causes of the illness and their concerns (worries) about each problem, for example the idea that taking medicines might make them dependent on and addicted to the medicine
- The effects on the patient's life of each problem, e.g. concern that a medicine may make them too drowsy to drive
- The expectations of the patient, e.g. that a medicine will instantly make them better
- The patient's feelings and thoughts about the problems, e.g. feeling that no medicine is strong enough to take away the symptoms.

The above are important and may indicate if a patient is unwilling to take, or is untrusting of, modern medicines. They may also indicate that a three times a day regimen and liquid oral medicine would be totally unsuitable for a patient and only a once a day regimen as a capsule would be appropriate. These are important issues for compliance and concordance (see Ch. 46).

Explanation and planning

This is the next stage of the interview, which has three areas, all of which are very appropriate to pharmacists (see Ch. 44):

To provide the correct amount and type of information

- To give comprehensive and appropriate information
- To assess each individual patient's information needs and to neither restrict nor overload
- To make information easier for the patient to remember and understand.

To achieve a shared understanding: incorporating the patient's illness framework (see Ch. 3)

- To provide explanations/plans that relate to the patient's perspective of the problem

- To discover the patient's thoughts and feelings about the information given
- To encourage an interaction rather than one-way transmission.

To plan: shared decision making

- To allow the patient to understand the decision-making process
- To involve the patient in decision making to the level they wish
- To increase patients' commitment to the plans made.

All of the above stages, although designed for medical interviews, are very relevant to pharmacists. Patients need to be involved in decisions about any treatment with medicines, and they need to be given sufficient information on what the medicine is used for and how to take it in a way that is achievable in their lifestyle. Also patients should be offered some information on side-effects so that they can make an informed choice. Chapter 46, on Concordance, clearly expresses this approach.

Closing the session

At the end of the session it is important to summarize what has taken place and the joint decisions made. The patient should also be informed about the next stage; for example this could be seeing how the medicine works and coming back to the pharmacy if the patient feels the medicine is not working. Ensure the patient knows what to do if the problem/symptoms do not resolve (e.g. go to see the doctor), and finally, check whether the patient agrees and feels comfortable with the chosen plan or needs to discuss any other issues.

Patterns of behaviour in communication

A number of terms are used in connection with behaviour during communication:

- *Assertive behaviour* may be defined as standing up for personal rights and expressing thoughts, feelings and beliefs in direct, honest and appropriate ways which do not violate another person's rights. Being assertive involves listening to others and understanding their feelings. An assertive communicator will find a mutually acceptable solution. An important part of being

Box 13.3

List of personal rights

- To state my own needs and priorities
- To be respected as an intelligent and capable equal
- To express my feelings
- To express my own opinions and values
- To say 'Yes' or 'No'
- To make mistakes
- To change my mind
- To say 'I don't understand'
- To ask for what I want (realizing that the other person has the right to say 'No')
- To decline responsibility for others' problems
- To deal with others without being dependent on them for their approval

assertive, therefore, is to formulate your aims and objectives clearly. People who behave assertively deal with other people as equals.

- *Aggressive behaviour* violates others' rights as the aggressive person seeks to achieve goals at the expense of others. Aggressive behaviour is often frightening, threatening and unpredictable. It will bring out negative feelings in the receiver and communication will be difficult.
- *Passive–aggressive behaviour* usually involves a person giving a mixed message; that is, he may agree with what you are saying but then raise his eyebrows and pull a face at you behind your back.
- *Submissive behaviour* is displayed by people who behave submissively, have very little confidence in themselves and show poor self-esteem. They often allow others to violate their personal rights and take advantage of them.

Assertiveness is a positive way of relating to other people – a means of communicating as effectively as possible, particularly in potentially awkward situations. Assertive behaviour is useful when dealing with conflict, in negotiation, leadership and motivation, when giving and receiving feedback, in cooperative working and in meetings. Assertive communication can give the user confidence, a clearer self-image and leads to a feeling of more control over situations, especially those of conflict.

People who behave assertively usually achieve what they set out to do. This does not necessarily mean that the other person does not also achieve what they set out to do. This is in comparison to those who

act aggressively, who think that they have achieved their goal, but this is usually at the cost of respect and loyalty from those around them. Submissive people rarely achieve what they want.

Part of assertiveness is recognition of personal rights and the rights of others. Box 13.3 lists examples of personal rights.

Techniques in assertive communication

Use of 'I' and 'You' statements

Using 'I' rather than 'You' in a statement places the responsibility with the asserter rather than attempting to place the responsibility on the other person. Use of 'I' statements can minimize negative reactions such as anger. For example, compare the following two statements which are effectively saying the same thing: 'You appear to have been arriving rather late for work recently' and 'I have noticed that you have been arriving rather late for work recently'. The first statement gives an impression of accusation while the second is more observational and less threatening.

Repeating the message

If a request for information is not being answered directly by the receiver, a useful assertive technique is to repeat the request. If this is done firmly and without aggression, the message can be repeated until a reply is obtained. However, there are situations when this technique would not be appropriate, e.g. when an answer to the request has been given, even though it may not be the desired response (as when children repeatedly ask for sweets and the parent has already said 'No!'). Repeating this request will not be helpful and will aggravate the situation.

Clear communication

To communicate we use both verbal and non-verbal language. Both are important and it is essential that they match or we will send mixed and confusing messages. An example of a mixed message in a community pharmacy may arise when asking a patient if she understands how to take her dispensed medicine. An affirmative reply may be given verbally by the patient but non-verbal signs such as close examination of the label and a creased forehead may indicate some confusion which would need to be clarified.

Extracting the truth

Strong emotions can get in the way of clear communication. Communicators who are angry or upset may cloud the message they are trying to convey with other issues. They may exaggerate or become emotional. It is important, as the receiver, to accept this in an assertive manner. Acknowledge true criticisms but do not be distracted by side issues.

Self-talk

In a situation of conflict we can often 'work ourselves up' to an angry or emotional state which can then lead to unclear and unsuccessful communication. If we use self-talk (i.e. talk to yourself) and clarify the issues in a situation, considering the points of view and rights of all those involved, not just ourselves, we can often defuse the situation inside ourselves. We can then be ready to undertake clear, unconfused communication which will lead to a more successful outcome. Self-talk does not have to involve 'giving way' to the other person. Rather it is a way of controlling naturally felt emotions and then, instead of 'letting fly', expressing yourself in a manner which is more likely to produce the desired result.

There are a number of steps which you could follow to increase your assertiveness:

- *Choose the right situation.* Choose situations where you believe you have a reasonably good chance of maintaining your assertion, and achieving a mutually acceptable outcome. Changes in behaviour come in small steps, e.g. making requests or giving praise.
- *Prepare for situations.* Spend a short time before an important situation working through the following steps: clarify your objectives, clarify your own and other people's rights, turn 'faulty' dialogues into sound ones, self-talk the assertive statements with which you want to start the interaction and consider your response to anticipated hassles.
- *Behave assertively during the situation.* To overcome unexpected hassles, buy brief thinking time, e.g. 'Have I got this right? What you're saying is . . . ', or 'I'd like to think about that for a moment'.
- *Review the situation afterwards.* Analyse what happened and learn from it. Be honest. Do not play down or exaggerate your success. Never berate yourself. Remember that some people may have a vested interest in your not becoming more assertive.

Empathy

Illness is often associated with different emotional aspects, like uncertainty, stress, fear and dependency. The ability to enter into the life of other people and accurately to understand both their meaning and their feelings is called empathy. It involves an accurate perception and identification of both the actual words and underlying feelings contained in what a person is saying. Pharmacists need the skill to respond in a way that communicates this understanding convincingly. Empathy is one of the cornerstones in communication skills and is an essential part of assertiveness. It is needed in information gathering, when interviewing customers and patients and when educating and counselling. Furthermore, the resolution of conflict situations requires empathic understanding. There are three elements to empathic communication.

Facilitating empathy

Being empathic requires that pharmacists are able to communicate their readiness and willingness to listen to other people and to establish a safe non-threatening atmosphere where they can express themselves. Much of this communication is non-verbal in nature, like eye contact, tone of voice and body posture. There is also a need to express respect and assurance that there is no need for embarrassment or fear of being criticized. People often speak intellectually about a problem rather than saying how they feel. Pharmacists should encourage them to describe their feelings. This does not mean that we should force people to say things they are not ready for.

Perceiving feelings and meaning

The correct identification of feelings and their meaning is important for pharmacists in their work. Patients often experience a combination of feelings, like being unfairly treated, hurt, depressed and angry. These need to be identified in order to respond properly. It is also important to pay attention to non-verbal communication and how closely it agrees with the verbal communication. Facial expressions and body movements may communicate more accurately how the person feels than is being verbally expressed initially. Some words commonly used to express different intensity of feelings are shown in Table 13.2.

Table 13.2 Feeling vocabulary

Feeling	Very strong	Strong	Moderate	Mild
Anxiety	Panic-stricken	Tense	Nervous	Worried
Fear	Terrified	Frightened	Fearful	Uneasy
Happiness	Elated	Joyful	Happy	Pleased
Depression	Suicidal	Depressed	Unhappy	Low
Sadness	Grief-stricken	Distressed	Sad	Sorry
Desire	Craving	Longing	Desirous	Wishful
Confusion	Chaotic	Disorganized	Bewildered	Uncertain
Confidence	Bold	Self-assured	Secure	Adequate

When trying to identify meanings and feelings of others it is necessary to be aware of our own personal biases, prejudices, stereotyped impressions or a pre-occupation with personal concerns. We have our own assumptions about how people, such as those with depression, feel and behave, or stereotyped views, e.g. that all drug addicts are the same.

Responding

The third component, responding, involves the verbal and non-verbal expression of how much we understood and that we are interested to hear more. Often, it may be tempting to just use the phrase 'I understand how you feel'. This may generate the answer 'No, you don't!' It is better to respond by restating and reflecting feelings, i.e. to restate what was said in slightly different words. Another way is to try to help people focus and clarify their own feelings on what is most important for them. You can also verbalize implied meanings or ask for further clarification.

How we communicate empathic listening is important. The most likely way to be effective is by understanding and focusing. Other helpful approaches include quizzing and probing, analysing and interpreting, advising, placating and reassuring. All of these include potential pitfalls but when used appropriately they can be effective. One technique that is rarely effective is generalizing the problem, e.g. when trying to give comfort you say that the problem is 'not serious' or 'everybody has it'. Other ineffective techniques include judging people or their actions, and warning or threatening them.

Just as with all other communication skills, some people are more empathic than others, but empathy and empathic listening can be practised and improved. This requires an active willingness to learn from experience and analyse different situations and our own actions and reactions with an open mind.

Barriers to communication

In a pharmacy setting there are a number of factors which can be of benefit to, or can detract from, the quality of any communication. Common barriers which exist can be identified under four main headings:
- Environment
- Patient factors
- The pharmacist
- Time.

Environment

Community pharmacies, hospital outpatient pharmacies and hospital wards are all areas where pharmacists use their communication skills in a professional capacity. None of these areas is ideal, but an awareness of the limitations of the environment goes part of the way to resolving the problems. Some examples of potential problem areas are illustrated below:

A busy pharmacy. This may create the impression that there appears to be little time to discuss personal matters with patients. The pharmacist is supervising a number of different activities at the same time and is unable to devote his full attention to an individual matter. It is important that pharmacists organize their work patterns in such a way as to minimize this impression.

Lack of privacy. Some pharmacies, both in the community and in hospital outpatient departments, have counselling rooms or areas, but many have not. Many hospital wards could be likened to a busy thoroughfare. For good communication to occur and rapport to be developed, ideally the consultation should take place in a quiet environment, free of interruptions. Lack of these facilities requires additional skills.

Noise. Noise within the working environment is an obvious barrier to good communication. People strain to hear what is said, comprehension is made more difficult and particular problems exist for the hearing impaired. The opposite may also be true, where a patient feels embarrassed having to explain a problem in a totally quiet environment where other people can 'listen in'.

Physical barriers. Pharmacy counters and outpatient dispensing hatches are physical barriers and also may dictate the distance between pharmacist and patient. This in turn can create problems in developing effective communication. A patient in bed (or in a wheelchair) and a pharmacist standing offers a different sort of barrier which will create a sense of inferiority in the patient. Ideally faces should be at about the same level.

Patient factors

One of the main barriers to good communication in a pharmacy can be patients' expectations. In today's world people have busy and hectic lifestyles. In many cases they have become used to seeing a 'good' pharmacy as one where their prescription is dispensed quickly. They are not expecting the pharmacist to spend time with them checking their understanding of medication or other health-related matters. However, once the purpose of the communication is explained, most patients realize its importance and are quite happy to enter into a dialogue.

Physical disabilities. Dealing with patients who have sight or hearing impairment will require the pharmacist to use additional communication skills. Practical suggestions on help which can be given to patients with sight impairment can be found in the chapter on counselling (see Ch. 44). Dealing with the hearing impaired is discussed in lates this chapter.

Comprehension difficulties. Not all people come from the same educational background and care must be taken to assess a patient's level of understanding and choose appropriate language. In some cases the lack of ability to comprehend may be because English is not the patient's first language. Pharmacists working in areas where there is a high proportion of non-English speakers may find it useful to stock or develop their own information leaflets in appropriate languages.

Illiteracy. A significant proportion of the population, both in the UK and in other countries, is illiterate. For these patients written material is meaningless. It is not always easy to identify illiterate patients as many feel ashamed and are unlikely to admit to it, but additional verbal advice can be given and pictorial labels can be used. For example the United States Pharmacopoeia has designed a range of pictograms for this purpose.

The pharmacist

Not all pharmacists are natural, good communicators. Identifying strengths and weaknesses will assist in improving communication skills. Some of the weaknesses which can be barriers to good communication are:

- Lack of confidence
- Lack of interest
- Laziness
- Delegation of responsibilities to untrained staff
- A feeling of being under pressure, especially time pressure
- Being preoccupied with other matters.

If any of these characteristics is present, the reason for it should be identified and resolved, if possible.

Time

In many instances time, or the lack of it, can be a major constraint on good communication. Try developing a meaningful conversation with someone who constantly looks at his watch! Similarly, if the person who has initiated the conversation is short of time, the wrong kind of questions may be used or little opportunity for discussion will be allowed. It is always worthwhile checking what time people have available before trying to embark on any communication. That way you will make the best use of what time is available.

Not all barriers to good communication can be removed, but an awareness that they exist and taking account of them will go a long way towards diminishing their negative impact.

Confidentiality

Matters related to health and illness are highly private affairs. Therefore it is important that privacy and confidentiality are assured in the practice of pharmacy.

According to the public, lack of privacy is one of the most important issues when developing pharmacy services. The public expects pharmacists to respect and protect confidentiality and have premises that provide an environment where you can communicate privately without fear that personal matters will be disclosed. There is a need to maintain the trust of the public by communicating in such a way that no doubts about lack of privacy or confidentiality arise. This concerns the whole staff of the pharmacy, not just the pharmacists.

Physical privacy can be assured by providing facilities (not necessarily always private counselling rooms) that allow communication without somebody else overhearing a private conversation. In addition there is a need to provide psychological privacy and this has much to do with how things are perceived. It is possible, by appropriate communication, to minimize the impact of distracting factors. The techniques are often non-verbal, such as proper use of the voice (not too loud, not too low), eye contact, leaning forward and concentrating on the person and their problem.

Ethical guidelines and privacy laws set the rules about confidentiality in pharmacy. Any information relating to an individual which the pharmacist or any other staff member acquires in the course of their professional activities has to be kept confidential. When communicating with other healthcare professionals it may be difficult to draw the line between what is acceptable and what is not acceptable. Without the consent of the person, only information to prevent serious injury or damage to the health of the person can be shared. We must act in the interests of patients and other members of the public. When communicating with patients/customers it is also important to respect patients' rights to participate in decisions about their care and to provide information in a way in which it can be understood.

Special needs

Patients with special needs must be considered carefully when adopting questioning skills. We need to be non-patronizing, avoid the use of jargon and adopt a procedure for obtaining information which is acceptable to the patient. Blind people will not be able to read any written material, unless it is in Braille. Special labels are available. They may also require some compliance aids to assist with measuring doses.

Many customers who come into pharmacies will suffer from a degree of hearing impairment. Studies have shown that one in six of the adult population in the UK has clinically significant hearing loss. By retirement age (61–70 years old), around 34% of people have significant hearing loss; this increases to 74% in people aged over 70. Considering that people in these age groups present the highest number of prescriptions, it is evident that pharmacists must implement appropriate communication skills.

Recognizing the profoundly deaf is usually simpler than recognizing those who have hearing impairment. The following guidelines may be useful for identifying these customers.

How to recognize the hearing impaired

A person with hearing difficulty is likely to do one or more of the actions listed in Box 13.4. Having recognized a customer with hearing impairment, the

Box 13.4

Actions usually associated with people with hearing difficulties

- Speak in an unusually loud or soft voice
- Turn their head to one side or cup a hand to their ear while listening
- Concentrate on lips while being spoken to
- Give inappropriate responses to questions
- Have a blank or confused expression during conversation
- Frequently ask speakers to slow down or repeat information
- Are unable to hear a conversation when they cannot see the speaker's mouth
- Are unable to carry on a conversation in a noisy environment

Box 13.5

Guidelines when speaking to the hearing impaired

- Ask them how they wish to communicate
- Make sure that background noise is at a minimum
- Look directly at the person and do not turn away
- Make sure sufficient light is on your face
- Do not hide your face or mouth behind hands, pens, etc.
- Do not shout
- Keep the normal rhythm of speech but slow down slightly
- Articulate each word carefully and exactly, particularly emphasizing consonants
- If a sentence is not heard, rephrase it or write it down
- Do not change the subject in mid-sentence

guidelines in Box 13.5 are helpful. Listening, and being able to demonstrate that you are listening, is very important using non-verbal responses for the deaf.

Difficult situations in pharmacy

There are times in all our lives when we have to deal with 'difficult situations'. Good communica-

tion skills may not always produce the perfect result but can help prevent making a situation worse. Further examples of difficult situations in pharmacy can be found in Table 13.1 and Example 13.2.

Conclusion

Good communication is not easy and needs to be practised. We all have different personalities and skills which means that we have strengths in some areas and weaknesses in others. If we can become aware of, and maximize, our strengths and work to minimize our weaknesses, we will become better communicators. Being articulate and able to explain things clearly is of great importance to a pharmacist. However, listening with understanding and empathy is of equal, and in certain situations of greater, importance. We may all hear the words being said, but are we really listening to the complete message?

This chapter has emphasized communication skills for pharmacists, particularly in the workplace, but remember, good communication is a life skill to be used at all times.

Example 13.2

Read through the following scenarios and think carefully how you would react and deal with such a situation in real life. Consider how the other person would be feeling. Remember, there is no one perfect answer. Discuss the scenarios with a friend or group of friends. This will also allow you to identify the different ways people react to the same situation.

1. A young girl returns to your pharmacy to purchase laxatives. You notice that she has been buying them fairly regularly, and decide to tackle the situation. How would you approach this as the pharmacist? How do you think the young girl will react?

2. A drug addict asks to purchase some 1 mL 'insulin' needles. You know that there is a needle exchange scheme at a pharmacy on the other side of town. How do you give this advice to the addict, or advise him on the safe disposal of the needles? How do you think the addict would react?

3. A hospital prescription for morphine, written for pain relief in a terminally ill patient, has been written incorrectly by a junior doctor. The doctor has already

been on duty for 8 hours. How do you approach her? How do you think she will react?

4. Worried parents ask for your advice as a pharmacist. They have found some tablets in their son's bedroom. You identify them, and they are drugs that have the potential for misuse and abuse. How do you handle this situation? How do you think the parents will react? Consider the feelings/reaction of the son. Where does confidentiality come into this?

5. A middle-aged man comes storming into your pharmacy. You have given him the wrong strength of tablets and he is very angry. What are you going to say to him and how? How do you think the man will react?

6. An older lady wishes to purchase some codeine linctus 'for someone else'. After much soul searching and questioning, you decide to sell her a 100 mL bottle. She returns 10 minutes later with a broken bottle (and not much evidence of codeine linctus). She claims she has dropped it, and wants a replacement. What are you going to say to her?

KEY POINTS

- Communication consists of both verbal and non-verbal communication
- After the spoken word, facial expression is probably the most important part of communication
- Eye contact must be maintained, but must not become a stare
- An awareness of personal space is needed to allow effective communication
- Assertive behaviour treats other people as equals, and is not to be confused with aggressive behaviour, which violates other people's rights
- Empathy (active listening) involves understanding other people's feelings and reflecting this back to them

- Questioning skills are important and may use different types of questions, e.g. open, closed
- Listening skills involve more than just hearing
- In the working environment there are many potential barriers to effective communication, including the environment, patient and pharmacist and the time implications
- Confidentiality must be assured in the practice of pharmacy
- Patients with special needs must be catered for in pharmacy and the development of good communication skills by pharmacists will be helpful
- Hearing loss is common in the elderly and will present a barrier to effective communication
- Pharmacists need to maximize their strengths and minimize their weaknesses of communication

14

Relationship with other members of the healthcare team

Felice S. Groundland

STUDY POINTS

- The other members of the healthcare team that work directly with the pharmacist
- The roles played by the other members of the healthcare team and how the pharmacist interacts with them
- The role of technicians, dispensers and medicine counter assistants and their qualifications
- The importance of leadership, delegation, negotiation and teamworking and how to achieve these

Introduction

There are seven principles in the Code of Ethics for Pharmacists and Pharmacy Technicians. These state that a pharmacist or pharmacy technician must:

1. Make the care of patients their first concern
2. Exercise their professional judgment in the interests of patients and the public
3. Show respect for others
4. Encourage patients to participate in decisions about their care
5. Develop their professional knowledge and competence
6. Be honest and trustworthy
7. Take responsibility for their own working practices

All the above principles have to be adhered to by all pharmacists and technicians. However, to achieve these principles, pharmacists cannot work in isolation if they are to provide the best service to the public. Nowadays most pharmacists work as part of a team with other healthcare workers. If

this team is to work efficiently to provide good pharmaceutical services to the public, then a good working relationship needs to be developed between all the members of the healthcare team. In many situations the pharmacist will be the manager/supervisor or responsible person for the team, as, for example, in a community pharmacy. In other situations the pharmacist may be part of a team but not responsible for the team, for example as a member of an ethics committee or team developing educational materials for use by ward staff in a hospital.

The relative position of the pharmacist in a team will determine the skills required to undertake an efficient role. If the pharmacist is the leader/manager/supervisor or responsible person for the team then the required essential skills will be leadership, managing/supervising and delegation. In order to delegate the pharmacist must be confident in the skills of the team and therefore may need to assess the training needs of the team members and organize any required training. Negotiating skills will also be needed but will be crucial if the pharmacist is part of, but not responsible for, a team. In such a situation the pharmacist must be a good teamworker.

What is teamwork?

Teamwork can be defined as the process whereby people work together cooperatively to deliver goals. The goals will vary depending on the type of team but it is essential that these goals are well defined. In any team it is important that each member knows the role they play and how they contribute to the goals. The introduction of standard operating procedures (SOPs; see Chs 7, 24, 43) has gone a long way in helping define each member's role and responsibility as well as fulfilling UK clinical governance criteria.

The following skills and attributes would be desirable for successful teamwork:

- *Listening skills* – within any team all members should be encouraged to speak out and offer suggestions for improvement which in turn may trigger other ideas from the other team members.
- *Questioning skills* – to always question why things are done the way they are and not to blindly accept something because that is the way it is always done.
- *Respect* – treat others as you would want to be treated yourself. This comes back to being an effective leader. Effective leaders command respect. However, all members of the team should be treated with respect for the role that they play in the team. After all, all members of the team and their role in the team are necessary for a productive, efficient team. All team members should treat each other with respect.
- *Helping* – this is the true essence of teamwork and ensures that everyone is involved in reaching the goals.
- *Sharing* – this means sharing ideas and information. If one person keeps important information to himself or herself, then the team will not function properly. Sharing also means that no one person should take the glory for the team's efforts as everyone has had a part to play.
- *Collaborating* – all members are encouraged to participate in the team and when there is a high level of collaboration then you will have an effective team. This requires elements of trust, shared goals and clarity of roles.
- *Communication* – a skill required in all areas and will involve communication on all levels, e.g. e-mail, meetings where face-to-face communication will be important or the written word. It is crucial not to be misunderstood at any level.

The healthcare team

The healthcare 'team' can be defined in a number of ways and will depend on the work environment of the pharmacist.

In community pharmacy the immediate team that the pharmacist works with on a day-to-day basis is made up of:

- Pharmacy technicians
- Accuracy checking technicians
- Dispensing/pharmacy assistants
- Medicines counter assistants or healthcare assistants/advisors.

The terminology will vary depending on the individual company or business.

The community pharmacist will also be involved with external people, depending on their job role – the extended 'team':

- A pharmacist providing services to residential or nursing homes will be in constant communication with the care home staff and a variety of clients, e.g. the elderly, children and psychiatric patients
- Communication will take place with the GP practices and their staff on a daily, weekly or monthly basis depending on requirements, e.g. receptionists, practice managers, practice nurses, practice physiotherapists, asthma and stoma nurses, etc.
- The pharmacist will also be in contact with healthcare professionals in the local area, for example community or district nurses, health visitors, psychiatric nurses, Macmillan nurses, physiotherapists
- The community pharmacist may liaise with the local drug misuse teams depending on the services provided in that pharmacy
- Other groups of professionals the pharmacist may have contact with include dentists, chiropodists and ophthalmic opticians and social workers
- Community pharmacists will have to work with the local primary care trust and its pharmacist representatives on clinical governance matters and contract negotiations.

This list is not exhaustive but gives an idea of the variety of people/professions the community pharmacist has to consider when providing expert patient care. They will interact on a daily basis when dealing with specific problems related to individual patients' care, selection of drugs by the healthcare professional, dealing with drug interactions, etc.

In a hospital pharmacy the pharmacist will also interact with pharmacy technicians but will have a closer working relationship with the nurses and doctors directly involved in the patients' care on a daily basis and with far more ease of contact than the community pharmacist has with the community GP. When dealing with the junior doctors and nursing staff in hospital the pharmacist will have a teaching/supportive role while assuming an advisory role on the use and side-effects of drugs when dealing with the more experienced consultants. Hospital pharmacists will also be in contact with other professionals with regard to discharging patients into the community, such as social workers, physiotherapists, occupational therapists, dentists and the local drug misuse team. Within the hospital environment the pharmacist may have to become involved with the various hospital committees, e.g. drug safety, ethics, general administration, formulary, etc. and interact with a range of professional as well as administrative roles. In addition, hospital pharmacists will be in contact with community pharmacists to ensure a seamless supply of medicines to those patients discharged from hospital on specialized drug regimens.

The changing role of the pharmacist as discussed in Chapter 1 has made it even more important that the pharmacist depends on their healthcare team to free up the time to allow them to deliver the various services required by the new pharmacy contracts. The pharmacist is moving further away from the traditional role of being 'counters and pourers and stickers and lickers' to advising patients and customers on their medicines, conducting medicine use reviews (MURs), promoting health advice, etc. (see Chs 5 and 47).

The community healthcare team

Medicines counter assistants/ healthcare assistants

From 1 July 1996 it has been a professional requirement that each member of staff whose work in a pharmacy will regularly include the sale of medicines must have completed a course or be undertaking an accredited course relevant to their line of work. The Royal Pharmaceutical Society of Great Britain's (RPSGB) requirement is that the courses should cover the knowledge and understanding associated with units 2.04 and 2.05 of the Scottish/National Vocational Qualification (S/NVQ) level 2 in Pharmacy Services. These are

entitled 'Assist in the sale of OTC medicines and provide information to customers on symptoms and products' and 'Assist in the supply of prescribed items (taking in a prescription and issuing prescribed items)'.

There is a requirement that the course should be completed within a 3-year time period and that the member of staff should be enrolled on such a course within 3 months of starting their role.

The following training programmes for medicines counter assistants/healthcare assistants have been accredited for the RPSGB by the College of Pharmacy Practice:

- AAH Retail Pharmacy
- Boots the Chemist
- Buttercups Training
- CMP Information Ltd.
- Moss Chemist
- National Pharmacy Association
- Superdrug
- Tesco Stores Ltd.

Medicines counter assistants/healthcare assistants will primarily be found in community pharmacy in residential areas and supermarkets. Their training usually takes the form of 'workbook-led on-the-job learning', meeting the above requirements for accreditation with the pharmacist acting as the tutor. This allows the relationship to develop and the pharmacist to realize the potential and limitations of these members of staff.

Dispensing/pharmacy assistants

The training required is much more in-depth than for the medicines counter/healthcare assistant to reflect the variation in role and responsibilities. The job title will vary depending on the sector of pharmacy the person works in and indeed the company/business they work for – dispenser, dispensing assistant, pharmacy assistant, assistant technical officer, etc. Whatever their title or sector of pharmacy they are working in, what they all have in common is that they are working under the supervision of the pharmacist.

From 1 January 2005 there is the professional requirement that these dispensing/pharmacy assistants are competent in the areas in which they are working to a minimum standard which is equivalent to the new

Pharmacy Services S/NVQ level 2 qualification or are undertaking such training.

This applies to staff working in the following areas:

- As for the medicines counter or healthcare assistants with units 2.04 and 2.05 qualifications (see above)
- The assembly of prescribed items including the production of labels
- Ordering, receiving and storing pharmaceutical stock
- The supply of pharmaceutical stock
- Preparation for the manufacture of pharmaceutical products, including aseptic products where relevant
- Manufacture and assembly of medicinal products, including aseptic products where relevant.

To fulfil this requirement a training programme relevant to the job needs to be completed within a 3-year time period and the member of staff should be enrolled on such a course within 3 months of starting their role. If a member of staff has not undertaken such a course but they fulfil the requirements of the 'grandparent clause' and a declaration of competence has been sent by their supervising pharmacist to the RPSGB during the 'grandparenting' period, then the member of staff does not need to undertake further study to remain a dispensing/pharmacy assistant. (The 'grandparent clause' recognizes that existing staff may already have completed an appropriate course and/or have relevant experience.)

The dispensing/pharmacy assistant is a key member of the healthcare team as they free up the pharmacist from the assembly processes involved in the dispensing of prescriptions.

Pharmacy technician

A pharmacy technician is someone who has undertaken a course that provides them with an S/NVQ Pharmacy Services level 3 qualification. The 'pharmacy technician grandparent clause' has allowed a number of other qualifications, formerly recognized as pharmacy technician qualifications, to be acceptable for registration purposes. Further details on these qualifications can be verified with the RPSGB.

Once qualified, the pharmacy technician may choose to join the register of technicians. This was a voluntary register opened by the RPSGB in January 2005 but registration is now a requirement for those wishing to use the title 'pharmacy technician' (this title is protected in law). By doing so they are bound by the Code of Ethics and must participate in continuing professional development – the same requirement as for pharmacists.

The pharmacy technician may work in hospitals, community pharmacy, health centres, primary care trusts, prisons and the armed forces and in the pharmaceutical industry. We will focus on community and hospital pharmacy.

Community pharmacy

Pharmacy technicians are required to make up the prescriptions issued by doctors. These are then checked by the pharmacist both for accuracy and to make sure that the dosage and treatment are safe for that patient, i.e. a clinical check.

The role of the technician involves:

- Reading prescriptions and translating doctor's instructions
- Counting tablets and measuring specific quantities of liquids
- Preparing accurate labels for medicines on the computer system which usually inform the patient what the drug is and how to use it
- Selling other medicines and other complementary preparations
- Referring to the pharmacist when appropriate
- Small-scale or individual preparation of extemporaneous products as requested by the doctor which are not supplied as ready to use by manufacturers
- Maintaining and managing stock within the pharmacy
- Record keeping and audit
- Being aware of the legal requirements relating to prescribing and supply of medicines.

As can be seen there is considerable overlap with the dispensing/pharmacy assistant role, but with additional responsibilities.

The pharmacy technician may choose to become an accuracy checking technician (ACT), which would require them to undertake a further period of study and development of a portfolio of evidence to demonstrate their competence in this area. The technician must have successfully checked 1000 items error free in a defined period of time (usually 4 weeks) while keeping a diary of all items checked and any errors made while checking or dispensing and completing any assignments required by the employer. They then have a final assessment which requires them to check the accuracy of a set amount of prescription items under timed conditions.

The checking technician plays an invaluable role. They will accuracy check the prescriptions once the pharmacist has clinically checked them. This has not only been shown to be more accurate than pharmacist checking but also, more importantly, it frees up the pharmacist to get on with the other new roles that are emerging, such as carrying out MURs in England, being involved in the electronic minor ailment scheme (eMAS) in Scotland, supplementary and independent prescribing, etc.

Hospital pharmacy

The work in the hospital pharmacy setting for a pharmacy technician has many similarities to that in the community sector. However, the work has greater variation due to the different areas for care within hospital. These include:

- Visits to the wards to take orders for medicines
- Preparation of radioactive materials or working on clinical trials
- Use of computers and robotics for purchasing, stock control and dispensing
- Production of medicines in special sterile units requiring specialist clothing and working in a sterile environment
- Working in manufacturing or production units in some hospitals.

Hospital pharmacy has also had the role of the ACT in place for a number of years now and the criteria for this role are similar to those described above for the community role.

Other members of the pharmacy team

There are other people who can play an important role in the pharmacy team but they are not present in every pharmacy team at all times. These are pre-registration pharmacy trainees and also pharmacy undergraduates either taking part in a period of vocational placement or working on a part-time basis in the pharmacy setting.

Pre-registration pharmacy trainees will have completed 4 years of study at university and obtained an accredited degree in pharmacy. In order

to become a pharmacist they are required to undertake a period of training, usually 1 year within a pharmacy setting, either community or hospital. Some may choose to enter industry and carry out a split placement between this sector and hospital but these only account for a small number of the graduates. At the end of the training period the graduate has a registration examination to undertake and pass before they can enter the pharmacy profession. During the training year the pre-registration pharmacy trainee becomes a valuable member of the team while turning their university knowledge into practical skills within the pharmacy. It is important that at this time the trainee has the end goal of pharmacist in mind and does not become absorbed into the day-to-day tasks of the job. The pre-registration pharmacy trainee is given guidance from their tutor throughout this period.

Pharmacy undergraduates join the pharmacy team at any time depending on the needs of the pharmacy setting. Some may work on a part-time basis at weekends, others for a period of time during the university breaks to gain experience in the different areas of pharmacy and decide where they will complete their pre-registration training.

Role of the pharmacist in teamwork

The role of the pharmacist, both in the primary and secondary care setting, is changing. No longer can the pharmacist work in constant isolation: they must learn to become integrated members of both their immediate and extended teams, and so it is essential for the pharmacist to recognize that team leading, delegation, negotiation and teamworking are essential skills that they must possess.

Leadership

There have been a lot of studies carried out to determine what it is exactly that makes good leaders. The majority of these studies lead to the conclusion that leadership is about the behaviour of the leader first and the skills that they possess second. It is about recognizing that people need to trust and respect you before they will listen and act on what you ask them to do.

In any one environment there can be a number of different teams working together, e.g. in the hospital setting or the community setting, and sometimes one particular team will outperform the others. Why is this?

In all cases it is attributable to the person leading the team and the fact that they possess such qualities as integrity, honesty, humility, courage, commitment, sincerity, passion, confidence, positivity, wisdom, determination, compassion and sensitivity. This makes their staff willing to go that 'extra mile' for them. Some people are naturally born with these behaviours already well developed but others, recognizing that these behaviours are important, can develop this side of their behaviours to achieve great leadership qualities.

A good leader will be able to use a number of different leadership styles depending on the situation they are faced with. Again some people have a dominant style of leadership, but to be truly great they need to look at all the other styles of leadership and develop these also.

As a pharmacist it is important to recognize that no matter what area of pharmacy you work in you will always be looked upon as the leader of that team, and it is crucial to know your own strengths and weaknesses and build on these. This is where continuing professional development (CPD) really comes into play. This is discussed in more detail in Chapter 10. CPD is the process whereby the pharmacist can effectively identify and plan what they need to address to develop their leadership qualities or indeed any area that will benefit their professional career.

The correct behaviour, especially towards your team, is the key to being an effective leader and the following are some tips towards being respected as a leader:

- Honesty and integrity – without this no one in your team will respect you
- Never shout at people no matter how angry you get as this only serves to break down the relationships built with the team ('praise loudly, blame softly' – Catherine the Great 1729–1796)
- Always lead by example – if you are not seen to be 'doing' then the message that sends to others is that it is not important to be hard working
- Recognize when you need to work with your team to get tasks done – nothing should be beneath you and you should never be afraid to 'get your hands dirty'
- You need to treat all members of the team fairly and based on merit, not singling people out

because they like the same football team, for example

- On the other hand you need to be seen to be dealing with any bad or unethical behaviour of team members. Ignoring this type of behaviour is giving out the message that you condone it
- Listen to your team and try to understand their point of view – it is sometimes important to place yourself in someone else's shoes to see their point of view. This does not mean you have to agree with everything but it will give you a better understanding of where they are coming from
- Accept the responsibility for when things do not go as planned – do not blame the team or individuals within the team
- Always give credit where credit is due even for your own successes, because you would never have got there without your team behind you ('Behind an able man there are always able men' – Chinese proverb)
- Provide support for the team so they know that they can trust you to act in their best interests
- Always ask for opinions and ideas from the team so that they feel that they are involved in the decisions you may make, especially if things need to change. It is easier to handle change if the team members have been involved from the beginning
- If you agree to do something then make sure you follow through – do not make empty promises as you will quickly lose the trust of your team
- Encourage the development of your team, giving them responsibility for certain tasks that stretch their abilities without putting undue pressure on them
- Be positive, even about things that have gone wrong – we can always learn from this and make things better the next time
- Have fun in the workplace – your staff should feel happy in the work they do and in the environment they work in as they spend so much time there; there is no point being miserable
- Smile!
- Remember why you are all there – what is the job in hand?
- Seek feedback from others to find ways you can develop and improve your skills and behaviours and recognize that we never stop learning.

No pharmacist can do all the tasks themselves so it is essential that they recognize that many tasks need to be delegated to the other team members.

Delegation

Good delegation will save you time, will develop your team and generally motivates all involved. It is not just a technique to free up time. Poor delegation will lead to frustration, demotivation among your team and failure of the task(s) involved so it is essential that delegation is effective.

When delegating tasks one should follow the SMARTER mnemonic. To ensure success on completion then all delegated tasks must be:

- *Specific* – if it is unclear what the task is, then how can it be completed effectively? Can this task, in fact, be delegated?
- *Measurable* – you have to be able to measure when the task has been completed to know that success has been achieved. What is the end goal or measure to demonstrate this? This needs to be clearly defined.
- *Agreed* – both parties must be in agreement to the task otherwise this is where frustrations and resentments start to form. Is the individual or team capable of doing the delegated task? Do they understand the bigger picture and where they fit in?
- *Realistic* – if the task is not achievable, either because of timescales or lack of the necessary skills or resources, then this will only serve to demotivate the person involved.
- *Timebound* – the task should not be so great that it cannot be completed in the timescales agreed, so this comes back to the task being realistic. If it is an ongoing task then specific review dates need to be in place and adhered to and agreed outcomes clearly defined, e.g. generation of reports, targets reached, etc.
- *Ethical* – you should not be asking your team to carry out a task that goes against their professional or moral ethics.
- *Recorded* – this is important to celebrate the successes of your team if you keep a record of the tasks that have been completed and it also helps to learn from tasks that have not been completed and enables you to provide constructive feedback to your team when things do not go as planned.

It is extremely important for the pharmacist to be able to delegate various tasks within the pharmacy to suitably trained persons because it is no longer cost-effective for the pharmacist to be carrying out tasks that others are more than qualified to complete. Thus this frees the pharmacist to get on with the job they were educated at university to do and leads to job satisfaction for all staff involved.

In order to get the members of the immediate and extended teams on board the pharmacist has to be aware of, and if necessary develop, their negotiation skills.

Negotiation

Negotiation is something that we do all the time in and out of the working environment and maybe do not realize it, e.g. deciding what to see at the cinema, where to go out to eat, where to go sightseeing on holiday, what shift someone should work and for how long, etc.

Negotiation is usually considered as a compromise between people to get what we want. To be really effective in the team environment the compromise should allow both parties to be satisfied with the eventual outcome. The only time you may want to consider the win–lose negotiation is if you do not need to have an ongoing working relationship with the other party. This is something that is going to be very unlikely in the pharmacy setting. If the pharmacist always negotiates to 'win' then the working relationship within the team will eventually break down and the working environment will suffer. Ultimately patient care deteriorates as no one works together.

Communication is the key link that will be used to negotiate and as such can be in a variety of ways – face to face, in writing, over the telephone, etc. (see Ch. 13). Body language is thus another area that the pharmacist may wish to develop as body language accounts for over 90% of a conversation.

For successful negotiation to occur the following should be considered:

- Goals – what do you need to get from the negotiation and do you know what the other party also wants? You need to be really clear why you are negotiating and think about what you will accept before entering into the negotiation.
- Separate people from the problem – do not get caught up in personalities and relationships and

focus on what the actual issues are. It will be a lot easier to justify a decision reached if the results are based on objective criteria.

- Generate a variety of possible solutions – no matter how ridiculous they might first sound – before going on to decide the best option to meet everyone's needs. Sometimes asking the other party 'What do you think?' might allow them to actually come up with a solution that you had not thought about but which fulfils everyone's needs.

Pharmacists in both the primary and secondary care sector are now required to work very closely together to deliver the government targets for access to health care, provision of services outside normal working hours in addition to the range of services and roles detailed in the new pharmacy contracts. As mentioned, pharmacists are dependent on the skills of their immediate teams to be able to fulfil these new roles and have to be able to demonstrate that they meet the clinical governance requirements. This requires a great deal of teamwork both within the immediate teams and the extended teams.

Conclusion

Pharmacists may work well in their immediate teams but if they are to embrace the changing role of pharmacy and health care then they need to extend their teamworking across a wide variety of healthcare professionals and embrace all the skills highlighted above.

It is essential that pharmacists start to maintain a formal record of all their contributions and interactions within the wide variety of teams to demonstrate their invaluable contribution to patient care.

KEY POINTS

- To meet their professional responsibilities pharmacists need to work with a wide variety of other healthcare staff
- A range of communication skills is required to be effective teamworkers together with the ability to respect, help, share and collaborate with others
- A healthcare team will be either an immediate or an external team
- In community pharmacy, the immediate team will be staff trained to carry out specific responsibilities
- External team members could include other pharmacists, doctors, nurses, health visitors, physiotherapists, drug misuse teams, dentists, chiropodists, opticians and administrators
- The exact role which the pharmacist has will depend on relative experience and knowledge
- There are detailed requirements for qualifications required of different levels of pharmacy support staff
- Some pharmacists will have to assume leadership roles, which requires a wide range of skills, some of which may have to be learned as part of CPD
- Delegation is often a necessity but has to be effective and achievable. The mnemonic SMARTER can be a useful guide
- Negotiation is frequently part of making progress in a healthcare team

15

Record keeping

Mary Zargarani

STUDY POINTS

- The types of records pharmacists keep and why they keep them
- How the law and the code of ethics affect pharmacists' record keeping

Introduction

Pharmacists are required to keep a number of different types of records within the pharmacy, the majority of them being legally required and some as good practice. With the evolving role of pharmacists, the need for and types of records to be kept are ever increasing. The aim of this chapter is to consolidate the different aspects and issues around record keeping in the pharmacy.

Why keep records?

There are many things that need to be recorded in the pharmacy. They can be categorized into three main groups; however, it should be noted that there can be considerable overlap between these groups:

- Records of supply, e.g. controlled drug register entry
- Clinical governance records, e.g. dispensing incident reporting and audit
- Consultation records, e.g. giving advice on weight loss to a diabetic patient.

Aside from the fact that many of these records are required legally or as part of the pharmacy's contractual requirements with the NHS, there may be different reasons why each type of record is made. The traditional records of supply and clinical governance are mainly kept for the purpose of invoicing and to provide an audit trail for monitoring standards, improving quality and ensuring safety.

Pharmacists may well be the only healthcare profession in the UK that has not documented their contribution to the health of the nation over the years. Therefore, unless the pharmacist develops the skills for and embraces record keeping, their role and future roles may be called into question. The reasons for record keeping have now taken on a new importance. Documentation can be used as justification for a pharmacist's decisions and judgment in difficult situations. Also pharmacists, like other professionals, have to justify their very role within the community. The records provide evidence and aid decision making. In addition, record keeping is an important form of communication between pharmacists and other healthcare professionals and can ensure continuity of care for a patient.

What to record?

In the majority of cases the information that should be recorded will be specified, or there may be a specific form to fill in. The traditional records of supplies and clinical governance are generally specified which makes this information relatively easy to record. The problem arises when there are no specified procedures to tell pharmacists what to record, e.g. consultation records. This is a relatively new area for the pharmacist. Before the changes to the pharmacy contract in 2005 they were not required to record

---

Box 15.1

Guide to the type of information to record in a consultation record

- Patients' identification details

  - Title
  - Name
  - Address
  - Age/date of birth
  - Telephone number
  - Identification numbers, e.g. NHS number, patient medication record number
  - Medical conditions
  - Current medication

- Date
- Time
- Who was involved, i.e. the pharmacist, GP, patient, nurse, etc.
- What was involved and the reason, e.g. identification of an overdose
- Outcome or proposed action, e.g. a dose reduction
- Possible follow-up
- Information sources used
- Name of person making the entry, if not the person involved

---

interactions with the public and information was provided on a daily basis without it being logged.

Consultation records should be written so that others can use the information provided and realize the same outcome as the person that made the record. The level of information recorded will depend on the situation. All records need to be concise, organized, factual and legible, and abbreviations should be avoided if possible unless clear and established. Beware of recording personal views and opinions about patients and their behaviour, unless it is relevant to the record, as according to the Data Protection Act (DPA) 1998 patients have the right to request their records. The list in Box 15.1 indicates the type of information to record if not specified.

Barriers to record keeping

There are two main barriers to record keeping, namely time and knowledge. The traditional records of supply and, to some extent, clinical governance are generally well kept and the time taken to carry out the

record is generally already built in to the procedures for the normal working day. Knowledge of the record, the procedure and location are also generally not an issue, as again the pharmacist is accustomed to the procedure. The problem arises with newer consultation records and some aspects of clinical governance that are not carried out regularly.

Knowing how to make the record can be a problem, especially for consultation records of which pharmacists in many cases will have no experience. Time can be a major issue for recording consultations, especially if the contact was opportunistic, which is often the case with the advice the pharmacist may provide. Is it feasible to record all of the information the pharmacist provides to patients on a day-to-day basis? The pharmacist cannot be expected to know the name of every person they give advice to concerning over the counter medicines, yet it may be necessary to record this interaction.

The sooner the record is made the better. Forgetting to record an opportunistic consultation is more likely if the pharmacist intends to 'come back to it later'. It may be helpful to have a logbook where a note can be kept and recorded appropriately later. Other healthcare professionals, such as GPs and nurses, leave themselves time after a consultation to record it straight away. Pharmacists may need to look at how these other professionals have overcome the barriers to record keeping in these new areas.

The future of records

The drive to keep records electronically is becoming more and more apparent. The benefits of keeping electronic records surround the potential for shared information between healthcare professionals and external audit purposes. For example, the Royal Pharmaceutical Society of Great Britain (RPSGB) inspectors or police may monitor an online controlled drug (CD) register without needing to attend the premises.

The advancement of electronic transfer of prescriptions (ETP) has led to the debate over the best method of access for pharmacists to view full patient medication records. This will enable the pharmacist to be better placed to intervene when necessary and may avoid unnecessary interruptions to the doctor. Medicines use reviews (MURs) can potentially be carried out more effectively and may reduce the likelihood of making recommendations that have already been tried or are inappropriate. Pharmacist prescribing will definitely require better access to records. Pharmacists are often required to make decisions without the full patient history. Improved access to records will save time and provide more efficient and effective outcomes for patients. Likewise other healthcare professionals involved in patient care need to know what input the pharmacist has made.

The Data Protection Act 1998

The Data Protection Act (DPA) was first introduced in 1984 as concern grew over the amount of personal information that was being held on computer. This act related only to data held electronically but in 1998 was updated to the current DPA which applied to data held in any format. Now in most cases the individual's permission must be sought before personal information can be stored, processed or used for direct marketing. Personal information is defined as any information that can be used to identify a living individual, such as name, address, date of birth, etc. Interestingly, there is no lower age limit that applies to the DPA, so as long as a child can understand their rights, their consent must also be sought.

The DPA requires explicit consent before the processing of personal data can take place. This is not the case for sensitive personal data when the processing is necessary for medical purposes. For consent not to be required, a healthcare professional or their staff, including pharmacists and their dispensing staff, must undertake the processing. Sensitive personal data relates to any information including opinions relating to the physical or mental health or condition of the individual. Processing of information means the use of this information in virtually any way, including destroying the information. All systems used to store information will need to be registered with the Information Commissioners Office which enforces the DPA, and this now includes electronic and written information. In the pharmacy, the patient medical record (PMR) system, prescription only medicine (POM) register, controlled drug (CD) register and any other method of data collection will need to be registered.

There are eight principles within the DPA. We will look at each principle in turn and how it applies to pharmacy.

1. 'Personal data shall be obtained and processed fairly and lawfully and shall not be processed at all unless certain conditions are met'

Generally permission must be sought from the individual before records are kept and they should under-

stand why the data are being collected, except for sensitive personal data which is included in PMRs which can be recorded without permission.

2. 'Personal data shall be obtained and processed for, or in ways which are not incompatible with, one or more lawful purposes'

Data cannot be collected without a lawful purpose. In the case of PMRs, clinical governance principles and the pharmacy contract require pharmacists to maintain PMRs. Guidance taken from the RPSGB states that if a patient requests the removal of their data from the PMR system and cannot be persuaded otherwise, they should be asked to sign a disclaimer. This does not apply to records made in the POM register or CD register as this is a legal requirement.

3. 'Personal data shall be adequate, relevant and not excessive in relation to that purpose or purposes'

PMRs should only contain information relevant for the purpose, e.g. notes on a patient's medical conditions and allergies would be relevant but information about their preferred brand of toothpaste would not be – unless it had implications for their medical care.

4. 'Personal data shall be accurate and kept up to date'

The data should be as accurate and as current as possible. Be aware that some of the information may change, such as the patient's exemption status, address, title, etc.

5. 'Personal data shall not be kept for longer than necessary'

If no longer required, generally data should be deleted or destroyed. In the case of PMRs, they may be kept for as long as necessary; however, with respect to the Consumer Protection Act where the PMR is the only record of supply, the record should be kept for 13 years.

6. 'Personal data shall be processed in accordance with the rights of the data subject (the individual) under the act'

The individual's rights are as follows:
- To know that their data are being processed
- To know exactly what data are kept, why and who will see them
- To prevent their data being used for marketing purposes
- To seek criminal proceedings or sue for compensation if their rights are disregarded
- To be provided with the details of the data being held on them within 40 days of the request

- The identity of the person requesting it must be verified as the individual himself or herself.

7. 'Personal data shall be protected against unauthorized or unlawful processing and against accidental loss, destruction or damage'

Only people that need access should have access. Dispensing staff will need access to PMR records to do their job, but a counter assistant would not. Staff with access to any personal data should also be trained with respect to the DPA. This also has implications for the layout of the dispensary workspace, in that customers should not be able to view the computer screens. All information must be backed up appropriately. Information can be passed on to others if the individual consents but this must be clarified. There are circumstances where information can be disclosed to a third party without the individual's consent. These include the following:

- Where a patient's health or age makes them incapable. In such cases it may be necessary to get someone else such as a parent, guardian or carer to make the decision to disclose information. However, information about an adolescent should not normally be disclosed to parents
- The third party is empowered by statute to require the disclosure
- Requested by a judge, coroner or crown prosecution office
- To a police or NHS fraud investigation officer who request in writing, confirming disclosure is necessary to prevent, detect or prosecute a serious crime
- When it is necessary to prevent serious injury or damage to the patient, a third party or the public.

8. 'Personal data shall not be transferred (with certain exceptions) outside the European Economic Area unless the recipient country operates the same controls on data protection as applies within the EEA'

Confidentiality

Confidentiality is protected by scores of pieces of legislation such as the DPA, the Human Rights Act 1998 as well as by common law. The NHS also has its own code of practice, as do pharmacists, and pharmacists must have systems that conform to all of the above. Confidential information includes both personal and medical details of patients and also information about other NHS employees such as a doctor's prescribing habits. In addition to the DPA, confidential information must be protected against improper disclosure during storage, removal, receipt or transfer. Also access control and data encryption are necessary. All confidential information must be disposed of so the information is irretrievable; in most pharmacies they will have a confidential waste bin.

Records of supply

The major examples of supply records made in the pharmacy and where they are kept are described below (this is not an exhaustive list).

POM register

The prescription only medicine (POM) register is possibly the most longstanding means of recording within the pharmacy. It is primarily used for recording the supply of POMs as a legal requirement of the Medicines Act 1968, but is also used traditionally by the pharmacist to record significant incidents occurring in the pharmacy for future reference. They are found in both the community and hospital pharmacy and must be kept on the premises for the specified time frame for the record made, generally 2 years from the date of last entry. They are used to record every sale or supply of a POM unless it is with relation to an NHS prescription or a prescription for a contraceptive. A record also is not necessary if the supply is by way of wholesale dealing where the invoice is retained or if a separate record has already been made in the CD register.

The supply of a POM may take many forms and each will require different information to be entered in the register and to be kept for a specified duration of time. This information may be found in the current edition of the Medicines, Ethics and Practice guide (MEP). The following list includes commonly made records of supply in the POM register:

- Private prescriptions
- Emergency supplies at the patient's or doctor's request
- Signed orders or supply to a person authorized to sell, supply or administer POMs
- Veterinary prescriptions (NB: it is not specified where the record is to be made but is traditionally made in the POM register).

CD register

This is probably the most important legal record in the pharmacy in relation to supply records. Not only the supply but also the receipt of all CD schedules one and two are recorded here as a legal requirement of the Misuse of Drugs Act 1971. Again, they are found in both the hospital and community pharmacy and must be kept on the premises for 2 years from the date of last entry. Discrepancies in the CD register can lead to serious consequences. If unresolved, there may be an investigation by the primary care organization (PCO) and the police. As a result of this, all written entries must be in indelible ink with no cancellations, alterations or obliterations. Any corrections must be made by a dated footnote to prevent unlawful supplies and create an audit trail. The legal requirements for the format of the register and information to be recorded can be found in the MEP.

Extemporaneously prepared medicines

Medicines are sometimes prepared and compounded by pharmacists in response to a prescription in the community or hospital pharmacy. This does not include the reconstitution of powders. The RPSGB has set out guidance in relation to this service which can be found in the MEP. This service is a type of manufacture which, in the case of pharmaceutical companies, is regulated by the Medicines and Healthcare products Regulatory Authority (MHRA). Pharmacists are not subject to these regulations as the manufacture is only small scale; however, the product must be prepared accurately and meet quality standards.

A product should only be prepared extemporaneously if there are no appropriate licensed products available. Records of the manufacture must be made, usually in a bound book used solely for that purpose. The record is made as an audit trail to be kept for a minimum of 2 years, but if possible 5 years, and should include the following:

- Formula
- Ingredients
  - o Quantities
  - o Source
  - o Batch number
  - o Expiry date
- The personnel involved in the manufacture
- The pharmacist taking overall responsibility

- Date of dispensing and patient's and prescription details if in response to a prescription

Supply of unlicensed medicinal products ('specials')

Some products may need to be compounded by a specials manufacturer, as there is a safety risk associated with the manufacture or if it is not possible to prepare the product accurately in the pharmacy. These products are referred to as 'specials'. The request for a special can only be made on the order of an appropriate prescriber, and they should be made aware that the product is unlicensed. The Medicines Control Agency (MCA) issued guidance in 2000 about the records the pharmacist should make with respect to the supply of specials. This is as follows:

- The source of the special
- The person to whom the product is supplied
- The date of the supply
- The quantity supplied
- The batch number
- Details of any adverse drug reactions.

These details should be kept for a period of 5 years and be available for inspection; however, the format or place of the record is not specified.

Poisons book

Pharmacists are able to supply non-medicinal poisons within the pharmacy. In law a poison is defined as a substance listed in the Poisons Act. It is not very common to supply poisons, but would be more likely in a rural pharmacy. The different poisons can only be supplied for specified purposes and the purchaser may need a certificate or form of authority and a signed order for the purchase of the poison. The pharmacist must keep a record of the supply in the poisons book and the signature of the purchaser is needed either in the register or on a signed order. The register must be kept for 2 years from the date of last entry, as must any certificates. The particulars to be recorded can be found in the MEP.

Clinical governance records

Clinical governance is the process by which professionals are accountable for continually improving the quality of their services and maintaining high standards. It relies on learning from experiences and therefore being open and honest is essential. It is a combination of a number of processes including accountability, audit, clinical effectiveness, patient and public involvement, remedying underperformance, risk management, staff management and continuing professional development (CPD). This process binds all professionals within the heathcare environment. Clinical governance is covered in more detail in Chapter 8; the focus here is on record keeping associated with clinical governance. Some examples are described below.

Audit

Audit is the process of systematic evaluation of work against set standards. In the pharmacy many processes will need to be audited and the results may be used internally or externally, e.g. by the PCO. The results of the audit need to be documented and may result in change in policies or standard operating procedures (SOPs).

PMRs

PMRs can be considered as records of supply as well as clinical governance records. Within clinical governance, PMRs enable pharmacists to be clinically effective. In order for PMRs to be useful to pharmacists they need to be up to date, accurate and contain as much detail as possible about the patient's medication history. The system used must have access control mechanisms, be able to identify drug interactions and highlight those that are more serious. There are minimum specifications for the contents of PMRs set out in the MEP with respect to identification of the patient, patient's GP and prescription details. However, the pharmacy contract requires more information about patients to be recorded with regards to advice and counselling given by pharmacists.

Risk management

Risk management can encompass many aspects of the service delivery and will apply to both hospital and community pharmacy. Examples of risk management procedures include:

Standard operating procedures (SOPs)

These documents should relate to all the work processes within the pharmacy and how they should be carried out to ensure the least risk and greatest effectiveness. The process should be portrayed in a stepwise manner and written so that even people with no experience can carry it out by following the SOP. All SOPs need to be signed by the accountable pharmacist and all staff working in the dispensary need to be trained regularly on the SOPs and a record of the training should be made in a training matrix.

Complaints procedure

There is an NHS complaints procedure and this applies to both hospital and community pharmacy. Complaints can be made orally or in writing. In the case of an oral complaint, a record of the complaint must be made including the name of the person making the complaint, subject of the complaint and the date on which it was made. If written, a record of the date on which the complaint was received must be made. A written response must be made within 2 days of the date of the complaint. The complaint should then be investigated and resolved appropriately. A record of all correspondence or phone calls to the complainant should be kept.

Error reporting and near misses

A near miss is defined as an error in the dispensing process which is identified before the medicine reaches the patient. All near misses should be logged and audited in line with company and RPSGB policy. The outcome of the audit should be implemented and a record should be made, and if it results in a change in procedure the SOPs must be updated. Any incident that results in patient involvement needs to be logged, and as of April 2005, reported to the National Reporting and Learning System (NRLS). The information should be logged on a reporting form that has the minimum information required by the NRLS. Serious incidents will be reported anonymously to the National Patient Safety Agency (NPSA) via the NRLS. Pharmacists need to demonstrate evidence of recording, reporting, monitoring, analysing and learning from patient safety incidents. The incident may be reported to the NRLS via the organization's risk management office (pharmacy superintendent office in large multiples), via the NPSA website or via the PCO.

Control of Substances Hazardous to Health (COSHH) Regulations 2002

All work places must conduct risk assessments and produce safety precautions with relation to dangerous substances. A hazardous substance includes anything that can cause risks to health and safety. There is no one list of substances. Common substances can be found in Health and Safety Executive (HSE) guidance documents and Chemicals Hazard Information and Packaging (CHIP) for Supply Regulations. Even dust can be classed as a dangerous substance if the concentration in the air exceeds certain limits.

In the pharmacy there will be a number of drugs or chemicals that are classed as dangerous substances, such as hydrogen peroxide and potassium permanganate. They can usually be identified by the warning labels on the packaging as directed by CHIP regulations. Some dangerous substances have their own regulations such as asbestos, lead and flammable chemicals and therefore COSHH does not apply. There are eight steps to carry out to comply with COSHH regulations which are listed in Box 15.2.

COSHH assessments can be recorded on paper or electronically. They should include why the risks identified are significant or not, the control measures and plans that apply to the substance. The COSHH assessment is a working document and should be updated every time there is a significant change, although most pharmacies will update the COSHH assessment once a year. External bodies such as health and safety officers may request records of COSHH assessment.

Box 15.2

Steps to carry out to comply with COSHH regulations

1. Assess the risks
2. Decide what precautions are needed
3. Prevent or adequately control exposure
4. Ensure control measures are used and maintained
5. Monitor exposure
6. Carry out appropriate health surveillance
7. Prepare plans and procedures to deal with accidents, incidents and emergencies
8. Ensure employees are properly informed, trained and supervised

CPD

This is a large part of clinical governance for which the pharmacist must take his or her own responsibility. Records tend to be kept at home and not in the pharmacy. The records may be kept on paper or electronically. Not only will a CPD cycle need to be completed, a portfolio of evidence supporting the cycle will also be required. More information about CPD can be found in Chapter 10.

Consultation records

Consultation records are a new concept for pharmacists and have come about as a result of the expanding role of pharmacists. The more services pharmacists provide, the more records they will need to keep. What to record may be specified and there may be a form to fill in but some of the time the pharmacist will need to decide what is relevant to record and where to record it. This section addresses the records kept for patient group directions (PGDs), services and the requirements of the pharmacy contract.

PGDs and services

Most PGDs and services that pharmacists can provide require some kind of training and accreditation by the PCO and involve the supply of a drug, usually a POM, to the patient under NHS payment agreements. All the terms of the service will need to be kept on the premises and this will specify the types of records required to provide the service. Each service will have its own requirements but they will encompass requirements of current legislation, namely the Medicines Act 1968. They may also require notes on the consultation in question, which may look more like a case history, much like doctors' notes.

The Pharmacy Contract 2005 in England

There are three tiers of services provided within this contract which are essential, advanced and enhanced services. The essential services include day-to-day dispensing, counselling and the provision of advice. These are services that pharmacists have already been providing. Now pharmacists need to provide evidence of this advice and counselling. MURs are currently the only advanced service to be introduced. An example of enhanced services is the provision of free emergency hormonal contraception via a PGD, and records of this need to be kept, as discussed above.

Any interventions made or advice and counselling given to patients known to the pharmacist that can be classed as clinically significant need to be recorded by the pharmacist in the PMR. Clinically significant could be described as when the action taken has a direct impact on patient care, which encompasses most counselling, advising and interventions made by pharmacists. The information recorded needs to be sufficient for another person to understand why, when, who and how this consultation took place. The following need to be recorded in PMRs for essential services:

- Supplies of medicines and appliances dispensed to patients
- Advice given and interventions made on prescribed medication
- Owed prescription medicines
- Advice given and interventions made on repeat dispensed medicines with clear audit trails
- Opportunistic advice on healthy living and public health, especially in patients with diabetes, coronary heart disease or high blood pressure and patients who smoke or are overweight
- Referrals to other health, social or support organizations using the signposting document given by the PCO
- Self-care purchases and referrals.

Some of these will also need recording on a specific form and be filed accordingly, such as the referral and intervention form, repeat dispensing cardex and owing dockets.

MURs and prescription interventions

More information about how to carry out a MUR or a prescription intervention can be found in Chapter 47. Here we will discuss the record keeping issues around MURs and prescription interventions.

There is a standard form to be filled in when carrying out a MUR. Care must be taken so that all information is neat, legible and understandable, not only for the healthcare professional but for the patient as well, since they should also be given a copy for their own reference. Abbreviations and jargon should be avoided where possible and statements that may alarm patients or damage relationships with doctors ought to be worded sensitively. Patient, doctor and pharmacist details should be written in capitals to avoid misinterpretation.

One copy of the form will need to be kept in the pharmacy for a minimum of 2 years and filled in an appropriate manner, and a summary should be entered in the patient's PMR. One copy will need to be sent to the GP, usually the top copy, so that they may be scanned onto the GP's patient records. The third copy should be given to the patient as a reminder of the issues discussed or to be taken to the GP as a discussion aid. Anonymized MURs and interventions may be requested by the PCO in order to check their quality and that they met the service specifications.

KEY POINTS

- There are three main types of records to be kept by pharmacists:
  - o Records of supply
  - o Clinical governance records
  - o Consultation records
- Some of the records may fit into more than one of these categories as the boundaries are not clear cut
- All record keeping must comply with the Data Protection Act
- Most records are legal requirements but the expanding role of the pharmacist means that, as a profession, we need to record more and more information for audit trail and to ensure clinical effectiveness
- It can be seen that record keeping is an important skill pharmacists must acquire
- This skill will need to be developed further in order to meet the demands of the expanding roles and clinical governance

Section Three

Pharmacy Prescribing and Selection of Medicines

Access to medicines and prescribing – introduction

Jason Hall

STUDY POINTS

- Independent and supplementary prescribing
- Patient group directions
- Minor ailment schemes
- What influences prescribing

Introduction

The legal constraints introduced in the United Kingdom to limit prescribing of certain medicines for humans to doctors and dentists remained largely unaltered until 1994 when suitably trained community nurses were added to the list of professions able to prescribe a limited range of medicines and appliances listed in the *Nurse Prescribers' Formulary* (NPF). Prior to the introduction of community nurse prescribing it was recognized that many district nurses were prescribing in all but name as they were instructing GPs what to prescribe and that much time was wasted waiting for GPs to write the prescription. The review of prescribing, supply and administration of medicines chaired by June Crown in 1999 recommended that there should be two types of prescriber: the independent prescriber and the dependent prescriber, although the term dependent prescriber has now been replaced by the term supplementary prescriber (Department of Health 1999). The independent prescriber is responsible for diagnosis and the supplementary prescriber is responsible for the ongoing care of the patient in line with an agreed clinical management plan (CMP). At the start of the 21st century there were significant changes to non-medical prescribing with the introduction of different classifications of

nurse prescriber and the extension of prescribing to suitably trained pharmacists and other healthcare professionals (Department of Health 2006).

Over the years there have been many reports from the Department of Health outlining the benefits of non-medical prescribing for patients, doctors and non-medical prescribers themselves (Department of Health 1999, 2006). Many of these benefits stem from having the healthcare professional responsible for the care of a patient's condition also writing the prescription (Box 16.1).

Independent prescribing

Independent prescribers (IP) are responsible for the diagnosis of the patient and can initiate prescriptions for patients without referring to other healthcare professionals. They have responsibility for monitoring and reviewing the patient's progress. The first group of independent non-medical prescribers were the community practitioner nurse prescribers. This was first introduced in 1994 in eight pilot sites. The scheme was extended nationwide in 1999. It is open to nurses holding a district nurse (DN) or health visitor (HV) qualification working in the community, and this includes a small number of practice nurses with a DN or HV qualification. Training consisted of 2 days of taught sessions in addition to an open learning package (approximately 15 hours of study material) followed by a written examination. This has now been incorporated into the DN and HV course. These prescribers prescribe from the NPF that can be found in the *British National Formulary* (see Box 16.2 for examples of items in the NPF).

Box 16.1

Anticipated benefits of non-medical prescribing

Patients

- Improved patient access to prescribers
- More accurate assessment of patient needs
- Better and quicker access to medicines

Doctors

- Saves time for doctors
- Clarifies professional boundaries

Healthcare professionals

- Improved use of healthcare professional's time
- Increased job satisfaction

Box 16.2

Examples of products in the *Nurse Prescribers' Formulary* (NPF) that can be prescribed by community practitioner nurse prescribers

Types of product that can be prescribed	Examples
Wound management products	Granuflex®
Catheter care products	Bard, Simpla, etc.
Analgesics	Paracetamol
Laxatives	Lactulose, phosphate enema
Skin preparations	Aqueous cream

In 2002 a new class of nurse prescriber was created; these were originally called extended formulary nurse prescribers. This opened prescribing to any registered nurse and it originally covered four main areas:

- Minor ailments
- Minor injuries
- Health promotion
- Palliative care.

Nurses that chose this route to becoming a prescriber were required to complete a training course which consisted of 26 taught days and 12 days learning in practice, which included prescribing under the supervision of a medical prescriber (Department of Health 2006). It should be noted that the taught element of the training programme did not include therapeutics, i.e. it did not cover what to prescribe for a particular condition; it did cover how to prescribe in a way that complied with legal requirements. In 2006 many of the previous restrictions on extended formulary nurse prescribers were removed and their name was changed to independent nurse prescribers. The independent nurse prescribers are able to prescribe any licensed medicine and some controlled drugs. Therefore there is no need for the extended nurse prescriber's formulary, which is no longer in existence. The changes in 2006 also paved the way for independent pharmacist prescribers. Independent pharmacist prescribers can prescribe any licensed medicine except controlled drugs.

Supplementary prescribing

Supplementary prescribing is viewed by the Department of Health as a voluntary partnership between the independent and the supplementary prescriber that has the agreement of the patient (Department of Health 2005). Therefore the patient must be informed regarding the underlying principles of the prescribing partnership by the independent prescriber and give their consent to the transfer of care to a supplementary prescriber (SP). The patient does not have to give written consent, but once consent has been given it should be noted in the patient's medical notes.

Providing the patient agrees, there is very little restriction as to what can be prescribed. The drugs that can be prescribed by supplementary prescribers include all 'prescription only medicines', 'pharmacy' medicines and 'general sales list' medicines, although the NHS prescribers cannot prescribe items listed in the Black List (Part XVIIIA of the Drug Tariff) at NHS expense. Controlled drugs and unlicensed medicines were added to the list of drugs that can be prescribed by supplementary prescribers in May 2005.

An independent prescriber, who must be a doctor or a dentist, makes the diagnosis. If the independent prescriber thinks that the patient can be safely managed by a supplementary prescriber then both the independent prescriber and supplementary prescriber agree a clinical management plan for the patient. However, the independent prescriber does not discard all their responsibility and must still review the patient at suitable intervals, which should rarely exceed a year (Department of Health 2005).

Name of patient:	Patient medication sensitivities/allergies:		
Patient identification, e.g. ID number, date of birth:			
Current medication:	Medical history:		
Independent prescriber(s) (IP): Contact details: [tel/email/address]	Supplementary prescriber(s) (SP): Contact details: [tel/email/address]		
Condition(s) to be treated:	Aim of treatment:		
Medicines that may be prescribed by SP:			
Preparation	Indication	Dose schedule	Specific indications for referral back to the IP
Guidelines or protocols supporting clinical management plan:			
Frequency of review and monitoring by:			
Supplementary prescriber:	Supplementary prescriber and independent prescriber:		
Process for reporting ADRs:			
Shared record to be used by IP and SP.			
Agreed by independent prescriber(s)	Date	Agreed by supplementary prescriber(s)	Date	Date agreed with patient/carer

Figure 16.1 • Clinical management plan used in supplementary prescribing.

The clinical management plan is central to supplementary prescribing in that it forms the agreement between the independent and supplementary prescribers that sets out what the supplementary prescriber is able to prescribe (Fig. 16.1). Each clinical management plan must be drawn up for a specific named patient. The nature of the clinical management plan can vary in terms of its detail and scope. At one end of the spectrum it could be very specific, allowing only relatively minor modifications to be made to the original prescription under specified criteria such as increasing the dosage of an antihypertensive drug in order to reduce blood pressure to a specified level. At the other end of the spectrum it could be very open, allowing the supplementary prescriber to prescribe a wide range of drugs in accordance with a clinical guideline such as the British Thoracic Society's guidelines for the management of asthma. The nature of the clinical management plan will depend upon the confidence and competence of the supplementary prescriber in each therapeutic area and also the willingness of the independent prescriber to delegate the responsibility. The plan also sets out the circumstances that would require referral back to the independent prescriber.

The patients most likely to benefit from supplementary prescribing are those with chronic conditions requiring ongoing care, such as diabetes mellitus, asthma or hypertension. In addition, those with uncomplicated conditions rather than those patients with multiple problems are likely to be the most suitable candidates for supplementary prescribing. In practice the supplementary prescriber is likely to continue prescribing the items initiated by the independent prescriber until there is a change in the patient's condition, provided such items have been included in the clinical management plan. A change in the patient's condition could involve a deterioration of a chronic progressive condition. An example of managing the deterioration is stepping up therapy by prescribing an additional item such as a steroid inhaler (preventer) to an asthmatic patient who is poorly controlled on a salbutamol inhaler (reliever) alone (see Ch. 37).

As supplementary prescribers do not diagnose conditions, one might assume that they would be unable to prescribe for patients presenting with acute conditions. However, they can prescribe items in response to changes in the patient's condition, provided such items have been included in the clinical management plan. A change in the patient's condition could involve an acute exacerbation of a chronic condition. An example is prescribing an antibiotic for a chest infection for a patient with chronic obstructive pulmonary disease (COPD).

Patient group directions

An alternative way of getting medicines to patients without writing a prescription involves the use of patient group directions (PGD). These allow pharmacists, or other healthcare professionals, to supply named products to patients that meet the inclusion criteria specified in the PGD (Department of Health 1998). The legal definition of a PGD is: 'A written instruction for the sale, supply and/or administration of named medicines in an identified clinical situation. It applies to groups of patients who may not be individually identified before presenting for treatment.'

Under a PGD, pre-packed licensed medicines can be supplied to patients who meet the appropriate inclusion criteria and do not meet any of the specified exclusion criteria. The PGD must state the qualifications and training required of the staff administering the PGD, and it must name the medicine(s) that can be supplied. It must also list any advice that should be given to the patient, describe the referral procedure and state the action that should be taken in the case of a patient suffering an adverse drug reaction (ADR). The PGD must be reviewed and approved by a team containing a doctor and a pharmacist.

The Department of Health has made it clear that the preferred route of getting medicines to patients is via the issuing of a prescription to a named patient by a trained and qualified prescriber and that PGDs should only ever be used where they offer clear advantages to patient care without compromising patient safety (Department of Health 1998). Situations that could be suitable for PGDs are those that involve one off or relatively short courses of standard treatment (i.e. the PGD operator does not have to select the drug, dose or formulation). An example of a PGD is the supply of emergency hormonal contraception through community pharmacies.

Over the counter medicines

Pharmacists have a long tradition of selling medicines over the counter to treat minor ailments. In some situations pharmacists might have a choice regarding the method of supply of a medicine to treat a patient. This could be via an over the counter sale, prescribing a medicine as part of a minor ailment scheme (see next section) or supply through a PGD. In some of these situations the exact same product could be supplied and the only differences between the different methods might be who pays for the treatment and whether records have to be made. The pharmacist's duty of care to the patient does not vary between the different methods of supply and pharmacists should not treat an over the counter purchase of medicine any differently than prescribing a medicine.

When recommending products to patients for over the counter purchase, the pharmacist is acting as an independent prescriber, although they can only recommend general sales list (GSL) medicines or pharmacy only (P) medicines. As an independent prescriber, the pharmacist must go through all the steps of the prescribing process (see Ch. 17). The steps include questioning the patient or their carer to ascertain signs, symptoms and relevant medical history including prescribed and purchased medicines that the patient is currently taking, to arrive at a working diagnosis. The patient should be involved in the decision-making process to achieve concordance, and appropriate advice given to allow the patient or their carer to monitor the progress of their treatment and to know when to seek further help or advice.

Minor ailment schemes

Minor ailments have been described as 'conditions that require little or no medical intervention' (see Box 16.3 for a list of minor ailments; Royal Pharmaceutical Society 2006). It has been recognized that treatments for minor ailments are responsible for considerable amounts of GP time and considerable amounts of NHS expenditure. Minor ailment schemes have been developed to allow patients to be seen by community pharmacists to ease the burden on GPs. There are many schemes in operation and each scheme is locally agreed by patients, practices,

Box 16.3

Minor ailments treated by pharmacists as part of minor ailment schemes in the UK

Athlete's foot
Bites and stings
Constipation
Contact dermatitis
Cough
Diarrhoea
Dyspepsia
Earache
Hay fever
Headache
Head lice
Mouth ulcers
Nasal symptoms
Sore throat
Teething
Temperature
Vaginal thrush
Viral upper respiratory tract infection (URTI)

pharmacists and primary care trusts and therefore there is no universally agreed minor ailment scheme. However, all minor ailment schemes should have a formal written protocol that sets out how the scheme should operate.

There are three main types of intervention that pharmacists can make when participating in a minor ailment scheme and schemes could involve one or more of these interventions. The first of these involves providing advice to the patient. The second involves the patient receiving a medicine and this could be via the pharmacist writing a prescription for a pharmacy only medicine or supplying a product via a patient group direction. When pharmacists prescribe medicines in a minor ailment scheme the medicine is usually from a locally agreed formulary. The third intervention is referral to a GP and many of the schemes include a fast track referral allowing patients who have been reviewed by a pharmacist to be seen more quickly by the GP should their condition warrant such speed. The arrangements for referral on to a minor ailment scheme also vary between different schemes with some schemes allowing self-referral by patients and others requiring referral from a healthcare professional or a practice receptionist.

The arrangements for payments for any product supplied via a minor ailment scheme vary between different schemes. In some schemes patients have to pay the full cost of the product but in others the costs are met by trusts for all patients and in some only for those patients exempt from the normal prescription levy.

Influences on prescribing

Prescribers must have an awareness of factors with potential to influence prescribing decision making and take steps to ensure that their decision making is not adversely affected by these influences. Researchers have been investigating medical prescribing decision making for many years and there is now an extensive amount of literature on the factors that can influence medical prescribing. By comparison there is much less written about non-medical prescribing, which means that we must consult the medical literature to review the factors likely to influence prescribing.

A number of patient factors have been reported to have an influence on medical prescribing decision making (Bradley 1992). The age of the patient has been reported to cause prescribers discomfort, with the very old and very young being responsible. In such cases prescribers should question whether they should prescribe for any group of patients where they lack experience. Patients who were well known to the prescriber were identified as a source of discomfort and these included frequent attenders at the practice and patients considered to be untrustworthy. Patients deemed untrustworthy by the prescriber, perhaps through the previous misuse of drugs, deserve the same consideration as other patients, although prescribers should be cautious regarding requests for items liable for misuse. The patient's social class, ethnic background and educational status were also reported to cause discomfort for some prescribers. It is obviously not acceptable to allow these factors to influence prescribing. It has been reported that patients affected prescribing decision making through demand for prescription items, although other researchers have suggested that doctors may overestimate this pressure to prescribe (Stevenson et al 1999). Prescribers should never assume patients want a prescription. They should explore what the patient feels about their condition as many patients visit healthcare professionals to receive reassurance that they do not have a serious problem rather than to get medicines to treat symptoms.

The characteristics of a product were also reported to influence prescribing decision making (Bradley 1992). Specific groups of products, such as antibiotics, benzodiazepines, cardiovascular drugs, non-steroidal anti-inflammatory drugs (NSAIDs), tranquillizers, antidepressants and sleeping tablets were reported to cause discomfort for prescribers. The important aspect for non-medical prescribers may not be the actual product that caused discomfort but rather the reasons for the discomfort. These included safety, their own expectations, appropriateness of treatment and uncertainty over diagnosis. Ensuring that prescribing decisions are based upon the best available evidence should help to minimize discomfort over the first three of these reasons. The last reason can be more difficult as there are situations, such as diagnosing mental health problems and diagnosing ailments in young children, where a suspected diagnosis is difficult to confirm or may not be confirmed until after a period of time, although the patient's symptoms are such that they require immediate management. Living with uncertainty can be difficult but informing the patient or their carer regarding the uncertainty and what action you recommend should help minimize its impact. A product's cost has been reported to have an impact on prescribing for some prescribers (Denig & Haaijer-Ruskamp 1995). The impact of cost on prescribing was related to the condition being treated such that the effects of cost on prescribing were greater for self-limiting conditions compared to conditions perceived to be serious.

The time available for a consultation with patients has been noted as a factor that can affect the volume of prescriptions written (Muller 1972). It has been suggested that having too little time with patients meant that it was easier to prescribe, rather than to explain why no prescription was required. This is obviously not an acceptable reason for prescribing. Prescribers must consider the time management of their consultations and determine strategies for eliciting patients' views on drugs and the management of their symptoms, as well as strategies to end a consultation without issuing a prescription.

Many studies have concluded that representatives from the pharmaceutical industry were the most commonly used source of information by prescribers when they were prescribing new drugs for the first time (McGettigan et al 2000; Prosser et al 2003). Interestingly, several studies that compared the quality of prescribing with the source of information used by the prescriber reported that poorer quality prescribing was associated with a higher use of information originating from the pharmaceutical industry (Haayer 1982).

Several studies have noted the influence of colleagues on medical prescribing decision making. It has been reported that hospital consultants are a major influence on the prescribing of GPs but fellow GPs are much less of an influence (Jones et al 2001). Colleagues can be a valuable source of information on developments in health care and sharing experiences with fellow professionals can aid the development of strategies to manage patient consultations discussed earlier. Establishing professional links with other prescribers – not just pharmacist prescribers but GPs, hospital medical prescribers, nurses and other non-medical prescribers – is to be encouraged.

Clinical governance in prescribing

Clinical governance is about regularly monitoring and continually updating services in a way that increases accountability for all activities with the overall aim of maintaining and improving standards of care. Prescribing is no different from any other pharmaceutical service and should comply with the principles of clinical governance. There should be clear lines of responsibility and accountability within organizations with regards to all aspects of prescribing so that prescribers and their managers are aware of their roles. Organizations should promote clinical audits and prescribers should participate in these audits where appropriate, as well as auditing their own prescribing performance against standards such as the National Prescribing Centre Competency Framework (see Ch. 17). Taking any drug will put a patient at risk of side-effects or adverse drug reactions. Prescribers must balance these risks against the potential benefits of the treatment. Organizations and individual prescribers must document errors and near misses so that all can learn and standards can be continually improved. Prescribers should have up-to-date therapeutic knowledge, be aware of national and local clinical guidelines and base their prescribing decisions on the best evidence available. Achieving concordance is key to ensuring effective treatment and prescribers must communicate the benefits and risks of the available treatment options to patients or their carers.

Code of Ethics

The Royal Pharmaceutical Society of Great Britain (RPSGB) Code of Ethics directs pharmacist prescribers to prescribe responsibly and in the patient's best interests. It provides further direction for pharmacist

Box 16.4

Code of Ethics and standards service specification for pharmacist prescribers

Limitations	Pharmacist prescribers must limit their prescribing to areas within their own professional expertise and competence
	Pharmacists should not normally prescribe for themselves, family or friends except in emergencies
	Pharmacists must only prescribe when they have adequate knowledge of the patient's health and medical history
Knowledge	Pharmacists must be aware of local and national clinical guidelines and take these into account when prescribing
Practicalities of prescribing	Pharmacists must make appropriate patient assessments and only prescribe when there is a genuine clinical need
	Where pharmacists can prescribe and dispense they must ensure that these roles are separated whenever possible
	This could be achieved by an accuracy checking technician or another pharmacist checking the final dispensed product
	Pharmacists must keep accurate and comprehensive records of the consultation with the patient and of the items that they have prescribed
Relations with other professionals	Pharmacists must refer the patient to another practitioner when appropriate
	Pharmacists must communicate effectively with other practitioners involved in the care of the patient

prescribers around limitations (what they can prescribe, who they should not prescribe for and the information they must have access to before they can prescribe), knowledge they should have, communication and the practicalities of combining prescribing and dispensing (Box 16.4).

KEY POINTS

- Some nurses became the first non-medical prescribers in 1994
- Independent prescribers are responsible for diagnosis and prescribing without reference to other healthcare professionals
- Supplementary prescribing is a voluntary partnership between prescriber and patients which is more beneficial in chronic conditions
- Diagnosis is made by an independent prescriber, then a clinical management plan is agreed between the independent and supplementary prescribers
- The clinical management plan is drawn up for a specific patient, but it can vary widely in detail and scope
- A patient group direction allows provision of named medicines in specific clinical situations, but not necessarily to a named patient
- Pharmacists may have the choice of over the counter sale, prescribing as part of a minor ailment scheme or supply through a patient group direction
- When recommending over the counter, the pharmacist is acting as an independent prescriber, but is restricted to GSL or P medicines
- Minor ailment schemes are locally agreed and vary widely
- In a minor ailment scheme, the pharmacist can give advice only, or supply, via a prescription or patient group direction, a prescription only medicine, or refer the patient to a medical practitioner
- A range of factors is known to affect doctor prescribing. These may also affect pharmacists
- Applying clinical governance and the RPSGB Code of Ethics to prescribing is a professional requirement

Chapter Seventeen

The prescribing process and evidence-based medicine

Jason Hall

STUDY POINTS

- The stages involved in the prescribing process
- Evidence-based medicine

Introduction

The prescribing of medicines is the most common medical intervention in patient care and drug costs are a major component of NHS expenditure. Ensuring optimum benefits for patients and value for money for taxpayers and other individuals and organizations paying for health care are priorities. A model of 'good prescribing' has been proposed that has four aims (Barber 1995). These aims are to: maximize effectiveness, minimize risks, minimize costs and respect patient choice. Maximizing effectiveness is about selecting a drug therapy that will achieve its therapeutic objective in a suitable timescale. Minimizing risks is recognizing that all drug treatments carry an element of risk of causing harm to the patient and that selection of the drug should be about managing the benefits and risks. The cost of therapy should also be taken into account by the prescriber (see Ch. 19). Such consideration should go beyond a simple review of the drug costs to also consider any costs of monitoring treatment such as blood tests, the length of treatment and any additional items that could be required, such as prescribing an additional drug to protect the gastrointestinal tract from adverse effects caused by the first drug. Establishing the views of the patient is a vital part of the process of assessing the relative importance of the first three aims in this model. Patients may differ in their views regarding managing the symptoms of a condition, living with the consequences of a condition, exposing themselves to risks of harmful effects and the amount of money they would be willing or able to pay for treatment. In addition, patients may wish product selection to take their lifestyle into account such that the frequency and route of administration of the selected product fits in with their daily routine. It is accepted that 'good prescribing' involves trade-offs between these four aims and that this often involves delicate balancing between each of the aims.

The prescribing process

The prescribing process will be considered under five headings, although there is some overlap between these and their sequence may not be the same in all cases. The first is concerned with all the things that must be in place before a prescriber can start to prescribe, the second with collecting information, the third with analysing the information and making the prescribing decision, the fourth with making appropriate records and plans for monitoring the patients progress; and the last with auditing and evaluating prescribing practice.

Prerequisites

Prescribing can only be carried out by healthcare professionals with appropriate prescribing qualifications and these will vary depending on the type of prescribing to be carried out. To prescribe prescription only medicines (POM), either on the NHS or privately, the prescriber must have successfully completed training to allow them to act as a supplementary or an independent prescriber (Department of Health 2006). The training course consists of a taught element (around 26 days) and learning in practice (around 12 days), which includes prescribing under the supervision of a medical prescriber. To participate in a minor ailment scheme and prescribe pharmacy only medicines (P medicines) at NHS expense the pharmacist will likely have had to complete appropriate accreditation set by the local primary care organization.

Patients who are to receive their prescriptions from a supplementary prescriber must give informed consent. Patients do not need to sign this informed consent but it is good practice to make a note in the patient's medical notes when informed consent was given. The exact nature of informed consent is difficult to define and it is likely that the input from the healthcare professional will vary between patients when obtaining consent. Observation of disputes between patients and physicians regarding whether informed consent was given shows that simply handing the patient a leaflet does not discharge the physician from their obligation to obtain informed consent. In any legal dispute it is up to the courts to decide which party they believe. However, the disputes that found in favour of the physician tended to be those where the physician was able to demonstrate that they had given the information to the patient because they had documented the advice they gave in the patient's medical records.

Prior to the patient consultation the prescriber should ensure that they are suitably prepared. Part of this preparation includes ensuring they have sufficient indemnity insurance that covers their prescribing and that their job description clearly shows that prescribing is part of their role. Another part of the preparation is acquiring the appropriate knowledge and skills (Box 17.1).

Consulting with the patient

Where possible, prescribers should familiarize themselves with the patient's medical history prior to the consultation. Obviously this would not be possible in minor ailment schemes as patients are likely to arrive without an appointment and their medical notes will not usually be available to the community pharmacist.

During the consultation, prescribers must take a full history of the presenting condition and any other factors such as other conditions the patient has and any other medications, including over the counter

---

Box 17.1

Checklist for knowledge and skills required by pharmacist prescribers

Legal restrictions affecting which medicines can be prescribed

Independent pharmacists can prescribe any licensed medicine except controlled drugs and supplementary prescribers can prescribe any licensed or unlicensed medicine including controlled drugs provided it has been specified in the clinical management plan

Professional restrictions affecting which medicines can be prescribed

It is vital that each prescriber prescribes only within their own area of competence. Knowing one's own limitations is a key skill for a prescriber. In addition, they must also have an appropriate level of experience dealing with the condition and it might be appropriate to refer a patient presenting with a condition rarely experienced to another prescriber for assessment and any prescribing if required

Administrative arrangements regarding payments for the service

The administrative arrangements regarding the prescribing process must be fully understood. In the case of minor ailment schemes, these arrangements could include a description of records that should be kept and how payment for the service is to be made. For NHS prescribing, the prescriber should be aware of the categories of patient that are exempt from NHS charges and what payments should be made by those that are not exempt

Patient confidentiality

Pharmacist prescribers must maintain patient confidentiality and take steps to ensure that no unauthorized personnel can gain access to patient medication records by securely storing the data either via lock and key or via appropriate electronic security measures such as passwords for data stored electronically

Ethics

Prescribers should be aware of the good practice guidance from the Department of Health and the Royal Pharmaceutical Society's statements on prescribing in the Code of Ethics before they start to prescribe. This guidance addresses prescribers not prescribing for themselves, not normally prescribing for members of their family, and also covers accepting gifts and hospitality for suppliers

Security

Prescribers must be aware of security issues surrounding prescribing and take steps to minimize the risks. Blank prescription forms could be used by drug misusers to try and obtain supplies of prescription medicines for abuse or to sell to others. Care must therefore be taken to ensure that the forms are securely stored. Personal security must also be considered if the prescriber is visiting patients in their own homes or other locations in the community

Therapeutic management of conditions

A pharmacist's knowledge and skills required for the management of a therapeutic area must be up to date and based upon the best evidence available at the time. The knowledge should extend to non-drug approaches to treatment as sometimes these could be the most appropriate intervention

Other members of the healthcare team

Prescribers should be aware of other professions they could refer patients to, e.g. general practitioner, the accident and emergency department in the hospital, dentists, the community nursing service (district nurses and health visitors), social services and self-help groups

medicines and complementary medicines, that the patient may be taking. It may be necessary to carry out further investigations such as measuring the patient's blood pressure. This information must be recorded in the patient's medical notes.

Before any prescribing can take place a diagnosis must be made. If the pharmacist is acting as a supplementary prescriber, the diagnosis will have been made by an independent prescriber, but the pharmacist should interpret the information obtained before and during the consultation to check that the patient's diagnosis remains valid. Independent prescribers must establish a working diagnosis based upon the information they have gathered on the patient. At this stage it may be necessary to request laboratory tests such as urea and electrolytes, red blood cell count and haemoglobin tests to help confirm the working diagnosis.

With increasing complexity of health care and increasing specialization of the roles of healthcare professionals there is a growing need for different professions to work together. Pharmacists must ensure that they are aware of the different professions they could call on for support or to refer patients to. Examples of referrals include the patient's general practitioner, the accident and emergency department in the hospital, dentists, the community nursing service (district nurses and health visitors), social services and self-help groups.

Where patient care is shared between healthcare professionals there is an obvious need for clear communication links, especially around monitoring and reviewing the patient's therapy. Clear communication links are particularly crucial in supplementary prescribing where two different professions can prescribe for a patient. There must be a clear description of the criteria that would require the supplementary prescriber having to refer the patient back to the independent prescriber. Examples of such referrals could be failure of the patient's condition to respond to the therapy outlined in the clinical management plan or the patient suffering an adverse drug reaction (ADR) to the prescribed medication. With supplementary prescribing, both independent and supplementary prescribers must have access to a common medical record.

Prescribing decision making

Upon analysis and interpretation of the patient's signs, symptoms and laboratory test results, the pharmacist prescriber must consider the treatment options, including the option of offering no treatment to the patient. The consideration of therapy options must include concurrent diseases and medication and the patient's lifestyle (would the treatment regime fit in with the patient's schedule or would side-effects of drugs affect their ability to perform their usual activities).

A key component of this phase is involving the patient in the decision making in order to achieve concordance. The prescriber must communicate the benefits and risks of the different treatment options to the patient or their carer. The principles of concordance dictate that patients should fully participate in the decision-making process, and a consultation style where patients are treated as equals and have the opportunity to ask questions and to raise any concerns or worries they might have is more likely to achieve this.

Following selection of the drug and its formulation, the dosage regime must be determined. The dosage guidance in the summary of product characteristics, *British National Formulary* or local and national clinical guidelines should be used to work out the dosage to be prescribed. In general, it is recommended that dosage be started at the lower end of the dosing schedule and that the dose should be gradually increased until the required therapeutic benefits are seen while minimizing side-effects. However, there are many exceptions to this, such as prescribing a loading dose for certain antibiotics or prescribing drugs where the therapeutic benefits are not obvious, such as drugs used in prophylaxis.

The prescriber must also indicate the quantity to be supplied on the prescription. The quantity to be supplied will depend upon whether the treatment is likely to be acute or chronic. If the treatment is acute then the quantity is likely to be enough for the recommended course of treatment. When determining the quantity to be supplied for a chronic condition, prescribers should bear in mind how often they would wish to review the patient, whether the patient has to pay for the item, the patient's ability to pay the prescription levy and whether there are any dangers from accidental or deliberate overdose. In general, smaller quantities offer the opportunity to review patient's therapy more frequently and reduce waste if patients are unable to take their medicine through the occurrence of troublesome side-effects or ADRs. However, smaller quantities can cause greater inconvenience as patients will have to visit their healthcare professional more frequently and will incur greater expense if they have to pay for their medication. Smaller quantities will also increase the prescriber's workload as they will have to write more prescriptions.

Recording and monitoring

It is important to realize that the responsibilities of the prescriber do not end with signing the prescription. The prescriber must make appropriate records of the medicine(s) prescribed and any advice given to the patient in the patient's medical notes. For paper held records, the prescriber will obviously have to write the name of the prescribed item, the formulation, the strength and the dosage instructions in the notes. In the case of electronic prescribing the details of what was prescribed, the date of prescribing and the directions will be stored automatically in the patient's records. However, there may be a need to record additional information such as when the patient should next be reviewed and the monitoring that is recommended.

All prescribing should be followed up with some monitoring although in some cases this may be left to the patient or carer to do themselves. Monitoring should address the anticipated benefits from therapy such as control of the patient's symptoms and harmful effects such as the patient suffering from adverse effects. In many situations the patient or their carer will be given advice regarding what to do should the beneficial effects not materialize or if the harmful effects are troublesome. However, there may be situations where these are not apparent, such as monitoring blood cell counts following administration of a drug known to affect blood cell formation. These patients should be informed when they will next need to have their therapy reviewed.

Prescribers must appreciate any drug can cause an ADR, but that certain drugs are more likely to cause an ADR. Therefore, they must be aware of the action required if patients suffer from an ADR. Minor ADRs that are known to occur with established medicines do not need reporting while serious suspected and actual ADRs for new and established medicines and all ADRs for new medicines should be reported via the yellow card reporting scheme (see Chs 19 and 47).

Auditing and evaluating practice

Like all areas of practice it is important that prescribers reflect upon their practice and use their continuing professional development (CPD) to develop professionally. Prescribing audits and prescribing reviews can assist the process of reflection. The availability of prescribing reviews will depend upon the area of prescribing practice and, to some extent, the location. The collation and analysis of prescribing data in secondary care is the responsibility of the trust and there is great variability in the availability of such data.

All parts of the UK produce prescribing reports for primary care prescribing although different organizations are responsible for these reports in different parts of the UK and there will be differences in the types of report produced. The majority of the reports are concerned with medical prescribing which is, perhaps, not surprising considering doctors are responsible for the majority of prescribing activity. Non-medical prescribing reports are produced locally by primary care organizations and therefore subject to greater variation between different localities. Prescribing data include the number of items prescribed and the cost of prescribing. It should be noted that these data allow questions for reviewing prescribing practice to be formulated but very rarely ever provide answers. There are many reasons why prescribing figures can be skewed one way or the other. These can make it difficult to make comparisons between practices. Examples of factors affecting prescribing rates include above average numbers of patients living in residential or nursing care or a practice being located in an area with a higher prevalence of disease such as a former coal mining area. Prescribing data do not contain any patient-specific data so it is not possible to differentiate 10 items prescribed for 10 different patients and 10 items prescribed for a single patient. Prescribing data do not contain any drug indications, which can make it difficult to review the prescribing of drugs with several indications. There are usually major differences between the case mix of different professional groups, which makes comparing prescribing across professional boundaries a particularly difficult task.

Evidence-based medicine

Evidence-based medicine (EBM) has been described as 'a means of closing the gap between research and everyday practice and ensuring that clinical decisions are based upon the best available scientific evidence' (MeReC Bulletin 1995). It allows healthcare professionals to compare the evidence for different treatment options. This comparison may sound straightforward but unfortunately the available evidence is frequently of variable quality and different studies may use different methodology or may measure different aspects of health, which makes comparisons difficult.

The process of EBM involves four stages (Eccles et al 1998). The first involves identifying the question to be answered, such as: 'Does treatment with

drug X prevent more cardiovascular events than treatment with drug Y?' The second stage involves searching the literature to find studies that have compared drug X with drug Y. The third stage is a critical appraisal of the studies that have been identified, which involves making judgments about the quality of the studies, comparing the evidence supporting drug X with that supporting drug Y and determining whether the balance of evidence favours one drug over the other. The final stage is applying the evidence to clinical practice, which could involve recommending one drug be prescribed by clinicians rather than the other.

Assessing the quality of the evidence involves comparing the studies reported in the literature (see Ch. 23). There is a hierarchy of type of studies in terms of quality with meta-analysis of more than one randomized controlled trial at the top, then single randomized controlled trials, then controlled trials without randomization, then descriptive or case control studies and finally reports from expert committees (Eccles et al 1998; see Table 17.1 for a description of these terms). A key point to note concerning the method used in the study is whether the study was double blind or not (double blind is where the researcher and the subjects did not know which treatments were given to the subjects). The review of a study should also consider whether there is a potential for bias in the study by considering who funded the study and the affiliations of the authors. It is important to review the doses of drugs used as some studies do not use equivalent doses of drugs, particularly where one drug is compared with a

Table 17.1 Studies investigating health care

Type of study	Description
Meta-analyses	A statistical method of combining the results of more than one trial
Double blind randomized controlled trial (RCT)	A study where one group of subjects is randomly assigned to receive one treatment and the other group to receive an alternative treatment or placebo. Double blind is where neither the researchers nor the subjects are aware of which group they have been assigned to
RCT	A study where one group of subjects is randomly assigned to receive one treatment and the other group to receive an alternative treatment or placebo
Case control studies	A study that compares one group of patients with another
Cohort studies	A study that follows the progress of a group of patients (a cohort) and compares their progress to the characteristics of the group members
Expert opinion	A report from an expert committee or opinions expressed by a respected group of experts

competitor's drug. The reviewers should consider whether the study used healthy volunteers or patients suffering from the condition and whether the demographic profile of the subjects was similar to the general population. Generally, the larger the study, in terms of the number of subjects included, the higher the quality of the study. However, the number of subjects needed to show an effect is dependent on the magnitude of the effect, with larger numbers needed to demonstrate smaller differences between the different arms of the study. The length of the study is another important consideration. This should be related to how the drug will be used in practice as the benefits reported in a study lasting 10 days would have more relevance to a drug used to treat acute short-term conditions compared to long-term chronic conditions where the benefits could wear off after the study ends. The review should consider the endpoint reported in the study (what was measured in the study) and whether the endpoint was the same as the intended outcome (e.g. the intended outcome of a treatment in a study could be a reduction in the incidence of cardiovascular events but the endpoint used in the study might just address one risk factor for cardiovascular events).

Information sources

The evolution of modern medicines and appliances has resulted in a tremendous increase in the range of products available on prescription and a corresponding increase in the amount of information available to support their use. This vast array of information originates from many sources including the pharmaceutical industry, academic institutions, professional bodies, government agencies and patient groups. Much of this information is aimed at prescribers and other professional groups, but, with the increased availability of this information through advances in information technology and the upsurge of public demand, many patients also have greater access to information about medicines. With such a variety of sources all competing for the attention of the prescriber there is a danger that they could be overloaded with information of variable quality and which is potentially conflicting.

Reports of studies published in the literature can be obtained by using online resources and archives such as Medline, Embase or PubMed, although it is likely that most searches will result in large numbers

of hits and reviewing the quality of such a large number of papers will be very time-consuming. Alternatively, there are several sources of evidence-based medicine reviews. The Cochrane Library is a collection of databases that contain evidence-based reviews and is available through the National Electronic Library for Health and University Libraries. Clinical Evidence from the BMJ Publishing Group provides a summary of the evidence available for managing a wide variety of conditions and includes an assessment of the quality of the evidence (see Ch. 23).

Guidelines

There has been a recent proliferation in the number of guidelines produced in developed countries to assist practitioners in a wide variety of clinical roles. They have been defined as 'recommendations on the appropriate treatment and care of people with specific diseases and conditions' (National Institute for Health and Clinical Excellence 2008). However, it should be noted that the foundations on which guidelines are based could range from guidance based on good quality evidence to those based upon expert opinion. The quality of guidelines can also vary and prescribers must decide whether a guideline is suitable for use in their practice. In addition, there are few, if any, guidelines that can provide guidance that is appropriate for 100% of patients. Prescribers should not follow guidelines blindly but consider in which situations the guideline should be used and those when it should not. If a prescriber decides to deliberately deviate from a guideline, they should document their reasons for deviation in the patient's medical notes.

The National Institute for Health and Clinical Excellence (NICE) is an independent organization responsible for providing 'national guidance on the promotion of good health and the prevention and treatment of ill health' (NICE 2008). NICE provides guidance to support the management of a wide range of clinical conditions. The Scottish Intercollegiate Guidelines Network (SIGN) produces evidence-based clinical guidelines for use by people working in the health service and for patients.

Computerized decision support

Software is available that can assist the healthcare professional with diagnosis and prescribing. Relevant patient information such as the age, sex, symptoms and any laboratory tests are entered on to the computer and this software compares these to information held on a database to suggest a diagnosis or further investigations that might be required. The NHS funds a service that helps 'health care professionals confidently make evidence-based decisions about the health care of their patients and provides them with the know-how to safely put these decisions into action' (Clinical Knowledge Summaries 2008). This service is called the Clinical Knowledge Summaries (CKS) service and is available through the National Library for Health on the NHS website. The CKS is replacing PRODIGY which was the original NHS decision support software. CKS also provides a clinical summary of recommendations for managing the patient's condition and information to enable the writing of a prescription, as well as providing access to patient information leaflets developed by NHS Direct.

Formularies

Drug formularies are lists of medicines that prescribers use (see Ch. 18). These range from personal formularies from an individual prescriber to formularies used by one or more general practices or one or more trusts. It has been claimed that formularies can improve prescribing by improving prescriber familiarity with medicines as they only need knowledge of a limited range of medicines. Formularies that span different organizations have the potential to improve consistency of prescribing across the primary–secondary care interface.

The process of producing a formulary can be very time-consuming but it can be educational for those contributing to the process. It provides organizations with the opportunity to compare different medicines within a class on the grounds of effectiveness, safety, patient acceptability and cost and to consider which medicines they wish to see prescribed by prescribers in their organization. Deciding whom to invite on to a formulary group to produce a new formulary is an important stage in the process. In small organizations, such as a general practice, it is likely that all prescribers would be involved in the selection of formulary drugs, but care should be taken to include the views of those affected by the formulary such as the practice nurse, health visitors, district nurses and community pharmacists. In larger organizations it would not be feasible to include everybody in the formulary group. Where

possible each section or department should send a representative who should be able to voice their views and provide feedback.

The methods used to inform prescribers regarding the formulary is another important step in the process, especially in large organizations as prescribers could be unaware of its existence. The cost of printing and distributing paper copies of the formulary will depend upon the quantity involved and type of binding that is used. These can range from a printed book to a ring binder with photocopied sheets. The formulary group should consider how often the formulary will be updated and how user friendly the format is to its prescribers, i.e. is it small enough to take on ward rounds or to visit patients in their home. With computer generated prescribing, the formulary medicines can often be highlighted or listed before non-formulary medicines.

In general, formulary groups should not expect 100% compliance with a formulary because there are always likely to be exceptional patients who do not respond to or have an ADR to certain drugs. The formulary group should therefore decide what level of compliance with the formulary they wish to see and also how they can monitor the actual compliance with the formulary. In some areas they will have no power to insist that formulary medicines are prescribed and they will have to persuade prescribers to consider formulary drugs first. If compliance with the formulary is particularly low then the formulary group should reflect on the suitability of the formulary (are the right drugs in the formulary?) and method of disseminating the formulary (are prescribers aware of the formulary and is it in a format they can use easily in their work?).

Competency framework

The National Prescribing Centre (NPC) is an NHS organization whose aim is 'to promote and support high quality, cost effective prescribing and medicines management across the NHS, to help improve patient care and service delivery'. The NPC has produced a competency framework which brings together the knowledge, skills, motives and personal traits that are considered to be required by a prescriber working effectively (NPC 2006). This framework should be used as a checklist by prescribers preparing to prescribe for the first time and also by prescribers reviewing their own practice as part of their CPD.

KEY POINTS

- Prescribing involves reaching a balance between risk and benefit. Cost and patient choice are both additional factors
- The prescribing process can be viewed as having five stages: having prerequisites, gathering information, analysis, records and monitoring, audit and evaluation
- Pharmacists, with appropriate training, can act as supplementary or independent prescribers
- Clear and complete records of all prescribing and instructions must be kept in the patient's medical record

- Evidence-based medicine closes the gap between research and clinical decision making
- There are four stages to evidence-based medicine: identifying the question, searching the literature, making a critical appraisal, applying the evidence to practice
- The quality of evidence can vary and must be appraised
- Useful information sources include: Medline, Embase, PubMed, Cochrane Library, NICE publications, clinical evidence, computer based clinical knowledge summaries, together with formularies
- The National Prescribing Centre has produced a competency framework

Formularies

Janet Krska

STUDY POINTS

- Different types of formularies
- The benefits of using a formulary
- Developing a formulary
- Formulary management systems

Different types of formularies

Formularies were originally compilations of medicinal preparations, with the formulae for compounding them. The modern definition of a formulary is a list of drugs which are recommended or approved for use by a group of practitioners. It is compiled by members of the group and is regularly revised. Drugs are usually selected for inclusion on the basis of efficacy, safety, patient acceptability and cost. Drugs listed in a formulary should be available for use. Information on dosage, indications, side-effects, contraindications, formulations and costs may also be included. An introduction, giving information on how the drugs were selected, by whom and how to use the formulary, is usually provided.

The most common formulary in use in the UK is the *British National Formulary* (BNF), which compiles details of all the drugs available for prescribing in the UK. It is produced by the Joint Formulary Committee, whose members include doctors and pharmacists as well as representatives from the Department of Health. It is revised every 6 months and is issued to all prescribers and registered pharmacies in both hospitals and the community. Formularies for dentists, the *Dental Practitioners' Formulary*, and for nurse prescribers, the *Nurse Prescribers' Formulary*, are also

included in the BNF. More recently a BNF for children was launched, in recognition of the need for different, more detailed information about prescribing in children.

Local formularies, or lists of recommended drugs, have been widely used in hospitals and increasingly in primary care throughout the UK for many years. Some are designed for small groups, such as one general medical practice, some are for all prescribers within a hospital; others may be intended for all prescribers within a large geographical area. The latter are often known as joint formularies, since they are compiled and intended for use by prescribers in both primary and secondary care. A recent survey found that 64% of primary care organizations have some sort of formulary and 47% are joint initiatives with secondary care. The increasing availability of a funded minor ailments service in community pharmacy, providing selected medicines free of charge to certain patients, has necessitated the development of formularies from which local pharmacists can supply the recommended products. Local formularies are usually developed and maintained by an Area Drug and Therapeutics Committee (ADTC). These committees involve pharmacists, hospital doctors, general practitioners and nurses who practise within a locality, and often also include management, public health and financial expertise.

Worldwide, formularies are a concept which is promoted by the World Health Organization (WHO). The essential medicines list (see Ch. 7) which is recommended as necessary for basic health care in developing countries is similar to a formulary. Any country can modify this list to meet its own particular needs and arrive at a 'national formulary'. The basis of any list is that the drugs it contains are of proven

Table 18.1 Examples of formularies

Purpose	Example formulary
General use	British National Formulary
Hospital formulary	University College London Hospitals NHS Trust Formulary
General practice	Cambridgeshire Primary Care Trust Formulary
Joint formulary	Tayside Area Prescribing Guide Lothian Joint Formulary
Specialist formulary	Palliative Care Formulary
Developing countries	WHO Essential Drug List

therapeutic efficacy, acceptable safety and satisfy the health needs of the populations they serve. Some examples of formularies are given in Table 18.1.

A formulary may be thought of as a prescribing policy, because it lists which drugs are recommended. Prescribing policies should, however, be much more detailed than a formulary, giving details of drugs which should be selected for use in specific medical conditions. Examples of prescribing policies in common use are antibiotic policies, head lice eradication policies and malarial prophylaxis policies.

Clinical guidelines contain more detailed information than a formulary about how a service should be delivered or patients treated and do not always specify the drugs to be used. Many are developed nationally, such as by the National Centre for Health and Clinical Excellence (NICE), Scottish Intercollegiate Guidelines Network (SIGN), British Thoracic Society, British Society for Haematology and so on. Local guidelines may be developed by ADTCs and are more likely to include recommendations which specify drugs included in the local formulary.

Benefits of formularies

Drug costs are a major component of the total cost of the NHS and are constantly rising. As the resources of the NHS are finite, it becomes increasingly necessary to contain the escalation in drug costs. Much evidence shows that drugs are not always prescribed appropriately. Therefore improving prescribing could reduce expenditure on drugs. Local formularies

which recommend specific drugs and exclude others are one means of achieving this. Prescribing policies assist prescribers in using the drugs in a formulary and specific treatment protocols make them even more useful. Clinical guidelines help to ensure that the treatment of patients is based on evidence of best practice. Used together, formularies, clinical guidelines and treatment protocols can ensure that standards of prescribing are both uniform and high quality. All these are tools used to promote rational and cost-effective prescribing.

Rational prescribing

Prescribing which is based on the four important factors of efficacy, safety, patient acceptability and cost should be rational. While many drugs may be available to treat any particular condition, the process of selecting the most appropriate one for any individual patient should take account of all these factors, plus other patient factors, such as concurrent diseases, drugs, previous exposure and outcomes. The four factors can also be applied to selection of drugs to treat populations of patients and it is for this situation that formularies are developed. Providing drug selection is based on good quality evidence of efficacy and toxicity, formularies then assist in making decisions regarding individual patients.

Cost-effective prescribing

Formularies often provide information on the cost of products to help users to become cost conscious.

Local formularies usually include only a small proportion of the drugs listed in the BNF, often between 200 and 500. If prescribers only use the range of drugs included in a local formulary, the range stocked by pharmacies can decrease, which reduces unnecessary outlay. Using a restricted range of drugs may allow pharmacists to buy these in bulk, further reducing costs. Formularies also encourage generic prescribing which may reduce costs even further. If fewer products are stocked, monitoring of expiry dates becomes easier and cash flow may improve. Any money saved on hospital or on GPs' budgets by using a formulary may be used to benefit patients in other ways. For example, reducing the prescribing of drugs which have little evidence of therapeutic benefit, such as peripheral vasodilators, could enable more to be spent on lipid-lowering drugs. Formularies may also recommend using more cost-effective alternatives to some expensive modified-release formulations. In addition, as safety is also a key factor in drug selection, formularies may contribute to reducing the incidence of adverse drug reactions, which often carry a high cost.

Educational value

Compilation of a formulary involves researching the literature to gather evidence of efficacy and toxicity. For those involved, this is a highly demanding task, but one which is of considerable educational benefit. There are also benefits for users of formularies. Prescribers who use a restricted range of drugs should know more about those drugs and their formulations through frequent use. Ultimately this should result in benefits for the patient, as prescribers' increased knowledge should reduce the risk of inappropriate prescribing, which could contribute to adverse effects, interactions or lack of efficacy.

Continuous care

A joint local formulary which covers both primary and secondary care encourages the same range of drugs to be prescribed, which makes continuing drug treatment across the interface easier. As patient packs are increasingly dispensed, patients are more likely to use their own drugs during a hospital stay. A joint formulary helps this, as there is less chance of drug therapy having to change to comply with a different formulary on admission to hospital.

Formulary development

Formularies take a very long time to produce: several years is not uncommon. Obtaining everyone's opinions and discussing the drugs to be included are the main reasons, for this prolonged time. A formulary then needs to be updated regularly if it is going to be useful, which is a further time commitment. There are two basic ways of producing a new formulary – either start from scratch or modify an existing one. Adapting another formulary to suit local needs is much less time-consuming than starting from scratch. Although much can be learned from looking at someone else's formulary, simply deciding to adopt it without any changes is not a good idea. Producing a formulary is an educational process, during which all concerned learn from each other's experience and update their clinical pharmacology and therapeutics along the way. Producing a formulary also brings a sense of ownership, which encourages commitment to it and increases the chance of it being used. Local needs should also be addressed by a local formulary, so copying someone else's may not be satisfactory.

A local ADTC is most likely to oversee the task of developing a formulary. Although the committee will include different healthcare professionals, pharmacists usually play a key role. Small subgroups of local experts may do most of the development work, but the opinions of potential users should also be sought. This is a very important point in formulary development. The people expected to use a formulary must have the opportunity to give their views on its content. If their opinions are not asked, they may feel that it does not apply to them and will be less likely to use it. Smaller formularies, such as for one general medical practice or ward, should be developed by all the prescribers working in that practice or ward together with a pharmacist. Such formularies may draw on the work of ADTCs and select even fewer drugs from the area formulary, but may add others. It is important that formularies reflect the needs of the population being treated. So obviously a formulary for a surgical ward will differ from that for a general practice, but both may be derived from the area formulary.

Content

The formulary should start with an introduction, giving the names of those who have compiled it, stating who is expected to use it and explaining its format (Fig. 18.1). It is important to state whether all the

(A)

Introduction

This pocket guide is designed to be a handy compact reference and includes the names of medicines recommended within the Tayside Area Prescribing Guide (TAPG). Where appropriate, medicines recommended as first choice are shaded in blue and those recommended for use in particular circumstances are in *italics*. First choice medicines are chosen on the grounds of efficacy, safety and cost-effectiveness and represent the best evidence-based and cost-effective choice for the majority of patients with a particular condition. Users should refer to the full document and the BNF for further detail and more specific information. This pocket guide is updated annually.

The most up to date version of the TAPG is maintained in electronic form at:
http://www.nhstaysideadtc.scot.nhs.uk/approved/formular/formular.htm
or on your local intranet under E-Health/Tayside Area Prescribing Guide.

For enquiries contact: kharknesst.glet@nhs.net
Tel: 01382 632351

Key

Drug name shaded blue: recommended first choice medicine
Drug name in *italics*: recommended only in particular circumstances
(see full TAPG)

(B)

3: Respiratory System

3.1 Bronchodilators
Beta₂-agonists
Short acting:
Salbutamol

Terbutaline

Long-acting:
Salmeterol

Formoterol

Antimuscarinic bronchodilators
Short-acting:
Ipratropium

Long-acting:
Tiotropium

Theophylline – prescribe by brand name:
Uniphyllin®

Compound bronchodilator preparations:
Combivent®

3.2 Inhaled corticosteroids
Beclometasone

Budesonide

Fluticasone

Ciclesonide?

Compound preparations:
Seretide®

Symbicort®

3.3 Cromoglicate related therapy and leukotriene receptor antagonists
Cromoglicate and related therapy:
Sodium Cromoglicate

Leukotriene receptor antagonists:
Montelukast

3.4 Antihistamines and allergic emergencies

Non-sedative antihistamines:
Cetirizine

Loratadine

Fexofenadine

Sedative antihistamines:
Chlorphenamine

Alimemazine

Allergic emergencies:
Adrenaline/Epinephrine

3.7 Mucolytics
Carbocisteine

Figure 18.1 ● Formulary introduction and formulary recommendations for respiratory drugs, illustrating presentation as a Pocket Guide (reproduced with permission from Tayside Area Prescribing Guide Pocket Guide 2007, copyright: NHS Tayside Drug and Therapeutics Committee).

drugs included are recommended for all users, and if not, how different recommendations can be distinguished. The BNF, for example, lists drugs the Joint Formulary Committee considers less suitable for prescribing in small type. The examples in Figures 18.1 and 18.2 illustrate how the recommended first choice drugs are highlighted. Local formularies may choose to place restrictions on some drugs, for use by specialists only, for certain indications only or in certain locations only. These drugs should also be easily distinguishable from the others in the formulary; in Figure 18.1 these are in italic. A list of contents and an index should be included to make the formulary easy to use.

Most UK formularies follow the BNF to classify medicines. Reference to the relevant BNF section is helpful if a local formulary is designed to be used in conjunction with it. Users can be directed to the monographs there for information on dosage, indications, side-effects, contraindications and precautions. Some formularies include all this information, but only for the recommended drugs. Other important information which may be given is local drug costs and the reasons for selecting the drugs included.

Drug costs are one of the factors taken into account when compiling a formulary (see below). The price of a drug can be expressed in several different ways. The prices given in the BNF are the prices of different pack sizes or for 20 doses of generics at drug tariff prices. The cost of a period of treatment may be more useful if comparisons are being encouraged. A suitable period may be 1 day, 1 month (28 days) or a standard course of treatment (e.g. 5 days for antibiotics). Since the price of the drug usually varies with the pack size, this may not be as easy to calculate as it first appears. A further complicating factor is the differing prices in hospital and community. If a formulary is designed to be used in hospital only, the hospital price may seem most relevant. However, the price of the drug may be different in general practice and patients may take the drug while living in the community for much longer than they take it in hospital. Therefore the price in the community is also of relevance, especially in joint formularies.

When large numbers of prescribers are to use a formulary, it is possible that not all of them will have been consulted about its content. If that is the case, providing explanations of how drugs have come to be included in a formulary is of particular importance. Many formularies state the general basis of drug selection as being efficacy, safety, patient acceptability and cost. Sometimes additional information is given about specific drugs, which can assist furthering drug selection. The BNF gives this type of information in introductory paragraphs to each section. An example is the statement that 'other thiazide diuretics do not offer any significant advantage over bendroflumethiazide and chlortalidone'. It may be desirable to reference the formulary to give readers the opportunity to see the evidence on which statements such as these are based. It may also be useful to explain local preferences, particularly in the case of antibiotic selection, which should take local microbiological sensitivities into account.

Some or all of the formulary may be presented as prescribing policies. While this is most likely for antibiotics, policies may be included for any group of drugs. If this approach is taken, details of which drugs are to be used in specific medical conditions should be given. It may be necessary to include alternatives and the particular occasions when they should be used. In a prescribing policy, details of the recommended dosage, route and method of administration and duration of therapy should also be included.

A local formulary may have sections relating to prescribing in certain types of patients, such as the elderly, children, those with renal or hepatic impairment, or in pregnancy and breastfeeding. As there is little point in reproducing the BNF, these too should reflect local recommendations.

Presentation of a formulary

The appearance of a formulary is an indicator of the importance attached to it by those who have produced it. If it is presented on a few tattered sheets of paper, those who are expected to use it are unlikely to have a great deal of respect for its content. This may lead to poor adherence to its recommendations. It is therefore worth creating a document which is attractive and looks professionally produced. It is also important to consider whether a paper or electronic format is desirable or whether both should be available.

Paper formats can be portable, making for ease of use in any clinical setting, from the hospital bedside to the patient's home. However, they are expensive to produce and still require regular updating. The size of the document is an important consideration. Ideally, it should be no bigger than pocket-sized, perhaps compatible in size with the BNF, to make it easy to use the two together. A simple list of formulary drugs is a useful option, such as that illustrated in Figure 18.1, produced by NHS Tayside Drug and Therapeutics Committee. This can be supplemented by a larger

(A)

Asthma: for management of asthma please refer to BTS / SIGN guideline No. 101 (revised May 2008) **COPD:** For COPD management please refer to NICE Clinical Guideline 12 (Feb 2004).
Although first choice drugs have been indicated where possible, for any inhaled treatment, choosing the most suitable device for the patient is the most important factor for ensuring effective therapy (see guidance). In general, patients are best treated with single-ingredient preparations so that the dose of each drug can be individually adjusted.

3.1 Bronchodilators

Beta₂ agonists
Short-acting

FIRST CHOICE: **SALBUTAMOL**

Salbutamol
Dose: (In asthma or COPD) By aerosol inhalation, 100–200micrograms (1–2 puffs), when required to relieve breathlessness.

Terbutaline
Dose: (In asthma or COPD) By inhalation of powder, 500micrograms (1 inhalation), when required to relieve breathlessness.

Long-acting

Salmeterol
Dose: (In asthma or COPD) By inhalation, 50micrograms (2 puffs or 1 blister) twice daily.

Formoterol (Eformoterol)
Dose: (In asthma or COPD) By inhalation, 6–12micrograms once or twice daily (dose depending on preparation used - see BNF). (Note: each metered 6 and 12microgram dose of Oxis® 6 and Oxis® 12 Turbohalers actually delivers 4.5 and 9micrograms respectively at the mouthpiece, each metered dose of Atimos Modulite® 12micrograms delivers 10.1micrograms)

☑ **Long-acting inhaled beta-2 agonists should not be used without inhaled corticosteroids in asthma;** they should be added to existing inhaled corticosteroid therapy and not replace it.

Click here for advice on the place of long-acting beta-2 agonists in the management of chronic asthma. Where adequate asthma symptom control is not achieved at the above doses of long-acting beta-2 agonists pease refer to algorithm click here and the BTS/SIGN asthma guidance for advice on maximising inhaled steroid therapy.

Antimuscarinic (Anticholinergic) bronchodilator
Short-acting

Ipratropium
Dose: (In COPD) By aerosol inhalation ▼, 20–40micrograms (1–2 puffs) 3–4 times daily.
(Ipratropium aerosol inhalation has had a black triangle status since it was changed to CFC-free).

Long-acting

(B)

Tiotropium
Dose: Inhalation in COPD only by dry-powder *HandiHaler®* device, 18micrograms once daily.
Dose: By inhalation in COPD only of *Respime®* aerosol ▼, 5micrograms (2 puffs) once daily.

5micrograms (2puffs) of the *Respime®* inhaler has similar lung deposition to 18micrograms (1 capsule) of the *HandiHaler®* device.

See COPD therapeutic notes. Do not co-prescribe tiotropium with a short-acting antimuscarinic (anticholinergic) bronchodilator, including compound preparations.

Theophylline - prescribe by brand name

Uniphyllin® m/r tablets 200mg, 300mg, 400mg
Dose: 200mg every 12 hours, increased gradually according to response to 400mg every 12 hours.

Note: there are other oral theophylline brands available. However, there are differences in bioavailability between them and dosages are not equivalent. Patients should keep with the same brand if changes in dose are made. Oral theophyllines are weak bronchodilators with a high incidence of side-effects and are now less commonly used with other drugs: some may produce theophylline toxicity (e.g. clarithromycin, erythromycin, ciprofloxacin, cimetidine), others may decrease plasma levels (e.g. anti-epileptics, rifampicin). See BNF for full interaction profile. Monitoring plasma levels of theophylline is not routinely necessary in stable patients but may be warranted in certain circumstances e.g. a change in clinical status, where toxicity is suspected or during concomitant use of ineracting drugs. Note: smoking cessation may increase theophylline levels. Seek advice if unsure. See MHRA Drug Safety Update Oktober 2008 for safety advice on theophylline containing medicines available over the counter from community pharmacists.

Compound bronchodilator preparations

In patients with severe COPD requiring regular nebulised bronchodilators, **salbutamol 2.5mg nebuliser solution and ipratropium 500microgram nebuliser solution** can be prescribed separately or as a combined product (**Combivent® nebuliser solution**).

Figure 18.2 • Formulary recommendations for bronchodilators, illustrating presentation as a detailed prescribing guide (reproduced with permission from http://www.nhstaysideadtc.scot.nhs.uk/TAPG%20html/Section%203/3-1.htm).

document in either paper or electronic form. If the formulary is only available as a large paper document which cannot be carried around, it is much less likely to be available when needed, which may mean its recommendations are ignored. Colour and a durable cover to withstand regular use can both add further to the appearance of a paper formulary, but also increase its cost.

Electronic formats are increasingly popular, but not all professionals use a computer when prescribing, so it may still be necessary to produce a paper version, even if this is only the list of drugs. A CD version is one option, but like a paper document, requires re-distribution whenever it is updated. Local organizations, such as hospital and primary care trusts, have an intranet, on which the formulary can be published. Linking the local formulary to electronic prescribing systems is perhaps the ideal option. Some prescribing systems incorporate decision support tools, which can include the formulary. Electronic versions may also make it easier to evaluate the formulary by examining prescribing adherence.

Ensuring that the formulary is up to date is extremely important and its presentation must allow for this. Loose-leaf binding will enable easy updating, but relies on everyone modifying their own copy. It is much easier to update an electronic version which is distributed via the Internet or intranet.

Whatever format is used, the formulary should be easy to use, to encourage prescribers to refer to it when necessary. This will be helped by a contents list, which for a paper version means the pages have to be numbered. Arranging the drugs in the same order as the BNF will also help to make the formulary easier to use, as prescribers should be familiar with this order. Using different typefaces and print size can make a formulary easier to use. Highlighting the drug names can be useful, as often the name of the recommended drug may be all that someone is seeking (see Fig. 18.1).

It may also be appropriate to provide access to the formulary for local patients. Increasingly, patients have access to clinical guidelines and are informed about what treatments are recommended for their medical problems. Providing a formulary has been developed using transparent methods and drugs selected on the basis of efficacy, safety, patient acceptability and cost, there is no reason to prevent patients from knowing of its existence. Access can be via the Internet, so need not add to publication costs.

Selection of products for inclusion

It is important to decide at the outset the range of indications which the formulary should cover. Some hospital formularies do not attempt to include drugs to treat all possible conditions. Some deliberately exclude certain drugs, such as those used in cancer chemotherapy and anaesthetics. These areas are extremely specialized, so drugs in these groups are never likely to be used by most prescribers. A formulary for use in general practice should aim to include enough drugs to treat between 80% and 90% of all common conditions which present to a GP. It is also useful to include emergency drugs, such as those which should be carried by GPs in their emergency bags. Clearly if a formulary includes all the available drugs, as does the BNF, it will not only be bulky, but also will not have many of the advantages that a local formulary can provide. It should be possible to cover most needs, either in hospital or general practice, with about 300–500 drugs. In selecting drugs for inclusion in a formulary, it is important to remember that recommendations are being made to treat the majority of the population. However, individual patients' needs and preferences should, where possible, be taken into account. This means that there may be individuals for whom the recommended formulary drug is not suitable, but the formulary should attempt to make provision for most commonly encountered situations. This usually means that, out of the range available, two drugs from a pharmacological class may be included rather than one.

While the four important factors are efficacy, safety, patient acceptability and cost, other factors are also usually considered (Box 18.1). Formulary drugs must be effective for whatever indications they are to be used, with minimal toxicity. Evidence of efficacy should be based on well-conducted clinical trials rather than anecdotal reports. Generally, prescribers' personal preferences are not a sound basis for selection of a particular drug or product. This is especially true when the formulary is to be used by many prescribers, as each may have their own preference. Occasionally there may be a range of similar drugs from which to select, but not all are licensed for all the indications the formulary is to cover. An example is beta-adrenoceptor antagonists, some of which have a range of licensed indications (Table 18.2). In this situation, selection of

Box 18.1

Factors influencing selection of drugs for inclusion in a formulary

- Efficacy for the indications to be included in the formulary
- Side-effect profiles and contraindications of individual drugs
- Interaction profile of individual drugs
- Pharmacokinetic profiles of individual drugs
- Acceptability to patients – taste, appearance, ease of administration
- Formulations available
- General availability, including generic availability
- Cost
- Usage patterns

the drug which covers most indications may be appropriate. Alternatively, separate drugs could be selected for different indications. This option results in difficulties when auditing adherence, as it is impossible to tell from looking at prescribing data only whether the drug is prescribed in line with the formulary recommendations.

If two drugs are equally efficacious, as is often the case within a group of pharmacologically similar drugs, the least toxic one is preferable. Any differences between the drugs in terms of their pharmacokinetics, contraindications, adverse effects and potential for interaction then become important.

Pharmacokinetic profiles of drugs are important in selecting drugs with an optimum half-life for their indications. It may also be possible to select drugs which are minimally affected by either liver or renal impairment. Among the benzodiazepine group, for example, those with short half-lives and which have no active metabolites are usually preferred as hypnotics, as they have no hangover effect. Differences in drug handling in children and the elderly may require different drugs to be recommended for use with these patients. Selection of drugs for use in pregnancy and breastfeeding will be influenced by their passage into the placenta and secretion into breast milk.

The range of contraindications, precautions and adverse effects may differ for drugs within a therapeutic class. While class effects are common, sometimes there are differences between individual drugs; again beta-adrenoceptor antagonists are a good example of this. Differences are most often found in the frequency and severity of adverse effects between drugs in a class. Where possible, formulary drugs should have the lowest frequency of, and least severe, adverse effects.

Table 18.2 Example using beta-adrenoceptor antagonists of how factors can be used to select drugs for a formulary

Factor	Examples of information to be taken into account	Examples of possible selection
Licensed indications	For hypertension there are many to select from	Atenolol, propranolol, metoprolol, etc.
OR	For arrhythmias, few are licensed	Sotalol, esmolol
Evidence of efficacy	For secondary prevention of myocardial infarction For heart failure	Atenolol injection, metoprolol, propranolol Bisoprolol, carvedilol
Toxicity	Water solubility results in less nightmares Intrinsic sympathomimetic activity causes less cold extremities	Atenolol, sotalol Oxprenolol, pindolol
Contraindications	Cardioselectivity is preferable in asthma and diabetes	Atenolol, bisoprolol, metoprolol
Pharmacokinetic profile	Long-acting drugs/products require fewer doses	Atenolol, modified-release propranolol
Generic availability	Usually reduces cost	Atenolol, propranolol, metoprolol, bisoprolol
Acceptability to patients	Once-daily doses, combination products may be useful	Atenolol, co-tenidone
Cost	Cheapest preferable if all other factors equal	Atenolol, propranolol, metoprolol

If drugs are similar in terms of efficacy and toxicity but have different potential for interaction, this could be a deciding factor. Drugs with fewer possibilities of interaction mean fewer problems in use.

Patient acceptability is an important factor, which will be affected by efficacy and toxicity. If drugs do not work, or if they cause side-effects, patients are less likely to take them. For orally administered drugs, palatability and ease of swallowing will contribute to acceptability. Other considerations may also be important, such as the extent to which a dispersible preparation actually disperses, or whether a modified-release tablet can be divided. Inhaled drugs are available in many different formulations and their selection will depend to an extent on what patients will or can use properly, to achieve maximum efficacy. For topical products, such as creams and ointments, patient acceptability is particularly important.

A local formulary may simply list drugs which are recommended or it may specify particular dosage forms of those drugs. Patient acceptability is likely to influence the different formulations selected for inclusion in a formulary more than the drug entities. However, the range of formulations available, which will in turn affect patients' acceptance of drug therapy, may be a factor in deciding which drugs to include. If a drug is available in a wide range of formulations, it may be a better choice than one which has very few. It is simpler for the prescriber to remember one drug name when a particular class of drug is required, rather than to have to choose different drugs because they come in different formulations.

Many formularies exclude all combination products which include two or more drugs in fixed ratio. This is because it is impossible to increase the dose of one drug without also increasing the dose of the other drug(s). Some patients may receive higher doses of one of the constituents than they require as a result. However, combination products are more favoured in primary care, where they are considered to improve patient compliance and also reduce prescription charges for the patient. Combination products may be useful if the pharmacokinetic characteristics of the components are compatible and it can be shown that patients require and obtain benefit from all the components individually, in the same ratio as the combination product. Unfortunately, very few combination products are used in this way. Their inclusion in a formulary will depend on local preferences and appropriate use will subsequently depend on individual prescribers.

Cost considerations are also important, but the aim of a formulary is to encourage rational and cost-effective prescribing, not primarily to save money. Cost-effective prescribing involves the use of the drug with the lowest costs which is also effective, has minimal toxicity and is acceptable to patients. The cheapest drugs may not be the most acceptable, or of adequate efficacy. For some groups of drugs, prescribing costs may actually rise as a result of using a local formulary, since the optimum drugs may be the most expensive. However, where efficacy, toxicity and patient acceptability are equal, cost should be the deciding factor in drug selection. As described above, both hospital and community costs of drugs should be considered when selecting drugs for a hospital formulary, as the bulk of the cost is likely to be borne by primary care. The purchase price of a drug may not be the only factor to be taken into account when considering costs. Pharmacoeconomic evaluations, which take account of the costs of the consequences of treatments, may also be necessary (see Ch. 19).

All drugs included in a formulary should be easily available, so 'specials', drugs available in hospital only, or on a named patient basis, should be avoided. Generic availability is a bonus, as it usually means costs are lower than for drugs which are only available as branded formulations. Most formularies specify that prescribing should be generic, where appropriate. The use of computer systems for prescribing, which automatically change prescriptions to the appropriate generic name, increases the proportion of generic prescriptions considerably. This should also reduce costs.

As part of their role in formulary development, pharmacists frequently provide unbiased information about any differences in efficacy, toxicity and cost between drugs. Some useful sources of information are the National Prescribing Centre in Liverpool or the Scottish Medicines Resource Centre in Edinburgh and Drug and Therapeutics Bulletin.

Use of prescribing data

All the factors mentioned so far can also be applied to the selection of drugs for individual patients. A further factor which may be considered when selecting drugs for populations is current prescribing habits. The main reason for this is that it is much easier to encourage use of a formulary if it involves few changes of habit. However, if the commonly prescribed drugs are not efficacious, or have a high incidence or severity of toxicity, it is better not to include them. Frequent use does not necessarily imply appropriate selection. Information about current prescribing is obtainable for either hospital or primary care prescribers. National databases on hospital prescribing are being developed, but prescribing data from computerized pharmacy supply systems are readily available which usually relate to wards or directorates. In primary care, data are available from the Prescription Pricing Division in England, Health Solutions in Wales, the Information and Statistics Division in Scotland and the Central Services Agency in Northern Ireland. The data can identify prescribing by an individual GP or by a practice.

From data on the frequency with which different products are prescribed it is usually possible to identify one or two drugs within each therapeutic class which account for the bulk of prescriptions. These should usually be considered for inclusion in a formulary, as little change in prescribing habits will be needed, providing they are efficacious and have minimal toxicity. It may be possible to include only these drugs in a formulary, or there may be a need for others to be included on a more restricted basis. If the commonly prescribed drugs are inappropriate on therapeutic grounds, alternatives may be required.

Formulary management systems

A formulary needs to be flexible and dynamic. A system must be devised which allows this. This is known as the formulary management system and it covers many other aspects of formularies.

Production, distribution and revision

Producing a formulary is a very time-consuming task which, although overseen by the ADTC, needs a driver to take responsibility for ensuring it is completed. Usually this is a pharmacist, who will be involved in collecting together the data on which the drug selection will be based (published evidence, prescribing data and expert or all group members' opinions), drafting material, reaching agreement on the format(s) and design to be used and seeing it through to production. The ADTC should consider who will need a copy and how it will be distributed. For paper versions, photocopying is cheapest for small numbers and can

still incorporate colour and be attractively bound for a professional appearance. However, if large numbers are required, printing becomes more economical.

Distribution by mail with a covering letter may be easiest for large numbers of people, but hand delivery, with verbal explanation, may help to encourage interest and therefore adherence to a formulary's recommendations. Launching of a new formulary (or indeed a revision) can usefully be accompanied by a meeting to explain its aims, describe how to use it and encourage discussion of its contents. Leaflets advertising the benefits of using the formulary and educational material may be usefully developed to encourage prescribers to learn about why they should consider using it.

Electronic versions can obviously be easily distributed within an NHS trust, but require just as much supplementary information to encourage their use. Specialist IT support to ensure that the formulary can be integrated with electronic prescribing systems is a key factor in their successful use.

After all the effort which goes into producing a new formulary has resulted in the final document, the thought of revising it is likely to be far from popular. However, because of the time taken to produce a new formulary, it will soon go out of date. If this is allowed to happen, respect for its content will decline. Adherence to its recommendations may follow suit. Revision should therefore be considered even before the formulary is finished. The BNF is revised every 6 months, but most local formularies cannot hope to achieve a similar frequency, because of the amount of work involved. Annual or biennial revision should be aimed at and specified at the launch. As new drugs are coming onto the market all the time, even 6-monthly revision will not be adequate to keep a formulary up to date. Some system, therefore, needs to be devised to allow new drugs to be considered for inclusion.

Responding to the needs of practice

Change is the norm in the world of drugs. New drugs are constantly becoming available, old drugs are removed from the market, new clinical trials provide evidence for efficacy of existing drugs in novel indications and post-marketing surveillance provides constantly changing data on adverse effect profiles. An awareness of all the facts this generates is essential, so that the formulary does not go out of date and can respond to the changes. In implementing a formulary, patients must not be deprived of the benefits of new information and drugs. There will also inevitably be an occasional need for patients to receive treatment outwith a formulary's recommendations, since a formulary cannot be expected to cover all possible situations. Methods are therefore needed to allow drugs to be considered for inclusion in the formulary, to allow drugs to be removed from the formulary and to supply non-formulary drugs when these are appropriate.

A method for allowing drugs to be considered for inclusion in a formulary should not be restricted to newly available drugs. It must allow any user of the formulary to propose a drug for consideration and should be able to provide an evaluated response within a reasonable time. Evidence of any advantages the proposed drug has over drugs already included, in terms of efficacy, reduced toxicity or cost, will be needed. This must be based on well-designed published clinical trials, the same basis as that used in the initial formulary development. Many formulary management systems require a form to be completed; an example is given in Figure 18.3. The person making the request must be informed as to whether the drug will be included and, if so, whether any restrictions will be placed on its prescribing. One option is to have

---

Request for inclusion of a new drug in a formulary

Drug name _____ Manufacturer _____

Formulations available _____

Indication(s) for which request is made _____

Usual dose and duration of treatment _____

Type of inclusion requested
☐ recommendation for general use
☐ specialist use only

If specialist use, which specialist(s)? _____

☐ restricted indication(s)
Reason for request
☐ novel therapeutic advance
☐ benefits over existing drug

Will the new drug replace an existing drug? Yes/No

If so, which? _____

Estimated number of patients per year who will receive drug _____

Estimated costs of treatment _____

Evidence provided in support of request:
☐ Summary of Product Characteristics
☐ Copies of RCTs, meta-analyses, review articles
☐ Pharmaco-economic evaluation

This request is supported by: (signatures required)

Consultant _____

Clinical Pharmacist _____

Trust Clinical Director _____

Figure 18.3 • Example of a form which could be used to request new drugs to be considered for inclusion in a formulary.

an appraisal period, say 6 months, during which prescribers can gain experience with a newly recommended drug. After this period the committee can then review the status of the drug.

If a drug is accepted onto an existing formulary between revisions, it is essential to inform all users of the change. One way of achieving this is to issue information bulletins, either by post or e-mail. A similar method can be used to inform users of any changes in the indications or doses of drugs which may also occur during the life of a formulary. Similarly, if drugs are to be withdrawn from the formulary, users must be kept informed. Regular bulletins issued by the ADTC are therefore an important feature of formulary management.

Withdrawals may occur because of manufacturers ceasing production, product licences being withdrawn or changes in manufacturers' recommendations. However, it may also be useful to consider withdrawing drugs from the formulary if they have not been prescribed for a long time. Again, 6 months would be a suitable time to study the prescribing of most drugs, except those whose use is seasonal. This could be done on a regular basis between major revisions, but would require consultation with prescribers before the withdrawal was implemented. The advantage of a practice such as this is that it helps to keep the number of drugs in the formulary to a minimum.

As there will be situations when a non-formulary drug is requested for a patient, it may be necessary to have a method of ensuring that the request is dealt with promptly. In primary care, there should be no problem in supplying a non-formulary drug, although there may be a delay if it is not stocked by local pharmacies owing to rare use. In hospital, however, pharmacies tend to stock only a limited range of drugs. Formulary drugs should always be easily available, but non-formulary drugs may need to be purchased specially. This will lead to delays in treatment. Some formulary management systems, usually in hospitals, require completion of a form for every non-formulary drug which is prescribed. The purpose of this is twofold: it acts as a deterrent to prescribing non-formulary drugs and also allows monitoring to see whether any drugs are frequently requested. Consideration may be given to including frequently requested drugs in the formulary. Usually forms require a senior medical staff signature, but there is a possibility that this requirement may be abused. Once a form with the appropriate signature is received, pharmacists should not simply assume that the request should be complied with. If this occurs, all that

has been achieved is an elaborate ordering system. For the formulary system to operate effectively, all prescribers requesting a non-formulary drug should be questioned to determine the reasons why a formulary drug is not suitable.

One of the most frequent reasons for requesting a non-formulary drug in hospital is that the patient was taking the drug prior to admission and prescribers are reluctant to change it. This can be viewed as an opportunity to review the medication, ensuring that it is appropriate for the individual patient. If it proves to be so, it may be possible to use the patient's own supply of the drug, providing there are systems in place to ensure this is indeed required and fit for use. If this is not an option, a decision must be made on whether the requested drug will be supplied from the pharmacy. The systems in place must ensure that this is a rapid process, particularly if a special purchase is required.

The most common reason for using non-formulary drugs in primary care is also that patients are already taking them and either they or their GPs are reluctant to change the prescription. Pharmacists can use the opportunity of conducting medication reviews to consider the appropriateness of any non-formulary drugs prescribed. Pharmacists also undertake regular review of repeat prescribing in many practices, using the techniques of drug utilization review, drug use evaluation and audit (see Ch. 19). Non-formulary prescribing can be assessed through these mechanisms and therapeutic switching undertaken to address any changes which would be of benefit.

The promotional activities of drug manufacturers' representatives will need to be controlled to prevent them from undermining the principles of a local formulary. Many NHS trusts have policies on which staff representatives are allowed to see and what they are allowed to supply. Manufacturers can be an extremely useful source of information on their products, but the inclusion of a drug in a formulary must be evidence based and unbiased. Making constructive use of the visit from a pharmaceutical company's representative can be a beneficial educational exercise to staff involved in using a formulary.

Clearly a lot of effort goes into operating a formulary and there are many advantages of a good formulary management system. The measure of success of any formulary is in the extent to which it is used or adhered to and the demonstration that prescribing is more rational. It may be possible to show improvements in efficacy and reduced toxicity and also cost savings, but these may be more difficult to achieve and to demonstrate.

Changing practice

Developing local formularies and treatment protocols encourages good relationships between prescribers and pharmacists. Building on this relationship is important to enable the changes to practice to be made which will be necessary in implementing these. Changing prescribing habits can be extremely difficult. Some prescribers dislike losing the freedom to prescribe as they choose and may reject a formulary and its concept. Often prescribers have developed personal drug preferences over the years and, even if they have no objection in principle to prescribing a different drug, may easily forget when actually writing prescriptions. Incorporating the formulary into electronic prescribing systems, which restrict choice or at least highlight formulary drugs as preferred, is therefore of great benefit. If agreement on what drugs should be used has been difficult to achieve, the resultant formulary may contain a large number of drugs. This can be more easily adhered to, but is less likely to achieve rational prescribing or to reduce drug costs. Conversely a formulary which is too restrictive is more likely to be difficult to adhere to.

When a formulary is introduced, some patients will be receiving medicines which are not included and they, too, may be resistant to change. The doctors who prescribe for these patients may also be unhappy about changing individual patients' drugs. This is especially likely if the patient is well stabilized on a particular drug, with little adverse effects. As drugs included in a formulary will have been selected on a sound basis, it could be more suitable for a patient than their current drug. Change may therefore be of benefit. Education of prescribers and patients may be necessary to convince them of potential benefits and can be supported by educational packages, as already mentioned. Pharmacists are often those most actively involved in educating and persuading prescribers to carry out changes. They are also well placed to implement formulary recommendations themselves within their roles as prescribers. Even without changing individual patients' drug therapy, if the drugs recommended in a local formulary are used for all patients starting new therapy, most prescriptions will in time include formulary drugs.

Research has shown that for clinical guidelines, visits to prescribers to provide education, involving local opinion leaders in educational meetings and interactive educational workshops are successful methods of changing behaviour. The same is likely to apply to formularies. A strategy should be developed which ideally includes a mixture of methods, because the more frequent the reminder, the more likely it is that practice will change. Constant reminders may be necessary to maintain prescribing within the recommendations of a formulary. However, feedback on adherence to the formulary is another important mechanism for reminding prescribers about it.

Auditing performance

Providing feedback to prescribers on whether they follow formularies is essential. Because formularies encourage rational prescribing, the extent of their use can be used as one indicator of the quality of prescribing. For other types of prescribing indicators, see Chapter 19. The simplest way to gauge whether a formulary is being used is to look at the same type of prescribing data used to help develop the formulary. Computerized prescribing data can easily be studied to assess whether formulary drugs are being prescribed. However, this type of data provides no information about the patients for whom the drugs have been prescribed. It cannot, for example, identify why patients have received prescriptions for non-formulary drugs. Nor can it be used to determine whether the formulary drugs were prescribed appropriately or whether formulary drugs were used within local guidelines or treatment protocols. For this, drug utilization review or clinical audit is required (see Chs 11 and 19).

For data to be of any use, they must be easy to interpret, accurate and up to date. They must also be of direct relevance to the prescriber to whom they are given and may allow comparison either to earlier prescribing or to the prescribing of others. Comparing the prescribing of several GPs or hospital doctors to each other is known as peer review. Comparison to a 'norm' of prescribing practice, or to the practices of others in the same peer group, often increases the desire of prescribers to conform to the 'norm' or the peer group. However, it is important to ensure that the 'norm' is desirable.

If hospital data generated by the pharmacy computerized stock control system refer to drugs issued to wards or directorates, care must be taken to determine whether this equates to drugs prescribed. Any drugs which were not issued through the computer system, such as patients' own drugs, may not show up in these data. Electronically incorporating the formulary into prescribing systems should make the measurement of formulary adherence relatively simple.

In primary care, prescribing data represent the number of prescriptions dispensed, excluding only prescriptions written which have not been presented to pharmacies and dispensed. They cannot, however, distinguish between formulary and non-formulary drugs. This must be done manually and a figure for adherence can then be calculated, again taking the quantities of each drug into account. Another source of data in primary care is the practice computer, which can again incorporate formulary drugs within its programs. However, if a practice does not generate or record all its prescriptions via the computer, the prescribing patterns obtained will not show the full picture. The number of prescriptions written usually differs from those dispensed, so a different picture of formulary adherence may be found if data from dispensed and written prescriptions are compared.

When providing feedback to prescribers based on prescribing data, care should be taken to ensure that the quantities of the different drugs used are taken into account in some way. For example, if 180 tablets of a formulary drug and 20 tablets of a range of four other non-formulary drugs are used, adherence should be quantified as 90% (180 out of 200 tablets used in total). It could also be calculated that adherence was only 20% if the range of drugs were used (one out of a range of five), but this would not be a reasonable representation of the overall prescribing.

Another source of valuable data for the formulary pharmacist is the request forms for non-formulary drugs, if they are used. Review of these can indicate the extent of non-formulary prescribing. These should also explain the reasons why non-formulary drugs were used. Records of clinical pharmacists' interventions made during routine prescription review or medication review which relate to non-formulary prescribing can also be studied.

Regular provision of information on performance is an essential part of formulary management. Any data which are presented to prescribers as a means of informing them of adherence to formulary recommendations will need to be attractive and easy to use, just like the formulary itself. Graphics and colour can be used to highlight important points. Finally, evidence of cost savings, if they have been achieved, may help to encourage use of the formulary. This is probably best expressed as actual expenditure compared to expected expenditure had the formulary not been used. If formulary adherence is found to be low, then this is an important result, which needs to be investigated to determine whether the formulary best serves the needs of the population or requires revision.

All this feedback should be provided in the same formats as the formulary – paper, electronic or both. It can be incorporated into regular published bulletins from the ADTC. This highlights the continuing importance of the formulary and should be an indication of the committee's willingness to update the formulary in the light of changing needs. Pharmacists can also use discussion of feedback information as another opportunity to market a formulary and gain the support of prescribers in its use.

KEY POINTS

- A formulary is a list of drugs which are recommended and available for prescribing
- A formulary may contain prescribing policies, which detail the use of drugs in specific medical conditions
- Local formularies are used in conjunction with clinical guidelines and treatment protocols to encourage rational and cost-effective prescribing
- Compiling a formulary is a valuable educational exercise
- Pharmacists should work with others to compile a formulary
- Drugs are selected for inclusion in a formulary on the basis of efficacy, toxicity, patient acceptability and cost
- Use of a formulary containing a restricted number of drugs may reduce the incidence of adverse drug reactions, interactions and lack of efficacy
- For a formulary to be accepted, there should be widespread consultation on its content
- A formulary should be easy to use, professionally presented in paper or electronic (or both) formats and revised at least every 2 years
- A formulary management system is required to provide systems for considering the inclusion of new drugs, deleting drugs and supplying non-formulary drugs
- Feedback information should be provided to prescribers on their adherence to a formulary to encourage its use
- Prescribing data can be useful in both developing a formulary and feeding back on performance
- Ideally a mixture of methods should be used to encourage use of a formulary

19

Drug evaluation and pharmacoeconomics

Janet Krska and Dyfrig A. Hughes

STUDY POINTS

- Safety, efficacy and economy
- Pre-marketing studies
- Post-marketing studies
- Pharmacoeconomic evaluation of medicines
- Drug utilization review and evaluation

Safety, efficacy and economy

The volume, complexity and costs of modern medicines are increasing. The need to compare the therapeutic efficacy (i.e. benefits) of medicines with their potential to cause harm (i.e. risks) and the economic implications of these is of paramount importance to the pharmaceutical industry, to healthcare providers and to society. Pharmacists play a major role in the evaluation of the safety, efficacy and economics of medicines use.

At a macro level, the pharmaceutical industry decides which line of drug development would best serve its financial and philanthropic interests. The few molecules out of the hundreds tested which show promise must be studied in clinical trials before they can be marketed as medicines. After products are licensed and marketed, society and its healthcare systems are then faced with difficult decisions on which specific patient populations to treat, or which new medicines to approve for use. Increasingly, decisions are based on economic evaluations, which attempt to calculate benefit:risk ratios for medicines in potential patient populations. In some countries, only medicines which have a clear cost-effective advantage over existing treat-

ment are funded by government. In the UK, various organizations work in differing ways to examine this aspect of medicine evaluation. At a micro level, clinicians (doctors, pharmacists or nurses) must then assess the relative risks and benefits of each medicine for individual patients. This involves consideration of factors which can affect drug disposition, efficacy and safety, such as concurrent disease states or other medicines, while also weighing up the risk of untreated disease and potential affordability. As pharmacists become more involved in selecting treatments, the importance of skills in evaluating all these factors to make individual clinical decisions increases. Furthermore, pharmacists are frequently required to evaluate the use of medicines in individual patients prescribed by others. This involves the further skills of drug use review and evaluation.

There are many techniques used in the evaluation of medicines for safety, efficacy and economy at pre- and post-marketing stages, as summarized in Table 19.1.

Pre-marketing studies

In most countries, evidence of safety, efficacy and quality must be presented to government-appointed regulatory authorities before a new product can be marketed. In the UK, this role is undertaken by the Medicines and Healthcare products Regulatory Agency (MHRA), who must be satisfied with such evidence before a marketing authorization (formerly called a product licence) can be granted. It is the responsibility of the MHRA to assure the public

Table 19.1 Methods of evaluating medicines in humans

Method	Subjects	Outcome
Clinical trials		
Phase I	Usually healthy volunteers ($\leq$60 adults)	Pharmacokinetics of drug Tolerability and toxicity profile (SAFETY)
Phase II	Selected and limited target patient population	Optimal dosage range (EFFICACY) Balance between safety and efficacy (THERAPEUTIC RATIO)
Phase III	Larger numbers of target patients (1000–2000 patients)	Comparative safety and efficacy of medicine Identification of common adverse drug reactions (<1:250 incidence)
Post-marketing pharmacoepidemiological studies		
Post-marketing surveillance (Phase IV)	Up to 10 000 patients	Less common and unpredictable ADRs Identification of patients at risk
Pharmacoeconomic evaluations	Variable numbers of patients using the medicine in routine clinical practice	Comparative cost minimization, cost-effectiveness, cost-utility or cost-benefit
Drug utilization studies or reviews	Variable numbers of patients using the medicine in routine clinical practice	Quantitative studies → patterns of drug use Some qualitative studies → appropriateness of drug utilization
Drug utilization review programme or drug use evaluation or clinical audit	Variable numbers of patients using the medicine in routine clinical practice	Clinical, social and economic consequences of drug utilization

that all medicines which reach the UK market have been assessed for safety, efficacy and quality. Cost issues are not taken into consideration. Efficacy has to be balanced against toxicity for each product and, while the MHRA's evaluation includes the active ingredients of a product and its formulation, final decisions must also take into account the nature of the disease to be treated and the duration of the treatment. What is an acceptable benefit to risk ratio may differ for a medicine used to prolong survival in terminal conditions compared to a prophylactic treatment which needs to be taken for life.

Prior to clinical trials in humans, the pharmacokinetics and pharmacodynamics of any new drug are studied in animals to indicate therapeutic and possible toxic effects. However, there are often substantial differences between species in drug handling and in drug response, so new drugs must be screened in more than one animal species. The poor relationship between the effects of drugs in animals and humans also means that great caution is needed before progressing to 'first time in man' trials.

Phase I trials

These first trials are carried out in healthy adult volunteers, to determine the drug's toxicity profile and to assess tolerability. A dosage range is tested initially with a stepwise increase in drug dose being given to successive volunteers. Subjects in Phase I trials are intensively monitored to determine the nature and severity of any predictable dose-related adverse effects. Pharmacokinetic data are usually generated from both single- and multiple-dose studies. These may be used to assist in deciding the best method of administration.

These trials provide only limited safety data, because the subjects are healthy adults and unlikely to have any compromised drug handling ability. Thus the potential risks of using the drug in patients at extremes of age, or in those with poor hepatic or renal function, are not known. There are also few subjects (e.g. 50–60), so only very common adverse drug reactions (ADRs) are detected.

Phase II trials

These commence while Phase I studies are still running. They are carried out in relatively small groups of target patients, usually within hospital departments specializing in particular areas of medicine. Their main aims are to establish efficacy and to confirm an effective dose in closely monitored and controlled conditions. Phase II studies give the first indication of the likely value of the drug in patients, i.e. its efficacy. There is less emphasis on safety assessments during this phase, but the results will enable a therapeutic ratio (i.e. the balance between efficacy and safety) to be determined. Double-blind randomized controlled trials use a control group with a matching placebo to assess the effectiveness of new therapies. Phase II studies also inform the design of Phase III studies which are more comprehensive. Phases II and III combined may study 1000–2000 patients. The regulatory authorities closely control Phase II and Phase III studies, for which clinical trial certificates or exemptions are required.

Phase III trials

These trials examine safety and efficacy. They are generally large-scale studies comparing a new medicine with other treatments or placebo. Where possible, they should have a randomized controlled design, which is generally accepted as the best method of conducting clinical research. Assigning each patient randomly to either the new treatment or control helps to prevent bias. For other aspects of the design of clinical trials, see Chapter 17.

Phase III trials are the main source of the information which appears in the summary of product characteristics (SPC) for the product. The conduct of clinical trials is subject to guidelines which cover ethical issues, the trial design, the roles of the various investigators and sponsoring company and the storage and analysis of data. For every clinical trial which takes place, approval must be obtained from either a local or a multi-centre research ethics committee. This committee will scrutinize the design of the trial, the information given to the patients and the procedures for obtaining consent, and that adequate compensation and insurance are available.

Safety is assessed by close monitoring of clinical signs and symptoms during scheduled clinical examinations and consultations, complemented by relevant laboratory investigations. Baseline pre-treatment data are compared with data obtained during periods of treatment with the study medicine. However, systematic assessment of symptoms experienced by the patients included in the trials is not always carried out and a systematic checklist for patients to complete has been suggested. Even with the numbers of patients involved in Phases II and III, these trials can only identify type A ADRs that affect 1 in ≥ 250 patients. Type B ADRs, which are neither pharmacologically predictable nor dose related, tend to be rare, so they are more likely to be detected in post-marketing surveillance studies.

Post-marketing studies

Once the MHRA is satisfied that a product is safe, efficacious and of suitable quality, it grants a marketing authorization, which means that the product can then be promoted to prescribers. This means that there is likely to be a large increase in the numbers of patients using the product and it is important that the authority continues to monitor its safety. The MHRA operates a system of post-marketing surveillance which involves spontaneous reporting of suspected ADRs, similar to that in many other countries. It is known as the Yellow Card system and all prescribers, pharmacists and patients can report suspected ADRs directly to the MHRA (see Ch. 47). Such schemes provide early warning signals of potential problems and can lead to hypotheses about associations between a medicine and an effect. These can then be tested using retrospective (e.g. case-control studies) or prospective studies (e.g. cohort studies). The main problems with spontaneous reporting schemes are under-reporting, difficulty in identifying new ADRs and the fact that incidence cannot be calculated, since there is no information on the number of patients exposed to the medicine. The benefits of patients reporting their ADRs to the MHRA are currently being evaluated, but in other countries it has been found that patient reports add to the usefulness of data obtained through reports submitted by healthcare professionals.

Case-control studies retrospectively identify patients who have developed a particular ADR and determine their level of exposure to the suspected medicine. This is then compared to a control group of patients without the ADR of interest. Case-control studies are smaller, much less expensive and generate results more quickly than cohort studies. They are used to investigate suspected ADRs identified by other means, e.g. cohort studies or spontaneous reporting, and are particularly useful for confirming type B ADRs. They are capable of establishing whether an ADR is caused by a medicine, but cannot measure the incidence of ADRs.

Cohort studies measure the incidence of ADRs in a group of patients exposed to a medicine over a period of time and compare this with the incidence in a similar control group who have not been exposed to the medicine. They are useful where a wide range of ADRs are associated with a single medicine, but are less useful for studying rare suspected ADRs. This is because large numbers of patients are required and must be followed up for prolonged periods of time, which is very expensive and may result in patients being lost to follow-up.

Safety assessment of marketed medicines (SAMM studies)

Formal studies to evaluate the safety of medicines which are sponsored by the pharmaceutical industry are known as SAMM studies. A SAMM study is defined as a formal investigation conducted for the purpose of assessing the clinical safety of marketed medicines in clinical practice. The conduct of these studies is also subject to guidelines. SAMM studies use the standard methods of case-control and cohort studies, but may also involve further randomized clinical trials.

Further clinical trials against other drugs/treatments

Most products are marketed having been subject to clinical trials in relatively few patients, which may have excluded certain patient groups. Furthermore, trials may have been conducted against placebo to demonstrate efficacy, but there may be no data on the comparative efficacy of a new product versus an existing treatment for the same condition. In addition, basic research may highlight new theories of how diseases may be treated which require older medicines to be tested for efficacy in conditions where they have not been used previously. Examples of this are the trials required to assess the efficacy of aspirin for prophylaxis against stroke and beta-adrenoceptor blockers in heart failure. As with any other clinical trial, the design is important and the randomized controlled design is considered the most appropriate.

Evaluation of medicines in children

While medicines used in adults must have undergone this rigorous testing before reaching the market and coming into widespread use, this is not the case for medicines used in children. Since there are many differences in both pharmacokinetic and pharmacodynamic aspects of medicines between children of different ages and adults, there are now increasing efforts to ensure that medicines to be used in children are also tested in children. This may involve production of specific formulations but should ensure the increased availability of medicines which have been specifically adapted and licensed for use in children, as well as providing more relevant information about efficacy and toxicity.

Herbal and homoeopathic medicines

Most herbal remedies are not licensed medicinal products and therefore no evaluation is required before they are marketed. Some, however, hold a marketing authorization similar to other medicines and so must have fulfilled the same criteria of safety, quality and efficacy (or effectiveness) and be accompanied by a patient information leaflet. A new process of regulation has recently been introduced covering 'traditional herbal medicines' which will assess safety and quality (see Ch. 20).

Homoeopathic remedies may be registered under a scheme which again only assesses quality and safety, and does not allow indications to be specified. A new scheme has recently been introduced which does permit indications (minor ailments only) to be included as part of the registration process for some products.

Pharmacoeconomic evaluation of medicines

Once a product is licensed, decisions must be made about whether it should be used. Local decisions may be made by drug and therapeutics committees (see Ch. 18). On a larger scale, decisions on whether new treatments should be available on the NHS in England and Wales are made by the National Institute for Health and Clinical Excellence (NICE) and the Scottish Medicines Consortium in Scotland.

Pharmacoeconomic evaluations play a central role in informing NICE's decisions, so pharmacists may conduct economic evaluations and certainly need to understand them. It is important to appreciate how NICE's work differs from the work of the MHRA, who decide whether products can be sold in the UK, by comparing benefits to risks. NICE considers whether medicines should be bought by the NHS, by comparing benefits to costs, i.e. whether they are cost-effective.

Estimates of cost-effectiveness are derived from economic evaluations, which are the comparative analysis of two or more alternative courses of action (interventions) in terms of their costs and consequences. Where the intervention is a medicine, the economic evaluation is called pharmacoeconomics. In an economic evaluation, cost refers to the sum product of the resources that are used and the unit cost of each item. Consequences are the health outcomes, for example the impact of therapy on mortality or quality of life (or both). An appreciation of the basic economic principles is necessary to understand the methods used and the basis for economic analyses.

Basic economic principles

Scarcity and choice

Resources such as land, labour and equipment are scarce (finite) compared to their possible uses, which are infinite. Therefore, no person or organization is capable of achieving all the good things they desire and some hard choices must be made. These choices may concern the fundamental direction of a person's career or an organization's responsibilities. They may also be choices about how best to achieve a particular goal. For a person, their salary is one measure of the resources available to them. They might not be able to afford both a new car and an exotic holiday, but must choose which they would get the most pleasure from (economists refer to this as utility).

An organization, such as the NHS, a hospital or a primary care organization, has a budget to fund new and existing activities. The use of this budget should be reviewed to make sure that patients' health gains from the mix of activities are maximized. The purpose of economic evaluations is to inform decision makers of the balance between costs and health gains in order that health outcomes are maximized at a population level.

Opportunity cost

When we make choices about personal or workplace activities, we usually spend money to engage appropriate resources. Considering only the amount of money spent as the 'cost' is a little narrow-minded. Economists would argue that the true cost (opportunity cost) of an activity is the utility from other activities that we can no longer afford. Thus, the opportunity cost of a person's car is not £10 000, but might be the pleasure of 2 weeks on an exclusive tropical holiday island which was not taken. Similarly, the opportunity costs of one coronary artery bypass graft might be two hip operations not performed. Acting to minimize opportunity cost, therefore, ensures that the utility we do obtain from using resources in a particular way is maximized. We call this efficiency, which is of two types: technical and allocative.

- Technical efficiency is about achieving particular goals on a fixed scale in the most appropriate way (e.g. comparing a range of interventions, including medicines and lifestyle changes, within a programme to reduce blood pressure)
- Allocative efficiency is concerned with choosing the right goals in the first place (e.g. coronary heart disease prevention or treating lung cancer) and the most appropriate scale for a healthcare programme.

Few diseases are left completely untreated (because it would not be fair or equitable) but normally efficiency demands that most of our scarce resources are used to maximize health gains for the greatest number of people. This philosophy is called utilitarianism. If people whose health status cannot be improved by health care are treated, there are fewer resources to help those who can benefit.

Supply and demand

Most people would not consciously consider 'minimizing opportunity cost' in their everyday lives. But they would usually try to get the most utility from the smallest amount of expenditure, which is the same thing expressed more simply. The price of goods and their availability are relied on as indicators of quality and desirability. The price mechanism for allocating resources works well if there are many buyers and sellers, each with similar accurate information about the goods and services on offer. However, the market for health care (unlike that for cars and package holidays) does not work very well. The reasons for this include:

- Health is demanded but cannot be directly provided
- The link between health care and improvements in health is uncertain
- We do not know when we will be ill
- Providers of health care have more information than consumers
- Insurance companies or governments usually pay for health care – not consumers.

When normal markets do not work well, economic evaluation can step in as a substitute for price to assist decision makers. The costs measured and valued in economic evaluation are analogous to the costs of production for a normal good or service. The consequences measured and valued in economic evaluation are analogous to the utility consumers enjoy when using a normal good or service.

Methods of economic evaluation

The basic steps in all economic evaluations are to:
- Clarify the economic question, with particular regard to technical or allocative efficiency, the interventions that will be compared and the population of interest
- Obtain the best clinical and economic evidence
- Identify and carry out the appropriate form of evaluation to answer the economic question
- Identify the key variables that influence the results of the evaluation and test the influence of any assumptions
- Present the results clearly and in a form that decision makers can easily interpret.

All the techniques of economic evaluation involve an explicit consideration and calculation of resource use, to ensure that healthcare expenditure has the maximum possible impact on health status. However, each method of evaluation handles consequences (or health effects) differently.

Principles of costing

The viewpoint (perspective) of an economic evaluation determines what should be included in measuring costs. Typical viewpoints are: a single healthcare organization, the whole healthcare system or society. For the same set of interventions, taking a different viewpoint can result in radically different economic conclusions. To give an example, the costs of drug therapy

for attention deficit hyperactivity disorder from a health system perspective is very different from the cost from a societal perspective, which may also consider the impact of treatment on education, social problems and crime.

Resources used directly in healthcare interventions may include:
- Skilled workers, e.g. doctors, nurses and pharmacists
- Equipment, e.g. computers, medical scanners and beds
- Space in which to work including heat, light and rent
- Consumables, e.g. medicines, diagnostic kits, syringes and dressings.

It is important to remember that it is not just the product acquisition cost that is used in economic evaluations, but the total costs related to treatment with that product, including for instance hospitalizations, blood tests, GP visits and so on.

Costs borne outside the healthcare system (e.g. by patients and carers, or in other sectors of the economy such as social care) may be less likely to have accepted and accessible market prices. Voluntary care costs, for example, might be valued using an average societal wage rate. Patients' public transport costs would be clear enough, but for car travel an appropriate mileage rate needs to be agreed or calculated. The productivity of patients going back to work should normally be excluded from costings. This is because any gains or losses in productivity flow from health status changes, which will be valued separately.

When identifying costs for groups of interventions that will be compared, any costs that are identical for all interventions can be safely ignored. This is because economists are more interested in marginal costs (e.g. the cost of one additional day in hospital) than average costs. Note that these may be very different. For instance, if a hospital operates at normal capacity, the average daily cost of a hospital bed will be similar to the marginal cost. However, if increases in local hospital catchment population required that a new ward needed to be built, then the marginal cost for the first patient admitted to that ward is substantially higher than the average cost (as it includes the cost of building the ward!). It is the costs of change and the differences between alternative interventions that are most relevant for practical and effective decision making.

Healthcare interventions often incur costs over a number of years and the duration of two alternative

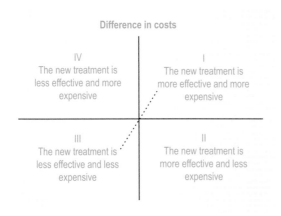

Difference in costs

IV	I
The new treatment is less effective and more expensive	The new treatment is more effective and more expensive
III	II
The new treatment is less effective and less expensive	The new treatment is more effective and less expensive

Figure 19.1 • Cost-effectiveness plane, illustrating where a new treatment is either less or more effective than current therapy (origin), and whether the costs associated with the new treatment are higher or lower. Decisions on treatments falling into the north-west and south-east quadrants are clear-cut. It is unlikely that treatments in the south-west will be adopted as they are less effective than available alternative therapy. Decisions on whether or not to approve treatments that are both more effective and more costly (north-east quadrant) require the use of economic evaluation, and a threshold cost-effectiveness ratio (represented by the diagonal line), below which treatments are deemed to be cost-effective.

interventions may be different. So timing is an important factor in many costings and is accounted for in a number of ways. First, all costs are counted in a base year, and are not inflated to account for price rises over the course of the interventions. This ensures that all costs reflect real resource use and not nominal monetary values. Second, capital costs (durable equipment) are apportioned over the lifetime of the equipment. This allows a fair comparison of interventions with different levels of up-front and recurring costs. Third, future costs are 'discounted' back to the base year. In general terms, this reflects a preference by people to put off costs rather than pay straightaway.

Whether consequences that occur in the future should be discounted in the same way as costs is open to debate. Without consistent discounting it is particularly hard to fairly compare health promotion interventions (with up-front costs and far-off consequences) with normal clinical treatments. NICE's current practice is to discount both costs and benefits, at a rate of 3.5% per annum.

Economic analyses are useful for informing decisions on allocating scarce healthcare resources. Occasionally, decisions are very straightforward and do not

require detailed economic analysis. These may include, for instance, examples where a new treatment is both more effective and less costly than existing therapy. Clearly in this situation, the new treatment is preferred, as this 'dominates' existing therapy. Conversely, a new treatment might be identified which is less effective yet more expensive. This would be dominated by existing therapy (Fig. 19.1).

The two logical alternative scenarios, where additional benefits come at additional costs and where fewer benefits are generated at reduced cost, can be represented by the north-east, and north-west quadrants of the cost-effectiveness plane, respectively (see Fig. 19.1). In the case of the former, the key question is whether the additional benefits justify the additional cost.

Types of economic evaluation

Cost-minimization analysis

Cost-minimization analysis (CMA) is only appropriate when there is robust evidence to show that two or more interventions have exactly the same health effects, i.e. are therapeutically equivalent in terms of health benefits and adverse effects. Interventions to be assessed by CMA fall on the vertical axis of the cost-effectiveness plane (see Fig. 19.1).

This is a question of technical efficiency and the intervention that costs the least is usually preferred, because spare resources can be used to treat more patients or be reallocated to other programmes. Choosing a more expensive option must be justified because using additional resources to achieve the same outcome takes resources away from other programmes where they might achieve something positive.

An example of CMA is the comparison by Lowson et al (1981) of different methods for providing domiciliary oxygen. The effectiveness of oxygen provided in cylinders or by concentrator was the same. Concentrators were cheaper for most patients despite high purchase and maintenance costs, but this result varied depending on the number of patients in an area who needed therapy.

CMA could also be used to compare branded and generic medicines, or different formulations of the same drug, but its practical applications are limited to cases where therapeutic equivalence has been demonstrated. Briggs & O'Brien (2001) argue that a lack of significance in the effect differences between interventions in a clinical trial is insufficient grounds for conducting a CMA.

Cost-effectiveness analysis

Cost-effectiveness analysis (CEA) is appropriate when the health effects of two or more interventions are not identical, but are measured in the same units, e.g. life years gained or symptom-free days.

This is a question of technical efficiency and is often appropriate within a particular healthcare programme, for example different interventions which all reduce myocardial infarction and stroke. However, CEA can only deal with one dimension of outcome at a time. Some other examples include: accidents prevented, decrease in blood pressure, deaths averted and strokes avoided. These measures are often clinical indicators or intermediate outcomes, e.g. blood pressure reduction is a predictor of subsequent effects such as stroke and health-related quality of life (HRQoL). The use of clinical indicators can be problematical, not least because the choice of indicator critically affects the results of an evaluation. The most appropriate indicator or outcome should be chosen before a study commences. Examples of CEA are shown in Box 19.1.

Cost-utility analysis

Cost-utility analysis (CUA) is the most useful form of economic evaluation and is appropriate when the health effects of two or more alternatives can be measured in terms of overall impact on quality and quantity of life.

CUA is a special form of CEA in which the consequences are measured in terms of quality-adjusted life years (QALYs). QALYs are calculated by estimating the total life years gained from a treatment and weighing each year (or part thereof) with a quality of life (utility) score. The utility value is 0 for 'dead' and 1 for 'full health'. Various methods can be used to measure and quantify quality of life, to provide a single summary score. The method pharmacists are most likely to be familiar with is a questionnaire such as the EuroQol-5D.

The advantage of the QALY is that it incorporates quality and quantity of life in a common currency that allows comparison of interventions from different clinical areas. So QALYs can be compared for very different interventions such as radiotherapy in advanced breast cancer, surgery for coronary artery bypass grafting and drugs for cardiovascular diseases. In

Box 19.1

Examples of cost-effectiveness analyses

- An economic analysis of the Heart Protection Study compared simvastatin with placebo in over 20 000 adults with vascular disease or diabetes over 5 years. The authors estimated the costs of preventing a major vascular event with 40 mg simvastatin daily was £11 600. However, this ranged from £4500 among participants with a 42% 5-year major vascular event rate, to £31 100 among those with a 12% rate.
- Abacavir is a nucleoside-analogue reverse transcriptase inhibitor used in combination with other antiretroviral therapy for the management of HIV. Unfortunately, it causes severe hypersensitivity reactions in about 4–8% of patients; however, HLA B*5701 is a known genetic risk factor for hypersensitivity reactions. Hughes et al (2004) conducted a cost-effectiveness analysis of testing patients for HLA B*5701 prior to initiation of abacavir therapy. The cost-effectiveness analysis demonstrated that, depending on the choice of comparator, routine testing for HLA B*5701 ranged from being a dominant strategy (less expensive and more beneficial than not testing) to an incremental cost-effectiveness ratio (versus no testing) of €22 811 per hypersensitivity reaction avoided. This means that compared with some antiretroviral therapies, the use of the test costs an additional €22 811 to avoid one hypersensitivity reaction.

contrast, a CEA measures consequences only in terms of quality or quantity: it is unidimensional. The advantage of CUA using QALYs is that it can answer questions of both technical efficiency and allocative efficiency in health care. For this reason, CUAs are the preferred form of economic evaluation for NICE appraisals.

Figure 19.2 presents a graphical representation of the impact of treatment, such as a medicine, on quality of life and life expectancy. The number of QALYs gained by one medicine over the other is the difference between the areas under the curves. In this figure, the disease is characterized by episodes of remission from symptoms, where quality of life is high, and relapses, where quality of life is low. Neither medicine A nor medicine B affects quality of life appreciably until the final stages of the disease where it is clear that medicine B is superior – both in improving health-related quality of life and in increasing life expectancy. For each medicine, QALYs are calculated

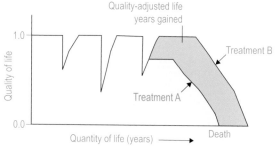

Figure 19.2 • A schematic representation of the impact of two treatments (A and B) on a chronic disease that is characterized by episodes of relapse and remissions. The area under the curves represents the total number of quality-adjusted life years (QALYs) associated with each treatment. The gain in QALYs is the shaded area between both curves.

as the area under the curves, so the shaded area represents the number of QALY gains achieved with medicine B compared to medicine A.

Now imagine that this lifetime QALY gain is equal to 1.0 QALY and that the total lifetime costs to the healthcare system associated with medicine A are £10 000 and with medicine B £20 000, but remember

that medicine B is more effective. The incremental cost utility ratio is calculated as the difference in costs divided by the difference in QALYs, which in this case equals £10 000 divided by 1.0 which equals £10 000 per QALY gained. The judgment as to whether this represents good value for money (and in which case whether it will be approved for use by the NHS) depends on whether or not £10 000 per QALY gained is considered acceptable. In practice, treatments and healthcare interventions that cost less than £20 000–£30 000 per QALY gained are considered cost-effective, and are likely to be approved for use.

Table 19.2 lists a range of cost-utility estimates from a selection of assessments conducted for NICE.

Cost-benefit analysis

Cost-benefit analysis (CBA) is the least common economic evaluation of health care because it is only appropriate when the benefits gained are expressed in monetary units. The term cost-benefit analysis is, however, sometimes used incorrectly in a general way to describe any form of economic evaluation.

Table 19.2 A list of cost-utility ratios (cost per QALYs) for a range of interventions that were appraised by the National Institute for Health and Clinical Excellence (NICE)

Treatment	Cost per QALY (£)
Methylphenidate for attention deficit/hyperactivity disorder	£5000–£28 000
Zanamivir for influenza	£38 000 for all adults
	£9300–£31 500 for at-risk adults
Laparoscopic surgery for inguinal hernia	£50 000 compared with open surgery
Riluzole for motor neurone disease	£34 000–£43 500
Donepezil, galantamine, rivastigmine for Alzheimer's disease	£0–£30 000 (limited to those with mini-mental state score >12)
Cox II inhibitors for OA and RA	>£30 000 for average risk OA and RA patients – dominant for high-risk patients
Beta-interferon and glatiramer acetate in MS	£35 000–£104 000
Sibutramine for obesity	£15 000–£30 000
Etanercept and infliximab for RA	£27 000–£35 000
Infliximab for Crohn's disease	£27 500

OA, osteoarthritis; RA, rheumatoid arthritis; MS, multiple sclerosis.

In CBA, the monetary units used to assess consequences reflect the value of health status improvement and not the cost of health care. The treatment offering the largest net consequence (value of consequences minus costs) is preferred. This technique can answer questions concerning allocative efficiency across the whole economy. In principle at least, the largest net consequence rule can help us decide whether to build a new hospital or a new road.

There are three ways to place a monetary value on consequences: implied values, the human capital approach and willingness to pay. Implied values are taken from insurance companies, court awards for accidents or risk premiums we pay people to do dangerous jobs. For example, travel insurance companies may state how much they will pay for the loss of an eye or limb. These values could be applied to the consequences of ophthalmic and vascular surgery respectively. Although implied values are one way to put a publicly acceptable monetary value on health effects, they do not exist for all possible consequences, may not be adjusted regularly and may be unpredictable.

The human capital approach places a value on human life that is equivalent to an individual's future income stream. This has the disadvantage of judging that the life of a managing director is worth more than that of a shop floor worker. This is unpalatable for most healthcare professionals and not widely applied. However, surveys do suggest that the general public values the lives of the very young and old less highly than the lives of productive workers with families. It has also been suggested that traditional societies tend to sacrifice weaker members first in times of hardship.

Willingness to pay (WTP) is the preferred way to place a monetary value on consequences. In a WTP survey, a description of the intervention and associated health effects is presented to disease sufferers or the general public. After reading the description, people are asked to place a monetary valuation on the scenario, which may incorporate preferences about the method of treatment, information provided by medical tests and actual clinical outcome. WTP may be related to income or ability to pay and this must be considered in any analysis.

Modelling and sensitivity analysis

More often than not, clinical trials do not capture all the data required for an economic analysis. Moreover, it is generally advisable to project the results of clinical

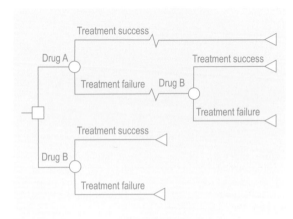

Figure 19.3 • An example of a decision tree as used in pharmacoeconomics.

trials beyond the time horizon of analysis, to capture lifetime costs and benefits. Economists use mathematical models to compile data from various sources, and to test the robustness of assumptions and uncertainties in the analysis. The most common forms of economic models are decision analyses (represented schematically as decision trees) and Markov models (Hughes 2004).

A decision tree maps out the alternatives being compared in as much detail as possible. Figure 19.3 shows the start of one possible tree, outlining various treatment options for use of a new medicine. The decision tree starts with a decision node (by convention a square). This is because most health care starts with a decision about whether one alternative or another is the most appropriate course of action. Subsequent probability nodes (by convention, circles) show the chances of each possible consequence occurring. At each probability node the sum of probabilities is 1, that is, a 100% chance that something will happen.

A range of interventions and their possible consequences can be mapped out clearly in a decision tree. Once the options are clear, probabilities can be attached to them using either new trial data or information from the existing literature. For each option we may also identify and state costs. At the end of each route through the decision tree there should also be a terminal node (by convention, a triangle) associated with a final outcome.

The expected costs and outcomes (e.g. QALY) for each initial decision can be calculated. For instance, if the probability of treatment success with medicine B (used first line) is 60%, and the costs associated with treatment success and failure are £1000 and £2000, respectively, then the expected cost is (60% × £1000) + (40% × £2000) = £1400. This means that, on average, the costs associated with medicine B, if used as first-line therapy, is £1400. We can calculate the incremental cost-effectiveness ratio by performing the same calculation to the costs and benefits for all the branches of the tree. Computer software to help draw and analyse decision trees makes their use particularly attractive for the comparison of multiple interventions.

Sensitivity analysis is the act of changing assumptions about the value or probability of costs and consequences, to determine whether or not the results of an evaluation are sensitive to such changes. Even without the help of a decision tree or computer software, evaluators should highlight any assumptions they make about costs and consequences and list the key variables that influence their recommendations.

Markov models are helpful for modelling the progression of chronic diseases. A disease is divided into health states (e.g. good health, bad health, death) and during a chosen period of time each individual is given a probability of moving from one state to another. Estimates of resource use and health effects are also attached to each state and transition. The model is then cycled to produce long-term estimates of cost-effectiveness in hypothetical patient cohorts.

Many healthcare professionals are distrustful of modelling and hypothetical data. However, in some cases it is the best information we have. These techniques should not be rejected out of hand, but instead questions asked about the assumptions made to produce the model and the accuracy of typical clinical scenarios. Better information is better than nothing at all and modelling can be a great deal better than a badly designed trial.

Appraising economic evaluations

During the process of making decisions about whether to recommend drugs for use in the NHS, NICE and other similar bodies assess the quality of research which has been carried out, using standardized methods. The quality of published clinical studies and economic evaluations in the medical and pharmacy literature is variable. For both, methodological details must be critically appraised to ensure the validity of the results prior to decision-making. Examples of checklists which can be used can be found in SIGN

Guideline 50 *A Guideline Developer's Handbook* (SIGN 2008).

Drug utilization review and evaluation

As well as their involvement in the evaluation of new medicines both before and after marketing, pharmacists play a large role in evaluating whether established medicines are being used appropriately. The proper (rational) use of medicines increases the quality of patient care and promotes cost-effective health care. The techniques used to do this are drug utilization review (DUR), drug use evaluation (DUE) and clinical audit. Audit is described in Chapter 11.

DUR is the assessment of patterns of drug use in a particular clinical context. DUE incorporates qualitative measures and emphasizes outcomes, including pharmacoeconomic assessment. DUE can identify problems in drug use, reduce ADRs, optimize drug therapy and minimize drug-related expenditure.

Selection of which drugs to study may be because of:

- High cost, for example gabapentin
- Wide usage or changes in usage, for example ulcer-healing drugs
- Known or suspected inappropriate use, for example clopidogrel
- Potential for improvements in patient care, for example bisphosphonates.

Some medicines will fall into more than one category, increasing the potential benefits of conducting DUR. Changes in legislation can result in changes in the way medicines are used, for example alteration of the legal classification. Usage patterns often also change when a new product is marketed. DUR can provide information on what these changes are and DUE can determine whether they are beneficial.

Drug utilization review

DUR developed in the 1960s and focused on describing which medicines were being used and their costs. It can involve the development of standards for the use of each medicine or group of medicines, which can be used as criteria against which the actual use of the medicines can be measured. This form of DUR is therefore very similar to clinical audit (see Ch. 11). The general study of patterns of medicines use and their associated costs is an important activity for pharmacists. This activity is used to identify therapeutic areas where drug choice requires review, more cost-effective therapy can be substituted or there is unexplained variation in prescribing between groups of prescribers or between populations. The subsequent activities which are undertaken to address these issues also often involve pharmacists. These may include medication review, medicine use review (MUR), prescription review, therapeutic switching programmes, clinical audit and DUE.

So that comparisons can be made between populations (such as those of different geographical areas or served by different prescribers), systems for classifying drugs and methods for quantifying their use are needed. The most widespread systems are the anatomical therapeutic chemical (ATC) system and the defined daily dose (DDD) which were developed by the Norwegian Medicinal Depot in the 1970s and were subsequently recommended by the World Health Organization (WHO) for international use. In the UK, the *British National Formulary* is more frequently used as a therapeutic classification for drugs than the ATC, but DDDs are widely used to quantify medicines use. There is a DDD for every drug on the market, based on the average recommended daily maintenance dose for the drug when used for its most common indication in adults. It is expressed in g, mg, microgram, mmol or units or as the number of tablets for combination products. The Nordic Council on Medicines sets the DDD for every drug in conjunction with the WHO.

While DDDs are used for this purpose worldwide, other methods of measuring prescribing are also used in the UK primary care setting. The average daily quantity (ADQ) has been developed for a number of drugs to reflect typical prescribing in England. To make comparisons between populations, a denominator is required, often 1000 patients. For example, the DDD of diazepam is 10 mg. It may be found that diazepam is used with a DDD of 2000/1000/year. This means that for every 1000 people, 2000 doses of diazepam were prescribed in a year. This is equivalent to 2 doses per person per year. By using DDDs, not only are quantities prescribed accounted for, but also an allowance is made for the frequency of administration. In order to enhance comparisons still further, a denominator which takes account of the differing needs of populations can be used. Examples of this are the ASTRO-PU (which accounts for the age, sex and temporary residential status of a population) and the STAR-PU which also accounts for variability within therapeutic groups.

Data can also be expressed in terms of cost, rather than quantity, again using this range of denominators. Thus it becomes possible to identify prescribing which is higher or lower than the norm for the actual population served in terms of either quantity or cost.

Drug use evaluation

Evaluating the use of medicines retrospectively and relating them to patient outcomes can be a valuable learning experience, but prospective DUE is much more beneficial to both prescribers and patients. If changes in prescribing are found to be necessary, these can be implemented after or even during the evaluation. As with clinical audit, the involvement of relevant prescribers is essential, to ensure benefits.

There are various levels at which the use of medicines can be studied. These range from very broad measures with little detail, usually obtained from routinely collected data, to more expensive methods, in which a great deal of useful information is obtained on individual patients. DUR studies which use only drug supply, purchase or prescribing records cannot be used to determine medicines use in relation to indication and outcome. The information which they provide is incomplete and any suggestions of prescribing being inappropriate based solely on this type of data should be made cautiously. Prescribing advisers do advocate the use of prescribing indicators, which are an indicative measure of the quality and cost of prescribing. They use the standard measures already described, but involve specific ways of combining data to enable more useful comparisons to be made. Some areas where prescribing indicators have been developed are listed in Box 19.2. The main purpose of prescribing indicators is to raise awareness of what is

Box 19.2

Examples of areas where prescribing indicators have been developed and are used to evaluate prescribing

Proportion of generic prescribing

Benzodiazepine prescriptions (ADQ per STAR-PU) should be minimal

Prescribing rate of atypical antipsychotics as a proportion of all antipsychotics

Prescribing rate of antibacterials (items per STAR-PU)

being prescribed and to highlight areas for more detailed methods of investigation, such as by examination of medical records.

Using purchasing records

The simplest level of information about which medicines are being used is obtained from purchasing records. Both hospital and community pharmacies use computerized systems for purchase, which means these data are readily available. This type of information allows comparison between pharmacies or over time, but provides no clues as to how the medicines are being used. It can point to potential areas which may need further investigation.

While DDDs can be used for the measurement of purchases, other measures such as cost, number of containers and number of dosage units may be more readily available.

Using issue records

A more detailed record of use can be obtained from the medicines issued from pharmacies, to individual patients via prescriptions or to wards in hospitals. The units used are the same as those of purchase. Again, computerization allows these data to be obtained easily.

In the community, the data are captured when the prescriptions are priced centrally. These data are issued to prescribers so they can evaluate their own prescribing. However, it is much more common for pharmacists to undertake this evaluation, using the techniques described here. Central data are available, such as those by the Prescribing Support Unit, which enable comparison of an individual's or a group's prescribing to the national 'norm'.

In some hospitals, it is possible to link data from pharmacy issues to individual clinicians. This will increase as electronic prescribing becomes more widespread. Even if the data can only be applied at ward level, this can still be helpful in developing and monitoring ward-based policies on medicines use.

Using prescription records

More detailed information from prescriptions, which includes the actual dose prescribed and the concurrent medication, can be obtained in community pharmacies from patient medication records. However, without patient registration and the recording of non-prescription medicines purchased, these are incomplete. In hospitals, this level of data is only easily obtainable with electronic prescribing. Manual data collection from prescriptions is time-consuming but provides information on the doses of drugs used, the extent of polypharmacy, prescribing errors and drug interactions.

Using medical records and trained investigators

In order to learn about the decisions behind the use of particular medicines and their effectiveness in patients, it is necessary to examine medical records. This requires expertise and time and can often be frustrated by the inadequacy of record keeping. Some hospital units and most general practices have computerized patient records, which allow links to be made to the drugs prescribed. In some hospitals, links are also available to computerized laboratory data. Many systems, however, are either undeveloped or, as with pharmacy-based patient medication records (PMRs), the records are often inaccurate or incomplete. Clearly, it is not possible to compensate for either a lack of data or inaccurate data. However, small studies undertaken manually can still be of considerable value in determining whether medicines are being used appropriately and effectively. These studies usually involve the use of trained investigators, such as pharmacists, reviewing medical records.

Pharmacists can undertake prospective DUE, which avoids the problem of inadequate records, by allowing data to be recorded and questions to be asked at the time of prescribing. This may help to improve the use of medicines through changing prescribing behaviour. It can also involve the patient, so providing a full picture of medicines use, including outcomes and compliance. While more expensive than DUR using purchase, issue or prescribing data, this may be regarded as part of the routine practice of pharmacists. Increasingly, national service frameworks and clinical guidelines specify, among other things, the treatments to be given to patient populations, emphasizing the importance of both DUE and clinical audit. The labour-intensive nature of these activities currently will be reduced when complete and accurate computerized data are available in patient records which are shared between healthcare professionals.

Evaluation of non-prescription medicines

Published information on the epidemiology of self-limiting minor illnesses is limited. Similarly, data on the pharmacoepidemiology of the medicines used in self-treatment of these minor illnesses is limited. The number of such medicines which can be bought from pharmacies or other outlets is constantly increasing, with many former prescription only medicines being re-regulated to allow their purchase. Manufacturers of non-prescription medicines collect data on sales, which provide a global overview of which medicines are being purchased. DUR requires similar methods to those used for prescription medicines, namely study of purchase or supply and data stored in community pharmacy PMRs. DUE of non-prescription medicines is increasing, with the development of patient questionnaire methods. Such studies do show that use is often inappropriate. However, currently these studies involve distribution from community pharmacies and therefore do not include the use of medicines purchased from other outlets. As increasing numbers of potent medicines become widely available without prescription, the requirement for a practical yet scientifically robust method of evaluating both the use of and adverse reactions associated with these medicines increases.

KEY POINTS

- Pharmacists have an important role to play in evaluating the safety, efficiency and economy of medicines' use
- The Medicines and Healthcare products Regulatory Agency (MHRA) requires evidence of safety, efficacy and quality before granting a marketing authorization for a new drug
- Clinical trials take place in three phases: Phase I determines the basic toxicity and tolerability, Phase II establishes efficacy and confirms the dosage, Phase III determines safety and efficacy on a larger sample using randomized controlled trials

- Post-marketing surveillance is required to establish many adverse reactions, particularly rarer ones
- Spontaneous reporting of adverse drug reactions (ADRs) to the MHRA is an important mechanism of post-marketing surveillance. Prescribers, pharmacists and patients can all report suspected ADRs directly
- Pharmacoeconomics applies the principles of economic evaluation to pharmaceuticals and pharmaceutical policies
- Some of the basic economic concepts are scarcity, choice and opportunity cost which can be applied to the medical field
- Application of the principles of costing may be straightforward but can be difficult, especially when trying to identify all the cost consequences related to a given treatment
- Cost-minimization analysis (CMA) may be applied (with caution) when outcomes are the same and relative cost is the variation
- Cost-effectiveness analysis (CEA) is applied when both outcomes and cost can vary, but outcomes are measured in common units
- Cost-utility analysis (CUA) incorporates quality of life and quantity of life into a single index, and is the most useful form of economic evaluation to assist in informing resource allocation
- Cost-benefit analysis (CBA) is complex, and is not used frequently for evaluating healthcare interventions
- To accommodate decision taking in health care, modelling and sensitivity analysis methods can be used
- Drug utilization review (DUR) is used to evaluate patterns of drug use within populations
- Drug use evaluation (DUE) relates drug use to patient outcome and along with clinical audit can be used to evaluate whether drugs are used optimally in practice
- Data which can be used for DUR and DUE include drug purchase records, drug issue records, prescription records and medical records

20

Complementary/alternative medicine

G. Brian Lockwood

- Types of complementary medicines and complementary therapies
- Extent and reasons for use of complementary/ alternative medicine (CAM)
- Regulation of CAM practitioners and complementary medicines
- The interrelationship between pharmacy and CAM

Introduction

Complementary/alternative medicine (CAM), originally referred to as 'fringe', 'holistic' or 'natural' medicine, was known as 'alternative' medicine in the 1970s and 1980s. Today it is increasingly called 'integrated' or 'integrative' medicine. Generally, it is referred to as complementary/alternative medicine, although the terms complementary medicine, alternative medicine and complementary therapies are used interchangeably. Zollman & Vickers' (1999) definition of CAM, which has been adopted by the Cochrane Collaboration (see Ch. 17), is given in Box 20.1.

Historically, CAM was the main form of medicine available to the world's populations, including those of Europe and the UK. In many parts of the world it still is today. What we now know as conventional or pharmaceutical medicine did not exist, hence the modern usage of the term. With the advent and expansion of discovery and production of mainly synthetic medicines by pharmaceutical companies, usage of mainly plant-based traditional medicines declined. These medicines are what we now refer to as CAM.

In essence, CAM is an umbrella term for a collection of different approaches to diagnosis and treatment. Over 50 diverse complementary therapies have been listed, some involving use of medicinal substances, while others use a range of therapeutic techniques. These range from homoeopathy (which involves the use of infinitely dilute preparations) to herbal medicine (the use of chemically rich plant material), and from acupuncture (the insertion of needles into specific points on the body) to therapeutic touch and spiritual healing (including 'distant' healing, which does not require the laying on of hands). Among the many forms of complementary therapies available, some use a variety of techniques but no medicinal products, some use only medicinal products, and there are also those which involve both medicines and techniques.

Some of the most well known complementary therapies, including those using medicinal products, are described in Box 20.2.

Several complementary therapies, such as herbalism, homoeopathy, aromatherapy and others, involve the administration of remedies, often in recognizable pharmaceutical formulations, e.g. herbal medicines, homoeopathic remedies and essential oils. These are collectively referred to as complementary (or 'alternative') medicines. As well as being used by some CAM practitioners in their practice, these types of products are widely available for purchase for self-treatment from pharmacies, health food stores, supermarkets, by mail order, via the Internet and from other outlets. Many of these are administered or recommended after consultation with therapists with varying range of abilities and qualifications, or simply bought by patients believing that they will be

Box 20.1

Definition of complementary and alternative medicine (Zollman & Vickers 1999)

'Complementary and alternative medicine (CAM) is a broad domain of healing resources that encompasses all health systems, modalities and practices and their accompanying theories and beliefs, other than those intrinsic to the politically dominant health system of a particular society or culture in a given historical period. CAM includes all such practices and ideas self-defined by their users as preventing or treating illness or promoting health and well-being. Boundaries within CAM and between the CAM domain and that of the dominant system are not always sharp or fixed.'

beneficial. In the UK, patients, the public, the media and many other groups consider the use of herbal medicines (whether prescribed by a herbalist or purchased over the counter) to be part of CAM. However, there is a view that herbal medicinal products with documented pharmacological activity and clinical efficacy lie alongside conventional medicines. Indeed, some herbal medicines, such as senna preparations, are conventional medicines.

This chapter discusses CAM, mainly from a UK perspective. In particular, the extent of use and regulatory aspects of CAM are considered, as well as issues of importance to pharmacy and pharmacists. There is a particular emphasis on complementary medicines, as these are widely available in pharmacies, and especially on 'European' herbal medicines, as these are

Box 20.2

Descriptions of complementary therapies common in the UK

Complementary medicines can be conveniently divided into three categories: those using only medicinal substances, those using a therapy without medicinal substances, and those using both.

A. Therapies using medicinal substances

Aromatherapy

The therapeutic use of aromatic substances, largely essential oils which typically contain numerous chemical constituents and are extracted from plants.

Aromatherapists believe that essential oils can be used not only for the prevention and treatment of disease, but also for their effects on mood, emotion and well-being. Aromatherapy is claimed to be a holistic therapy in that practitioners will select an essential oil or combination of essential oils to suit each client's symptoms, personality and emotional state. The most common method used for application of essential oils is massage using a carrier oil; other methods include the addition of essential oils to baths and footbaths, inhalations, compresses and use in aromatherapy equipment, e.g. burners and vaporizers.

Flower remedies and essences

Developed in the UK by Dr Edward Bach, who believed that physical disease was the result of being at odds with one's spiritual purpose, i.e. negative states of mind induce illness. His approach to health focused only on the mental state of the patient. He identified 38 negative psychological states of mind (e.g. jealousy, guilt, hopelessness) and developed a remedy designed to be used for each of these emotional states. The Bach collection comprises 39 remedies, 37 of which originate from flowers/trees, one from natural spring water, and 'Rescue Remedy', a combination of five of the other 38 remedies. Flower remedies are extremely dilute preparations, but are not homoeopathic remedies.

Many countries have their own collection of flower remedies/essences based on native plants/trees, e.g. Australian Bush Essences.

Herbalism

Traditional herbalism had a historical basis, partly based on the galenical model of the four 'humours' and the belief that an excess of any of the humours leads to disease. Today treatment is aimed at 'restoring balance' and 'strengthening bodily systems'. Herbalists aim to treat patients in a holistic way by selecting a herb or combination of herbs to treat a particular person and his/her unique set of symptoms. One of the principal tenets is that the whole plant extract, and not an isolated constituent, is responsible for the clinical effect. It is claimed that herbal constituents, and even combinations of herbs, work synergistically to achieve benefit and reduce the possibility of adverse effects.

Rational phytotherapy/phytomedicine (science-based herbal medicine) has an entirely different approach to that of traditional herbalism. It involves the use of specific plant (or plant part) extracts standardized to specific constituents (where possible) with documented pharmacological activity for the treatment of specific clinical conditions. In this regard, phytotherapy has a similar approach to that of conventional medicine.

Herbalism involves preparations made from plants or plant parts. In some instances (e.g. use by herbalists), a crude drug (e.g. dried leaf) is used. Manufactured products use extracts of plants or plant parts, formulated as, for example, tablets, capsules, creams and tinctures. They may contain a single or multiple herbal ingredients, obviously including numerous single chemical entities.

Homoeopathy

The use of highly dilute, succussed substances to stimulate the body's own healing activity (the 'vital force'). One of the key principles is 'like cures like' – a substance which in large doses causes a set of symptoms in a healthy person can be used to treat such symptoms in an ill person, e.g. homoeopathic preparations of coffee (Coffea) are used to treat insomnia. Treatment is holistic – two patients with the same set of symptoms may be given different remedies depending on their personal characteristics, physical appearance, mental and emotional state, etc. Although there are several hypotheses, there is not yet a plausible explanation for the mechanism of action of homoeopathy. Furthermore, on balance, rigorous clinical trials do not show an effect for homoeopathy over that of placebo.

Homoeopathy uses highly dilute preparations which may be of plant, animal, mineral, insect, biological, drug/chemical or other origin. Formulations include tablets, pillules, creams/ointments, liquids and injections.

Nutritional medicines

Nutraceuticals and food supplements are preparations of substances commonly found in the diet, e.g. fish oils, or occurring naturally in the body, e.g. co-enzyme Q10. In the UK, many herbal products, e.g. garlic tablets, are sold as dietary/food supplements.

Traditional Chinese medicine (TCM)

An ancient Chinese method of health care which coexists alongside orthodox medicine today. TCM includes a range of therapies, such as Chinese massage, but is best known for the practices of traditional Chinese acupuncture (see Acupuncture) and traditional Chinese herbal medicine (CHM). The basic concepts of TCM ('yin-yang' and the 'five elements') apply to CHM. The fundamental principle of treatment is to restore 'balance and harmony'. Medicinal substances are classified as having particular attributes, e.g. hot, cold, tonifying, moistening, and it is the consideration and combining of these attributes during therapy that is thought to bring about balance to patterns of clinical dysfunction. For example, 'cooling' herbs would be used to treat a patient whose pattern of illness is described as 'hot'. Usually, herbal formulae comprising around 4–12 different medicinal substances are used to treat specific clinical patterns. Substances used as part of TCM may include animal as well as herbal material.

B. Therapies not using medicinal substances

Acupuncture

This involves insertion of needles into a specific point or set of points on the body for the treatment of specific conditions. Various forms exist, such as auriculoacupuncture (needling of specific points on the ear) and electroacupuncture (electrical stimulation of inserted needles). The two main types practised in the UK are described below.

- *Medical acupuncture*: usually practised by doctors who have trained in acupuncture and who use the therapy alongside conventional medicine. Insertion of needles is given as far as possible according to the principles of neurophysiology and anatomy (i.e. directed at stimulating nerve endings).
- *Traditional Chinese acupuncture*: part of the broader system of TCM. Uses concepts of 'yin-yang' and the 'five elements' to explain the physiological functioning of the human body and the development of medical disorders in order to guide diagnosis and treatment. Traditional Chinese acupuncturists aim to restore the balance of energy in the body by 'unblocking meridians' (pathways along which life energy is believed to flow) by inserting needles strategically in specific points along meridians.

Chiropractic

Chiropractors believe that misaligned or maladjusted vertebrae ('subluxations'), caused by accidents, strains, poor posture, innate skeletal distortions, etc. affect the spine and surrounding muscles, nerves and ligaments. This is believed to result in local or radiating pain, affecting joint movement, and causing swelling or weakening of muscle groups, thereby contributing to the disease process. There is, as yet, no clear explanation from current knowledge of spinal mechanics and neurophysiology as to how this might happen.

Chiropractic diagnosis includes physical examination, palpation of the vertebral column, assessment of posture, etc. and often the use of X-rays to examine bone alignment and to detect conditions such as osteoporosis which would contraindicate manipulative treatment. The principal technique used in chiropractic is a series of short sharp thrusts aimed at restoring normal joint motion, correcting subluxations, improving posture and/or removing painful stimulation to the nerves. Generally, chiropractors manipulate the neck and spine, but may also use techniques such as massage and even dietary and lifestyle advice as part of a holistic approach. McTimoney chiropractic uses lighter movements than does standard chiropractic.

Healing

A transmission of 'therapeutic energy' between healer and patient, which may or may not be associated with particular religious beliefs. It can be performed at a distance ('distant healing') or by laying on of hands ('therapeutic touch').

Osteopathy

Osteopaths believe that a wide variety of disorders can be traced to disorders of the musculoskeletal system, particularly the spinal vertebrae, but also to dysfunction in certain muscle groups. Manipulative techniques are used to correct these joint and tissue disturbances to restore normal bodily function. Osteopaths use a detailed medical history, physical examination, assessment of posture, observation of patient movement, etc. and, occasionally, X-rays in diagnosis. Direct techniques (soft tissue and joint movement, and high-velocity thrusts) and indirect techniques (positioning-type techniques where the joints are moved without force) are used in treatment. Generally osteopaths use more rhythmical and gentler pressure on the whole body, including the spine, whereas chiropractors tend to use more sharp, short, thrusting pressure on the spine (see Chiropractic).

Reflexology (also known as reflex therapy)

A form of treatment and diagnosis which involves massage of specific points on the feet (mainly on the soles but also on the tops and sides – maps of the areas of the feet corresponding to different areas/organs of the body have been drawn up). It is based on the belief that there are reflexes in the feet for all parts of the body. Reflexologists claim to be able to identify sites of tenderness and 'lumps' or granules of crystalline material, which, in reflexology, are taken to represent remote organ disease. Manual stimulation of the reflex points is believed to break down the deposits so that they can be eliminated, and to increase the flow of 'healing energy' through 'channels'. At present, these theories are unsubstantiated.

C. Therapies using both medicinal substances and other treatment

Anthroposophical medicine

A philosophical vision of health and disease based on the work of Rudolf Steiner who explored how man's soul and spiritual nature relate to the health and function of the body. Steiner viewed each person as having four 'bodies' or 'forces': physical; etheric; astral; spiritual. Practitioners of anthroposophy aim to understand illness in terms of how these four elements interact; the aim of treatment is to stimulate the natural healing forces of the body. The anthroposophic approach is a holistic one; practitioners may use a range of therapies including diet, therapeutic movement (eurhythmy) and artistic therapies as well as anthroposophic medicines in an integrated therapeutic programme. The medicines are derived mainly from plant and mineral sources; many are combinations of herbal ingredients. Particular attention is paid to the source and methods of farming used in growing raw plant materials for preparing anthroposophic medicines (e.g. organic culture only).

Ayurvedic medicine

The traditional system of medicine of India. Its essence is to achieve and maintain balance between the 'elements' and 'energies'; illness is believed to result from imbalance. Ayurvedic diagnosis is based on physical observation and questioning. Treatment usually involves Ayurvedic herbal remedies as well as dietary modifications, meditation, exercise, massage. The medicines are herbal/mineral preparations; heavy metals (e.g. lead, arsenic) are sometimes used in the manufacturing process.

ﾭ

among the most widely used 'complementary medicines' in the UK. Also, from a biomedical perspective, herbal medicines (rather than for example homoeopathic remedies) are likely to have the greatest potential in terms of both benefits and risks.

Extent of use of CAM

The use of CAM is a popular healthcare approach in developed countries, and there is evidence that use of complementary therapies and complementary medicines is increasing. For example, data from nationwide surveys involving US adults indicated that the use of CAM was increasing (Eisenberg et al 1998). Use of at least one of 16 complementary therapies in the previous year had risen significantly from 33.8% of the sample in 1990 to 42.1% in 1997. Self-treatment with herbal medicines was one of the therapies showing the greatest increase over this period (2.5% of sample in 1990 compared with 12.5% in 1997).

Reliable estimates of CAM use among adults in England come from a postal questionnaire survey involving 5010 adults (response rate = 59%) carried out in 1998 by Thomas et al (2001). The study found that within the previous 12 months, approximately 10% of the sample had used at least one of six complementary therapies (acupuncture, chiropractic, homoeopathy, medical herbalism, hypnotherapy or osteopathy), and that approximately 22% had purchased over the counter (OTC) homoeopathic or herbal medicines in the previous year.

Market research carried out by Mintel International (2005) estimated that retail sales of herbal medicines alone were worth £87 million in 2004, representing growth of 16% since 2002, whereas total sales of herbal medicines, homoeopathic remedies and essential oils have risen to £147 million by 2004. Around 50% of sales of herbal medicines and homoeopathic remedies are made in pharmacies. Mintel have estimated that 33% of the UK population have taken CAM during 2004, but only 4% have visited a CAM practitioner for their medicine. Self-treatment using CAM remedies raises the issue of the cause of any beneficial effects, as many of these are practiced as holistic therapies, which is not the case when simply purchasing medicinal products.

The use of CAM is not limited to the private sector – in some cases, the NHS funds access. For example, there are five NHS homoeopathic hospitals in the UK to which GPs can refer their patients. Also, GPs can prescribe homoeopathic preparations on NHS prescriptions. In 1998, over 150 000 homoeopathic items were dispensed against NHS prescriptions; data from the Prescription Pricing Authority show that the net ingredient cost for these was £927 600. Since that year there appears to have been an unexpected downward trend in NHS dispensing (Table 20.1). Furthermore, a survey reported by Thomas et al (2001) estimated that in 1998 there were over 2 million visits to complementary therapists funded by the NHS, and that the NHS expenditure on CAM was £50–£55 million per year. However, it has been claimed that many people who might like to take advantage of a wide range of CAM are prevented from doing so by lack of resources, as only 10% of CAM is currently provided by the NHS (Foundation for Integrated Health 2007).

Table 20.1 Trends in homoeopathic prescribing on the NHS

Year	Number of items	Net cost (£)
1998	150 000	927 000
2004	94 500	661 400
2005	83 000	593 000
2006	63 000	442 700

http://www.ic.nhs.uk/statistics-and-data-collections/primary-care/prescriptions

Reasons for use of CAM

Symptoms and conditions

Complementary medicines are used by the general public and by patients both for general health maintenance and for the relief of minor, self-limiting conditions. For example, studies involving pharmacists and consumers have suggested that herbal products to help relieve stress and sleep problems are those most frequently requested by pharmacy customers and 'recommended' by pharmacists to consumers following consultations regarding symptoms.

Use of complementary medicines is not necessarily limited to symptoms or conditions suitable for OTC treatment. Indeed, many patients use complementary medicines and complementary therapies for symptom relief in, or treatment of, serious chronic illnesses, such as cancer, HIV/AIDS, multiple sclerosis, rheumatological conditions, asthma, depression,

Table 20.2 Levels of use of a number of herbal and nutraceutical products for treating a range of medical conditions

Medical condition	Use among participants (%)	Herbal/nutraceutical product
Prostate cancer	4.5	Saw palmetto
	1.2	Lycopene
	0.7	DHEA
Enlarged prostate	18.3	Saw palmetto
	1.6	Lycopene
	1.4	Cranberry
Osteoarthritis	28.7	Glucosamine
	19.9	Chondroitin
	6.2	MSM
Bladder infections	5.8	Cranberry
Neck, back or joint pain	16.6	Glucosamine
	10.5	Chondroitin
	4.5	MSM
Depression	5.8	St John's wort
Lactose intolerance	0.9	Lycopene
Degenerative eye conditions	4.2	Lutein
Perimenopause	4.9	Black cohosh
	1.7	Dong quai*
	6.7	Soy products
Stress	3.2	St John's wort
Memory loss	9.6	Ginkgo biloba
	7.1	Fish oil
	6.0	Coenzyme Q10
Insomnia	3.6	Melatonin
Diabetes	0.2	Dong quai*
	0.3	Lycopene
High blood pressure	0.3	Dong quai*

Reprinted from Gunther S, Patterson RE, Kristal AR, Stratton KL, White E 2004 Demographic and health-related correlates of herbal and specialty supplement use. Journal of the American Dietetic Association 104(1):27–34, with permission from American Dietetic Association.
DHEA, dehydroepiandrosterone; MSM, methylsulfonylmethane
*Angelica sinensis root

gastroenterological disorders, skin conditions and so on. Use of CAM is usually (but not always) to supplement conventional health care, rather than to replace it. Special patient groups also use CAM, including the elderly and women who are pregnant or breastfeeding. It is also used by some parents/guardians for children in their care.

A number of surveys of CAM users have been carried out; frequently females have been shown to have higher use than males, and usage tends to be greater between 35 and 64 years, and in higher social classes (Ernst & White 2000). A survey on the use of herbal products and nutraceuticals in over 60 000 elderly patients revealed extensive use for a range of medical conditions, a number of which would normally be expected to be treated by conventional medicines (Table 20.2).

Beliefs, perceptions and attitudes

There are numerous reasons why people choose to use complementary medicines and therapies. They include dissatisfaction with conventional medicine in terms of effectiveness and/or safety, satisfaction with CAM and the perception that it is 'safe'. There are also more complex reasons that are associated with cultural and personal beliefs, views on life and health and experiences with conventional healthcare professionals and CAM practitioners.

An individual's choice to use CAM approaches is tied in with 'healthcare pluralism' – people may use any of several treatment options, such as taking advice from family and friends, consulting a CAM practitioner and consulting a pharmacist, GP or other healthcare professional. Related issues include whether individuals disclose CAM use to conventional healthcare professionals and whether there is better compliance with CAM treatment regimens than with conventional drug regimens.

Regulation of CAM

CAM practitioners

There are around 40 000 complementary practitioners in the UK, according to a 1997 survey of CAM organizations commissioned by the Department of Health (Mills & Peacock 1997). These practitioners are using either medicinal products, alternative techniques, or both.

With the exception of osteopaths and chiropractors (the General Osteopathic Council and the General Chiropractic Council were established by acts of parliament to regulate their respective disciplines), CAM practitioners are not legally required to undertake any training before practising. While most CAM practitioners will have trained in their chosen therapy, others may not, or they may have trained in one complementary therapy but practise several. Furthermore, there is wide variation in the level of training and methods of assessment. For the major therapies – acupuncture, homoeopathy, herbal medicine, osteopathy and chiropractic – training is generally highly developed, with many institutions having university affiliation and offering courses at degree level. However, training for other complementary therapies is less intensive and more disparate.

The estimate of numbers of CAM practitioners given above is based on membership of CAM organizations, but cannot be precise as some practitioners are registered with more than one organization and some are not registered at all. Generally,

practitioners are members of a registering or accrediting body, although criteria for membership vary widely. Also, many complementary therapies have several registering organizations, although some disciplines are taking steps to become unified under one regulatory body.

The practice of complementary therapies is not limited to CAM practitioners – some conventional healthcare professionals, including pharmacists, practise CAM. Some institutions offer specialized courses for conventional healthcare professionals, and there are registering organizations which represent state-registered healthcare professionals who have undertaken training in and practise certain complementary therapies. For example, the British Medical Acupuncture Society represents medically qualified individuals with training in acupuncture.

Against this background, the House of Lords (2000) report on CAM included several recommendations regarding training and regulation of CAM practitioners, including conventional healthcare professionals who practise CAM. In summary, these recommendations were:

- Regulatory bodies of healthcare professionals should develop guidelines on competence and training in CAM
- Statutory regulation of CAM practitioners, particularly acupuncture and herbal medicine, and possibly non-medical homoeopathy; a Herbal Medicines Regulation Working Group has been set up to take the process forward for herbal medicines
- Training for CAM practitioners should be standardized, independently accredited and include basic biomedical science.

The issue of training also relates to staff employed in retail outlets, e.g. health food stores which sell a vast range of complementary medicines, who sell or advise on complementary medicines. A small study has suggested that information and advice given by health food store staff may not always be appropriate.

Complementary medicines

The majority of complementary health products are not licensed as medicines. Therefore, the competent authority, which, in the UK, is the Medicines and Healthcare products Regulatory Agency (MHRA), has not assessed evidence of their quality, efficacy and safety.

Herbal medicines

Herbal products are available on the UK market as licensed herbal medicines, herbal medicines exempt from licensing and unlicensed herbal products sold as food supplements (Barnes et al 2007). In several cases, the same herb is available in all three categories. Potentially hazardous plants are controlled as prescription only medicines (POMs) and certain others are subject to dose (but not duration of treatment) and route of administration restrictions, or can only be supplied via a pharmacy and by, or under the supervision of, a pharmacist.

Most licensed herbal products were initially granted a product licence of right (PLR) because they were already on the market when the licensing system was introduced in the 1970s. When PLRs were reviewed, manufacturers of herbal products intended for use in minor self-limiting conditions were permitted to rely on bibliographic evidence to support efficacy and safety, rather than being required to carry out new controlled clinical trials, so many licensed herbal medicinal products have not necessarily undergone stringent testing.

Herbal products exempt from licensing are those:

- Compounded and supplied by herbalists on their own recommendation
- Consisting solely of dried, crushed or comminuted (fragmented) plants (i.e. they must not contain any non-herbal 'active' ingredients) sold under their botanical name and with no written recommendations for use
- Made by the holder of a specials manufacturing licence.

This was initially intended to give herbalists the flexibility to prepare remedies for their patients. However, manufacturers can legally sell products under this exemption. Furthermore, at present, there is no statutory regulation of herbalists in the UK, although this is under review.

The majority of herbal products are sold as food supplements without making medical claims and are regulated under food, not pharmaceutical, legislation. In the UK, the MHRA has the statutory power to decide whether a specific product satisfies the definition of a relevant 'medicinal product' and, therefore, is subject to the provisions of regulations relating to Medicines for Human Use Regulations (1994, 2000, 2005). If a product is determined to be a relevant medicinal product, and if it does not meet criteria for exemption, then the manufacturer is required to submit an application for a full product licence and/or remove the product from the market. The procedure allows for the company to request a review of the decision. In this case, the views of an independent panel, the Independent Review Panel on Borderline Products, are taken into consideration.

Manufacturers of licensed medicines, including licensed herbal products, are required to satisfy the MHRA that their products are made according to the principles of good manufacturing practice (GMP). While some established manufacturers of unlicensed herbal products also manufacture their products to GMP standards, others do not. There is no guarantee that such products are of suitable pharmaceutical quality. The quality of plant raw materials can be affected by several factors and, therefore, it is important that finished (marketed) herbal products are of suitable quality. The *European Pharmacopoeia* (5th edition, 5.1–5.8, 2005–2007) contains over 100 monographs on herbal drugs, and further examples are in preparation.

'Ethnic' medicines available in the UK include traditional Chinese medicines (TCMs) and Ayurvedic medicines (see Box 20.2). Such products are subject to the same legislation as 'western' complementary medicines. In the UK, there are further restrictions on certain toxic herbal ingredients, namely *Aristolochia* species, found in some TCM products, and on other herbal ingredients that may be confused with toxic herbal ingredients. In addition to containing non-herbal ingredients such as animal parts and/or minerals, some manufactured ('patent') TCM products have been found to contain conventional drugs as listed ingredients, some of which (e.g. glibenclamide) may have POM status in the UK. Non-herbal active ingredients of any type cannot legally be included in unlicensed herbal remedies, and inclusion of drugs with POM status represents an additional infringement of UK medicines legislation. For some ingredients, such as certain animal parts, restrictions under the Convention on International Trade in Endangered Species (CITES) of Wild Fauna and Flora also apply.

Prior to 2004 it was widely considered that the system of licensing for herbal medicines did not give consumers adequate protection against poor-quality and unsafe unlicensed products. Nor did it allow manufacturers to provide appropriate information to inform consumers' choice of products. Against this background, a new European Union (EU) directive (2004/24/EC) was proposed which aims to establish a harmonized legislative framework for authorizing the marketing of traditional herbal medicinal products. The directive requires EU member states to set up a specified simplified registration procedure for traditional herbal medicinal products which could not fulfil full medicines licensing criteria. Under this EU directive, all manufactured traditional medicinal herbal products are required to be registered under the Traditional Herbal Medicines Registration Scheme (THMRS). This directive has been in force from October 2005, but there is a transition period of 5 years from that date for manufacturers to meet the requirements. Some of the main features of this scheme are that manufacturers will be required to provide:

- Evidence that the herb has been used traditionally in the EU for at least 30 years (15 years' non-EU use will be taken into account)
- Bibliographic data on safety with an expert report
- Quality dossier demonstrating manufacture according to principles of good manufacturing practice (GMP).

Under this directive, it is not possible to make claims about the product's efficacy, but only regarding its traditional use. The new directive is not a route to licensing for herbal POMs or for traditional herbal medicines that can be licensed by the conventional route. As it stands, the proposed directive would accommodate ethnic medicines that have been used in the UK (or any other EU member state) for at least 15 years. This directive also lists problematic consequences of imported US products and restricted herbs.

EU Directive 2004/24/EC also gives guidance on permitted medicinal indications. Labelling may also be covered by the Joint Health Claims Initiative (JHCI), which restricts excessive claims.

Homoeopathic remedies

In the UK, homoeopathic remedies are subject to medicines legislation. A simplified registration scheme (Simplified Scheme) exists in the UK (and the rest of the EU) for homoeopathic medicinal products which:

- Are intended for oral or external use
- Are sufficiently dilute (usually a minimum dilution of 1 in 10 000)
- No medical claims are made.

Since 1 September 2006, new homoeopathic products may be registered under the National Rules Scheme. For such products, manufacturers are required to demonstrate quality and safety, and efficacy, together with appropriate product labelling and literature. Manufacturers of homoeopathic medicinal products which are administered parenterally, are below the minimum dilution, or make efficacy claims are required to substantiate this in the same manner as is required for conventional drugs.

Other complementary medicines

Products marketed as food or dietary supplements include non-herbal substances, such as glucosamine, vitamins, minerals and fish oils. These products are sold under food legislation and are marketed without medical claims. Such products may be deemed by the MHRA to be a relevant medicinal product (see 'Herbal medicines' above). Some 'supplements' are subject to stringent restrictions on their use. Melatonin is a POM, available on a 'named patient' basis only as there are no licensed melatonin products in the UK. However, in the USA, melatonin is sold as a food supplement. A new draft EU directive is aimed at harmonizing the marketing of food supplements in member states.

Gamma linolenic acid (GLA), widely available as unfractionated evening primrose oil, was widely used as a supplement, principally for premenstrual syndrome, but later obtained a full product licence for the two conditions of psoriasis and mastalgia, although these were withdrawn in 1995.

Essential oils used by aromatherapists in their practice for medicinal purposes are considered to be medicinal products, but are exempt from licensing provided they meet certain criteria (see 'Herbal medicines' above). Aromatherapy products sold through retail outlets are not subject to licensing regulations unless they are marketed as medicinal products. Some essential oils are available as licensed medicinal products, e.g. peppermint oil capsules, although such products are conventional medicines, not aromatherapy products. These examples highlight the possible confusion for both pharmacists and patients.

Pharmacy and provision of CAM

Pharmacies and pharmacists have several roles in the provision of CAM. Community pharmacies are a major source of complementary medicines for people who purchase and self-treat with these products. Pharmacists may also be asked for information and advice on self-treatment with complementary medicines. In addition, community pharmacists may be presented with NHS (FP10) prescriptions for homoeopathic medicines. Some independent pharmacies provide consulting rooms that are available for use on a sessional basis by CAM practitioners, and a similar initiative was recently adopted by some branches of a large multiple, which offered consultations with practitioners of several CAM therapies, including homoeopathy, herbalism and osteopathy. Also, there are several community pharmacies which specialize in CAM, e.g. homoeopathic pharmacies which offer professional homoeopathic pharmaceutical services.

Pharmacists' involvement with CAM is not limited to the community. Pharmacists employed in NHS homoeopathic hospitals provide pharmaceutical services in the pharmacy and on the wards. Pharmacists employed in conventional NHS hospitals may be involved with the supply of certain complementary medicines.

Pharmacists' training in CAM

In September 1999, the Science Committee of the Royal Pharmaceutical Society of Great Britain (RPSGB) set up a working group on complementary and alternative medicine to examine issues in this area of importance to pharmacy and pharmacists.

Pharmacists' involvement in the provision of CAM at any level raises several issues, particularly with regard to pharmacists' knowledge of and training in CAM, their professional accountability and the quality, safety and efficacy of complementary medicines sold or supplied. The RPSGB Code of Ethics states that pharmacists providing homoeopathic or herbal medicines or other complementary therapies have a professional responsibility:

- To ensure that stocks of homoeopathic or herbal medicines or other complementary therapies are obtained from a reputable source of supply
- Not to recommend any remedy where they have any reason to doubt its safety or quality
- Only to offer advice on homoeopathic or herbal medicines or other complementary therapies or medicines if they have undertaken suitable training or have specialized knowledge.

Almost all pharmacies sell complementary medicines, particularly herbal medicines and homoeopathic remedies. The majority of pharmacists are asked for and 'recommend' specific complementary medicines. However, the extent of teaching on pharmacognosy (the scientific discipline which covers the chemistry, biological and clinical effects of natural products, particularly plants) and herbal and complementary medicines in the MPharm programme is limited and varies between schools of pharmacy. Furthermore, the majority of practising pharmacists have not undertaken or received training in areas of CAM, although Centre for Pharmacy Postgraduate Education (CPPE) training manuals are freely available in England.

Pharmacists' training in CAM should not be limited to complementary medicines. It should include an awareness of the background to, evidence for and safety concerns with regard to complementary therapies such as acupuncture. This is because patients' use of such treatments may have implications for pharmaceutical care. For example, research involving community pharmacists in the USA has suggested that some patients with chronic conditions temporarily or permanently use complementary therapies instead of their prescribed medicines. This has also been shown to have an effect during surgical operations (Ang-Lee et al 2001).

Pharmacists' professional practice

At present, pharmacists' professional practice with regard to complementary medicines is not optimal. Many pharmacists do not routinely ask customers and patients specifically about their use of complementary medicines, nor record such use on patient medication records. Pharmacists are encouraged to apply principles of good professional practice with regard to complementary medicines, and to be aware that patients' use of complementary medicines may have implications for pharmaceutical care. For example, it is possible that patients may use complementary medicines in addition to, or instead of, conventional medicines, without telling their doctor or pharmacist. The concurrent use of complementary medicines, particularly herbal medicines, and conventional drugs is of concern as there is a potential for interactions to occur. For example, important interactions have been documented between St John's wort and certain prescribed medicines, including warfarin, digoxin, theophylline, ciclosporin, HIV protease inhibitors, anticonvulsants and oral contraceptives. Many other examples have been reported.

The role of the pharmacist in reporting suspected adverse drug reactions (ADRs) associated with herbal medicines has been recognized by the MHRA. In November 1999, the MHRA Yellow Card scheme for ADR reporting was extended to include reporting by all community pharmacists (hospital pharmacists were granted reporter status in April 1997) (see Ch. 47). Community pharmacists are asked by the MHRA to concentrate on areas of limited reporting by doctors, namely conventional OTC medicines and herbal products. The Yellow Card scheme also applies to unlicensed herbal products. While the MHRA does not formally request reports of suspected ADRs associated with other types of unlicensed products, it is unlikely that the MHRA would ignore a genuine report of a serious suspected ADR associated with a non-herbal unlicensed product.

Efficacy and safety of CAM approaches

It is beyond the scope of this chapter to consider evidence for the efficacy and safety of individual complementary medicines and complementary therapies. Evidence from randomized controlled trials for the efficacy of complementary therapies for specific conditions is rare, but a search of the Cochrane Library database reveals varying evidence of efficacy for a range of CAM products.

This is not to say that such approaches are not efficacious, rather that for many, rigorous research has not been carried out. There are several reasons for this, including a lack of research funding for and research infrastructure in CAM.

Similarly, CAM is often assumed to be 'safe', but this assumption is not based on appropriate studies. In fact, some complementary therapies have been associated with serious adverse effects. In addition, formal spontaneous reporting schemes (i.e. similar to the MHRA Yellow Card scheme for ADR reporting) do not exist for 'manual' complementary therapies, such as acupuncture, chiropractic and osteopathy.

The relative lack of research in CAM means that there is also a lack of evidence-based information on which to base treatment decisions for specific patients. Nevertheless, there are several sources of information in CAM, including specialist databases and specialist fields within established databases. Several reference texts written by pharmacists have summarized and critiqued the available evidence in areas of CAM (see Appendix 5 for further reading suggestions). An MHRA document, 'Safety of herbal medicinal products', lists intrinsically toxic constituents of herbal ingredients, a number of quality related issues, herb–drug interactions and precautions in specific patient groups.

The future for complementary medicines

On the basis of current trends in market research data, it has been predicted that sales of complementary medicines will continue to increase (Mintel International 2005). Longitudinal data on the utilization of complementary therapists are not available for the UK, although increasing numbers of such practitioners may suggest increasing public demand for holistic treatment with these therapies. In addition, the increasingly widespread marketing and sale of these products demonstrates the interest of large sections of the public to control their health by using these products.

With the EU directive on traditional herbal medicinal products, the future is set to bring improved quality standards for these preparations – manufacturers will need to meet standards for GMP, or remove their products from the market. Initiatives involving ethnic medicines are also aimed at improving quality standards for these preparations. However, as this sector is less developed in the UK, it is likely that improvements in the quality of ethnic medicines will be seen over a longer time period.

Improvements in quality standards, together with other requirements in the traditional herbal medicinal products directive, will put an increased emphasis on manufacturers to provide evidence supporting the safety of their products. At the same time, the increasing use of herbal medicines, particularly by patients using conventional drugs and those with serious chronic illness, may result in the emergence of new safety concerns, such as indications of uncommon ADRs, those occurring with long-term use and interactions with conventional medicines.

Against a background of widespread and increasing use of CAM, it is recognized that CAM practitioners need to be regulated, and that conventional healthcare professionals need to be knowledgeable about complementary medicines and therapies. The House of Lords Select Committee on Science and Technology's (2000) report on CAM made several recommendations with regard to statutory regulation of those who practise CAM (see above), and these recommendations were accepted by the government (Department of Health 2001). Thus, in the future, conventional healthcare professionals should have a basic knowledge of complementary medicines and therapies, and doctors, pharmacists and others may interact with state-registered CAM practitioners.

In its response to the House of Lords' report, the government stated that if a therapy gains a critical mass of evidence, the NHS and the medical profession should ensure that the public has access to that therapy. Thus, in addition to homoeopathic treatment, which is already available through the NHS, certain complementary therapies and licensed complementary medicines with a sound evidence base may also be available on NHS prescriptions.

In the long term, the future for 'complementary medicines', particularly herbal medicines and nutraceuticals, may lie with pharmacogenetics and pharmacogenomics. These relatively new fields of research are widely held to be central to the discovery of new drugs and to the future of therapeutics. Yet the pharmacogenetics of ADRs, and optimizing treatment on the basis of a patient's genotype, has not been discussed in the context of herbal medicines. It is reasonable to assume that individuals with a different genetic profile will have different responses to complementary medicines as well as to conventional drugs.

The distrust of traditional CAM in the 1970s and 1980s has of course been followed not only by increased public awareness of their possible benefits, but also by major investigation by pharmaceutical companies, and by government and institutional researchers. This has led to recent (in terms of the historical development of conventional medicine) development of single product plant medicines, such as galantamine (*Narcissus cultivars*), atracurium (intermediate from *Leontice leontopetalum*), artesunate and artemether (*Artemesia* spp.), and taxol (*Taxus* spp.), with the prospect of more chemical entities being derived from CAM.

KEY POINTS

- The use of complementary/alternative therapies, particularly herbal medicines, is widespread and appears to be increasing
- Most community pharmacies sell complementary medicines, particularly herbal medicines and nutraceuticals, and many pharmacists are asked for advice on such products
- Hospital pharmacists may also encounter patients who use complementary medicines
- The use of complementary medicines may have implications for pharmaceutical care, e.g. drug interactions can occur
- Most complementary medicines currently are sold as unlicensed products, so evidence of their quality, safety and efficacy has not been assessed by the MHRA
- Other than for osteopaths and chiropractors, there is at present no statutory regulation of practitioners of complementary therapies, including those using medicinal substances

21

Routes of administration and dosage forms

Arthur J. Winfield

STUDY POINTS

- The different routes of administration of drugs
- The advantages and disadvantages of each route
- The types and uses of dosage forms

Introduction

Following the administration of a medicine, the drug has to reach its site of action or receptor in order to produce an effect. How this is achieved is often a complex process affected by many factors. The first stage will be the release of the drug from the dosage form, to be followed by absorption into the body (unless it is for a surface effect at the site of administration). There is then a distribution process, usually in the blood, which will take the drug to the site of action. As soon as it is in the body, metabolic processes, especially in the liver, will start to change the drug and the elimination process will also commence. A detailed discussion of these processes is outside the scope of this book, although it does have a significant impact on the choice of both the route of administration and the actual dosage form. There is a growing awareness that the correct choices can have an important impact on therapeutic outcomes for the patient. Further details about biopharmacy can be found in Aulton (2007) and on pharmacokinetics in Walker & Wittlesea (2007). This chapter will review the various routes of administration used for drug delivery and discuss some of their advantages and disadvantages. Brief details of a variety of dosage forms are also given. Figure 21.1 illustrates the principal routes of administration.

Routes of administration

The oral route

The oral route can produce either a systemic or a local effect. For a systemic effect the drug, formulated in either a solid or a liquid form, is absorbed from the gastrointestinal tract (GIT). This is the most commonly used route for drug administration. There are several reasons for this:

- From a patient's point of view it is the simplest route
- Self-administration of drugs can be carried out
- If used properly, it is also the safest route.

However, there are disadvantages which should be borne in mind:

- The onset of action is relatively slow
- Absorption from the GIT may be irregular
- Some drugs are destroyed by enzymes and other secretions found in the GIT
- Because the blood supply from the GIT passes through the liver via the hepatic portal system, it is subject to hepatic metabolism before it enters the systemic circulation. This is called first pass or presystemic metabolism
- Drug solubility may be altered by the presence of other substances in the GIT, e.g. calcium
- Gastric emptying is very variable and can be influenced by factors such as food, drugs, disease state and posture. Not only does it affect the onset of action, but if it is extended it may cause a drug to be inactivated by gastric juices owing to prolonged contact

1 Buccal (inside mouth)
2 Oral (swallow)
3 Sublingual (under tongue)
4 Nasal
5 Rectal
6 Vaginal
7 Inhalation (to lungs)
8 Eye
9 Ear

10 Parenteral
  a Intravenous
  b Subcutaneous
  c Intramuscular
  d Intraspinal
Topical – skin (any site)

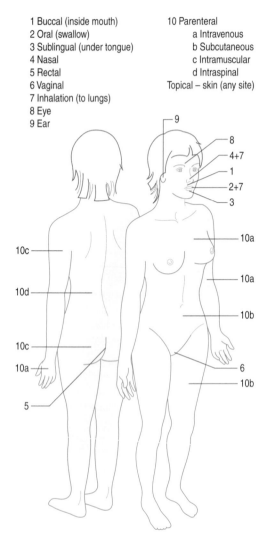

Figure 21.1 • Diagrammatic representation of the main routes of administration.

- It is an unsuitable route of administration in unconscious or vomiting patients and for immediate pre- or postoperative use.

The buccal routes

A drug is administered by these routes by being formulated as a tablet or spray and is absorbed from the buccal cavity. The highly vascular nature of the tongue and buccal cavity, and the presence of saliva which can facilitate the dissolution of the drug, make this a highly effective and useful route for drug administration. It can also be used for a local action.

Two sites are used for absorption from the buccal cavity:

- For sublingual absorption, the area under the tongue is used. This gives a very fast onset of action of the drug but duration is usually short
- For buccal absorption, the buccal sulcus is used. This is the area between the upper lip and the gum. Tablets formulated for absorption from the buccal sulcus give a quick onset of action but will also give a longer duration of action than the sublingual route. This route can also administer drugs with a longer half-life for an extended duration of action.

It is important that patients are made aware of the difference between the two sites and they should be given full instructions on how to administer their tablets, to ensure maximum benefit. For details of suitable patient instructions, see Chapter 36.

The advantages of the buccal route are:

- There is a relatively quick onset of action
- Drugs are absorbed into the systemic circulation, thereby avoiding the 'first pass' effect
- Drugs can be administered to unconscious patients
- Because the tablet is not swallowed, antiemetic drugs can be given by this route.

The rectal route

For administration by this route, drugs are formulated as liquids, solid dosage forms and semi-solids (see Ch. 34). The chosen preparation is inserted into the rectum from where the drug is released to give a local effect or it may be absorbed to give a systemic effect.

The rectum is supplied by three veins, namely the middle and inferior (lower) rectal veins which drain directly into the systemic circulation and the upper rectal vein which drains into the portal system which flows into the liver. This means that, depending on the position within the rectum, only some of the drug absorbed from the rectum will be subject to the first pass effect. Bioavailability, therefore, may be less than 100% but may be better than obtained from other parts of the GIT.

The amount of fluid present in the rectum is small, estimated at approximately 3 mL of mucus. This affects the rate of dissolution of the drug released from the suppository. However, there is also muscular movement which spreads the drug over a large area and promotes absorption.

The advantages and disadvantages of this route of administration are as follows.

Advantages

- Can be used when the oral route is unsuitable, e.g. severe vomiting, unconscious patient, with uncooperative patients such as children, elderly or mentally disturbed and patients with dysphagia
- Useful when the drug causes GIT irritation
- Can be used for local action.

Disadvantages

- Absorption can be irregular and unpredictable, giving rise to a variable effect
- Less convenient than the oral route
- There is low patient acceptability of this route in the UK. A wider acceptance is found in other parts of the world.

The vaginal route

For administration by this route, drugs may be formulated as pessaries, tablets, capsules, solutions, sprays, creams, ointments and foams which are inserted into the vagina. Most often this route is used for a local effect. However, drugs absorbed from the vagina are not subject to the first pass effect and can give systemic bioavailability better than with the oral route.

The inhalation route

Drugs are administered usually by inhalation through the nose or mouth to produce either local or systemic effects. This route is used predominantly for local administration to treat respiratory conditions such as asthma. For this, drugs are delivered directly to the site of action, i.e. the lungs. A variety of dosage forms are used, from simple inhalations consisting of volatile ingredients such as menthol to sophisticated inhaler devices (see Ch. 37). A major benefit of the inhaled route is that the drug dose required to produce the desired effect is much smaller than for the oral route, with a consequent reduction in side-effects. Because of the high blood flow to the lungs and their large surface area, drug absorption by this route is extremely rapid and can be used to give systemic action.

The nasal route

The nasal cavity has been traditionally used for producing local effects using solutions as drops or sprays. More recently it has been used for systemic action because of its good vascular supply which avoids first pass metabolism, although it does have some local enzymic activity.

The topical route

In the topical route the skin is used as the site of administration. This route is most commonly used for local effects using liquid and powder dosage forms in addition to the traditional ointments, creams and pastes (see Ch. 33). The skin has a natural barrier function, but specialized dosage forms have been developed which, when applied to the skin, allow the drug to pass through and produce a systemic effect. This avoids first pass effects and can produce close to zero-order kinetics over prolonged time intervals. A more detailed discussion of this route of administration can be found in Chapter 33.

The parenteral route

This is the term used to describe drug administration by injection. Within this general term there is a variety of different routes. The main ones are:

- *Intravenous route*, where drugs are injected directly into the systemic circulation. This produces a very fast onset of action
- *Subcutaneous route*, where drugs are injected into the subcutaneous layer of the skin. This is the easiest and least painful type of injection to administer
- *Intramuscular route*, where drugs are injected into muscle layers. This method can be used to produce a fairly fast onset of action when the drug is formulated as an aqueous solution. A slower and more prolonged action will occur when the drug is presented as a suspension or in an oily vehicle.

These and other specialized types of injection are discussed more fully in the chapter on parenteral products (see Ch. 38).

Dosage forms

Drugs are presented in a wide variety of dosage forms. How a drug is formulated is dependent on a variety of factors and the same drugs may be presented in several different dosage forms. It is important for pharmacists to appreciate the different properties of the varying dosage forms in order that the most appropriate or most acceptable formulation is given to the patient. This section gives brief information on the different types of dosage forms. Additional, more detailed, information is found in the chapters dealing with specific formulations (see Chs 30–39) and in Aulton (2007).

Aerosols

These consist of pressurized packs which contain the drug in solution or suspension and a suitable propellant. They are most commonly used for their local effect in the treatment of asthma. These devices are fitted with a metering valve which allows a known dose of drug to be delivered each time the device is fired. Some aerosols are for topical use, particularly in the treatment of muscle sprains and injuries. These may contain substances such as non-steroidal anti-inflammatory drugs or counterirritants.

Applications

This is the name given to solutions, suspensions or emulsions which are for topical use. They contain substances such as ascaricides or antiseptics.

Capsules

These are solid dosage forms, generally for oral use. Some drugs formulated as capsules are intended to be inhaled. It is therefore important to inform the patient on their appropriate use. For both types of capsule, the drug is contained in a gelatin shell, usually as a powder or a liquid. Modified-release preparations are available where the drug is presented in the gelatin container as small pellets with different coatings.

Collodions

These are liquid preparations for external use. The liquid is painted on the skin, where it forms a flexible film. They contain substances such as salicylic acid which is useful in the treatment of corns.

Creams

These are semi-solid emulsions for external use. Because of the water content they are susceptible to

microbial contamination and either include a preservative or are given a short shelf life. Creams are easier to apply and are less greasy than ointments, so patients often prefer them.

Dusting powders

These are finely divided powders for external use. Their main uses are as lubricants to prevent friction between skin surfaces and for disinfection and antisepsis in minor wounds.

Ear drops

These are used topically to treat a variety of ear problems. The drug, or mixture of drugs, is presented as a solution or suspension in a suitable vehicle such as water, glycerol, propylene glycol or alcohol. The drops are inserted into the ear, using a dropper. Some vehicles, such as alcohol, may cause a degree of stinging when applied to the ear. Ensure that the patient is aware of this and is assured that it is a normal sensation. If patients find the degree of stinging unacceptable they may have to be given ear drops with an aqueous vehicle. Oils such as almond or olive are often recommended for the alleviation of impacted earwax. It is usually suggested that such oils, before being dropped into the ear, should be warmed. This must be done very carefully and only minimal heat applied, i.e. the oil placed on a warm spoon. Excessive heat will have serious consequences for the integrity of the ear.

Elixirs

An elixir is a solution of one or more drugs for oral use. The vehicle generally contains a high proportion of sucrose or, increasingly nowadays, a 'sugar-free' vehicle such as sorbitol solution, which is less likely to cause dental caries. The therapeutic action of drugs presented as elixirs varies widely and includes antihistamines, antibiotics and decongestants.

Emulsions

These are mixtures of two immiscible liquids, usually oil and water. When the term 'emulsion' is used this refers to a preparation for oral use.

Enemas

An enema is an oily or aqueous solution which is administered rectally. A variety of drugs are formulated as enemas and are used to treat conditions such as constipation or ulcerative colitis. They are also used in X-ray examination of the lower bowel and for systemic effects, such as the use of diazepam in status epilepticus and febrile convulsions.

Eye drops

These are sterile preparations used to administer drugs to the eye.

Gargles

Gargles are aqueous solutions used to treat infections of the throat. They are often presented in a concentrated form with instructions to the patient for dilution. Gargles should not be swallowed but held in the throat while exhaling through the liquid. After a suitable time period, usually a minute or so, the patient should spit out the gargle.

Gels

Gels are semi-solid dosage forms for topical or other local use. They are usually transparent or translucent and have a variety of uses. Spermicides and lubricants are often presented in a gel form. Preparations containing coal tar or other drugs used in the treatment of psoriasis and eczema are also presented in this form. Many patients prefer this formulation because it is non-greasy.

The term 'gel' is also used to describe colloidal suspensions of drugs such as aluminium and magnesium hydroxides.

Granules

This term is used to describe a drug which is presented in small irregularly shaped particles. Granules may be packed in individual sachets containing a unit dose of medicament or may be provided in a bulk format where the dose is measured using a 5 mL spoon. Some laxatives are among the drugs currently presented as granules.

Implants

This term refers to solid dosage forms which are inserted under the skin by a small surgical incision. They are most commonly used for hormone replacement therapy or as a contraceptive. Release of the drug from implants is generally slow and long-term therapy is achieved. In the case of the contraceptive implant the effect continues for up to 3 years. A testosterone implant used in the treatment of male hypogonadism will maintain adequate hormone levels in the patient for 4–5 months. Implants must be sterile.

Inhalations

These are preparations which contain volatile medicaments which may have a beneficial effect in upper respiratory tract disorders such as nasal congestion. Some inhalations contain substances which are volatile at room temperature and the patient can obtain a degree of relief by adding a few drops to a handkerchief or a pillowcase and breathing in the vapour. Other inhalations are added to hot water and the impregnated steam is then inhaled. Many users of the latter type of inhalation use boiling water. Pharmacists should advise against this, as the steam produced is too hot and can damage the delicate mucous membranes of the upper respiratory tract. Overuse of this type of preparation should also be avoided as it may cause a chronic condition to develop. The use of these strong aromatic decongestants is contraindicated in children under 3 months owing to the risk of apnoea.

Injections

These are used parenterally and are sterile (see Ch. 38).

Insufflations

This term is used to describe drugs presented in a dry powder form, usually in a capsule, which is inserted into a specially designed device where the capsule is broken, the contents released and the patient inhales the powder. Today, the most common use being made of insufflations is in the treatment of asthma. Some patients find these 'breath-actuated' devices easier to use than aerosol devices.

Irrigations

These are sterile solutions most commonly used in the treatment of infected bladders. Sterile solutions of sodium chloride 0.9% (physiological saline) are used to treat a wide range of common urinary tract pathogens. Antifungal drugs such as amphotericin and locally acting cytotoxics, e.g. doxorubicin and epirubicin, are introduced into the bladder, as irrigations, to treat mycotic infections and bladder tumours, respectively.

Linctuses

A linctus is a viscous liquid for oral use, the majority being for the relief of cough. The viscous nature of the preparation coats the throat and helps to alleviate the irritation which is causing the problem. Previously, many linctuses contained a high level of sucrose; however, many have been reformulated as 'sugar-free' products to reduce the risk of dental caries. Because the viscous nature of linctuses is beneficial, they should not be diluted prior to administration.

Liniments

These are liquids for external use. They are used to alleviate the discomfort of muscle strains and injuries. Because of the rubefacient nature of some of the ingredients, some sportsmen will use them prior to starting a sporting activity in an attempt to avoid any muscle damage. Examples of active ingredients found in liniments are turpentine oil and methyl salicylate.

Lotions

These are liquids for external use and may be solutions, suspensions or emulsions. They have a variety of uses which include antiseptic, parasiticidal and soothing. Care should be taken when recommending lotions for the treatment of head lice. Those which have an alcohol base should be avoided in asthmatics and young children, as the alcoholic fumes may cause breathing difficulties. Aqueous-based products should be advised.

Lozenges

These are large tablets designed to be sucked and remain in the mouth for up to 15 minutes. They do not contain a disintegrant and the active ingredient is normally incorporated into a sugar base, such as sucrose or glucose. The main use of lozenges is in the treatment of mouth and throat infections.

Mixtures

This is a generic term which is used for many liquid preparations for oral use.

Mouthwashes

These are similar to gargles but are used specifically to treat conditions of the mouth. The active ingredients are usually antiseptics or bactericidal agents.

Nasal drops and sprays

These are isotonic solutions used to treat conditions of the nose. Locally acting decongestants are commonly presented as nose drops. The container includes a dropper device to allow the patient to deliver the appropriate dose into the affected nostril(s). Overuse of nose drops is common as patients find it difficult to judge the number of drops being delivered. Other preparations for both local and systemic use are presented as sprays (metered or pump).

Ointments

Ointments are semi-solids for topical use.

Paints

Paints are solutions for application to the skin or mucous membranes. Those used on the skin are often formulated with a volatile vehicle. This evaporates on application and leaves a film of active ingredient on the skin surface. Paints to be used on the throat and mucous surfaces normally include a viscous vehicle such as glycerol, which enables the preparation to remain in contact with the affected area. Paints are used for their antiseptic, analgesic, caustic or astringent properties, and should be supplied with a brush to assist application.

Pastes

These are semi-solids for external use. They differ from creams and ointments in that they contain a high proportion of fine powder, such as starch. This makes them very stiff and means they do not spread readily over the skin's surface. Corrosive drugs such as dithranol are often formulated as pastes so that paste applied to the psoriatic lesion will not spread onto healthy skin and cause irritation.

Pastilles

Pastilles are for oral use and, like lozenges, are designed to be sucked. They contain locally acting antiseptics, astringents or anaesthetics and are used to treat, or give symptomatic relief of, conditions affecting the mouth and throat. They have a jelly-like consistency produced by their basis of gelatin or acacia.

Pessaries

Pessaries are solid dosage forms for insertion into the vagina. They are used for both local and systemic action.

Pills

Pills are a moulded oral dosage form which has been superseded by tablets and capsules. The term is still used by the general public, incorrectly, to describe any solid oral dose form.

Powders (oral)

These occur as both bulk and divided powders. Bulk powders usually contain non-potent active ingredients such as antacids. The dose is measured using a 5 mL spoon.

Individual powders are used for more potent drugs where accuracy of dosage is more important. An individual dose is packaged separately, either in a sheet of paper or in a sachet.

Suppositories

These are solid dosage forms for insertion into the rectum. They are used for both local and systemic actions.

Suspensions

Suspensions are liquid dose forms where the active ingredient is insoluble. Suspensions are available for both oral and external use.

Syrups

These are concentrated aqueous solutions of sugars such as sucrose. The term 'syrup' is frequently, but incorrectly, applied to certain sweetened liquids intended for oral use. The term 'syrup' should nowadays only be used to refer to flavouring vehicles. Sucrose is being replaced by sorbitol as the sweetening agent in many preparations to give 'sugar-free' syrups to reduce the risk of dental caries.

Tablets

This is the term used to describe compressed solid dosage forms generally intended for oral use, although some pessaries are tablets for vaginal use. As well as the standard tablet made by compression, there are many different types of tablet designed for specific uses, e.g. dispersible, enteric- coated, modified release or buccal.

Transdermal delivery systems

This term is used to describe the adhesive patches which, when applied to the skin, deliver a controlled dose of drug over a specified time period to produce a systemic effect.

KEY POINTS

- The route can be chosen to give local or systemic effects, fast or slow onset, and is influenced by biopharmacy and pharmacokinetics
- The oral route is the most commonly used route
- Gastric emptying, stability and other materials present in the GIT may limit availability of drug from the oral route
- Sublingual absorption gives a short, fast-onset activity
- Buccal absorption takes place between the gum and lip
- Buccal routes of administration can be used with unconscious patients and to avoid first pass metabolism
- Rectal absorption partially avoids first pass metabolism
- Rectal administration is useful for nil-by-mouth patients and in cases of gastric irritation. However, it is poorly accepted in the UK
- Vaginal administration can give systemic effects avoiding first pass metabolism
- Inhalation requires a much lower dose than the oral route, with a rapid onset

- Administration to the skin may be used for both local and systemic effects
- Injections can give the fastest onset of action but prolonged action is also possible using oily intramuscular injections

- A wide range of different dosage forms have been devised which have different properties and uses
- The same drug may usefully be used in different formulations to assist different types of patients

22

Prescribing for minor ailments

Paul Rutter

STUDY POINTS

- The growth of self-care and the increased access to medicines
- The key skills required to arrive at a working diffential diagnosis for a minor ailment
- Getting information from patients who present at the pharmacy with symptoms or conditions
- Techniques to make questioning more effective and how to pick up on non-verbal cues
- Full assessment of patient's symptoms in order to provide treatment and/or advice for minor ailments

Introduction

The community pharmacist plays an essential role in providing patient care. In most western countries, a network of pharmacies allows patients easy and direct access to a pharmacist without an appointment. Without pharmacists, general medical services would be unable to cope with patient demand. In effect, pharmacists perform a vital triage role for doctors by filtering those patients who can be managed with appropriate advice and medicines and referring cases which require further investigation. This has been a central role of community pharmacists for many decades, but over the last 20 years the role has taken on greater significance as there has been a shift in global healthcare policy to empower patients to exercise self-care. For pharmacists to safely, effectively and competently manage minor ailments requires considerable knowledge and skill. It involves having the underpinning knowledge on diseases and their clinical signs and symptoms, the ability to apply this knowledge to an individual patient and use problem solving to arrive at a working differential diagnosis. This has to be combined with good interpersonal skills such as picking up on non-verbal cues, asking appropriate questions and articulating clearly any advice which is given. This chapter attempts to provide the contextual framework behind the growing prominence of the pharmacist in managing minor ailments and the key skills required to maximize performance.

The concept and growth of self-care

The concept of self-care is not new. People have always treated themselves for common illnesses and pharmacists have always provided an avenue for people to practise self-care. Self-care does not mean individuals are left on their own and means more than just looking after themselves. It includes all the decisions and actions people take in respect of their health and covers recognizing symptoms, when to seek advice, treating the illness and making lifestyle changes to prevent ill health. The expertise and support provided by healthcare professionals, such as pharmacists, is crucial to making self-care work. The profile of self-care has dramatically increased in recent years and is largely government driven, consumer fueled and professionally supported.

Government policy

The creation of national healthcare schemes, such as the NHS has encouraged the general population to become more reliant on institutional bodies to look after their health. This has led to increased demand on services provided by these bodies, including the management of minor illness. For example, more than one in three GP consultations are for minor illnesses and an estimated 20–40% of GP time could be saved if patients exercised self-care. Similar findings have been recorded for patients attending hospital emergency departments. This dependence by patients on bodies such as the NHS has led to government policies which encourage and facilitate self-care. In the UK, the government agenda for modernizing the NHS was spelled out in its White Paper The NHS Plan (2000). Within this document the government made its intention clear to make self-care an important part of NHS health care. It stated that the front line of health care was in the home. Since that time the government has published numerous papers detailing why and how maximizing self-care can be achieved. The prominence placed on this government strategy is evidenced by the Department of Health having a dedicated website on self-care (http://www.dh.gov.uk/en/Policyandguidance/Organisationpolicy/Selfcare/index.htm). Included in these policy documents are specific papers looking at the role of pharmacy (e.g. A Vision for Pharmacy in the New NHS, 2003; Choosing Health through Pharmacy, 2005). It is clear that UK government policy centres on patient empowerment and utilizing all healthcare professionals to encourage patient self-care.

Widening access to self-care

The guiding principle of NHS modernization is to provide services that are best suited to the needs and convenience of patients. With regard to self-care, this can be achieved by encouraging patients to practise self-care themselves or by making better use of other healthcare professionals' skills.

NHS walk-in centres and telephone help lines

The UK government has been proactive in facilitating self-care, most obviously by the formation of NHS walk-in centres and the telephone help lines NHS Direct (England and Wales) and NHS 24 (Scotland). The aim of walk-in centres is to improve access to health care that supports other local NHS providers. The service is nurse led but some employ doctors to work at particular times. The first NHS walk-in centre opened in 2000 and there are now approximately 90 operating in England. The Department of Health states that over 5 million people have used a walk-in centre with the main users being young adults. NHS Direct, launched in March 1998, has seen remarkable government investment and rapid and widespread expansion. It is a 24-hour nurse led service that receives over 500 000 calls per month. Although originally designed as a telephone help line service, NHS Direct now also offers an online service and direct interactive digital TV plus the publication of its self-help guide.

Deregulation of medicines

Less obvious, but arguably more important, has been the expansion of medicines available without prescription (Table 22.1). This has direct impact on

Table 22.1 Chronological history charting prescription only medicine (POM) to pharmacy (P) and P to general sales list (GSL) deregulation

Year	POM to P	Examples	P to GSL	Examples
1983	3	Oral ibuprofen Loperamide Terfenadine[1]	0	
1984–86	0		0	
1987	3	Hydrocortisone	0	
1988	2		0	
1989	2		0	

Continued over

Table 22.1 *(Continued)*

Year				
1990	0		0	
1991	2	Nicotine gum	0	
1992	8	Vaginal imidazoles Nicotine patches	0	
1993	5		0	
1994	17	H$_2$ antagonists Minoxidil Beclometasone nasal spray	2	Effervescent aspirin and lidocaine
1995	7		2	Oral ibuprofen
1996	3		2	Clotrimazole
1997	3		8	Loperamide
1998	5		3	
1999	3		2	Nicotine gum
2000	4	Terbinafine	2	Famotidine
2001	5	Emergency hormonal contraceptives Prochlorperazine	5	
2002	2		0	
2003	1		5	Minoxidil Beclometasone nasal spray
2004	3	Omeprazole Simvastatin	3	Terbinafine
2005	2	Chloramphenicol	3	
2006	2	Sumatriptan Amorolfine	1	
Total	82		38	
2007	5		5	
2008	3		7	

[1] Terfenadine reverted back to POM control in 1997 following serious adverse events in America and was subsequently withdrawn by the manufacturers.

community pharmacists and represents one of the major ways in which pharmacy can contribute to self-care. Widening access to medicines previously only available via prescription supply is a global phenomenon and not unique to the UK.

The switching of prescription only medicines (POMs) to pharmacy (P) status is now well established. Loperamide and ibuprofen were the first POMs to be switched in 1983. The rate of POM to P deregulation after the initial two switches was slow, with only nine medicines deregulated between 1984 and 1991 (see Table 22.1). This was in part due to the bureaucratic process in place at the Medicines Control Agency (MCA; now known as the Medicines and Healthcare products Regulatory Authority, MHRA). In 1992 the MCA changed the process by which medicines were deregulated. Under the new system, changes to the product's legal status could be made without requiring amendments to the POM Order, thus speeding up the process. This change was effective, with no fewer than 30 medicines being deregulated over the next 3 years.

Further streamlining took place in 2002 to encourage manufacturers to switch medicines from both POM to P and P to general sales list (GSL). At approximately the same time, the White Paper Building on the Best (2003) set a target of 10 medicine switches each year (both POM to P and P to GSL) which was endorsed in The NHS Improvement Plan (2004). Between 1983 and 2008, over 80 POM to P and 40 P to GSL switches were made, although, the target of 10 switches per year from 2004 has yet to be met.

More recent POM to P switches have seen new therapeutic classes deregulated (e.g. proton pump inhibitors, triptans) and further deregulation of medicines from different therapeutic areas seems likely. The profession has played its part in this process, with the Royal Pharmaceutical Society of Great Britain (RPSGB) producing a consultation document on future candidates for POM to P switching (2002), some of which are now deregulated or being considered (e.g. tranexamic acid in 2007). Perhaps the largest area for future growth of deregulation centres on chronic disease management. Government policy toward self-care now embraces both acute and chronic illness (Supporting People with Long Term Conditions to Self Care: A Guide to Developing Local Strategies and Good Practice, 2006) and in 2004, the deregulation of simvastatin paved the way for further medicines to be available to manage chronic illness. This now enables UK consumers to purchase a medicine which government agencies have declared too low a priority to fund on the NHS (coronary heart disease risk of 10–15% over 10 years). This move therefore puts the emphasis squarely on the shoulders of the consumers to decide for themselves whether they want to initiate primary prevention.

Medical opinion on deregulation

Medical opinion is important in non-prescription use of medicines by patients. Doctors may advise patients to take them, prescribe them or dissuade their patients from using them. Relatively few studies have been conducted over the period of deregulation in the UK to ascertain GPs' attitudes towards the move for greater access to previously POMs. Around the time of the first deregulated POM, loperamide, Morley et al (1983) found GPs were generally against potential switches. Not until 1992 was further work published on GPs' attitudes to deregulation of medicines. Spencer & Edwards asked respondents their opinion on pharmacists managing 14 conditions treated at the time with POM medicines. Mixed results were found, ranging from the majority of doctors (87%) in agreement for pharmacists to use co-dydramol for toothache to almost no support (11%) for cimetidine to be given for dyspepsia. Erwin et al in 1996 and Bayliss et al in 2004 repeated the same questions. Over this 20 year period there is evidence that the attitudes of British GPs towards greater availability of medicines have become more positive. Bayliss et al hypothesized that this change in attitude is in part due to the length of time a product has been available without prescription and is supported by a 1999 Finnish study that found doctors were moderately positive, but more reserved towards those drugs only recently given over the counter (OTC) status. Results from all studies, except Bayliss et al, only considered acute conditions. When GPs were asked about management of chronic conditions, their opinions were strongly against such a move, yet opposition to the management of chronic illness might lessen in time, as it has with acute conditions.

Minor ailment schemes (MAS)

One barrier to patient self-care is the NHS system itself. Over 85% of prescriptions dispensed are exempt from the prescription charge (NHS statistics 2004). Therefore patients entitled to free prescriptions are likely to seek a doctor when they have minor illness, as any prescription issued will be free of charge in contrast to purchasing potentially the same product from the pharmacy. In response to this, a scheme dubbed 'Care at the Chemist' was established in Merseyside in 1999. It involved eight pharmacies and one GP practice and allowed patients free access to medicines through the pharmacy to treat 12 self-limiting conditions. Of the 1522 patients who used the scheme, only 21 patients were referred back to the GP. A 30% reduction in GP workload was observed for the 12 conditions included in the scheme. The scheme was subsequently replicated elsewhere and similar findings were observed. Consequently, the government called for widening participation of

MAS, and the new pharmacy contract for England and Wales has seen MAS incorporated into the enhanced service specification and in Scotland it is included as a core service. MAS are designed to meet the needs of the local patient population. Consequently, different models exist throughout the country although many bear much similarity to the 'Care at the Chemist' scheme. However, there are some primary care trusts and health authorities that now use a common scheme and there is growing support for a national scheme to be implemented in England. In some schemes, patient group directions (PGD) have been incorporated to allow pharmacists to prescribe POMs to treat conditions such as urinary tract infections and impetigo. A useful resource is the National Prescribing Centre (NPC) website (http://www.npc.co.uk/mms/SIGs/minor_ailments/#HELP).

The public's view on self-care and access to deregulated medicines

The public's attitude toward self-care and its actual actions are contradictory. A King's Fund study (2004) found that almost 90% of respondents believed they were responsible for their own health and a Mintel report (2004) found that 8 out of 10 people said they had to be 'really ill' to visit a doctor. However, it is estimated that upwards of 40% of GP time is spent dealing with patients who present with minor illness and only 25% of people who suffer minor illness self-treat with a purchased non-prescription medicine. It appears then that the government's message on promoting self-care is understood by people but is not being translated into action. Of some comfort to the government are findings from 2003 and 2004 Mintel lifestyle surveys that show increasing numbers of people consulting a pharmacist while the number of GP consultations is slowly falling. These latter studies cite convenience as a major contributory factor to pharmacy consultation rather than waiting for a GP appointment. However, patient attitudes over being questioned before medicines are sold are seen as a barrier. A study by Morris (1997) found most consumers had a degree of awareness of why pharmacy staff might require information but almost two-thirds had expected to make their most recent purchase without being questioned. Cantrill et al (1997) also found that pharmacists reported more than 10% of consumers unwilling to answer questions.

It appears that some sectors of the public are unhappy to be questioned by pharmacy staff. This group poses difficulty for pharmacy staff but asking questions ensures responsible purchasing of OTC medicines by consumers. There is also a small body of research both in the UK and USA that indicates that the public regards OTC medicines as inherently 'weaker' than prescription medicines. OTC status in itself may lead to a perception that the medicine cannot be harmful. For example, 40% of people in a US study believed that OTC medicines were 'too weak to cause any real harm' (Roumie & Griffin 2004). That doses of medicines switched from POM to P may be lower than those used on prescription is likely to reinforce such beliefs and could influence why people believe that they should not be questioned.

Getting information from the patient

As healthcare professionals, community pharmacists are in a unique position. Patients have free and easy access to their advice. Not only do patients take advantage of this but they value it. Surveys have shown that the general public believes pharmacists to be one of the most trusted occupations. It is important that the faith the general public has in pharmacists is maintained and enhanced. Ensuring that you are competent to handle minor ailments is one way to do this. The following steps highlight the key considerations you should think about when someone asks for your advice about a particular symptom or condition they have.

First impressions

It is said that you never get a second chance to make a first impression. When we meet somebody for the first time we make assumptions about that person. We often put people into categories and the assumptions lead to expectations of their behaviour, jobs and character. This initial judgment of a person is often based purely on what we see and hear and includes appearance, dress, age, gender, race and physical disabilities. It is important that we are aware of these assumptions in order to avoid stereotyping people. For example, the impression we have of a person wearing a denim jacket may be very different from our impression of the same person wearing a suit. As you get to know a person better, initial impressions are either reinforced or discarded, but in the context of dealing with patients who want advice about minor illness, this could be the first and last time you see them. This first impression works both ways and pharmacists who create a friendly approachable impression are more likely to find patients receptive to what they say.

From the perspective of deciding what the patient's problem is, this 'first impression' can be very helpful in giving you clues to their state of health. Assessment of the patient begins the moment the patient enters the pharmacy. Most pharmacists will probably do this at a subconscious level but what is important is to bring this to the conscious level and build it into your consultations. Many visual clues will be apparent if they are actively looked for. How old are they? Many conditions are age-related and this will help narrow down the number of conditions that need to be differentiated from one another. What is their physical appearance? Is the patient overweight or showing signs of being a smoker? Are there any signs of confusion, pain or systemic illness? For example, does the patient look well or poorly? For people who appear in discomfort or look visibly poorly, this might influence your decision to treat or refer – they might have a self-limiting condition such as viral cough but have marked systemic upset which necessitates referral. How did the person present to the pharmacy counter? Did they walk over in a normal manner or did they appear nervous, shy or reluctant? It might mean that the person who appeared nervous wants advice but is embarrassed to ask or they are intimidated by the environment and atmosphere. These 'cues' can be picked up by the pharmacist and appropriate action taken to make the person more at ease. The key is to observe your patient. Take time to assess what they look like, how they move and how they behave. This initial assessment will provide useful information which shapes your thinking and actions and is the first step to reaching a differential diagnosis.

Questioning

Arriving at a diagnosis is a complex process. In medicine it is based on three kinds of information: patient history; physical examination; and the results of investigations. Currently, physical examination and using diagnostic tests are rarely used in community pharmacy practice. Pharmacists rely almost exclusively on questioning patients when deciding whether to offer treatment or perhaps refer the patient for further evaluation. Studies have shown that an accurate patient history (gained from asking questions alone) is a powerful diagnostic tool. Supplementary examinations and diagnostic testing do improve the odds of reaching a correct diagnosis, but only by 10–15%.

The pharmacist's diagnosis will, in many cases, be a differential one; the signs and symptoms are suggestive of a particular condition but it is difficult with absolute certainty to label the exact cause. For example, someone who presents with acute cough is likely to have a viral self-limiting cough but it could possibly be bacterial in origin. Advice and treatment might well be the same but an exact diagnosis cannot be made. Of course, in certain circumstances this can be done, for example head lice, eczema caused by a watchstrap or psoriasis on a knee, etc.

The ability to ask good questions to gain the appropriate information is therefore critical. The type of question and the way in which it is asked will dictate the level of response given.

Use of open and closed questions

There are two main types of questions: open and closed. A closed question is one which is direct and close-ended. It requires the respondent to give a single word reply such as 'yes' or 'no'. They can be very useful when asking for specific information or to test understanding. Examples of closed questions are:

- Are you taking any medicines from the doctor?
- Have you ever had this rash before?
- Do you suffer from hay fever?
- Have you changed your washing powder?
- Is the pain worse in the mornings?

Open questions are open ended and allow people to respond in their own way. They do not set any 'limits' and generally allow the person to provide more detailed information. Open questions encourage elaboration and help people expand on what they have started to say. Examples of open questions include:

- Describe your symptoms to me.
- Tell me where the pain is.
- How do you relieve the symptoms of headache?
- What do you do when that sensation occurs?

The above examples show that open questions are often built around words like 'what' and 'how' and generally allow an element of 'feeling' to be introduced by the patient in the reply. Open-ended questions are not without their problems. Some patients when asked an open-ended question will launch into a detailed explanation of their symptoms and it can be difficult to pick up on the important information that is mixed in with irrelevant facts. This can be time-consuming, which can make pharmacists reluctant to use open questions.

Choosing the correct type of question can prove to be difficult, particularly in a busy pharmacy where other patients are waiting for prescriptions or advice. It is tempting to ask a number of closed questions which will provide information, albeit limited to what can be gleaned from one word answers. However, this could result in the patient being 'bombarded' with many questions and make them feel as if they have been through an interrogation. Pharmacists must learn to develop good questioning skills to enable them to build up an accurate picture of the patient's condition. In most consultations a mixture of closed and open questions will be needed. It also allows patients time to elaborate certain points and builds their confidence in the pharmacist.

As previously mentioned, how patients react to being asked questions in the pharmacy has been subject to some research. Findings have shown that some people feel it is not the legitimate business of pharmacy staff to ask what they may view as 'personal' questions about why the medicine is needed. It is therefore important to ensure that those people who are less responsive to being asked questions are dealt with in an appropriate way. This is usually done by explaining why questions have to be asked and using non-verbal communication. Position, posture and eye contact are important to give a relaxed, open appearance. Avoid using a counter or desk as a barrier or getting too close and invading a patient's 'intimate zone' (see later).

Drawing together information

It is important that pharmacists are sensitive to the needs of their patients when asking questions. If the patient indicates they wish to speak privately or you notice they appear uncomfortable, then every effort should be made to provide a quiet area for conversation. With the new community pharmacy contract now in place, most pharmacies have consultation rooms which provide areas for this purpose. The pharmacist must tailor their questioning strategy to each patient. It is also important that each question is asked with a purpose. There is little point asking a question if nothing is done with the answer. A number of techniques have been advocated to maximize information gathering from patients. These include the use

of acronyms, the funnelling technique and clinical reasoning.

Acronyms

Acronyms have been developed to help pharmacists remember which questions should be asked. WWHAM (Who is the patient? What are the symptoms? How long have the symptoms been present? Action taken? Medication being taken?) is the best known and simplest acronym to remember and has been advocated by many as a useful tool in gaining information from patients. Other acronyms have been subsequently developed and include ENCORE, ASMETHOD and SIT DOWN SIR. The difficulty with using acronyms is that they are rigid and inflexible – a 'one size fits all' approach. In addition, there is a tendency to ask questions for no reason – it is part of the acronym so the question has to be asked even though there might be no relevance or underpinning reasoning for asking the question. This is especially true of WWHAM, and because it is simple to remember it also means it provides the least information. Other acronyms do provide more information but because they are longer they become almost impossible to remember. Acronyms can be helpful in gaining some information from the patient but pharmacists should not rely solely on them. Each patient is different and it is unlikely that an acronym can be fully applied, and more importantly, it might miss vital information.

Current prescription workload and staff skill mix in most pharmacies makes pharmacist intervention in requests for advice or product selection impossible on every occassion. Up to 75% of patients are first seen by a counter assistant. The standardization of their questioning by using an acronym via a standard operating procedure (SOP) might be appropriate to ensure basic information is obtained from all patients.

The funnelling technique

A funnelling technique can be used to allow direction and focusing of ideas on a specific topic. This involves initially asking background open questions to provide basic information, then asking specific closed questions to provide specific detail and clarify points. In these circumstances, it can be useful to paraphrase comments made, to ensure that the understanding of the information being obtained from the patient is accurate. This checking procedure allows the pharmacist to check understanding and minimizes misinterpretation. It is possible during any one conversation to use more than one 'funnel', e.g. establishing a patient's current medical condition, then going on to suggest appropriate action or medication available. In a pharmacy setting, where time can be a limiting factor, using the funnelling technique can be useful for directing and focusing a conversation to enable an end point to be achieved more quickly.

Clinical reasoning

Clinical reasoning relates to the decision-making processes associated with clinical practice. It originates from medicine in determining the best way physicians solve diagnostic problems. It is a thinking process directed towards enabling the practitioner to take appropriate action in a specific context. Based on these principles, the encounter with a patient in a community pharmacy is no different. It fundamentally differs from using acronyms or the funnel approach in that it is built around clinical knowledge and skills which are applied to the individual patient. Various models have been used to explain the process and include hypothetico-deductive reasoning and pattern recognition.

Hypothetico-deductive reasoning

This is a process in which a number of hypotheses are generated which are then used to guide subsequent information retrieval from the patient. Each hypothesis can be used to predict what additional findings ought to be present if it were true. Very early in a clinical encounter and based on limited information, practitioners will arrive at a small number of hypotheses. The practitioner then sets about testing these hypotheses by asking the patient a series of questions. The answer to each question then allows the practitioner to narrow down the possible diagnosis by either eliminating particular conditions or confirming their suspicions. Hypothesis generation and testing involves both inductive (moving from a set of specific observations to a generalization) or deductive reasoning (moving from a generalization to a conclusion in relation to a specific case). Therefore, induction is used to generate hypotheses and deduction to test hypotheses.

Pattern recognition

Pattern recognition relies more on inductive processes than deduction. For example, take a newly qualified pharmacist and a very experienced pharmacist who

has been qualified 25 years. If they both see the same patient with the same problem, they both might arrive at the same conclusion, but how this was achieved will probably be different. This is because not all cases seen by more experienced practitioners will require applying a hypothetico-deductive model. For example, impetigo has a very characteristic appearance. Once a pharmacist has seen a case of impetigo, it is a relatively straightforward task to diagnose the next case by recalling the appearance of the rash. Therefore much of daily practice will consist of seeing new cases that strongly resemble previous encounters. For this reason, expert reasoning in non-problematic situations tends to be drawn from pattern recognition from previous stored knowledge and clinical experience.

Whether we are conscious of it or not, most people will use a combination of hypothetico-deduction and pattern recognition when dealing with patients. Neither model provides an error-proof strategy and error rates of up to 15%, especially in difficult cases in internal medicine, have been reported in the medical literature. However, these models of 'responding to symptoms' are more likely to gain the correct diagnosis compared to using acronyms and the funnel method because acronyms and the funnel method tend to just gather information without having a hypothesis in mind. Example 22.1 highlights the clinical reasoning approach.

A further hypothesis to test in Example 22.1 would now be sputum production. Knowledge of the conditions listed indicates that postnasal drip, allergy and medication are not associated with sputum production. As these are the three conditions which we have doubts over from the first question, it seems a good follow-up question to ask if the patient is producing sputum; if so, then these three conditions can be eliminated.

The patient tells you that there is a bit of phlegm but they haven't really looked at the colour. This now means you are left with six possibilities. To differentiate between them, further distinguishing questions need to be asked. Some chronic cough conditions tend to show periodicity during the day, either being better or worse in the morning or evening. From our remaining conditions we know that generally:

- Chronic bronchitis is worse in the morning
- Asthma is worse in the evening
- Bronchiectasis is worse in the morning and evening
- Tuberculosis shows no variation
- Cancer shows no variation
- Nocardiosis shows no variation.

Example 22.1

A man in his early sixties (slightly overweight) wants something for his cough.

Step 1: Visual clues: age, sex and overweight
Step 2: Conditions to consider

Based on epidemiology, the most likely cause of cough in any age patient is viral infection, yet many other conditions can cause cough. These can be categorized by their prevalence within the population and give the pharmacist clues to the magnitude of likeliness that the person will have that condition and should be borne in mind during consultation.

Likely	Postnasal drip, allergies, acute bronchitis
Unlikely	Croup, chronic bronchitis, asthma, pneumonia, angiotensin converting enzyme inhibitor
Very unlikely	Heart failure, bronchiectasis, tuberculosis, cancer, pneumothorax, lung abscess, nocardiosis

In this case our patient is approximately 60 years old so certain conditions can be eliminated (e.g. croup) and others are less likely (e.g. pneumothorax tends to occur in young people, heart failure and lung abscess tend to occur in the elderly). This leaves a possible 12 conditions which could present to the community pharmacy which have cough as the primary symptom.

Step 3: Formation of hypotheses

The initial question needs to narrow down the number of conditions that must be considered. A number of questions are relatively discriminatory, such as duration of cough, sputum production and presence of systemic symptoms. If we take duration (he has had the cough for 4 or 5 weeks) then this should eliminate acute causes of cough (up to 3 weeks' duration) and leaves us with a list of nine possibilities, although three of these, post-nasal drip, allergy and medication, can be either acute or chronic:

- Chronic bronchitis
- Asthma
- Bronchiectasis
- Tuberculosis
- Cancer
- Nocardiosis
- Postnasal drip?
- Allergy?
- Medication?

Our patient says that the cough is always worse after getting up in the morning. This therefore tends to point to a diagnosis of chronic bronchitis. Obviously, the diagnosis is very tentative and we can now ask supplementary questions (generally closed questions) which should support the differential diagnosis. For example, our hypothesis would be that the person is a smoker or ex-smoker; we would expect them not to have any marked systemic symptoms; and we would expect that the person has a history of repeated episodes of cough. These confirmatory questions should be all positive and support our initial suspicions. If the patient responds in a different way to that which we anticipated then the differential diagnosis would need to be revised and hypotheses reconstructed to establish the cause of the cough. In this example the patient has to be referred.

This example illustrates the principle of hypothetico-deductive reasoning and the process behind it. In this instance, if an acronym, for example WWHAM, was used, the same outcome of referral would have been reached, as the 'H' question – how long have symptoms been present? – would have alerted the pharmacist to the chronic nature of the cough (all pharmacy text books on this area recommend referral for chronic cough). However, the information gained would have been superficial, which would not give you an idea of its cause and it would also ask irrelevant questions, such as who it was for (we already knew) and what medication they had tried.

For pharmacists, pattern recognition does play a part in shaping the above process but if the outcome is referral then clinical experience with the condition can be limited. Unless the patient returns or you follow up the case with the doctor, it is rare that pharmacists get feedback on the outcome of the referral. This therefore means that clinical experience of that symptom or condition is not consolidated by being given feedback on the diagnosis. Unfortunately, this means that if similar cases present again then pattern recognition can be used, but the level of knowledge remains at the same level as the outcome is always referral. Pharmacists should try to find out the outcome of referrals so that clinical experience increases and pattern recognition is improved.

Physical examination

Within the confines of a community pharmacy the type and extent of physical examination that can be performed is naturally limited and the majority of pharmacists will have received no formal training on how to conduct physical assessment. Examples of physical assessments that are suitable within the pharmacy include eye and ear examinations, assessment of skin disease and general inspection of the oral cavity. These examinations require little training but will improve the odds of making a correct diagnosis. This is one area where pattern recognition is very important – for example looking at a person's skin rash will always be better than getting an explanation from the patient.

Picking up on non-verbal cues

The meaning of what a person says is made up of several component parts. These are the words which are spoken, the tone of voice used, the speed and volume of speech, the intonation and a whole range of body postures and movements. It is generally agreed that in any communication the actual words convey only about 10% of the message. This is called verbal communication. The other 90% is transmitted by non-verbal communication which consists of body language (about 50%) and how it is said (about 40%).

Body language

Body language can be broken down into several component parts which include gestures, facial expression, eye contact, physical contact, body posture and personal space. It is the combination of all these components which gives the overall impression. It is important to ensure that they are all compatible. If a mixture of messages is portrayed it will cause confusion to observers.

Gestures

Hand gestures in particular are useful when emphasizing a point or to help to describe something. Used appropriately, they can greatly enhance communication and improve understanding. Observing the patient's gestures can give useful information on how concerned they might be or where the problem is. For example, someone presenting with abdominal pain might say they have stomach ache but point to the lower abdomen. In these cases, the non-verbal hand clue is much more informative than the spoken word. Also the person might point to a specific region, as the pain is very localized (e.g. appendicitis), or they

might move their hand over a larger area (e.g. irritable bowel syndrome).

Gestures are also useful for the pharmacist to use as they can emphasize or reinforce a point or describe a particular procedure. However, it is important not to overuse them, as this can detract from the spoken word and become a distraction to the listener. Do some 'people watching'. It is amazing how much information about people you can pick up just by quietly observing their gestures.

Facial expression

Facial expressions are a very important part of communication. Facial expression says a lot about mood and emotion, with the eyes and the mouth giving the dominant signs. As well as ensuring that facial expression is encouraging and welcoming, it is important for pharmacists to be able to read the meaning of facial expressions. In this way important points regarding a patient's level of comprehension or receptiveness can be judged.

Eye contact

Avoiding eye contact is a very successful way of avoiding communication. This can be very well illustrated by observing a class of students who have just been asked a question by a lecturer!

The maintenance of eye contact during a conversation is vital to ensure the continuation of the process, because it indicates interest in the subject and is also useful as a means of determining whose turn it is to speak. However, care must be taken. Holding eye contact for too long can be off-putting and will reduce the success of the communication. Anyone who has been stared at will know how uncomfortable this can be.

Body posture

We can usually control the words we say, but it is more difficult to control our body language. It is possible, therefore, to send out mixed messages by having a positive verbal message but a negative body posture. This will only serve to confuse the patient and it is likely that the outcome of the interaction will be poor. There are several classic body postures which have been identified as having significant meanings:

- *The closed position*. A person standing with their arms folded would illustrate this. This is seen as a rather negative posture and is unlikely to encourage communication
- *Feet position*. It is often found that a person's feet will be pointing in the direction in which he wants to go. This can be used to check whether the patient is interested or would rather be elsewhere
- *Positive body posture*. Leaning towards the person who is talking or sitting in a relaxed fashion are both examples of non-verbal language which can encourage good communication.

Physical contact

This is an important aspect of any communication process and can be used to enhance verbal communication. A sympathetic touch on an arm can often say far more than any number of words. However, physical contact is governed by broad social rules which vary greatly between cultures. The British are identified as one of the least 'touching' nations, while in many cultures touching between the sexes is unacceptable. An awareness of this is important for pharmacists who will come into contact with people from a wide variety of social and cultural backgrounds. What is considered acceptable behaviour in one culture could be unacceptable in another.

Personal space

We all have our own space in which we feel comfortable. Personal space varies between cultures and its extent depends on the situation. An awareness of personal space is important for pharmacists as it can play an important role in the success or otherwise of communication. If you carry on a conversation with someone at too great a distance it may be difficult to build up any rapport. However, if you are so close to people that they feel uncomfortable and threatened, no meaningful dialogue will occur. The different space zones are generally divided into four main areas.

General area

This is approximately 3 m or more. This is the space we would normally prefer to have around us if we are addressing a group of people or are working alone.

Sociable area

This is approximately 1–3 m and is the type of distance used when communicating with people we do not know very well.

Personal area

This is approximately 0.5–1 m. This is the space we would normally feel comfortable with when at a business or social meeting with people we know reasonably well. It is sufficiently close to allow friendly and meaningful communication without any individuals feeling threatened by having their intimate zone invaded.

Intimate area

This is usually 0–50 cm. This space is reserved for people we know very well. Husbands, wives, children, close friends and family are examples of the kind of people with whom we would be comfortable at these distances. If anybody else enters this so-called 'intimate zone' we feel threatened and will generally withdraw into ourselves. However, this is the space that pharmacists must enter if they are to perform physical examinations. This is why it is essential that pharmacists, if performing an examination, must gauge the level of acceptance by the patient by asking permission to perform the procedure and explaining what is involved.

Vocal communication

Vocal communication, sometimes called paralanguage, concerns the vocal characteristics, the quality and fluency of the voice. The quality of the voice refers to the tone, pitch, volume and speed. Tone in particular can convey more meaning than actual words. 'Thank you for asking the question' said in a harsh voice contradicts the words and indicates that it is not meant. The same words in a warm tone show sincerity. The volume must be adjusted to the circumstances and can emphasize key words. The speed of speaking must enable the listener to understand. Varying the speed and pitch can make the words more interesting and hold the listener's attention. Effective use of vocal communication requires that we become proficient at speaking with a warm confident tone of voice at an appropriate speed and volume and without interruptions or vocal mannerisms.

Outcomes from the consultation

The final step in prescribing for minor ailments is telling the patient what course of action you feel is most appropriate. This could be a combination of referral to another healthcare professional, giving advice or supplying a product. It is important that you give the patient as much information as they want or need and this draws on your skills of counselling (see Ch. 44).

Timescales

One of the key things a patient needs to know is what is the best course of action to take. Obviously this will depend on a number of factors including the patient themselves, the differential diagnosis and the severity of the condition. As a general rule, all patients should be advised on a timescale when they need to consult further medical help, whether they return to the pharmacist or see another healthcare practitioner. This allows the patient to understand the nature of the problem and know when they should seek further help. This will have to be gauged on a person-to-person basis. For example, take three patients all presenting with viral cough. Although the condition is self-limiting the timescales given to each patient can vary. If the first person presents after 7–10 days then you might tell them to see the doctor in the next 5–7 days if symptoms do not improve. The second patient has only had symptoms for 2 days, in which case you would give them a longer timescale. The third person might have had symptoms for 5 days but compared to the first two patients they have severe symptoms which would warrant automatic referral for a second opinion. This process is known as a conditional referral.

Treatment and advice

Once a full assessment of the symptoms has been made, and a decision made that the patient does not require immediate referral, appropriate recommendations should be made. Selection of an appropriate treatment for a condition involves application of pharmacology, therapeutics and pharmaceutics knowledge. The first step will be to choose an appropriate therapeutic group to recommend. The next step would be to assist the patient in the choice of product within the therapeutic group. For many therapeutic groups there is a wide variety of products available, often in various combinations. The pharmacist should take into account the efficacy, potential side-effects, interactions, cautions

and contraindications. With regard to efficacy, pharmacists should be aware that many OTC medicines have little or no evidence base. This does not necessarily mean they are not effective, but in today's climate of evidence-based health care then products with proven efficacy should constitute first-line treatment.

The difficulty in establishing efficacy has many explanations and includes: products that are available OTC predating clinical trials, a general lack of trial data or poorly conducted trials, the placebo effect seen with some OTC medicines and the nature of self-limiting conditions – is it the medicine working or the symptoms resolving on their own? Despite this, patient demand for a medicine to treat their symptoms is strong. Recommending an OTC medicine despite inadequate evidence of its efficacy is justifiable because many patients have a desire to try something to give them symptomatic relief. A negative or dismissive response by the pharmacist to a request from a patient can be harmful in that such patients may lose faith in the pharmacist and exercise self-care elsewhere where there is no qualified person to assess their symptoms. When selecting a product, the patient's needs should be borne in mind. Factors such as prior use, formulation and dosage regimens should be considered. For example, antacids are available in both tablets and liquid form. Liquids tend to have a quicker onset of action than tablets but can be inconvenient for a patient to carry around with them or take to work.

Non-drug treatment should also be offered where appropriate. For example, providing medication for motion sickness can be supplemented with advice on how to reduce symptoms, for example focusing on distant objects, not overeating before travel or sitting in the front seat in car journeys will help to reduce symptoms. Advice on increasing dietary fibre and fluids is an essential part of the management of conditions such as constipation and haemorrhoids. Certain situations where pharmacists are being consulted by patients for advice on symptoms are ideal opportunities to promote health education (see Ch. 5). For example, someone who is asking for advice about a cough could be asked about their smoking habits.

Children and the elderly

These two patient groups have the highest usage of medicines per person compared with anyone else. Care is needed in assessing the severity of their symptoms as both groups can suffer from complications. For example, the risk of dehydration is greater in children with fever or the elderly with diarrhoea. Invariably, lower doses are used in children, and because the elderly suffer from liver and renal impairment they frequently require lower doses than younger adults. Children should be offered sugar-free formulations to minimize dental decay and elderly people often have difficulty in swallowing solid dose formulations. It is also likely that the majority of elderly patients will be taking other medication for chronic disease and the possibility of OTC–POM interactions should be considered.

Pregnancy

The potential for OTC medicines to cause teratogenetic effects is real. The safest option is to avoid taking medication during pregnancy, especially in the first trimester. Many OTC medicines are not licensed for use in pregnancy and breastfeeding because the manufacturer has no safety data or it is a restriction on their availability OTC. Table 22.2 highlights those medicines where restrictions apply.

Table 22.2 Medicines to avoid during pregnancy

Medicine	Advice in pregnancy
Antihistamines – sedating	Some manufacturers advise avoidance, although chlorphenamine and triprolidine are classed by Briggs et al[1] as being compatible
Antihistamines – non-sedating	Manufacturers advise avoidance as limited human trial data, but animal data suggest low risk
Anaesthetics – local (benzocaine, lidocaine)	Avoid in third trimester – possible respiratory depression
Bismuth	Manufacturers advise avoidance
Crotamiton (e.g. Eurax)	Manufacturers advise avoidance
Fluconazole	Avoid
Formaldehyde (e.g. Veracur)	Manufacturers advise avoidance
Ocular lubricants (e.g. hypromellose, carbomer)	Manufacturers advise avoidance as safety has not been established
H_2 antagonists	Avoid
Hyoscine	Manufacturers advise avoidance as possible risk of minor malformations
Migraleve (opioid component)	Avoid in third trimester
Iodine preparations	Avoid
Midrid	Avoid
Minoxidil (e.g. Regaine)	Avoid
Monphytol paint	Manufacturers advise avoidance
Posafilin	Avoid
Selenium (e.g. Selsun)	Manufacturers advise avoidance
Systemic sympathomimetics	Avoid in first trimester as mild fetal malformations have been reported

[1] Briggs GG, Freeman RK, Yaffe SJ 2008 Drugs in pregnancy and lactation: a reference guide to fetal and neonatal risk, 8th edn. Lippincott Williams & Wilkins, Philadelphia. (This is one of the standard reference texts used by medicine information centres in answering medicine suitability during pregnancy.)

Table 22.3 Interactions of OTC medicines with POMs that can be significant

Medicine	Possible interactions	Outcome
Antihistamines – sedating	Opioid analgesics, anxiolytics, hypnotics and antidepressants	Increased sedation
Antacids (containing calcium, magnesium and aluminium)	Tetracyclines, quinolones, imidazoles, phenytoin, penicillamine, bisphosphonates, ACE inhibitors, angiotensin II	Decreased absorption
Aspirin	NSAIDs and anticoagulants Methotrexate	Increased risk of GI bleeds Reduced methotrexate excretion, toxicity
Bismuth Chloroquine	Quinolone antibiotics Amiodarone, sotolol, antipsychotics	Reduced plasma quinolone concentration Increased risk of arrhythmias
Fluconazole	Anticoagulants Ciclosporin Carbamazepine and phenytoin Rifampicin Atorvastatin	Enhanced anticoagulant effect Increased ciclosporin levels Increased levels of both antiepileptics Decreases fluconazole levels Increased atorvastatin levels that can lead to muscle pain/myopathy NB: Seriousness of the possible outcome would mean it is good practice to avoid all statins with fluconazole
Hyoscine	TCAs, and other medicines with anticholinergic effects	Anticholinergic side-effects increased
Ibuprofen	Anticoagulants Lithium Methotrexate	Enhanced anticoagulant effect Reduced lithium excretion Reduced methotrexate
Opioid-containing products	Alcohol, opioid analgesics, anxiolytics, hypnotics and antidepressants	Increased sedation
Prochlorperazine	Alcohol, opioid analgesics, anxiolytics, hypnotics and antidepressants	Increased sedation
St John's wort	Anticoagulants SSRIs Phenytoin, phenobarbital, carbamazepine Oral contraceptives Antivirals, ciclosporin, digoxin	Reduced anticoagulant effect Potential serotonin syndrome Reduced antiepileptic serum level Reduced efficacy of contraceptive Reduced plasma concentrations
Systemic sympathomimetics, including isometheptene (ingredient in Midrid)	MAOIs and moclobemide Beta-blockers and TCAs	Risk of hypertensive crisis Antagonism of antihypertensive effect
Topical (nasal or ocular) sympathomimetics	MAOIs and moclobemide	Risk of hypertensive crisis
Iron salts	Tetracyclines, quinolones, penicillamine	Reduced absorption if taken at same time

ACE, angiotensin converting enzyme; GI, gastrointestinal; MAOI, monoamine oxidase inhibitor; NSAID, non-steroidal anti-inflammatory drug; SSRI, selective serotonin reuptake inhibitor; TCA, tricyclic antidepressant.

Interactions of OTC medicines with other drugs

Medicines that are available for sale to the public are relatively safe. However, there are some important drug–drug interactions to be aware of when recommending OTC medicines. These are listed in Table 22.3.

Providing advice (patient counselling)

The service specifications of the pharmacists' Code of Ethics provides some guidance on the content of the counselling role of pharmacists. The specification on the supply of dispensed medicines states 'Pharmacists must ensure that the patient receives sufficient information and advice to enable the safe and effective use of the medicine'. The sale of OTC pharmacy medicines is similarly covered by the service specifications and the pharmacist is required to provide 'advice relevant to the product and the intended customer'.

Counselling should take place in a thoughtful, structured way. Pharmacists must have the ability to explain information clearly and unambiguously and in language the patient can understand. The counselling process should not be a monologue by the pharmacist giving a long list of information points. To be successful, it must be a two-way process. There should be ample opportunity for the patient to ask questions. Rapport is built up between the pharmacist and the patient and a much more meaningful dialogue can take place. What information to give to the patient will vary from case to case and will depend on a number of factors such as prior use and knowledge, the age of the patient and their comprehension level. However, as a general summary, patients should know:

- How to take or use the medicine
- When to take or use the medicine
- How much to take or use
- How long to continue to take or use
- What to expect, e.g. immediate relief, no effect for several days
- What to do if something goes wrong, e.g. if a dose is missed
- How to recognize side-effects and minimize their incidence
- Lifestyle or dietary changes which need to be made, if appropriate.

Aids to counselling

Patient information leaflets, warning cards and placebo devices are all useful aids when giving advice to patients. Most OTC medicines provide product information, often as a patient information leaflet (PIL). These PILs, where appropriate, can be used during counselling and important points highlighted. Placebo devices, e.g. inhalers, drops, patches, etc. can be used to demonstrate a particular administration technique and also to check a patient's ability to use the product. Leaflets on how to use ear drops, eye drops, eye ointment, pessaries, suppositories, etc. are available. Having given the information, it is then of major importance to check if the counselling has been successful. What does the patient understand, and do they have any problems? Watching the patient's body language and maintaining eye contact can give useful clues as to whether the message is being understood and whether compliance is likely.

Conclusion

In conclusion, the pharmacist plays a pivotal role in helping patients exercise self-care and provides an effective screening mechanism for doctors. The continued deregulation of medicines to pharmacy control will mean that pharmacists over the coming years will be able to prescribe more medicines from more therapeutic classes. This necessitates that all pharmacists have up-to-date clinical knowledge and can competently perform the role. This might require many to acquire new skills (e.g. physical examinations) and take a much more active role in monitoring and following up the patient after advice and products have been given.

KEY POINTS

- Pharmacists have a traditional role in assisting patients with self-care
- Recent increases in patient self-care are government driven, consumer fuelled and professionally supported
- It is estimated that 20–40% of GP consultations are for conditions which are suitable for self-care
- Since 1983 there has been a policy of re-regulation of medicines, mainly POM to P, providing the public with access to a wider range of medicines
- Minor ailment schemes, linked to PGDs, enable pharmacists to prescribe a range of medicines on the NHS

- While public opinion supports pharmacists supplying medicines for self-care, there is resistance to being questioned by pharmacy staff
- Pharmacists require effective communication skills in order to be effective in advising patients
- The first impression of the patient and by the pharmacist can be vital
- Medicine recognizes three inputs in reaching a diagnosis – patient history, physical examination and test results. Only the first, and occasionally the second are available to pharmacists
- Using open and closed questions, the relevant medical history of the patient can be obtained, but the pharmacist must be sensitive to the patient's wishes
- Various techniques can be used to improve the efficiency of the process, including the use of acronyms, the funnelling technique, clinical reasoning and pattern recognition

- Non-verbal cues are often more important than the words used
- Important parts of body language include gestures, eye contact, body position, personal space and physical contact
- Vocal communication is important for understanding and rapport
- When prescribing, first-line treatment should have proven efficacy
- Non-drug advice is also appropriate
- Special considerations apply to children, the elderly and women who are pregnant or breastfeeding
- Patient counselling is a requirement and aims at ensuring the patient knows how, when and how much medicine to take, how long to take it for, what to expect, and what actions to take if something is wrong

23

Information retrieval

Parastou Donyai

STUDY POINTS

- How to categorize health- and medicine-related information
- Relevant search and retrieval processes including essential preparatory and analytical elements
- Organizations that can help with information retrieval
- How practically to apply the suggestions in this chapter to enable you to practise and perfect the art of information retrieval

Introduction

The current era is characterized by man's ability to store, retrieve and transmit large volumes of information using computer technology. Albert Einstein proposed that the secret of success is 'to know where to find the information and how to use it'. Most pharmacists would probably agree. This chapter aims to provide the reader with a theoretical understanding of how to source health- and medicines-related information in the present information age. While the quality of retrieved information is also considered, guidance on the detailed evaluation of what is known broadly as 'clinical evidence' is found elsewhere (see Ch. 19).

The new Code of Ethics and Standards for pharmacists and pharmacy technicians lists seven principles with supporting explanations that together define what it means to be a registered pharmacy professional. For example, pharmacists must have the appropriate knowledge and competence for their work and they must also adhere to types of action and behaviour that uphold the reputation of the pharmacy profession. In the Code of Ethics and Standards, the knowledge and provision of health- and medicines-related information specifically is considered in the following manner. In relation to their own knowledge and competence, pharmacists must develop their skills in line with their area of expertise, keeping up to date with relevant progress through continuing professional development (CPD). In some instances, for example with pharmacist prescribers, pharmacists must also have access to a wide range of medicines-related information, and their practice, wherever possible, must be evidence based and in accordance with relevant national and local guidance. Decisions must be based on clinical and cost-effectiveness and pharmacists must recognize and avoid potentially biased information. In relation to the provision of medicines-related information to those who want or need it, pharmacists are expected to be able to provide accurate, reliable, impartial, relevant and up-to-date information on a wide range of issues in a manner which recipients can easily understand.

Yet with thousands of medicinal products, dressings and appliances on the UK market, pharmacists are highly unlikely to hold in-depth knowledge of all health- and medicines-related issues at all times. Periodically all pharmacists will need to supplement their knowledge either proactively or reactively, for CPD purposes or to address practice-related queries. Therefore, the ability to retrieve relevant health- and medicines-related information in a timely and efficient manner becomes central to the practice of all pharmacy professionals (Box 23.1). One particular group that benefits specifically from a good working knowledge of information retrieval is pharmacists involved in research, be it in academia or in practice.

> **Box 23.1**
>
> ### Pharmacy activities that might involve information retrieval
>
> - Solving patient-specific clinical problems
> - Critical evaluation/appraisal of the literature
> - Preparation of a scientific paper
> - Effective provision of verbal and written information to the public
> - Clinical guideline development
> - Drug policy management (e.g. formulary management, drug use evaluation or audit)
> - Preparation of bulletins and newsletters
> - Managing the entry of new drugs into health care
> - Adverse drug reaction/event management
> - Continuing professional development

Where does information exist and how can it be retrieved?

Information retrieval is the tracing and recovery of stored information. Health- and medicines-related information can range from patient information to drug monographs to more sophisticated health technology assessments. It can exist in many forms from the archives of a drug company to the World Wide Web (the web). To acquire the art of information retrieval one must ultimately appreciate the range of relevant information that exists, where it exists and how it might be sourced.

Some years ago traditional scholars would have discounted the web as an appropriate first topic for discussion. Not so today. Most present-day pharmacists sourcing health- and medicines-related information are likely to use the Internet (the net) at some point during their search, if not to begin with. The expanse of information posted on the web and its apparent accessibility has integrated the Internet into most work routines. While on the whole the seemingly endless material may not suit most pharmacists' information needs, there are specific online resources that pharmacists can browse in order to look for health- and medicines-related information. These include official websites operated by governments, professional, practice, regulatory or academic bodies as well as websites belonging to patient groups and the pharmaceutical industry. We will deal with some of the well established sites. However, the fluid nature of the Internet, the vast array of information available,

plus the variable nature of each query will probably also involve the information-seeking pharmacist in some degree of Internet searching. This necessitates a fuller discussion of search engines and search strategies. A myriad of specialized scientific databases and other portals are also accessible via the net. Some databases are also available on CD-ROM. These act as directories for scientific papers and other publications and as such can be used to search for available material. Searching databases and the material they contain is considered separately.

Before widespread use of the Internet, the principal source of health- and medicines-related information was the printed book. Books still contain a vast array of indispensable information and, arguably, reputable ones play a vital role in information management. Although individual pharmacies may not keep the full range of essential books, specialist centres will have access to these and to other resources. The topic of books and that of organizations that help with health- and medicines-related queries are covered in the later parts of this chapter.

The Internet

The World Wide Web is less than 20 years old at the time of writing this book. Yet it contains several billion pages and has become woven into the fabric of everyday life, especially in the developed world. The Internet in its current form came into being in 1983. The web took form around 1989/90, was launched in 1991 and came into widespread use from 1993 onwards. From the beginning it acted as a place where large numbers of files and documents could be stored for download, circulation, discussion and communication. These days many thousands of documents and other items are added to the web every hour. Consequently it is not possible to categorize all available websites in order to create a comprehensive directory of the web. Most people create their own directory of useful websites or search the Internet for the information they need.

The web address

The term website is used to denote a set of themed, linked web pages, usually accessed via a 'homepage'. Web pages are written in hypertext mark-up language (htm). A web page is a collection of text, graphics, sound and/or video that corresponds to a single window of scrollable material. Web pages are stored on a web server, a program that hosts the website and 'dispenses' the pages in response to a web browser. The web browser displays web pages after communicating with the server. There are a large number of browsers in existence, although currently the majority of users in the western world employ either Internet Explorer® or Netscape Navigator®.

Each page on the web has a distinct web address known as the uniform resource locator (URL), sometimes referred to as the uniform resource identifier (URI). The URL can be a good clue as to the quality of the information found on a website; this is covered in detail, below. The 'locator' in URL can also give an indication of where one is within a website; for example, on the homepage or further in. The locator can also indicate the source of the information being viewed; for example, whether it is from the Department of Health or a pharmaceutical company.

A web address or website name appears on the address bar. All website names are part of the domain name system (DNS) and look similar to this: http://www.dh.gov.uk/.

Box 23.2 breaks down this address and examines the individual parts. In summary, the web address

http://www.dh.gov.uk/Publicationsandstatistics/index. htm is showing: protocol://server.name.domain. country/pathname/document name.file extension.

Directory of useful websites

This section provides a list of some of the more established health- and medicines-related websites with the proviso that any printed list can become quickly outdated (Table 23.1). Web addresses or pathnames can change or more useful sites can be created. Each record in the catalogue of websites in Table 23.1 represents an electronic resource that can be browsed or searched for relevant information by pharmacy professionals. To help order the directory, a classification scheme has been followed with subheadings to group similar websites together. A short description of each site is provided and, where applicable, tips on some useful sections have been included. The list is not exhaustive and it should be used as a starting point by readers to create a personalized catalogue of essential health- and medicines-related information websites.

 Box 23.2

Individual components of a typical domain name system
The web address http://www.dh.gov.uk/Publicationsandstatistics/index.htm

PROTOCOL. http:// shows us that we are looking at a website with http meaning 'hypertext transfer protocol', the set of rules used by the computer to access and deliver web pages. The variation https:// indicates a secure connection (secure http) to the site in question

SERVER AND ORGANIZATION'S NAME. www.dh informs us that we are viewing a website held on a computer or a web server known as www belonging to an organization called 'dh', in this instance the Department of Health. Although quite often a web server computer is called www, some websites have dispensed with www and some use different server names such as 'news' or 'staff' or 'students'

DOMAIN AND COUNTRY. .gov.uk tells us that we are looking at the website of a governmental institution in the UK. This part of the web address is the 'domain', other examples of which are .edu (educational); .com (commercial); .co (a company); .ac (academic); .org (non-governmental, non-profit making organizations). Sometimes domains are followed by a country code that indicates the location of the computer holding the website, for example .uk, but some websites, especially those originating in North America, omit this information

PATHNAME AND DOCUMENT NAME. Beyond the homepage of an organization's website, other pages are ordered in a hierarchy of folders in which the various information can be found. In this example, Publicationsandstatistics indicates we are looking at a folder in which we will find an index page .index.htm, stored as a htm file

FILE EXTENSION. The file extension usually identifies the type of data found in the file. For example, the extension .htm (or .html) indicates a file that contains code expressed in the hypertext mark-up language used to develop pages that are to be placed on the web. There are countless other examples; the extension .txt indicates a file containing textual data; the extension .pdf indicates a file in portable document format, widely used for Internet publication of official documents because it allows exact reproduction of printed text

Table 23.1 Directory of 'established' websites that can be accessed via the Internet for health- and medicines-related information. Each subsection is arranged in alphabetical order. These websites should form the basis of an individual's database of useful websites

Name of website and web address	Brief description of content and tips on useful subsections
Governmental and regulatory bodies	
Department of Health http://www.dh. gov.uk/	Contains material produced by and for the Department of Health, of relevance to health professionals. Visit and bookmark letters and circulars: http://www.dh.gov.uk/en/ Publicationsandstatistics/Lettersandcirculars/index.htm Visit and bookmark the Orange Guide on Drug Misuse and Dependence – Guidelines on Clinical Management: http://www.dh.gov.uk/assetRoot/04/07/81/98/04078198.pdf
European Medicines Agency http:// www.emea.europa.eu/	Website of the European Union body responsible for issuing European marketing authorization and for regulating the safety, quality and efficacy of medicinal products
Medicines and Healthcare products Regulatory Agency http://www.mhra. gov.uk/	Information about the regulatory processes for medicines and medical devices in the UK, including news about initiatives in Europe and beyond. Allows online reporting of safety problems. Visit and bookmark drug safety updates: http://www.mhra.gov.uk/mhra/ drugsafetyupdate Find and bookmark news on Safety of Herbal Medicines, and Drug Analysis Prints (DAPs) – a complete listing of the suspected adverse drug reactions (ADRs) through the Yellow Card scheme
United States Food and Drug Administration http://www.fda.gov/	American counterpart to the MHRA, the FDA is responsible for ensuring safety, quality and efficacy of medicines and medical devices as well as other items such as foods, cosmetics and radiation-emitting devices in the US
NHS bodies, evidence-based medicine and guidelines	
AHFS Drug Information	Drug information provided by the American Society of Health-System Pharmacists; electronic access available via Medscape: http://www.medscape.com Search the Drug Reference section. Visit http://www.medscape.com/druginfo/
All Wales Medicines Strategy Group http://www.wales.nhs.uk/sites3/ home.cfm?OrgID=371	Provides advice on strategic medicines management and prescribing, a conduit through which consensus is reached on medicines management issues, especially those affecting both primary and secondary care in Wales. Click on 'AWMSG finalized documents'
Bandolier http://www.medicine.ox.ac. uk/bandolier/	Academic department providing collection of abstracted evidence (systematic reviews of treatments, of evidence about diagnosis, epidemiology or health economics) under various subheadings. Visit and bookmark the learning zone: http://www.medicine.ox.ac.uk/ Bandolier/learnzone.html
British National Formulary http://www. bnf.org/bnf/	The BNF provides UK healthcare professionals with authoritative and practical information on the selection and clinical use of medicines in a clear, concise and accessible manner. Visit BNF Extra for access to various 'calculators'
Centre for Reviews and Dissemination http://www.york.ac.uk/inst/crd/index. htm	Academic department that undertakes systematic reviews related to health and social care interventions and delivery and organization of health care. Produces three databases: NHS Economic Evaluation Database (NHS EED); Database of Abstracts of Reviews of Effects (DARE); Health Technology Assessment (HTA) Database. Visit the databases: http://www.crd. york.ac.uk/inst/crd/crdweb
Clinical Management Plan Library Online http:// www.cmponline.info/	Relatively recent repository of clinical management plans for use by supplementary prescribers

DIAL www.dial.org.uk	Website of an information service, based at Royal Liverpool Children's NHS Trust (Alder Hey), offering advice on the use of medicines in children, to healthcare professionals working in the UK and Eire
Drug and Therapeutics Bulletin http://www.dtb.org.uk/	Subscription-based publication of the British Medical Journal group providing independent evaluations of, and practical advice on, individual treatments and the overall management of disease for healthcare professionals. Articles based on synthesis of evidence with opinions from a wide range of specialist and generalist commentators
DrugScope http://www.drugscope.org.uk	Independent centre of information and expertise on drugs of abuse in UK
Health Protection Agency http://www.hpa.org.uk/infections/	Provides support and advice to various bodies and NHS professionals to protect UK public health. Remit includes communicable disease surveillance and microbiology, radiation, chemical and environmental hazards as well as major emergency response. Try index of topics: http://www.hpa.org.uk/topics/index.htm
Health Technology Assessment programme http://www.ncchta.org/	Independent research into the effectiveness, costs and broader impact of healthcare treatments and tests for those who plan, provide or receive care in the NHS. Visit research projects: http://www.ncchta.org/research/index.shtml
HIV Drug Interactions http://www.hiv-druginteractions.org	Educational HIV pharmacology resource providing specific advice on HIV drug interactions
Immunization Against Infectious Diseases (the Green Book)	Provides the latest information on vaccines and vaccination procedures for all the vaccine-preventable infectious diseases that may occur in the UK Access http://www.dh.gov.uk/ then Home >> Public health >> Health protection >> Immunisation >> Green book Free paper copy from 0845 954 0000 or greenbook@broadsystem.com on leaving name, occupation, address & RPSGB registration number
Indiana University cytochrome P450 website http://medicine.iupui.edu/flockhart/	Information about drug interactions that are the result of competition for, or effects on, the human cytochrome P450 system
IPPF Directory of Hormonal Contraceptives http://contraceptive.ippf.org	Website of International Planned Parenthood Federation, recommended and used by the RPSGB Information Service to identify foreign contraceptive pills. Free registration
NHS Immunisation Information http://www.immunisation.nhs.uk	NHS website providing a comprehensive, up-to-date and accurate source of information on vaccines, disease and immunization in the UK
Malaria Reference Laboratory http://www.malaria-reference.co.uk	Based at the London School of Hygiene and Tropical Medicine, the Malaria Reference Library provides an integrated service for public health in relation to malaria. Visit Malaria prevention guidelines for British travellers under Advisory service
National Horizon Scanning Centre http://www.pcpoh.bham.ac.uk/publichealth/horizon/	Based at the University of Birmingham, the centre provides advanced notice to the Department of Health and national policy makers in England of selected key new and emerging health technologies that might require urgent evaluation, consideration of clinical and cost impact or modification of clinical guidance around 2–3 years prior to launch on the National Health Service
The National Institute for Health and Clinical Excellence http://www.nice.org.uk/	The independent organization responsible for providing national guidance on the promotion of good health and the prevention and treatment of ill health, produces guidance on areas of

Continued over

Table 23.1 *(Continued)*

	public health, health technologies and clinical practice. Visit and bookmark guidance: http://www.nice.org.uk/guidance/index.jsp
National Library for Health http://www.library.nhs.uk/	NHS electronic library. Aims to be the best, most trusted health-related knowledge service in the world. See other evidence-based sites and links included in this table. Visit and bookmark Clinical Knowledge Summaries for 'minor-ailment' type guidance (formerly Prodigy guidance): http://cks.library.nhs.uk/home Visit and bookmark National electronic Library for Medicine (formerly DrugInfoZone): http://www.nelm.nhs.uk/en/ and, for example, search for Patient Group Directions; find and bookmark the online Dictionary; find and bookmark information on pre- and post-launch reviews
National Poisons Information Service: Toxbase® http://www.toxbase.org/	A clinical toxicology database, freely available to UK NHS hospital departments and general practices, NHS Departments of Public Health and HPA Units
National Prescribing Centre http://www.npc.co.uk/	Part of the NHS, the NPC aims to promote and support high-quality, cost-effective prescribing and medicines management to improve patient care and service delivery. Visit and bookmark Current Awareness Bulletins: http://www.npc.co.uk/ecab/ecab.htm. Visit and bookmark MeReC Bulletins: http://www.npc.co.uk/merec_bulletins.htm
National Travel Health Network and Centre (NaTHNaC) http://www.nathnac.org/	Funded by the Department of Health, the centre has been created to promote clinical standards in travel medicine with the goal of *protecting the health of British travellers*
Netting the Evidence http://www.shef.ac.uk/scharr/ir/netting/	Academic department bringing together various organizations and learning resources related to evidence-based medicine
Palliative drugs.com http://www.palliativedrugs.com/	Created by palliative care practitioners, the website aims to promote and disseminate information about the use of drugs in palliative care. It features a Palliative Care Formulary but some areas are password protected
Prescription Pricing Authority (Division) http://www.nhsbsa.nhs.uk/prescriptions	Provides pricing information for NHS prescriptions dispensed in England and related services with associated usage statistics. Monthly NHS electronic drug tariff available on this site
Pro-File Database http://www.pro-file.nhs.uk	Tool designed to help NHS pharmacy staff to identify and source unlicensed 'special' medicinal products needed to treat individual NHS patients whose clinical needs can't be met by use of (a) licensed medicine(s)
NHS Purchasing and Supply Agency (PASA) http://www.pasa.nhs.uk/PASAWeb	Website of executive agency of the Department of Health concerned with getting the best value for money for NHS purchased goods and services. Visit 'Pharmaceuticals' under 'Products and Services'
Royal College of Obstetricians and Gynaecologists http://www.rcog.org.uk/index.asp?PageID=8	Makes available a range of guidelines on women's health. Visit Faculty of Sexual and Reproductive Healthcare: http://www.ffprhc.org.uk/
Scottish Intercollegiate Guidelines Network http://www.sign.ac.uk/	SIGN develops and disseminates national clinical guidelines containing recommendations for effective practice, based on current evidence. Visit and bookmark guidelines: http://www.sign.ac.uk/guidelines/index.html
Scottish Medicines Consortium http://www.scottishmedicines.org.uk/	Provides advice across Scotland to NHS Boards and their area drug and therapeutics committees about the status of new medicines, formulations or major new indications for established medicines. Contains searchable database of reviews

Solutions http://www.uclhsolutions.com/	UK National NHS Shortages Database focusing on communication and management of pharmaceutical supply problems
Surgical Materials Testing Laboratory http://www.smtl.co.uk/	Website of NHS laboratory for testing and evaluation of surgical dressings and medical disposables. Click on site map for layout of content. Visit and bookmark dressing data cards: http://www.dressings.org/dressings-datacards-by-alpha.html
Travax http://www.travax.nhs.uk/	An interactive online database providing up-to-the-minute travel health information for healthcare professionals
UK Medicines Information (UKMi) http://www.ukmi.nhs.uk	The website hosts UKMi strategy, policies, clinical governance standards and training materials, together with minutes of meetings of the UKMi Executive and its working groups. Some areas are password protected
Welsh Medicines Resource Centre http://www.wemerec.org/	Website providing independent information on prescribing for healthcare professionals working in Wales
Pharmacy organizations and associations	
National Pharmacy Association http://www.npa.co.uk/	Trade association for UK community pharmacy owners. Provides professional and commercial support and represents community pharmacy at national negotiations. Try searching for the quarterly Pharmacy Flyer
Royal Pharmaceutical Society of Great Britain http://www.rpsgb.org.uk/	The professional and regulatory body for pharmacists in England, Scotland and Wales, it also regulates pharmacy technicians, currently on a voluntary basis. Go to Download Society Publications, find the latest copy of Medicines, Ethics and Practice and search 'Section 1.3 Alphabetical list of medicines for human use' to find legal classifications of medicines
Continuing professional development	
Centre for Postgraduate Pharmacy Education http://www.cppe.manchester.ac.uk/	The CPPE is funded by the Department of Health to provide continuing education for practising pharmacists and pharmacy technicians providing NHS services in England
The College of Pharmacy Practice http://www.collpharm.co.uk/	A limited company and registered charity, aiming to promote continuing education and training in pharmacy. Try searching for 'Competency Frameworks' under the Faculty of Prescribing and Medicines Management
NHS Education for Scotland http://www.nes.scot.nhs.uk/	Educational solutions for NHS Scotland staff. NHS Education for Scotland (Pharmacy) is the National UK Centre for Continuing Pharmaceutical Education in Scotland. Visit and bookmark: http://www.nes.scot.nhs.uk/pharmacy/default.asp
Welsh Centre for Post-Graduate Pharmaceutical Education http://www.cf.ac.uk/phrmy/WCPPE/index.html	Provides continuing professional development service to all pharmacists and their support staff in Wales
Pharmaceutical industry	
The Association of the British Pharmaceutical Industry http://www.abpi.org.uk/	Trade association for UK companies producing prescription medicines. Also represents companies engaged in the research and development of medicines for human use. Visit and bookmark interactive educational pages: http://www.abpischools.org.uk/
Electronic Medicines Compendium http://emc.medicines.org.uk	Associate website of the ABPI. Provides electronic copies of Summaries of Product Characteristics (SPCs) as well as patient information leaflets (PILs) for members' products

Continued over

Table 23.1 *(Continued)*

	licensed in the UK. Continuously updated with new and revised SPC and PIL information after approval by licensing authorities
The Proprietary Association of Great Britain http://www.pagb.org.uk	Trade association for UK producers of over-the-counter medicines and food supplements. Visit and bookmark the Consumer Health Information Centre: http://www.chic.org.uk/ Visit and bookmark the Medicine Chest, a directory of medicines and food supplements are available over the counter: http://www.medicinechestonline.com/
Patient information	
Best Treatments http://www.besttreatments.co.uk/btuk/home.html	Website produced by the BMJ Publishing Group based on clinical evidence in a patient-friendly format. Also accessible via NHS Direct website. Subscription-based
Family Planning Association http://www.fpa.org.uk	Website of Family Planning Association, a leading sexual health charity
Medicines Guides http://medguides.medicines.org.uk/	Produced by an independent not-for-profit group, the Medicine Guides are being developed in partnership with NHS Direct to provide people with information about medicines, conditions and different treatment options
Medline Plus® http://medlineplus.gov/	American health information website for patients with medicine-related information, illustrated medical encyclopaedia, interactive tutorials and health news. Belongs to the US National Library of Medicine (http://www.nlm.nih.gov/), and the US National Institutes of Health (http://www.nih.gov/). Visit and bookmark the interactive tutorial homepage: http://www.nlm.nih.gov/medlineplus/tutorial.html
NHS Direct http://www.nhsdirect.nhs.uk/	Official NHS website for 24-hours delivery of information and advice about health, illness and health services to the public. Can search for a local health service or visit and bookmark interactive tools and healthy living zones
Netdoctor http://www.netdoctor.co.uk	Collaboration of UK and European healthcare professionals. For information about drugs, search the Medicines section only: http://www.netdoctor.co.uk/medicines/
Patient UK http://www.patient.co.uk	Authored by GPs, the website aims to provide non-medical people in the UK with good quality information about health and disease
Talk to Frank http://www.talktoFrank.com	Independent government funded website providing information on drugs of abuse

Bookmarking

Readers are encouraged to set up their own bespoke directory of health- and medicines-related websites that they can update as required. Once a number of relevant websites have been identified and authenticated for inclusion, a simple way of starting the collection is to store the directory as a saved text file, using hyperlinks to connect each typed URL address in the document to the address bar on the browser and therefore the desired web destination. Hyperlinks are usually in a different colour to the rest of the document or are underlined and can be activated by a mouse click.

Hyperlinks also provide a useful way of finding and bookmarking other useful websites from existing ones. Websites normally have a directory of related websites as 'links'. By clicking on a link, a request is sent to the computer that holds that information, asking it to send it to your screen. Following these links on the screen is known as 'browsing', sometimes referred to as 'surfing'.

A well-accepted method of bookmarking relevant pages is to use an Internet browser with functions such as 'Favourites', 'Bookmarks' or 'Hot List'. A marker points at a website which then enables the user to quickly return to that site without having to remember and type in its URL. In this way, the

'Favourites'-type function acts like a conventional bookmark. Browsers usually offer the facility for organizing the bookmarks into folders and subfolders.

There are also innovations such as the social bookmarking website http://del.icio.us, which provides a means of storing personal bookmarks online instead of within the browser, thus enabling bookmark information to be accessed and shared online.

Searching the Internet

Accessing a list of useful websites and following the links therein is one approach to finding health- and medicines-related information on the Internet. Browsing the net in this way is likely, however, to be unproductive unless the query falls specifically within the remit of a known website. With the web estimated to contain around 40 billion pages, at some point it is likely that the website containing the required information is simply unknown to the user and it has not been possible to reach it via 'browsing' the Internet. For that reason, it is essential to have a good appreciation of Internet search options.

Commercial search engines

The Internet is not controlled or owned by any individual or organization in particular. Unlike a catalogue, which is normally a well thought out record created and maintained for a purpose, the Internet plays host to a multitude of material with limitless authors. The Internet is vast but far removed from a library of approved and organized material. The manner in which information is stored on, and then retrieved from, the Internet is quite unique. There is no central catalogue of the Internet and no 'people' physically vetting the web to create large-scale records. Instead, computers are used to create indexes of the web.

A variety of websites concentrate on providing Internet search facilities. Some are set up as web portals with the aim of providing a complete resource for everything on the web that they consider to be worthwhile. Portals display their own editorial material, news headlines and other up-to-date information, as well as links to commercial partners and paid advertisements. They are good for general or commercial information but most will fail to identify websites for non-profit organizations such as the NHS. Web portals also provide a search facility. Examples of web portals include Yahoo®, MSN® and AOL®. Other websites concentrate purely on providing a search facility; examples include the search engines Google™, Altavista® and Ask™. Search engines attempt to search all the text on all the pages of the web. They use software to seek out and index web pages, storing the results in sizeable databases. Essentially they are clusters of powerful computers, endlessly navigating the web and building indexes of pages based on words and links found on those pages. When a user types a query, the search engine searches its database for pages that contain words matching the query and displays the results as a list of links. Box 23.3 gives a more detailed explanation of search engine components. Each search engine ranks results according to its own criteria and so different search engines can give different results for the same query. Search engines are useful for finding obscure information or for some research-type activities. They may, however, retrieve a multitude of items that are of little or even no relevance to the search activity.

Box 23.3

Search engines are essentially made up of three interconnected parts: the crawler, the indexer and the query processor

THE CRAWLER (SPIDER)	This is a specialized program, a form of robot that constantly travels the web similar to a browser, following links with absolute diligence, returning a copy of each page it finds for the indexer
THE INDEXER	This program maintains an extremely large database of computerized records. For any given website, the index will list all the pages on that site alongside other relevant information. The database is then inverted so that a typed phrase will lead to relevant URLs. Indexes are analysed in a manner that ranks the search results, giving preference to what are thought to be web pages more relevant to the user's inquiry. Tagged and analysed pages are ultimately handed over to the query processor
THE QUERY PROCESSOR	This program moves between the user interface and the indexer. The query processor is designed to make it user-friendly, and to enable it to make an intelligent guess about the user's intentions in making their query. The query processor also finds a way of dealing with misspellings, for example by relating them to past misspellings

Effective use of search engines

An informed approach to using search engines for health- and medicines-related information starts from an insight into the workings of these, as detailed above. Before beginning a new search, the user should take time to consider what they already know, the knowledge gaps and the types of information required. It is always advisable to have a plan so as to focus the search. The user should carefully select a set of keywords that best reflect the information need and narrow the search to a particular subject or topic. Any subsequent search results should be compared to the original information need. If appropriate material is found on the first page of the search, the activity need go no further. It is especially important to know when to stop searching, especially when there is a time limit on the search activity.

When, however, the results do not match the information need, for whatever reason, it is advisable to pause and reflect. The user should take time out to consider what they are searching for; can the search be refined, by changing keywords, perhaps adding, taking away or replacing them? The keywords must match the information need. One additional approach is to subtract any redundant words from the search query. These include words such as 'a', 'an', 'the', 'and', 'in', 'any', 'my', etc. It might also be helpful to re-arrange the search so that the more important search terms are placed first, to give more influence when the results are ranked.

Most search engines provide guidance on their specific 'operators'. For example, Google™ provides a list of its most popular tools for refining searches under its 'cheat sheets'. Boolean terms for academic databases are described in more detail in the sections below. In Google™, the Boolean terms AND and NOT are not used in the traditional sense. Google™ will automatically link a series of words using the AND operator. Instead of NOT, to eliminate a word from the results, a space should be left after the word that is needed and a minus sign (−) should be typed immediately before the word that is to be excluded. The term OR can, however, be used in Google™ by typing OR between the words. Google™ can also be forced to link words by using a plus sign (+), especially where one of the words is a common word that might normally be ignored. The search engine can also be asked to search for a string of words in a particular order, for example 'Community-acquired pneumonia'. The user should examine search engine tools to make the most of any advanced features beyond the basic search box. Sometimes, the search engine itself may need to be changed or the basis of the search re-examined.

It is important to recognize that search engines do not necessarily index the whole of each document they retrieve. A search engine may upload each page in full, but it may only use the first few thousand characters for indexing. Therefore, should the vital information exist further down the web page, beyond where the robot will read, it will escape being indexed. Where a search engine does return a link to a site, sometimes it is not possible to access the content if the user is behind their organization's 'firewall'. This is because some organizations either block content from a list of undesirable websites or will only allow content from a list of desirable websites. Also, search engines do not locate everything on the web first-hand. It might be that a general search engine finds another site that is a more appropriate starting point, for example a health services directory. In that way, the search is narrowed automatically from a general search engine to a topic-specific one.

Some public web pages are protected from search engines through use of a file (robots.txt) that blocks access to the robot. This normally relates to personal, sensitive, interactive, timely or premium (subscription, or paid for) content. The robot is excluded from a page, the search engine does not get to index that page, and thus will not return it as a result. Another place that search engines cannot always reach is commercial data collections, or collections of valuable, copyrighted content, such as subscription-based academic journal databases and other specialized databases, information in professional directories, patents, and news articles.

Assessing the quality of information on the web

There is no restriction on what is placed on the web, by whom or from which geographical location. There is certainly no process of editorial or peer review for material placed on the web. No UK organization is currently responsible for regulating health- and medicines-related information on the Internet. Under these conditions, there is always the danger that an Internet site contains incomplete, inaccurate, irrelevant, obsolete or even hoax information. As a result, the utmost care should be taken in making use of health- and medicines-related information from the

Table 23.2 Evaluating the quality of an Internet-based website for health- and medicines-related information

Activity	Purpose
Follow internal links	To find out as much as possible about the resource. For example: the scope of the material; the intended audience and the intended coverage; the origin of the information; who owns the website and who is responsible for the content; the provenance of the website; involvement of others in the production of material; any access restrictions; frequency of updates
Analyse the URL	To find out where the information comes from and to judge if they are qualified to provide the information. For example the individual or group that has taken responsibility for the website, relevant contact details and specifically all involved in the production and dissemination of the information, including the author, webmaster or equivalent, copyright owner, publisher, sponsor
Examine the information contained	To find out the subjects and types of materials covered; comprehensiveness of coverage; notable omissions; audience and level of detail if explicitly stated; notable indicators of accuracy (e.g. potential for bias, ability to e-mail corrections); editorial or refereeing procedures; research basis to the information; 'main creation date'; the frequency and/or regularity of any updating
Consider the presentation	To find out if the resource is frequently unavailable or noticeably slow to access; any access restrictions (e.g. by geographical region, hardware/software requirements); whether there is a registration procedure and whether this is straightforward; whether the available content is free or subscription based; the copyright statement and copyright restrictions; notable design features and facilities and whether these are particularly good or bad; appropriateness of images and/or advertising; whether the site is particularly difficult or easy to use; presence or absence of user support facilities and/or help information; and particularly good or bad help information or support services
Obtain additional information	To find out if an individual or group has taken responsibility for the website; whether they are qualified to provide this information; whether the resource is well known (e.g. recommended via links), reviewed and/or heavily used
Compare to other similar websites	To find out if a resource is unique in terms of content or format and any differences between mirror and original sites for the same materials

Internet. An informed approach must include a system for evaluating the quality of the information found against the intended use of that information. No single quality indicator exists; the user must piece together a variety of indicators to assess the value of the website on its merits. Factors listed below can all affect the quality of an information source; they are not mutually exclusive and must be considered in combination. Table 23.2 provides summary guidance on evaluating the quality of a website.

Context of the website

The user must identify the scope of the website (i.e. what it aims to cover) as well as the intended audience (i.e. at whom the information is aimed). Knowledge of URL nomenclature helps to contextualize information found; the organization's name, domain and country all give discernible clues. For example, although accurate, information on a product licensed in the USA may not be applicable in the UK market.

The user should also assess the authority and reputation of the author(s) and website providing the information. Authority is based primarily on the perceived knowledge, qualifications and expertise of the author(s) as well as the reputation of the parent organization; for example, an author writing in their capacity as a lecturer at a university and a healthcare professional writing as an employee at an NHS hospital both offer acceptable credibility.

Reputation is created when others endorse the value of a website by using it. The user should consider and draw inferences from the popularity of a website. Establishing the provenance of a source can also help assess its potential quality, for example knowing when the website, including any preceding material (e.g. CD-ROM), was first established. A final consideration is how the website compares with rival material and whether it offers anything unique. This is especially important with 'mirror sites', which are essentially copies of existing websites. Mirror sites exist to enhance efficiency; for example a UK mirror site from a US-based pharmaceutical company provides a faster service to European users than the original US site. However, although mirror sites are expected to cover the same information, there may be a time lag in updating the material compared to the original website.

Content of the website

The reputation and popularity of a site, or even the expertise of an author, do not guarantee the quality of content. Here, the key questions relate to the accuracy, currency and coverage of the health- and medicines-related information found. The likely accuracy of a website is inextricably linked to its perceived authority. Users will rely on a number of markers to judge accuracy, including: whether the information has been edited or peer reviewed; the basis of the information (e.g. whether evidence based or arising from research); possible bias (e.g. ulterior motives for dissemination of the information and whether that can impact on accuracy); and the overall impression provided by a website (e.g. presence of typographical errors – see also 'Format of the website' below).

In relation to currency, it is important to find out when the information found was produced (and updated) and if the user is planning on consulting the website again, whether the frequency of updates can provide up-to-the-minute information. A final consideration is the coverage provided by material found on the website. The relevance of this factor depends very much on the user's information needs. The quality of coverage includes the comprehensiveness of a resource, links to further information, the range of topics covered and any retrospective coverage in the form of archived material.

Format of the website

As well as a marker of immediate usefulness, the format of a website is important when considering its potential use in the future, for example when deliberating whether or not to include a website in a bespoke directory. Three distinct factors can be considered here, namely accessibility, presentation and usability. In relation to accessibility, as previously indicated, some resources are simply not available to the public. However, of the 'available' websites, some require special software or hardware for accessing content; some require subscription, or at least registration; some websites contain material with copyright restrictions; and some are not written in English or are available only as an English translation. Also, overwhelming demand, server unreliability and heavy use of graphics can all impede access to an otherwise good website. These factors can all be considered when judging accessibility of a website as a marker of its quality and future usefulness.

Most probably users will also intuitively form an impression of a website based on its design and interface. This might be based on such factors as sensible use of hypertext links and other navigation aids, indexes, menus and search facilities, consistency of screen design, font sizes used, appropriateness of imagery, the level of advertising and other markers of functionality and professionalism. Usability is, of course, related to accessibility and presentation. A good website should allow the user to navigate the site and find the required information; help and support facilities, contact information, training material and user support groups also contribute to usability.

User-generated content

Recent times have seen an upsurge in what is known as user-generated content on the Internet. Whereas previously, a relatively select group of publishers and editors determined the kinds of 'content' that would be made available, nowadays anyone can create content. Users have no difficulty publishing their output if they can find a way to put it on the Internet, where it is instantly available to a global audience and where it can be found by search engines. Many kinds of user-generated content exist. A particular example is a wiki, a type of website that allows the visitors to easily add, remove, edit and change some available content, sometimes without the need for registration. An important example is Wikipedia, marketed as a free encyclopaedia. This is a vast online reference work that is written and edited by its users. For this reason, it has also been the subject of endless debate. If it can be changed at will by (literally) anyone, how can it be an authoritative reference source? Yet, because it is easily accessible and provides wide coverage, students will (sadly, erroneously) use websites such as Wikipedia in preference to good, authoritative textbooks.

The sequence of information

Information is often repackaged, re-versioned and developed for different audiences and different uses. Whether available on the Internet or elsewhere, health- and medicines-related information has by tradition been categorized on the basis of an accepted chronology of inception and development. As such, information is labelled, on an ordinal scale, as belonging to a primary, secondary or tertiary reference source depending on its position in the information supply chain. Primary reference sources are those in which new information is published, usually in the form of research, such as papers in biomedical journals. Secondary reference sources, such as academic databases, act to index and/or abstract literature from primary sources. Tertiary sources provide an overview of a topic in a condensed readable form and include textbooks, drug compendia and formularies; with authors drawing on the primary literature for material. An awareness of the chronology and origin of information can help pharmacists identify where to look for the most appropriate type of information for their particular information needs. Table 23.3 lists the advantages and disadvantages of each category of information.

Primary reference sources

The primary literature is the basis of the information hierarchy, leading to the development of secondary and tertiary literature, although with variable time lags. The term primary literature is used in essence to refer to original publications and normally entails research papers published in journals, although it can include other material such as case reports, case series, editorials and letters to journal editors. Preliminary research findings are sometimes presented at conferences in the form of poster or oral presentations. A record of these is normally published in the conference abstract book

Table 23.3 Advantages and disadvantages of primary, secondary and tertiary reference sources

Source	Advantages	Disadvantages
Primary	Contains current, original and 'cutting-edge' information	Potential for bias and not guaranteed to be without errors Interpretation and critical appraisal required by readers Time lag from publication to widespread acceptance
Secondary	Rapid access to the primary literature	Time period between article publication and inclusion in secondary sources (lag time) varies between databases (e.g. weeks to months) User needs to have access to primary sources
	Large spectrum of information on specific topics Journals covered generally of a high standard	The number of journals indexed by each system depends on the scope of the database
	Ability to link concepts to perform complex searches	Command language varies between databases
	Most resources have a facility for provision of routine updates on selected topics (selective dissemination of information)	The user needs to be familiar with a particular database's structure and terminology and to have proficient search skills in order to search effectively (training) Need for user to be proficient in sifting through the sources listed on a particular subject to find the most relevant information Not suitable for browsing Can be expensive to access relative to tertiary sources
Tertiary	Present users with a manageable digest of a vast amount of published information Easy to handle, readable, contain concise information and indexed	Out of date almost as soon as published – exceptions include electronic books with frequent updates Information in textbooks sometimes not comprehensive Poorly referenced Opinion of author

Table 23.4 Reporting guidelines for specific study designs

Initiative	Type of study	Source
CONSORT	Randomized controlled trials	http://www.consort-statement.org
STARD	Studies of diagnostic accuracy	http://www.consort-statement.org
QUOROM	Systematic reviews and meta-analyses	http://www.consort-statement.org
STROBE	Observational studies in epidemiology	http://www.strobe-statement.org
MOOSE	Meta-analyses of observational studies in epidemiology	http://www.consort-statement.org

or the conference website. Sadly, conference abstracts are the only place that some research ever materializes in an original form; this is especially so for some pharmacy practice research.

The publication of research papers

Primary research enters the public domain once the researchers write and submit their work to a primary reference source, such as a journal publication. To this end, authors aim to create accurate, clear and easily accessible reports of their studies that can be considered for publication by a journal editor. Authors are generally considered to be those who have made substantive intellectual contributions to the paper. This includes conception and design, or acquisition of data, or analysis and interpretation of data, drafting the article or revising it critically, for important intellectual content and final approval of the version to be published. Each journal is headed by an editor who is the person responsible for its entire editorial content, although some journals also have an independent editorial advisory board to help establish and maintain editorial policy.

Most health- and medicines-related research papers based on empirical methods such as observational and experimental studies follow a conventional style such as that advocated by the International Committee of Medical Journal Editors (ICMJE). The text of these papers is usually divided into sections with the headings Introduction, Methods, Results and Discussion, and sometimes Conclusion. This so-called 'IMRAD' structure is not an arbitrary publication format, but rather a direct reflection of the process of scientific discovery. Other portions of published papers include the title, abstract, keywords, acknowledgments, references, and individual tables, figures and legends. Other types of articles, such as case reports, reviews and editorials, usually

follow other formats. Specific research designs have additional reporting requirements (Table 23.4).

Abstracts and keywords merit a special note, since abstracts are the only substantive portion of articles indexed in many electronic databases and the only portion many readers read. Keywords assist indexers in cross-referencing the article. Abstracts should reflect the content of the article accurately and provide the context or background for the study, stating the study's purposes, basic procedures (selection of study participants, observational and analytical methods), main findings (giving specific effect sizes and their statistical significance, if possible) and principal conclusions. The abstract should emphasize new and important aspects of the study or observations. Some journals request that, following the abstract, authors identify 3–10 keywords or short phrases that capture the main topics of the article. The keywords may be published with the abstract. Terms from the medical subject headings (MeSH) list of Index Medicus should be used (see sections below); if suitable MeSH terms are not yet available for recently introduced terms, current terminology may be used.

Once a manuscript is received, a process known as 'peer review' is used by editors to help decide which manuscripts are suitable for their journals. Peer review also helps authors and editors in their efforts to improve the quality of reporting. Peer review is the critical assessment of manuscripts submitted to journals by experts who are not part of the editorial staff. Unbiased, independent, critical assessment is an intrinsic part of all scholarly work and peer review is considered to be an important extension of the scientific process. It can also be a time-consuming process. A peer reviewed journal is one that has submitted most of its published research articles for outside review. However, even the 'best' journals contain some material, such as letters and short reports, that have not been refereed.

The quality of health- and medicines-related journals is variable. Some journals do not adopt a peer-review process and can publish studies that are not scientifically robust. Even the process of peer review cannot be guaranteed to pick up some things such as a methodological flaw or investigator bias. Citation indexes and impact factors can be used to help assess the quality of a publication (see below). High-impact factor journals such as the *British Medical Journal*, *The Lancet*, the *New England Journal of Medicine*, *Nature* and the *Journal of the American Medical Association* are considered prestigious publications. Primary reference sources of particular relevance to pharmacy practice include the *Pharmaceutical Journal*, *International Journal of Pharmacy Practice* and the *American Journal of Health-system Pharmacy*.

Because a primary reference source presents the paper in its original form, the reader has the opportunity to critically appraise and analyse the study or article in order to develop a conclusion on its merits. However, this does necessitate a degree of critical appraisal skills and, for example, some knowledge of scientific methods and statistics.

Open access academic information

The traditional way in which research is published, as described above, can be summarized as follows: the authors write up their research into a paper and submit it to a journal, the paper is peer reviewed to ensure quality, the publisher then publishes the paper in the journal. The costs are normally paid for through the income generated by subscriptions to the journal. An alternative to this model now exists in the form of open access publishing. In the open access publishing model, the authors make the research available on the web, via a repository or in a freely accessible journal, with authors paying for this privilege and the process bypassing the publisher completely. Some journals following the 'traditional' model of publishing will also make papers available to all in an open access style provided the authors meet the costs. Understandably, academics and publishers often have differing views on whether open access publishing is a good thing or not.

Additionally, all universities in the UK are now expected to maintain an open archive of the peer-reviewed literature they have produced. Some may also use this archive to store internally produced technical reports that have not been published elsewhere (or that may be undergoing the review process or are 'in press'). Many researchers, academics and academic research groups also maintain web pages listing their publications. A good strategy for locating papers written by a particular academic author or their affiliation is to try and find their personal, departmental or research group web page. There is often a link to their publications, sometimes with full text available.

Secondary reference sources

Secondary information sources can be used to locate primary literature. In general, secondary reference sources are searchable resources that index and/or abstract from the primary literature. Some are equipped with alerting systems, which scan selected journals as soon as they are published and send summarized abstracts directly to users to help them maintain a knowledge – albeit superficial – of new developments from a large pool of journals. Nowadays, the data format used for providing users with frequently updated content is known as a web feed. A recent addition to web feeds is the RSS (really simple syndication) feed, which contains either a summary content from an associated website or the full text. RSS can be read using software called RSS reader or feed reader. The user subscribes to a feed by entering the feed's link into the reader or by clicking an RSS icon in a browser that initiates the subscription process. The reader checks the user's subscribed feeds regularly for new content, downloading any updates that it finds.

Secondary reference sources are generally searchable electronically but may also be available in hard-copy format. Secondary reference sources include commercial academic databases, resource gateways (collections of sites that have been reviewed and in some sense approved by the gateway maintainers) as well as the more recent academic search offerings of Internet search engines such as Google™ Scholar and Microsoft® Live Academic.

Academic databases

Unlike the Internet, which as discussed above is effectively an uncontrolled repository for a large assortment of material, an academic database is a well-designed catalogue created and maintained by trained personnel. A database, in essence, is a set of searchable records, with each record describing an item in an organized collection. Nowadays records are commonly maintained as a set of virtual cards in a computer database. Two main categories of academic database exist: the 'bibliographic' database contains information in summary form (the abstract) about journal articles, books and other materials; the 'full-text' database provides access to electronic versions of the full text of documents. The abstract in theory provides the most important information about the item to enable the user to make a quick and informed decision as to whether they need to look at the full text. Bibliographic databases cover a greater amount of material compared to full-text databases, thus offering a way of pinpointing hard-to-find papers from the vast amount of published literature.

The purpose of an academic database is to enable users to systematically search the records so that specific search terms can ultimately 'unearth' relevant items. In the case of a scientific paper, for example, its record might contain details of title, authors, journal name, date of publication, page numbers, subject classification, keywords, abstract and so on. Each of these categories in a database is called a 'field'. The record then is a collection of several fields of information about the item, be it a book or a journal article. The process of creating and adding records to an academic database is known as indexing and each record is called a citation.

Some journals ask for submitting authors to provide a set of keywords, usually corresponding to MeSH headings, for the purpose of indexing and classification. MeSH is the National Library of Medicine's controlled vocabulary thesaurus. It consists of sets of terms naming descriptors in a hierarchical structure that permits searching at various levels of specificity. MeSH descriptors are arranged in both an alphabetical and a hierarchical structure. At the most general level of the hierarchical structure are very broad headings such as 'Anatomy' or 'Mental Disorders'. More specific headings are found at more narrow levels of the eleven-level hierarchy, such as 'Ankle' and 'Conduct Disorder'. There were 24 767 descriptors in the 2008 MeSH. There are also over 97 000 entry terms that assist in finding the most appropriate MeSH heading; for example, 'Vitamin C' is an entry term to 'Ascorbic Acid'.

Many academic databases now exist, and although their search interfaces might at first look very different, similar tools are usually found on each. To the novice user, academic search interfaces can appear somewhat intimidating; the form looks quite complex and appears as an advanced search screen. But the format of the academic database search screen enables the user to simultaneously search for something specific (e.g. the keywords) in any of the database's fields. Sometimes each text entry box

Box 23.4

Checklist for exploring the search interface and other features of an academic database new to the user

The user should take the time to find out:

- How to combine keywords
- How to search in different fields
- How to limit searches
- How to keep track of useful citations
- How to export citations
- What format the information can be viewed in
- How the items might be retrieved
- Whether full text is available
- Whether there is a browse feature for scanning specific journals
- Whether an article's references are also available as links or in full text
- Whether there is a 'cited by' option
- How easy it is to move between articles

in the interface corresponds to a field. Sometimes the user has to use Boolean operators (see below). At times the user has to employ some complex syntax to link keywords to the required search fields. Not all the fields need be searched during a particular search exercise but combining search terms and using the fields wisely does enable the user to better pinpoint records. For example, restricting the keywords to particular fields such as the title or abstract can help focus the search by returning only those articles where the keywords are a prominent feature. A new database resource can be explored by examining helpful features that enhance efficiency (Box 23.4).

Boolean logic defines logical relationships between terms in a search. The conventional Boolean search operators are **and**, **or** and **not**. They can be used to create a very broad or very narrow search (Box 23.5). To make better use of Boolean operators, one can use *parentheses* to nest query terms within other query terms. Search terms and their operators can be enclosed in parentheses to specify the *order in which they are interpreted*. Information *within* parentheses is read *first*, followed by the information *outside* the parentheses. For example, when one enters (aspirin OR ibuprofen) AND analgesic, the search engine retrieves results containing the word aspirin or the word ibuprofen together with the word analgesic in

Box 23.5

Boolean operators that can be used when searching academic databases

And   Combines search terms so that each search result contains all of the terms. For example, pharmacy and education finds articles that contain both pharmacy and education

Or   Combines search terms so that each search result contains at least one of the terms. For example, medicine or drug finds results that contain either medicine or drug

Not   Excludes terms so that each search result does not contain any of the terms that follow it. For example, painkiller not paracetamol finds results that contain painkiller but not paracetamol

the fields searched by default. If there are nested parentheses, the search engine processes the *innermost* parenthetical expression first, then the next, and so on until the entire query has been interpreted. For example, ((aspirin OR ibuprofen) AND analgesic) OR painkiller.

Once a search is conducted and results returned, most databases offer a facility for marking and exporting useful records. Users can then decide which references are worth retrieving as full papers. Most databases traditionally classified as bibliographic will automatically help retrieve the full paper through icons such as 'Check for Full Text' and 'View Full Text'. This is because databases can link up with the other subscribed resources available to users who might be logged in as members of a library or similar information service. If a subscription is in place for a particular item, and the full text of the particular article is available within the database, a link to the full-text item will be automatically inserted into the page at the appropriate point. Thus access to the full text of the article can be virtually seamless for the user. This makes the boundaries between full-text and bibliographic resources now somewhat blurred. Full-text resources, as the name suggests, provide access to full papers. They come from individual publishers, as individual titles, or through subscription agents, who provide a single point of access to electronic journal titles from different publishers and disciplines.

Citation indexes and impact factors

As referred to above, citation indexes and impact factors can be used to help assess the quality of a publication. A citation in a paper is the formal acknowledgement of intellectual debt to previously published research. It generally contains sufficient bibliographic information to uniquely identify the cited document. An obvious example of a citation is a reference listed at the end of a scientific research paper. Commercial databases such as the Science Citation Index® (SCI) (covers 3700 journals) and the more comprehensive Journal Citation Report® (JCR) (covers more than 7500 journals) use software to track the total number of times that a journal has been cited by all journals included in the database to return 'total cites' for each journal. In addition they calculate article counts for each journal covered in the database, each article being a significant item (e.g. a research paper) published in the journal.

Citation and article counts are taken to be important indicators of how frequently current researchers are using individual journals. From such information, SCI and JCR can then return the impact factor for a journal in any specific year. The impact factor in brief is the average number of times that articles from the journal published in the preceding 2 years have been cited by others. In this way, SCI and JCR are considered to provide a systematic way of evaluating the world's leading journals and their impact in the global research community. The notion, well accepted in the scientific community, is that the higher the impact factor, the 'better' the journal. What then is the implication for journals with a low impact factor (true of a number of pharmacy publications)? Readers should note that a number of pharmacy journals, although well used in the pharmacy research community, are not included in large academic databases and thus neither indexed nor rated for their impact.

Box 23.6 lists the main health- and medicines-related databases.

Tertiary reference sources

Information from primary reference sources, perhaps retrieved using a secondary reference source, can in due course come to be included in textbooks and similar tertiary publications. As mentioned above, tertiary reference sources provide an overview of a topic in a condensed readable form with authors drawing on the primary literature for material. Examples are textbooks, drug compendia and formularies. A wide range

Box 23.6

Secondary reference sources for health- and medicines-related publications. Each database may be searchable via a number of interfaces such as CD-ROM and the Internet

BioMed Central provides full access to its portfolio of 186 'open access' journals

The Cochrane Library is part of the Cochrane Collaboration, an international not-for-profit and independent organization, dedicated to making up-to-date, accurate information about the effects of health care readily available worldwide. There is a collection of databases to search. The Cochrane Database of Systematic Reviews (CDSR) represents a high level of evidence on which to base clinical treatment decisions. In addition, there is Database of Abstracts of Reviews of Effects (DARE; other reviews); Cochrane Central Register of Controlled Trials (CENTRAL; clinical trials); Cochrane Methodology Register (CMR; methods studies); Health Technology Assessment Database (HTA; technology assessments); NHS Economic Evaluation Database (NHSEED; economic evaluations)

CrossFire is a chemical information solution, covering over 200 years of primary literature. The two databases, Beilstein (organic) and Gmelin (inorganic), collectively contain data on structures, reactions, facts and citations for more than 11 million organic, inorganic and organometallic compounds

DrugDex® provides monograph-type drug information on FDA-approved, non-US, over the counter and investigational medicines

Embase is a major biomedical and pharmacological database, produced by Elsevier Science. It indexes over 5000 biomedical journals from 70 countries. Coverage dates back to 1974 and it includes over 11 million records. There is particular emphasis on European literature and it is renowned for extensive coverage on drug research, pharmacology and pharmaceutics. The controlled vocabulary for searching (using Emtree) is distinct from that used by Medline. More than 80% of recent records include full author abstracts. The database is updated daily and the lag time between publication and database entry is generally shorter than with Medline

International Pharmaceutical Abstracts (IPA) is a comprehensive collection of pharmacy literature including information on drug use and development, pharmacy practice and education. IPA is produced by an information company called CSA and offers coverage of pharmacy literature from 1970, covering 800 health journals published worldwide. The scope of the database ranges from clinical pharmacy to legislation, sociology, economics, ethics and information processing and literature

Intute: health and life sciences is a free online service providing access to 'best' web resources for education and research, evaluated and selected by a network of subject specialists. The 31 000 resource descriptions listed are freely accessible for keyword searching or browsing

Iowa Drug Information Service (IDIS) indexing/full-text system is a bibliographic database produced by University of Iowa, USA. It is an indexing service for 200 premier English language medical and pharmaceutical journals but only those articles relating to drug therapy in humans are indexed

Medline is widely regarded as the premier database for bibliographic and abstract coverage of biomedical literature. It is created by the US National Library of Medicine (NLM®), and uses MeSH (medical subject headings) indexing with tree, tree hierarchy, subheadings and explosion capabilities to search citations from approximately 5000 current biomedical journals. Coverage dates back to 1966. Most records are from English language sources or have English abstracts. Medline is the largest component of **PubMed**, the freely accessible online database of biomedical journal citations and abstracts also created by the US. PubMed contains a number of additional services to Medline

Natural Medicines Comprehensive Database provides evidence-based, clinical information on natural medicines

Pharm-line® is a database for medicines management, pharmacy practice and prescribing produced by medicines information pharmacists at Guy's and St Thomas' Hospital, London. It started in 1978 and comprises more than 180 000 abstracts from over 100 major English language pharmaceutical and medical journals. About 11 000 new records are added each year. The abstracts are indexed using keywords from the specially developed Pharm-line Thesaurus, also used by many medicine information pharmacists to index their in-house information. All medicines information centres in the UK have access to Pharm-line and to the user guide that gives detailed search instructions

Science Direct contains over 25% of the world's science, technology and medicine full-text and bibliographic information. It offers a journal collection of over 2500 titles. In addition, the 'Backfiles' program offers the ability to search a historical archive of over 6.75 million articles from the desktop, to Volume 1, Issue 1. The collections contain 4 million articles prior to 1995, and 2.75 million articles from after 1994

TICTAC is a visual drug identification database provided by Virtual Health Network. It covers medicines, illicit drugs, veterinary products, vitamin and food supplements, herbal remedies and products that might be mistaken for drugs such as confectionery. It contains detailed information on over 23 000 tablets and capsules or related products with over 65 000 high-quality images of those products

Web of Science® consists of five databases of information gathered from scholarly journals, namely: Science Citation Index Expanded; Social Sciences Citation Index; Arts & Humanities Citation Index; Index Chemicus; and Current Chemical Reactions. *Science Citation Index Expanded* is a multidisciplinary index to the journal literature of the sciences, fully indexing over 6650 major journals across 150 scientific disciplines. It includes all cited references captured from indexed articles. In addition, the *Science Citation Index Expanded* provides access to current information and retrospective data from 1900 to the present

of tertiary reference sources covering all aspects of health- and medicines-related topics exist. Key publications include *Martindale: The Complete Drug Reference*, and the *British National Formulary* (BNF). There are also textbooks covering specific subject areas such as drug interactions, adverse drug reactions, pharmaceutical compatibility and stability, complementary medicines and drug use in specific patient populations (e.g. children, the elderly, renal impairment, pregnancy and breastfeeding). Table 23.5 lists some of the key tertiary drug information resources for practising pharmacists in the UK.

Textbooks are important for locating established knowledge or information that is not rapidly changing. The information in a tertiary source is updated against new information or knowledge documented in the primary literature only once every 3–4 years, when the book is updated and published as a new edition. Thus it can take 5 or more years for new research findings to filter into medical textbooks. In addition, most books are out of date almost as soon as they are published. Time constraints in editing and publishing mean that it takes a year or more between the author's submission of a manuscript and actual publication of the textbook.

Table 23.5 Key tertiary drug information sources for pharmacy inquiries (further details available on publishers' websites)

Type of resource	Authors/editors	Publisher
Core resource		
Martindale: The Complete Drug Reference	Sweetman S	Pharmaceutical Press; http://www.pharmpress.com
British National Formulary	Mehta DK	Jointly by British Medical Association and the Royal Pharmaceutical Society of Great Britain; http://www.bnf.org
Monthly Index of Medical Specialities	N/A	Haymarket Business Subscriptions; http://www.haymarketbusinesssubs.com/
The OTC Directory	N/A	Proprietary Association of Great Britain; http://www.pagb.co.uk/
Chemist & Druggist Directory	N/A	CMP Medica; http://www.chemistanddruggist.co.uk/
Therapeutics		
Goodman and Gilman's Pharmacological Basis of Therapeutics	Brunton L, Lazo J, Parker K	McGraw Hill; http://www.mcgraw-hill.co.uk
Avery's Drug Treatment	Speight TM, Holford NHG	Blackwell Publishing; http://www.blackwellpublishing.com/
Clinical Pharmacy and Therapeutics	Walker R, Whittlesea C	Elsevier; http://www.elsevier.com
Applied Therapeutics: The Clinical Use of Drugs	KodaKimble MA, Young LY, Kradjan WA, Guglielmo BJ	Lippincott Williams & Wilkins; http://www.lww.co.uk/
Therapeutic Drugs	Dollery C	Churchill Livingstone; http://www.elsevierhealth.com/

Continued over

Table 23.5 *(Continued)*

Clinical Medicine	Kumar PJ, Clark ML	Saunders Ltd.; http://www.elsevierhealth.com/
Oxford Textbook of Medicine (3 vols)	Warrell DA, Cox TM, Firth JD, Benz EJ, Weatherall D	Oxford University Press; http://www.oup.co.uk/
Oxford Handbook of Clinical Medicine	Longmore M, Wilkinson IB, Turmezei T, Cheung CK	Oxford University Press; http://www.oup.co.uk/
Merck Manual of Diagnosis and Treatment	Porter RS	Merck and Co.; http://www.merck.com/
Adverse drug reactions		
Meyler's Side-Effects of Drugs: The International Encyclopaedia of Adverse Drug Reactions and Interactions	Aronson JK, Dukes MNG	Elsevier; http://www.elsevier.com
Meyler's Side Effects of Drugs Annuals	Aronson JK	Elsevier; http://www.elsevier.com
Adverse Drug Reactions	Lee A	Pharmaceutical Press; http://www.pharmpress.com
Children's doses		
British National Formulary for Children	Mehta DK	British Medical Association, Royal Pharmaceutical Society of Great Britain, Royal College of Paediatrics and Child Health; http://www.bnfc.org/
Neonatal Formulary: Drug Use in Pregnancy & the First Year of Life	Northern Neonatal Network (Ed)	Blackwell Publishing; http://www.blackwellpublishing.com/
Paediatric Formulary	Guy's, St Thomas' and Lewisham Hospitals	Guy's, St Thomas' and Lewisham Hospitals
Complementary therapies		
Herbal Medicines	Barnes J, Anderson LA, Phillipson JD	Pharmaceutical Press; http://www.pharmpress.com
Homeopathic Pharmacy: Theory and Practice	Kayne SB	Churchill Livingstone; http://www.elsevierhealth.com/
Dietary Supplements	Mason P	Pharmaceutical Press; http://www.pharmpress.com
Contraception		
Contraception: Your Questions Answered	Guillebaud J	Churchill Livingstone; http://www.elsevierhealth.com/
The Pill and Other Forms of Hormonal Contraception: The Facts	Guillebaud J	Oxford University Press; http://www.oup.co.uk/
Cytotoxics		
Cytotoxics Handbook	Allwood M, Stanley A, Wright P	Radcliffe Medical press; http://www.radcliffe-oxford.com/
Cancer Principles & Practice Of Oncology	DeVita VT, Hellman S, Rosenberg SA	Lippincott Williams & Wilkins; http://www.lww.co.uk/
Diagnostic tests		
Special Tests: The Procedure and Meaning of Some of the Commoner Tests in Hospital	Evans D	Elsevier; http://www.elsevier.com

Interpretation of Diagnostic Tests	Wallach JB	Lippincott Williams & Wilkins; http://www.lww.co.uk/
Oxford Handbook of Clinical and Laboratory Investigation	Provan D	Oxford University Press; http://www.oup.com/uk

Dictionaries

Medical Abbreviations and Eponyms	Sloane SB	Elsevier; http://www.elsevier.com
Stedman's Concise Medical Dictionary	Stedman T	Lippincott Williams & Wilkins; http://www.lww.co.uk/

Drug abuse

Drugs of Abuse	Wills S	Pharmaceutical Press; http://www.pharmpress.com

Drug administration

Handbook of Drug Administration via Enteral Feeding Tubes	White R, Bradnam V	Pharmaceutical Press; http://www.pharmpress.com
Administering Medicines through Enteral Feeding Tubes	Royal Hospitals, Belfast	Royal Hospitals, Belfast
NEWT Guidelines for Administration of Medicines to Patients with Enteral Feeding Tubes or Swallowing Difficulties	Wrexham Maelor Hospital	North East Wales NHS Trust
Handbook on Injectable Drugs	Trissel LA	American Society of Health-System Pharmacists; http://www.ashp.org
The Syringe Driver: Continuous Subcutaneous Infusions in Palliative Care	Dickman A, Schneider J, Varga J	Oxford University Press; http://www.oup.com/uk

Drug interactions

Stockley's Drug Interactions	Baxter K	Pharmaceutical Press; http://www.pharmpress.com
Drug Interactions, Analysis and Management	Hansten PD, Horn JR	Facts and Comparisons; http://www.factsandcomparisons.com

Evidence-based medicines

Clinical Evidence	Young C	BMJ Publishing Group; http://www.bmj.com/
Evidence Based Medicine	Straus SE, Richardson WS, Glasziou P, Haynes RB	Churchill Livingstone; http://www.elsevierhealth.com/

Legal and ethical

Dale and Applebe's Pharmacy Law & Ethics	Applebe GE, Wingfield J	Pharmaceutical Press; http://www.pharmpress.com
Medicines, Ethics and Practice – A Guide for Pharmacists	Royal Pharmaceutical Society of Great Britain	Royal Pharmaceutical Society of Great Britain; http://www.rpsgb.org.uk

Palliative care

A Guide to Symptom Relief in Palliative Care	Regnard C, Hockley J	Radcliffe Medical Press; http://www.radcliffe-oxford.com/
Palliative Care Formulary	Twycross R, Wilcock A, Charlesworth S, Dickman A	Radcliffe Medical Press; http://www.radcliffe-oxford.com/

Continued over

Table 23.5 *(Continued)*

Pharmacokinetics		
Basic Clinical Pharmacokinetics	Winter ME	Lippincott Williams & Wilkins; http://www.lww.co.uk/
Pregnancy and lactation		
Drugs in Pregnancy and Lactation	Briggs GG, Freeman RK, Yaffe SJ	Lippincott Williams & Wilkins; http://www.lww.co.uk/
Medication and Mothers' Milk	Hale T	Hale Publishing
Handbook of Obstetric Medicine	Nelson-Piercy C	Taylor & Francis Ltd; http://www.taylorandfrancis.co.uk/
Drugs During Pregnancy and Lactation	Schaefer C, Peters PWJ, Miller RK	Elsevier; http://www.elsevier.com
Prescribing in Pregnancy	Rubin P, Ramsay M	Blackwell Publishing; http://www.blackwellpublishing.com/
Therapeutics in Pregnancy and Lactation	Lee A, Inch S, Finnigan D	Radcliffe Medical Press; http://www.radcliffe-oxford.com/
Psychiatry		
Psychotropic Drug Directory	Bazire S	Healthcomm UK Ltd; http://healthcomm-uk.com/
Maudsley Prescribing Guidelines	Taylor D, Paton C, Kerwin R	Taylor & Francis Ltd; http://www.taylorandfrancis.co.uk/
Case Studies in Psychopharmacology	Taylor D, Paton C	Taylor & Francis Ltd; http://www.taylorandfrancis.co.uk/
Renal impairment		
Drug Prescribing in Renal Failure: Dosing Guidelines for Adults	Brier ME, Aronoff GR	American College of Physicians; http://www.acponline.org/
The Renal Drug Handbook	Ashley C, Currie A	Radcliffe Medical Press; http://www.radcliffe-oxford.com/
Surgery		
Oxford Handbook of Clinical Surgery	McLatchie G, Borley N, Chikwe J	Oxford University Press; http://www.oup.com/uk
Wound management		
Formulary of Wound Management Products	Morgan D	Euromed Communications; http://www.euromed.uk.com/

Because the knowledge base in many areas of therapeutics is rapidly changing, the information contained in textbooks may be too old to be useful. This problem does not apply, however, to those textbooks available in electronic full text as these can be more regularly updated, usually every few months. Another important exception is the BNF, which is updated and published as a new edition every 6 months.

Tertiary references should be the first port of call when trying to find background information on a subject. With the advent of the electronic age, it is easy to forget that information can be found quickly and easily in the humble book. Books are easy to handle, readable, contain concise information and are indexed.

Having said that, the reader must also be aware that the information presented in a textbook is subject to the opinion, evaluation and bias of the author. It is often assumed that what is written in a textbook must be accurate; in fact, the author(s) may not have comprehensively searched, analysed or interpreted all information. The information contained in textbooks may also not be as comprehensive as the reader would like. This may be due to factors such as restriction on chapter length or the degree of emphasis that the author has placed on each topic. Because they cover topics very broadly, textbooks are often poorly referenced, indicating only the most significant papers to support or refute a stated case. A reluctance to use textbooks is especially evident in the newer generation of pharmacy students used to the immediacy of information on the Internet. But especially in comparison to user-generated websites such as Wikipedia, good textbooks are an important and reliable resource and they should not be overlooked.

Organizing and citing references

For academic work, it is often necessary to store a relatively large number of retrieved citations. It is always advisable to implement some system for keeping track of the information amassed. A number of bibliography management systems exist for this purpose. Examples include RefWorks, EndNote®, Reference Manager® and ProCite®. These products help users create personal databases. They enable users to import, organize, manage and export citations, to create reference lists and bibliographies for written academic work such as projects, reports and papers.

A number of referencing styles exist for citing retrieved information. Most academic institutions and publications have standardized requirements. Some of the more widely used citation styles are listed in Box 23.7. Whatever style is used, accuracy, clarity and consistency are the key factors when citing information sources. Guidelines for citing electronic sources are not yet fully standardized because these sources, which include the Internet, are constantly changing

 Box 23.7

Common citation styles

- American Medical Association (AMA) style
- American Psychological Association (APA) style
- Chicago: author-date style
- Chicago: humanities style
- Harvard style
- Modern Language Association (MLA) style
- Vancouver/ICMJE style

Box 23.8

Some general formats for references including punctuation

Journals

Donyai P, O'Grady K, Jacklin A, Barber N, Franklin BD. The effects of electronic prescribing on the quality of prescribing. Br J Clin Pharmacol. 2008 Feb; 65(2):230–37.

Books

Rees J, Smith I, Smith B. Introduction to pharmaceutical calculations. 2nd ed. London: Pharmaceutical Press; 2005. p 240

Dissertations and theses

Pannala Venkata AS. Peroxynitrite induced oxidative modification of low density lipoprotein [dissertation]. London University of London; 1998. p 250

Papers and poster sessions presented at meetings

Van den Berg M, Donyai P. How is the language of medicines use review leaflets symbolizing the service? Paper presented at: 13th Health Service Research and Pharmacy Practice Conference; 2007 April 2–3; Keele, UK.

Journals on the Internet

Wright JR, Kowaleski B, Sussman J. What constitutes a clinical trial: a survey of oncology professionals. Trials [internet]. 2008 March 3 [cited 2008 March 14];9 (12). Available from http://www.trialsjournal.com/content/9/1/12

Websites

PJOnline [Internet]. London: The Pharmaceutical Journal; c1999–2008 [cited 2008 March 14]. Available from: http://www.pjonline.com/

and citation formats have to adapt to these changes. See Box 23.8 for some general reference formats. Most biomedical journals now follow the Vancouver/ICMJE referencing style. Readers are directed to the website of the International Committee of Medical Journal Editors for more detailed guidance (http://www.icmje.org/).

Avoiding plagiarism

As discussed, a citation is the formal acknowledgement of intellectual debt to previously published research. Therefore, referencing is a way of ensuring that due credit is given to other people's work. It is sometimes easy to copy and paste from journal articles and web pages into one's own work. While common knowledge does not need a citation or reference, taking someone's work and not indicating where it came from is termed plagiarism and is regarded as an infringement of copyright. To attempt to pass off such work as one's own is considered cheating. This is not appreciated in any field of work. Plagiarism is considered a serious matter and higher education institutions invest in plagiarism detection software to scan assessment material.

Information services

Pharmacists are expected to be able to provide accurate, reliable, impartial, relevant and up-to-date information on a wide range of issues. Sometimes pharmacists themselves need help with answering health- and medicines-related queries. A number of organizations exist to help. Unlike libraries which normally provide information in an unprocessed manner, pharmacy information services can provide tailor-made answers to specific enquiries using analysis and interpretation. In the UK, the best known facility is the Medicines Information service based in NHS pharmacies.

Most information services will work to standardized procedures to ensure quality in enquiry answering. Pharmacists working in any sector of the profession should follow similar methods. The same basic information should be collected from the enquirer, to include: the enquiry, the name and contact details of the enquirer, the urgency of the enquiry, the purpose and sources already used. Ideally the full manner in which enquiries are handled should be documented to provide an audit trail for quality assurance purposes. Clear and comprehensive documentation is necessary for legal and ethical reasons, in order to ascertain exactly what information was provided, by whom and what resources were used. Appropriate documentation also ensures that an enquiry can be located at a later date, to save time in dealing with future enquiries. See Box 23.9 for the type of information that needs to be documented in relation to each enquiry.

Medicines information services

The NHS Medicines Information service is provided by a network of 250 local Medicines Information centres based in the pharmacy departments of most

Box 23.9

Headings for documenting medicines information enquiries

- Full name and contact details of enquirer
- The date and time the enquiry was received
- Full identity of the person receiving the enquiry
- Mutually realistic agreed timescale for provision of answer
- Enquirer's preference for method of reply
- Clear account of the enquiry describing the question and the background information in sufficient detail to allow a third party to tackle the enquiry without further contact with the enquirer
- All relevant background information for patient-specific enquiries to include patient age, sex, weight; medication (including dose and duration of therapy); diagnosis, relevant medical history; liver and renal function; history of adverse drug reactions; whether pregnant or breastfeeding
- Annotation of enquiry at various stages with the date and signature, e.g. annotate the search with the date and identity of the researcher
- The search itself in the order the resources have been searched with clear identification of resources
- Evaluation of the information, consideration of practicality of advice and detail of answer
- Consideration of method of communication
- Summary of answer given (including further points discussed)
- Completion date and/or time
- Full name of person who handled the enquiry
- All other relevant information
- Descriptive title for the enquiry
- Relevant keywords

hospital trusts as well as 14 regional centres and two national centres (Northern Ireland and Wales). The aim of Medicines Information is to support the safe, effective and efficient use of medicines through the provision of evidence-based information and advice on therapeutic use of medicines. The centres are staffed by pharmacists and technicians with clinical expertise, and particular skills in locating, assessing and interpreting information about medicines. Local and regional medicines information centres provide an enquiry answering service, to patient and healthcare professional enquirers, on all aspects of drug therapy. Over half a million enquiries are handled by the service each year.

In addition, the UK Medicines Information (UKMi) network produces a range of resources available through its own Internet site (www.ukmi.nhs.uk) or that of the National electronic Library of Medicines (NeLM) (http://www.nelm.nhs.uk/en/). They include the UKMi new medicines portfolio which comprises early horizon scanning information on drugs in clinical development through to evaluations of medicines once marketed. Via NeLM, UKMi also provides a comprehensive daily news service that includes in-depth assessments of key published clinical studies (known as In-Focus). The news service generates RSS feeds for a number of specialist libraries hosted by the National Library for Health. In addition, a number of UKMi specialist advisory services make their material available through NeLM, for example the drugs in lactation database. UKMi also produces 'Pharm-Line', a bibliographic database focusing on medicines management, prescribing and pharmacy practice (subscription based).

Royal Pharmaceutical Society of Great Britain information centre

There is an information centre based at the Royal Pharmaceutical Society headquarters in London comprising the Library and Technical Information Service. The information pharmacists in the Technical Information Service can help answer scientific and technical questions relating to pharmacy practice or continuing education from members of any branch of pharmacy. The subject scope includes advice on the usage and availability of proprietary and other medicinal products, adverse drug reactions and interactions, and the identification of medicines from overseas. The Royal Pharmaceutical Society Library in Edinburgh specializes in pharmaceutics and quality control. The pharmaceutics information service is provided by the society's fellow in pharmaceutics. It is a problem-solving and advisory service on matters that relate to pharmaceutics, pharmaceutical technology and the practical aspects of pharmacy. Areas of expertise include the application of physical, chemical and biological sciences to the formulation, design, stability, preparation and presentation of dosage forms. Enquiries about pharmaceutical packaging, especially child-resistant packaging, are also handled.

National Pharmacy Association information services

The National Pharmacy Association (NPA) has an information service for members only. The department is a complete reference centre, skilled at assisting members with a wide range of pharmacy practice-related questions such as drug information, NHS matters and law and ethics. It also publishes leaflets and resources on practice and legal issues, and community pharmacy-focused news updates. In addition, the NPA information department includes a specialist library of British and foreign reference books and a range of technical CD-ROMs. Further details can be found at http://www.npa.co.uk.

The pharmaceutical industry medical information departments

All pharmaceutical companies are able to provide certain types of information on their products. This source of information can be particularly important for new products, when there is often a lack of published information.

Conclusion

The ability to retrieve relevant health- and medicines-related information in a timely and efficient manner is central to the practice of all pharmacy professionals. The advent of the electronic age and the expanse of available information can make information retrieval appear a daunting task. However, categorizing information, developing an understanding of search and retrieval processes, knowing who to approach for help as well as groundwork and deliberation can all help facilitate the process. Of course, practice makes perfect and it is only through the practical application of the advice given in this chapter that the art of information retrieval can be truly accomplished.

KEY POINTS

- As part of their work, pharmacists handle a large amount of information. In order to do so efficiently they must know how to find and evaluate information sources

- While the Internet gives access to a vast resource, but of variable reliability, printed books still play an important role
- A web address (URL) gives useful information about the likely validity of the site content
- Pharmacists need to develop some form of bookmarking for sites relevant to their area of work
- Commercial search engines give access to web pages, but to use them effectively it is necessary to understand their operators; this often involves Boolean logic or something similar
- No search engine will give access to all relevant websites
- There is no control over material placed on the web, so its reliability must be evaluated by the user, for which guidance is available including authority, reputation, currency, peer review, etc.
- User-generated websites, such as Wikipedia, are less reliable
- Information sources are classified as primary, secondary or tertiary
- Primary reference sources are original research publications which normally follow a conventional layout style – called IMRAD – together with other useful information including an abstract and keywords

- There are many full-text journals available online
- The quality of journals is reflected in their impact factor
- Secondary sources are searchable indices or abstracts which lead to primary sources
- Keywords are often used for searching, especially in academic databases
- Tertiary sources present an overview of a topic and include textbooks, compendia and formularies, providing access to other sources
- Textbooks are quick and easy to use, but are inevitably out of date and may be subject to bias or be incomplete
- Bibliographies are created using recognized citation styles and are often stored using special software
- NHS information services are based, mainly, in hospital pharmacies in the UK. They use standardized procedures to ensure quality and efficiency in answering queries
- The UK Medicines Information (UKMi) network produces resources which are available through its website and the NeLM, including horizon scanning, medicines evaluations and specialized databases

Section Four

Dispensing and Related Pharmaceutical Practice Activities

The prescription

Ian Smith

STUDY POINTS

- The information required on a prescription
- The different types of prescriptions presented at a pharmacy
- The routine procedure for checking and dispensing prescriptions
- Information sources required for prescription dispensing

Introduction

The access to medicines by the general public varies dependent on the laws of each country. In the UK, the Medicines Act 1968 classifies medicines into three categories, namely:

- General sales list (GSL)
- Pharmacy medicine (P)
- Prescription only medicine (POM).

GSL medicines are available for sale to the public through many retail outlets. These medicines are for the treatment of minor ailments or conditions and have a history of being safe and effective for patients when they self-medicate with these products. P medicines are available only from pharmacies and are sold under the supervision of a pharmacist. Some P medicines are those that have recently been 'deregulated' from the POM classification. Other P medicines are restricted in their supply to the public due to the nature of the condition they are intended to treat or because they have a greater tendency to be misused or abused compared to GSL medicines. POM medicines are normally

supplied to a patient after they have received a prescription from an authorized prescriber. In the past the authorized prescribers were doctors, dentists and veterinary surgeons but recently more professions have been authorized to write prescriptions, including nurses and pharmacists (see Chs 2, 14).

A prescription is a paper or electronic document detailing the medicine or medicines to be dispensed for an individually named patient and issued by an authorized prescriber. The medicine can be any of the above three legal categories. A prescription item is one named medicine on a prescription, e.g. aspirin tablets. A prescription may contain more than one prescription item, e.g. aqueous cream, pholcodine linctus and aspirin tablets (three prescription items), in which case the prescription may be referred to as a multiple item prescription. In addition to medicines, a prescription may contain other items or appliances required by the patient for their treatment, e.g. wound dressings, elastic hosiery, blood glucose monitoring equipment, needles and syringes, nutritionally complete feeds and gluten-free foods.

In the UK, a state-funded National Health Service (NHS) and a private system of health care run alongside each other. Prescriptions can be provided to patients by prescribers in both systems. In the NHS system, not all medicines or appliances available can be prescribed. Limiting the access to medicines and appliances has been used as a method to reduce the cost to the government of providing the NHS (see Ch. 6).

POM medicines can, under certain criteria, be supplied without a prescription to the public by way of an emergency supply or through a patient group direction (PGD). PGDs are used for the supply of POM and P medicines by designated healthcare professionals to individual patients, subject to any exclusion stated in the PGD. PGDs are written directions signed by a doctor or dentist and by a pharmacist relating to the supply and administration, or administration only, of certain POM and P medicines. The particulars to be included in a PGD are detailed in Box 24.1. Records of supply to individual patients are required as part of the PGD process (see Ch. 16). PGDs have been used in pharmacy for the supply of a number of different types of medication such as emergency hormonal contraception, nicotine replacement therapy and head lice treatments.

Although at present the majority of prescriptions are produced on paper, there will in future be a continued move towards electronic prescriptions in both the community and in hospitals. Electronic prescriptions have the same legal force as prescriptions signed in writing. The benefits of electronic prescriptions include patient convenience, easier ordering of repeat prescriptions and more complete information about prescribing. The production of electronic prescriptions might in the future mean an end to incomplete and illegible prescriptions. Although electronic prescriptions will become the norm in the NHS, private prescriptions will, for the foreseeable future, remain as paper documents. This chapter will concentrate on paper prescriptions in use at the time of writing. The information contained on both paper and electronic prescriptions and the method of dispensing and recording is essentially the same.

Information required on a prescription

When producing a prescription, the prescriber is giving information and instructions to the person who will supply the medicine to the patient. A prescription is in effect three types of document in one, in that it is a clinical document, a legal document and an invoice. Law may require some of the information on the prescription and some of the information is required to ensure the patient receives the correct medicine. The dispenser will also have to take payment for the medicine from the patient or send the prescription to the appropriate body for them to pay, hence it is also an invoice.

The information and instructions that are required as a minimum are detailed below.

Box 24.1

Particulars to be included on a patient group direction

- Time period the PGD is in force
- Class of medicine
- Restriction on quantity to be supplied
- Clinical situation
- Clinical criteria
- Class of persons excluded
- Circumstances when advice from a doctor is required
- Pharmaceutical form
- Strength or maximum strength
- Applicable or maximum dosage
- Route of administration
- Frequency of administration
- Minimum or maximum period of administration
- Relevant warnings
- Details of follow-up action
- Arrangements for referral for medical advice
- Records to be kept

Name and address of the prescriber

This identifies who the prescriber is and informs the pharmacist where to contact the prescriber should there be an issue related to the prescription. A telephone number on the prescription is helpful, but if the pharmacist suspects the prescription is a forgery this number should not be used as there have been cases where the telephone number has been changed so the pharmacist has contacted someone who has then pretended to be the prescriber.

Date of the prescription

This identifies when the prescription was written. The law usually defines the length of time from being written that a prescription remains valid. In the UK, all NHS prescriptions should be dispensed within 6 months of the date on the prescription except for certain types of controlled drugs where the requirement is they are dispensed within 28 days.

Name of the medicine (with strength and dosage form, if relevant)

Dose and dosage regimen

Directions should be as specific as possible. Ideally, the amount to be used and the number of times a day that it should be taken should be stated. Vague directions – in particular 'Take as directed' – are of little value to the patient and should be avoided. It such situations the pharmacist will have to ensure that the patient is clear about how to use or take their medication.

Total amount to be dispensed or length of treatment time

This can be stated in a number of ways as detailed below.

Directions for use

The directions for use will include the dose and dosage regimen but the prescriber may include additional information about the product. This can include how to use (e.g. spread thinly, dissolve in water), where to use (e.g. in the eye, in the ear, on the scalp), why they are using it (e.g. for pain, for sleeping). The prescriber may also indicate a maximum amount that should be taken, particularly if the medicine is dosed on a 'when required' basis.

Name and address of the patient

This identifies the patient who is to receive the medicine. The age of the patient would also be useful to enable the pharmacist to check the dose of the medicine, particularly if the person is very young or very old.

Prescriber's signature

This is usually a legal requirement of prescriptions.

The above details are not totally inclusive, depending on the prescription type and the legal requirements of the country.

It is important that the person dispensing the product is aware of the information they require and is able to take the appropriate action to clarify and complete any missing or ambiguous information.

A number of specific terms, for example 'dose', 'dosage regimen', etc. are used in the above list and are often confused. These terms are explained below and Example 24.1 demonstrates the terms using an extract from a prescription.

Example 24.1

Examine the following details which have been abstracted from a prescription:

Brufen® tablets 200 mg
Two tablets to be taken three times a day
Send 84 tablets

Using the above prescription as an example, the dosage form, strength, dose, dosage regimen, total daily dose, total amount, proprietary name, generic name and length of treatment are:

Term	Example
Dosage form	Tablets
Strength	200 mg
Dose	400 mg (2 tablets of 200 mg)
Dosage regimen	400 mg three times a day
Total daily dose	1200 mg
Total amount	84 tablets
Proprietary name	Brufen®
Generic name	Ibuprofen
Length of treatment	14 days

Dosage form

The term dosage form refers to the type of formulated product. Examples of different forms would be tablets, capsules, creams, ointments, ear/eye/nasal drops, aerosols, suppositories, vaginal pessaries and creams, mixtures, linctuses and patches and these are discussed in the following chapters. Each dosage form may also be presented in a number of specialist forms. For example, tablets are available as modified-release, enteric-coated, dispersible, buccal, soluble, and chewable. The dosage form should be stated on the prescription if there is more than one form available. For example, glyceryl trinitrate is available as tablets, modified-release tablets, a pump spray, an aerosol spray, an injection, ointment and patches. The prescriber will need to state the precise form to ensure that the required product is supplied.

Strength

Strength refers to the amount of drug in the dosage form or a unit of the dosage form (e.g. a capsule, a tablet, a patch). The strength of a dosage form can be expressed in a number of ways. For example, the strength of oral liquids is usually expressed as the amount of drug per usual dose volume (e.g. ampicillin suspension is available as 125 mg/5 mL and

500 mg/5 mL) or the strength may be expressed in units (e.g. nystatin suspension is available as 100 000 units/mL). External liquids, topical preparations and injections are usually expressed as an amount per millilitre or gram (e.g. naloxone hydrochloride injection 400 micrograms/mL, nystatin cream 100 000 units/g, terbutaline sulphate nebulizer solution 2.5 mg/mL) or as a percentage (e.g. chloramphenicol eye drops 0.5%, ketoconazole cream 2%, benzyl benzoate application 25%, lidocaine injection 0.5%). Single-dose unit forms, e.g. tablets or suppositories, are usually expressed as the amount of drug in one dose unit, e.g. diclofenac sodium suppositories are available in 12.5 mg, 25 mg, 50 mg and 100 mg strengths.

Dose

This is the amount of drug taken at any one time. This can be expressed as the weight of drug (e.g. 500 mg) or volume of drug solution (e.g. 5 mL, 2 drops) or as the number of dose unit forms (2 capsules, half a tablet, 1 sachet, 1 patch) or some other quantity (2 puffs, 1–2 inches of ointment).

Dosage regimen

Dosage regimen refers to the frequency of administration or the number of times the dose is to be taken in a period of time. Examples include: 5 mL twice a day; use the cream night and morning; 1 injection every 4 weeks; 3 tablets three times a week.

Total daily dose

The total daily dose can be calculated from the dose and the number of times per day that the dose is taken. Some maximum doses of drugs are expressed in terms of per day rather than each separate dose (e.g. the total daily dose for paracetamol by mouth in the *British National Formulary* (BNF) is 4 grams).

Total amount to be supplied

This refers to the total amount of the medicine to be supplied to the patient. This can be expressed as a number of units (e.g. 21 tablets, 12 suppositories), as a volume (e.g. 100 mL of mixture, 5 mL of eye drops) or as a weight (e.g. 30 g of cream) or as a single pack size or multiple thereof (e.g. 1 tube of ointment, 2 inhalers). It may mean that the person dispensing the prescription may have to calculate the total amount if the prescriber states a dosage regimen for the preparation and a number of days of treatment (e.g. one to be taken three times a day for 28 days).

Generic name

The generic name is also known as the approved name. All drugs are given an approved name which is usually related to their chemical structure and the medical classification of the drug. This name is adopted by the World Health Organization and is known as the recommended international non-proprietary name (rINN). In the UK these names are usually co-opted as a British approved name (BAN). European law (92/27/EEC) requires that only the rINN be used and as a result some BAN names have been modified to the rINN (e.g. frusemide has changed to furosemide). Prescribers in the UK are encouraged to use generic names for cost-saving reasons as generic products are usually less expensive than the equivalent proprietary product (see below) and hence the generic name is the most commonly used name on prescriptions. If the prescription is written by the generic name, in the UK, any equivalent product can be supplied even if it also has a proprietary name. The person who dispensed the prescription may lose money if they supply a more expensive proprietary product when the prescription is written generically.

Proprietary name

This can also be referred to as the brand name, manufacturer's name or trade name. The company that first produces and markets a drug will give it a proprietary name. The company will apply for a trademark in respect of the proprietary name. The granting of a trademark means that no other company can use that name. Usually proprietary names are short, distinct and easy to remember and write. They may reflect the name of the company or the condition the medication is being used to treat or the type of medication. After expiry of the patent (in the UK, 20 years from first date of discovery or, under a certificate of supplementary protection, 15 years from the date of first marketing) the drug may be produced by other companies using the approved (or generic) name. Drugs may be prescribed by their proprietary name. If the prescriber, in the UK, states the proprietary name or the manufacturer of the product, this product or the product manufactured by the stated manufacturer must be supplied.

Length of treatment

The length of treatment may be stated on the prescription (e.g. use for 1 week) or it may be possible to calculate the length of time from the amount prescribed and the dosage regimen (e.g. 21 capsules to be taken 'one three times a day' will be sufficient for 7 days' treatment).

Types of prescription forms

As stated previously, in the UK there are two providers of health care: the private sector and the NHS. Concomitantly there are two categories of prescriptions, namely private prescriptions and NHS prescriptions. Additionally, prescriptions may be provided in both the primary care sector (e.g. community) and the secondary care sector (e.g. hospitals). The format of prescriptions in these two sectors will be different.

Private prescription forms

Private prescriptions do not have a standard format and can, in fact, be a piece of paper containing all the required information. Normally some of the information, such as the name, the address and qualifications of the prescriber, are pre-printed on the paper. The symbol ℞ is often used on private prescription forms to indicate that the form is a prescription. Changes in the law relating to controlled drugs in the UK have led to the production of a standard form for private prescriptions for controlled drugs for human use. All veterinary prescriptions are private prescription.

NHS prescription forms

NHS prescriptions should only be issued to NHS patients. There are a number of different types of NHS prescription forms available in the UK that may be dispensed at any community pharmacy. Each type of prescription form is given a different number and colour and might have a different format depending on where in the UK they originate from and the type of prescriber who generated the prescription.

Hospital prescription forms

There is no standard form for hospital prescribing for patients staying in hospital, and the actual format and design will depend on the individual hospital trust. However, the forms usually contain much of the same information. They usually have space for the prescription details, as well as space for confirmation of the administration of the medicine by nursing or other staff. For convenience, most hospital forms are divided into three separate areas, namely medicines to be administered on a regular basis, medicines to be administered once only and medicines to be administered on an 'as required' basis. Some forms may also have an area for listed medicines that can be administered by nursing staff at their discretion. Such medicines may be simple analgesics, sore throat lozenges, laxatives, etc. In addition all hospital prescription forms will require space for identification of the patient and will also have room for important details about the patient such as if they are allergic to any medicines.

Routine procedure for dispensing prescriptions

The dispensing of prescriptions requires a logical and very thorough approach in order to ensure the patient gets the right product in the right form, at the right dose with the right advice. It is imperative that the pharmacist conducts a thorough check of the prescription to ensure that it is complete and clinically acceptable. The product should then be assembled and labelled in a manner that ensures the product and all the information is accurate and that it is professional in its appearance. All stages involved in the dispensing process should be covered by a standard operating procedure.

The stages involved in dispensing a prescription are:

- Receiving the prescription
- Clinical and legal checking of the prescription
- Assembly of the product and labelling
- Accuracy checking the product against the prescription
- Delivery of the product to the patient with the appropriate advice about the product.

Receiving the prescription

It is important at this stage that the person receiving the prescription has checked the patient details so that:

- The appropriateness of the prescription for that patient can be assessed
- Any required records can be completed correctly

- The product can be labelled for that patient (see Ch. 28)
- If necessary the prescription can be delivered to the correct patient at the correct address
- The patient can be contacted, if necessary, even after the medicine has been dispensed and supplied to the patient.

The full name of the patient should be ascertained to ensure that the medicines reach the person for whom they are intended. The information should also include the sex of the patient, if it is not given elsewhere on the prescription. The sex of the patient may be necessary in the assessment of the appropriateness of the medicine for the patient (see Example 24.2).

The full address of the patient is also checked and completed if required. It may be possible that two patients have the same name and so the address will identify the patient. If two patients have the same address and name, then it is helpful if the age or date of birth of the patient is stated. The age of the patient if they are under 12 years old is a legal requirement on prescriptions in the UK. Since the advent of computer-generated prescriptions and with electronic prescriptions, the date of birth of the patient is being supplied on most prescriptions. On private prescriptions, the age of very young children may be expressed as a fraction. If the age is expressed in days, weeks or months, then the denominator is 7, 52 and 12, respectively. For example, an age of 3 days may be abbreviated to 3/7, an age of 3 weeks may be abbreviated to 3/52 and an age of 3 months to 3/12.

As well as checking patient details, the person taking the prescription in should also be able to check if the product is available in the pharmacy or whether it needs to be ordered and, if so, how long it will take to arrive. This information is useful in advising the person collecting the prescription how long it will take before it is ready for collection.

The person taking in the prescription may also have to take payment for the prescription. They should understand how to calculate the cost of the prescription and may be required to understand the rules about who pays for their prescriptions and what checks may be required to ensure the patient is making a legitimate declaration of exemption.

Clinical and legal checking of the prescription

This is an essential role of the pharmacist to ensure that the prescription is legally complete and clinically correct for the patient. The pharmacist should check that all the information required to select and dispense the right product is available on the prescription. Any information which is missing or ambiguous will require the pharmacist to take some action before the prescription can go to the next stage in the dispensing process. If information is not present the pharmacist should ascertain this information and the prescription might have to be sent back to the prescriber for the prescription to be completed or altered. In the UK, if it is not possible to get the prescription back to the prescriber or the prescriber cannot be contacted, the pharmacist can add information relating to the dose, strength and quantity to be

---

Example 24.2

Examine the following details found on a prescription:

Mrs Joyce Hind
2 High Street
Mediton
Hytrin tablets starter pack
To be taken as directed
Send 1 pack

Hytrin is the proprietary name for terazosin, an alpha-adrenoceptor blocking drug which is used for the treatment of urinary retention in benign prostatic hyperplasia and for the treatment of mild to moderate hypertension. It is available as two starter packs with different numbers of different strength tablets in them. In the above prescription the patient is female and the drug is most likely to be prescribed for the treatment of hypertension. Thus an indication of the sex of the patient is useful to the pharmacist in this case, since it would indicate that the patient should receive the starter pack for hypertension. However, it would still be important to check with the prescriber that this is the case.

supplied using the endorsements 'prescriber contacted' and 'prescriber not contacted' as outlined in the BNF.

The pharmacist should also check that the prescription is appropriate for the patient and that it will be of benefit and not cause the patient harm. A number of court cases have identified that the pharmacist has a responsibility for what they have supplied under the directions of the prescriber. Therefore, in addition to ensuring the prescription is legal and complete, the pharmacist should be checking the clinical elements of the prescribing and contacting the prescriber to discuss any issues they have identified.

One suggested way to do this review is by using the mnemonic IDEAL CASE, as follows:

I – nteractions

D – ose

E – vidence of harm/benefit

A – ppropriate (and here is where we make a CASE for the medication)

L – egal and complete

C – ost-effective

A – cceptable to the patient

S – afe

E – ffective

Interactions

Does the drug interact with any other items the patient is taking or with the patient's condition? Many of the programmes which are used to produce labels and store a patient's medication record in the pharmacy have the functionality that will identify possible interactions. The information is normally highlighted on the computer screen in the pharmacy with an indication of the possible importance of the interaction. The pharmacist needs to be able to interpret this information and, using any other information they have, decide what action would be appropriate to ensure that no harm comes to the patient.

Dose

Is the dose and dosage regimen appropriate for the patient and their condition? (See Example 24.3.) This is more significant when dealing with drugs that have a narrow therapeutic window (i.e. the dose difference between the therapeutic dose and the toxic dose is small) and when using medication in the very young or very old patient. Being able to calculate the appropriate dose for the patient is a key skill and will sometimes require knowledge about the weight of the patient. Doses should be checked against the maximum dosage information contained in the BNF in the UK. The BNF states maximum doses in a number of ways:

- A specific dose per day – e.g. 200 mg per day
- A specific dose per day for a specific time – e.g. 200 mg per day for 7 days
- A specific dose for a specific number of times per day – e.g. 200 mg three times daily
- A combination of the above – e.g. 200 mg per day, in divided doses, for 15 days

---

Example 24.3

Look at the following details which are written on a prescription:

Elizabeth Riley
2 Black Avenue
Mediton
Bendroflumethiazide tablets 5 mg
1 tablet to be taken at night
Send 28 tablets

On the above prescription there is no indication of the age of the patient. It cannot be assumed that the patient is an adult. If the patient is a child, then the dose may be inappropriate and the BNF for children would have to be consulted. Bendroflumethiazide is usually taken in the morning, not at night, but night workers may take the tablets at night. In this case it is essential to check with the patient and the prescriber for the correctness of the prescription. If the patient is taking the medication for hypertension then the normal dose would be 2.5 mg each morning and increasing the dose will have little enhanced effect, and this too may need to be discussed with the prescriber.

- An initial dose – e.g. 200 mg initially, then ...
- A dose per kg of body weight – e.g. 250 micrograms per kg
- A dose per square metre of body surface – e.g. 25 mg per metre squared
- A maximum dose – e.g. do not take more than 2 tablets at any one time; do not take more than 8 in 24 hours.

If the strength or dose and dosage regimen is missing or incorrect on the prescription, the pharmacist will have to calculate an appropriate strength, dose or dosage regimen. The pharmacist will then have to discuss this with the prescriber to ensure that this meets the patient's requirements.

The dose and dosage regimen of the medication may be affected by other medication on the prescription, or the conditions the patient may be suffering from. This is particularly true if they have any degree of kidney failure, as these are the main routes of excretion of drugs from the body.

Evidence of benefit/harm

Is there any evidence the patient is benefiting from the treatment? Do they believe it is working and is there any evidence that their condition is improving? Could it be causing them any harm? Are they suffering from any adverse effects? Is another treatment on the prescription being used to treat these side-effects? (See Example 24.4.)

Appropriate

Is the product the most appropriate medication available for the patient and their condition? This leads into the use of the mnemonic CASE, which helps to look at the specifics of the drug in terms of its cost, its acceptability to the patient and its safety and efficacy.

Legal

Check the prescription complies with any laws related to the supply of medicines. The legal requirements will be dependent on the legislation in place in the individual country at the time of writing the prescription. For example, the *Medicines, Ethics and Practice* guide covers the legislation relating to prescriptions generated in the UK adequately for most purposes. However, the legal requirements are likely to require the prescription, at the very least, to be signed and dated by the prescriber. Clearly it is the responsibility of the pharmacist to check that the signature is genuine and the date correct.

Cost-effective

Is there a more cost-effective product? Does this treatment offer the most cost-effective option? This might be worth considering if a cheaper medication has the same evidence of safety and efficacy (e.g. comparing the use of simvastatin and atorvastatin). Sometimes the prescriber prescribes a dose of two

---

Example 24.4

Examine the following details which are written on a prescription:

Elizabeth Riley
2 Black Avenue
Mediton
Ibuprofen tablets 400 mg
1 three times a day
Send 84
Simvastatin tablets 40 mg
1 tablet to be taken at night
Send 28 tablets

On the above prescription you may find after talking to the patient that the ibuprofen is being prescribed to treat muscle pain. Muscle pain is a recognized adverse drug reaction (ADR) of a statin which the prescriber may have missed. You would then need to discuss with the prescriber the possibility that the symptoms may be due to an ADR to the statin. This would enable the prescriber to decide on an appropriate course of action to take which could mean undertaking further tests on the patient to establish if it is a true ADR.

10 mg tablets when it would be cheaper to provide one 20 mg tablet.

Acceptable to the patient

Ask the patient if they can take or use the medication? Ask if they are able to take their medication as they are directed to take it? Try and find out if they take their medication all the time and investigate how concordant they are. If the patient does not or cannot take the medicine, there is little reason for it to be dispensed in the first place. Some of the considerations might be, for example, can they swallow tablets or would a liquid or soluble product be more acceptable? Or, can they use their inhaler correctly? If the patient cannot use the inhaler after effective counselling then they should be considered for an alternative device which they might find easier to use. Can they get into child resistant containers? If not, could the medicine be supplied in a device that the patient can get into?

Safe

What do I have to do to ensure the product is safe for this patient? Which possible side-effects might they suffer? What should they do if they suffer from these side-effects? In some cases this will mean that they have to return to the prescriber, but should they stop their treatment or keep taking it until they can see the prescriber? Do I need to tell them about any cautions when taking the medication? (This might be telling them about driving or operating machinery or taking alcohol when taking their medicine.) Does the treatment need to be monitored? If so, when, how often and how should it be monitored? When should the treatment be reviewed and stopped? When would I be justified in looking for a safer alternative treatment? If the patient is currently on a treatment dose, when can that be reduced to a maintenance dose or even stopped?

Evidence based

Is the treatment the most effective treatment available? Is the treatment evidence based? Does the treatment concur with any available guidelines or protocols (see Chs 17 and 18)?

The use of this mnemonic and considerations of the questions should help the pharmacist to clinically and legally review the prescription and thereby to ensure that the patient is being treated optimally. The phar-

macist should then deal with any issue. Some issues will prevent the prescription from being dispensed, such as missing information, a potential overdose and a serious interaction. These will mean the pharmacist has to contact the prescriber before the prescription is sent to the next stage in the dispensing process. Some issues can be raised with the prescriber after the prescription has been dispensed, such as issues about the cost-effectiveness of the treatment. Ensuring the patient gets adequate counselling when the medicine is delivered to the patient might be enough to satisfy some of the issues, particularly in relation to information about possible side-effects and cautions in using the medication.

Assembly of the product and labelling

This stage involves producing a label for the product, selecting the product from where it is stored in the pharmacy and doing any assembly work and putting the label onto the product. Usually trained pharmacy technicians carry out this stage in the process and some pharmacies have introduced dispensing robots to select the products. The assembly work can range from picking a patient pack from a shelf to making the product from its ingredients. Accuracy in this stage of the assembly process is paramount in ensuring that the patient gets the product ordered on the prescription. Picking the wrong strength or form, or even the wrong product, are errors that can occur at this stage. The dispenser needs to take great care in selecting the products because many drugs have similar names, as outlined in Box 24.2 or they may be in containers with a similar appearance (see Ch. 9).

Box 24.2

A few products with similar names

Aldactide	Aldactone
Betnesol	Betnelan
Co-amilofruse	Co-amilozide
	Co-amoxiclav
Cardene	Codeine
Daonil	Danol
Gliclazide	Glipizide
Nicardipine	Nifedipine
Promazine	Promethazine
Zocor	Zoton

At this stage of the process the dispenser may be required to make records, either for legal purposes such as completion of a controlled drugs register, or as good practice, such as adding information to a patient medication record (PMR). The prescription may need to be priced if it is a private prescription or endorsed as required if it is an NHS prescription.

Accuracy checking the product against the prescription

This final accuracy check is present to ensure that there has not been an error in the dispensing process. It is an important stage in minimizing risk to the patient. The person involved in carrying out this check needs to work in a structured and methodical manner without interruption to have the best chance of working effectively. Until recently the pharmacist exclusively did the final check, but more and more accredited checking technicians are being trained to perform this task. This will free up the pharmacist to carry out other tasks which better match their skills, e.g. the delivery of medicines usage reviews (MURs) to patients (see Ch. 47).

Delivery of the product to the patient with the appropriate advice about the product

The final stage is to hand the product to the patient. This stage can be done by a pharmacist or can be delegated to another member of staff. It is important that whoever gives the medicine to the patient ensures the patient has all the advice they need. The pharmacist must be confident that the patient can take or use their medication correctly. The patient should be able to identify signs to tell if the medicine is having the desired effect or is causing a problem and they should know what to do about it. Once the prescription has been handed to the patient, the prescription form will be filed or sent to the appropriate place so the pharmacy receives payment.

Information sources

When dealing with a prescription it is important that the pharmacist knows where to look for

up-to-date information relating to different aspects involved in checking the prescription. Drugs are continually being introduced to the market and the indications for some drugs change, as do doses, dosage regimens and formulations. In addition, some drugs are removed from the market for a variety of reasons. Prescribers will need independent, accessible and unambiguous reviews of effective treatments when writing prescriptions, while pharmacists will require similar information to clinically check the prescription and advise the patient. In addition the dispenser will also need information relating to the cost of the medication to the patient and any rules which they must apply to ensure appropriate remuneration and reimbursement, as well as information about the availability and where to order the products. Some of the most useful information sources in the UK are listed in Box 24.3 (see also Ch. 23 for more detailed information).

The BNF is published and updated every 6 months and lists the products available for dispensing in the UK. It is sent to all doctors, pharmacists and prescribing nurses in the NHS. The *Nurse Prescribers' Formulary* and *Dental Practitioners' Formulary* are included in the BNF and are also published as separate booklets. There is also a BNF for Children which has been produced to provide sound up-to-date information on the use of medicines for treating children. The BNF is the major source of easily available information on the characteristics of individual medicines, including proprietary and generic formulations, strengths, dose and dosage regimens, drug side-effects and

> ### Box 24.3
>
> **Some of the reference sources most frequently used in dispensing**
> British National Formulary (BNF)
> Medicines, Ethics and Practice Guide
> Stockley's Drug Interactions
> Drug and Therapeutics Bulletin
> Drug Tariff
> MeReC Bulletin
> Effective Healthcare
> Prescribers' Journal
> Pharmaceutical Codex
> Current Problems in Pharmacovigilance
> Martindale: the Extra Pharmacopoeia

drug interactions. The most recent copy should always be used. For more comprehensive information about medicines you should refer to Martindale.

The Royal Pharmaceutical Society of Great Britain (RPSGB) produces the *Medicines, Ethics and Practice guide*. It outlines the legal requirements for the sale and supply of medicines and poisons in the UK and contains the RPSGB Code of Ethics for Pharmacists and Pharmacy Technicians.

The Drug Tariff is the resource which details the rules for the NHS remuneration and reimbursement for pharmacy contractors in the UK and contains information on what is or is not allowed on NHS prescriptions.

If the pharmacist cannot find the information that they require in the reference sources they have available, they can contact the local medicines information department which will be listed in the BNF, or the manufacturer of the product where appropriate.

KEY POINTS

- Prescriptions are paper or electronic documents issued by an authorized prescriber for an individual patient
- Prescriptions detail the medicinal treatment required for the patient and may be paper based or electronic
- Prescriptions can be written by a number of people and may be private or NHS prescriptions and may be for GSL, POM or P medicines
- Prescriptions can contain more than one prescription item
- Prescriptions must contain adequate information before they can be dispensed
- All prescriptions should be checked for clinical and patient appropriateness before assembly and dispensing
- This is best achieved by working methodically to ensure no items are overlooked
- Access to reference sources is often required

25

Dispensing techniques (compounding and good practice)

Judith A. Rees

STUDY POINTS

- Good dispensing practice to ensure quality
- The working environment and procedures
- Extemporaneous dispensing equipment and its correct use, including:
  - Weighing equipment
  - Measuring liquids
  - Mixing and grinding equipment
  - Heating equipment
- Manipulative techniques used in dispensing and compounding
- Ingredients and their selection
- Problem solving in extemporaneous dispensing
- Methods of counting tablets and capsules

Introduction

This chapter deals with some of the practical aspects of good pharmacy practice. It will concentrate on the small-scale manufacture of medicines from basic ingredients in the community or in hospital pharmacy. This process is called compounding or extemporaneous dispensing. In addition, good practice which applies to all aspects of dispensing will be considered.

In modern practice, most medicines are manufactured by the pharmaceutical industry under well controlled conditions and packaged in suitable containers designed to maintain the stability of the product (e.g. sealed in an inert atmosphere). Therefore, extemporaneous dispensing, which cannot be as well controlled, should only be used when such products are unavailable. Reasons for unavailability of products may include:

- Non-licensed products
- Products no longer on the market or unavailable from the manufacturer, e.g. due to low demand or superseded by newer formulations/drugs
- Products requiring an individualized dose, e.g. paediatric or geriatric patients
- Products requiring an individualized formulation for a patient, e.g. the replacement of arachis oil by an inert oil for a patient allergic to arachis (peanut) oil or the removal of certain ingredients such as colouring agents
- Veterinary products, e.g. special formulations for different species.

The pharmacist undertaking extemporaneous dispensing has a responsibility to maintain equipment in working order, ensure that the formula and dose are safe and appropriate and that all materials are sourced from recognized pharmaceutical manufacturers. There are also requirements concerning calculations, maintaining good records and labelling regulations. Any staff involved in the process should be adequately trained. These requirements should all be incorporated within standard operating procedures (SOPs).

It is important to remember in any dispensing process that the end product is going to be used or taken by a person or an animal. It is therefore important that the medicine produced is of the highest achievable quality. This, in turn, means that the highest standards must be applied during the preparation process. If we expect quality assurance procedures to be important in the pharmaceutical manufacturing industry then the same careful attention to detail must be applied to small-scale production, i.e. extemporaneous dispensing.

The working environment and procedures

Organization

The working environment has a considerable influence on a worker's efficiency. However, an individual worker, such as a dispenser, can improve efficiency and safe working by developing a tidy and organized method of working. For example, a dispensing bench cluttered with several containers all containing different ingredients makes selection of the correct ingredient more difficult and more prone to error. Ingredients should always be returned to their appropriate shelf/cupboard when the required quantity has been measured out. Thus a safe system of working is essential for a dispensary and the development and use of SOPs should be followed. Additionally, health and safety regulations must be applied in the dispensary.

Cleanliness/hygiene

The dispensing bench, the equipment and utensils, and the container which is to hold the final product must all be thoroughly clean. Lack of cleanliness can cause contamination of the preparation with other ingredients. For example, a spatula which has been used to remove an ingredient from one container will adulterate subsequent containers if not washed before being used again. Cleanliness will also minimize microbial contamination.

Similarly dispensing staff should have a high standard of hygiene and hand washing facilities should be readily available. Hence, a clean white overall should be worn and be kept fastened up since open overalls are a potential safety hazard. Open overalls may result in clothes becoming stained if any spillages occur. Hair should be tied back and preferably covered with a disposable hat/cap and any skin lesions covered with a dressing. Disposable gloves should be worn during preparative work and discarded afterwards. Consideration should be given to the use of masks if volatile substances or fine powders are to be handled.

Documenting procedures and results

Keeping comprehensive records is an essential part of the dispensing process. Records must be kept for a minimum of 2 years (ideally 5 years) and include the formula and any calculations, the ingredients and quantities used, their sources, batch numbers and expiry date. All calculations or weights/volumes should be checked by two people and recorded. Any substances requiring special handling techniques or hazardous substances should be recorded with the precautions taken. The record for a prescribed item should also include the patient and prescription details and date of dispensing. A record must be kept of the personnel involved, including the responsible pharmacist.

All SOPs should be available and adhered to. Any deviations from a SOP should be recorded.

Equipment

Not only is the selection of the correct equipment or 'tools' for the job essential, but the tools must also be used in the correct way and maintained in good order to ensure performance is unimpaired.

Weighing equipment

Nowadays, weighing equipment can be divided into non-automatic and automatic weighing equipment. Non-automatic weighing equipment requires an operator to place and/or remove the items from the balance pan. Such weighing equipment can be a mechanical beam balance, which has a pan on one end of the beam for weights and a pan on the other end of the beam for the material to be weighed (Fig. 25.1) or it can be an electronic top-pan balance, in which case the substance to be weighed is placed on the pan and an electronic display gives the weight. Automatic weighing equipment is designed to automatically fill a package to the required weight without the intervention of an operator. Such equipment is used in the pharmaceutical industry, but unlikely to be used for extemporaneous dispensing. Whichever type of weighing equipment is used, it must be suitable for its intended use and be sufficiently accurate. In the UK, weighing equipment must be calibrated in metric units and must be marked with maximum and minimum weights that can be weighed.

General rules for the use and maintenance of weighing equipment

Balances can give incorrect readings because of poor practice or misuse. The following points are important to ensure accurate weighing:

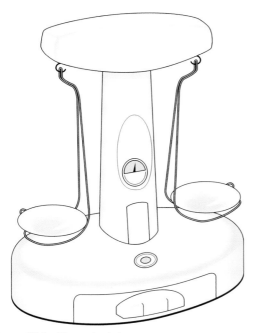

Figure 25.1 • Dispensing balance.

- It is important to use balances on a level surface: most will incorporate a level indicator device, so make sure it reads level before trying to adjust for a zero balance display.
- Balances must be correctly balanced before use, with any indicators reading zero. On electronic balances the display should indicate zero, not be blank. If zero is not indicated then incorrect readings, and hence weights, may be obtained.
- Strong draughts, caused by air conditioning or a breeze as a result of doors or windows being open, can affect some balances and make a correct reading impossible. Therefore always site a balance in a draught-free area.
- Always keep the balance pan clean and free from debris underneath the balance pan itself. Build-up of debris can interfere with the weighing operation.
- Regular checks with stamped weights should be made to ensure the balance is working correctly.
- If possible keep a record of when, and by whom, the check was carried out as well as the result.
- Never weigh less than the declared minimum weight or more than the maximum weight declared on the balance.

Use of a beam balance

As well as the above, the following 'rules' apply to the use of a beam balance:

- Ensure that the balance and pans are clean.
- Check that the pointer is swinging freely.
- Remove the appropriate weights, using the tweezers provided, and place them on the left-hand pan. (Never handle weights, as this will affect their accuracy and risks contamination.)
- Immediately close the lid of the weight box or close the drawer containing the weights after removal of the weights. If it is left open there is a possibility that ingredients to be weighed will fall into the box/drawer, contaminating the weights and affecting their accuracy.
- A solid material to be weighed should then be placed carefully onto the right-hand scale pan. Do not weigh ingredients on a piece of paper as this introduces a potential inaccuracy. The exception is when weighing greasy or semi-solid materials, e.g. white soft paraffin, when a counterbalanced piece of paper should be used.
- When the correct weight has been achieved the pan should be carefully removed from the balance and the material transferred to a suitable container.
- Errors in this transference stage may occur if care is not taken to ensure that all the weighed material has been removed from the scale pan. If the drug is to be dissolved or incorporated into a suspension, it can be washed from the scale pan using some of the appropriate liquid vehicle.
- Tapping the glass pan against the side of the container can cause it to become chipped. This will affect the accuracy of the balance and slivers of glass will not improve the health of the patient!
- The balance pan should then be washed and dried thoroughly, before any further substance is weighed. A second substance must never be weighed on the remains of the first.
- The weights should be returned to the box/drawer.

Use of top-pan balance

- Ensure that the balance is level, in a draught-free environment and working properly.
- Place an appropriate container (such as a weighing boat) or piece of paper on the pan and use the auto-zero to cancel its weight.
- Add the material to be weighed until the correct weight is shown on the display.

- Carefully remove the weighed material as above.

In addition to using the balance correctly there are one or two other rules which should be observed when weighing, to ensure good dispensing practice. These are:

- If using a solid material that requires size reduction by grinding or sieving, always ensure that this procedure is carried out before weighing the required quantity. If a quantity of powder is weighed and then size reduced by grinding in a mortar or sieving, there is a strong possibility that some of the material will be lost in the process and the final preparation will not contain the correct proportions of ingredients. The best approach is to roughly weigh an excess quantity, grind or sieve it as required, then accurately weigh off the required quantity.
- As far as possible never split quantities and do two weightings, as this will increase the inaccuracies.
- If a quantity less than the legal minimum is needed, it is necessary to weigh the minimum weight allowable (or more) and make an excess of the product or prepare it by trituration (see Ch. 35).

Measuring liquids

Liquid measures

All measures for liquids must comply with current weights and measures regulations and should be stamped accordingly. Traditionally, conical measures (Fig. 25.2) have been used in dispensing, although, if not used carefully, they can be less accurate than cylindrical measures.

Whichever type of measure is chosen, always ensure the following:

- The level of liquid is read to the bottom of the meniscus.
- The measure is vertical when reading the meniscus. If this is not done, considerable errors in quantities can occur, especially with conical measures, where the error increases with height because of the slope of the sides.

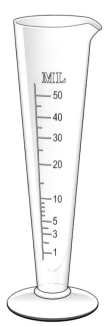

Figure 25.2 • Conical dispensing measure.

- The measure is thoroughly drained. Even if the ingredient is only slightly viscous, it is amazing how much can be left in the measure.
- As far as possible, never use more than one measure. Splitting the volume between two measures increases the potential for error.
- Always select the smallest measure which will hold the desired volume, because this gives the greatest accuracy. For example, use a 10 mL measure to measure 5 mL; do not use a 20 mL measure.
- If the substance being measured is so viscous that it would be very difficult to drain the measure effectively, then the volume should be measured by difference. This is done by pouring an excess into the measure and then pouring off the liquid until only the excess volume remains (see Example 25.1).

When measuring liquids it is important to observe two simple rules which ensure good dispensing practice:

Example 25.1

25 mL of glycerol is required.
Because of the viscosity it is difficult to remove it completely from the measure.

It is therefore advisable to measure, say, 35 mL and pour off the 25 mL required, ensuring that 10 mL is left in the measure. Remember to allow sufficient time for the liquid to drain back down.

- Always hold the liquid container with the label uppermost so that you pour away from the label. This ensures that any liquid which runs down the side of the bottle will not affect the label by obscuring the label. This is especially true for highly coloured substances (such as amaranth solution) or corrosive substances (e.g. acids). Replace any damaged label immediately.
- If possible, when pouring liquids, hold the cap of the container in your hand, preferably between the fourth finger and the palm of your hand. It is possible you may be measuring more than one liquid and if caps are left lying on the dispensing bench it is easy to mix them up and place the wrong one back on the container.

Measuring small volumes

It is important to select the correct equipment when measuring. The minimum measurable volume for a 10 mL conical measure is 1 mL. Graduated pipettes can be used for volumes from 5 mL down to 0.1 mL. For volumes smaller than this, a trituration should be made. The viscosity of the substance being measured should also be considered.

Correct use of pipettes

Pipettes can be either the 'drainage' or 'blow-out' variety. A rubber bulb or teat should be used. Never use mouth suction.

- A bulb or teat should be placed over the mouth of the pipette, taking care not to push it down too far.
- The container of the substance to be measured should be ready on the bench.
- The top of the container should be removed and held in the hand, between the fourth finger and the palm of the hand.
- The pipette should be put into the container, taking care that only a short length of the pipette is immersed. If a quantity of liquid is allowed to collect on the outside of the pipette, the accuracy of the measuring will be affected.
- The correct amount of liquid should then be drawn up the pipette. Take care at this stage as the liquid may shoot up the pipette into the bulb.
- If a pipette bulb is being used, the appropriate valve is pressed to prevent the liquid running out of the pipette, the pipette is removed from the container and the liquid then released into the desired container.

- If using a simple teat, this should now be flicked off with the thumb and a finger placed firmly over the top of the pipette, taking care not to allow any liquid to be lost. The pipette can then be withdrawn from the container and the liquid measured out by removing the finger from the top of the pipette.

Nowadays, semi-automatic pipettes can be used for dispensing.

Mixing and grinding

Mortar and pestle

The mortar (bowl) and pestle (pounding device) are used to reduce the size of powders, mix powders, mix powders and liquids, and make emulsions. Two types, each available in a range of sizes, are used.

Glass mortar and pestle

These are generally small and therefore cannot be used for large quantities of material. The smooth surface of the glass reduces the friction which can be generated, so they are only suitable for size reduction of friable materials (such as crystals). They are useful for dissolving small quantities of ingredients, for mixing small quantities of fine powders and for the mixing of substances such as dyes which are absorbed by and stain composition or porcelain mortars.

Porcelain or composition mortars and pestles

These are normally larger than the glass variety and have a rougher surface. They are ideal for size reduction of solids and for mixing solids and liquids, as in the preparation of suspensions and emulsions.

Size reduction using a mortar and pestle

Selection of the correct type of mortar and pestle is vital for this operation. A flat-bottomed mortar and a pestle with a flat head should be chosen. A flat-headed pestle in a mortar with a round bottom, or vice versa, will mean a lot of wasted effort.

Using a mortar and pestle for mixing powders

Adequate mixing will only be achieved if there is sufficient space. Overfilling of the mortar should therefore be avoided. The pestle should be rotated in both right and left directions to ensure thorough mixing. Undue pressure should not be used, as this will cause impaction of the powder on the bottom of the mortar.

Table 25.1 Filter paper characteristics

Number (Whatman series)	Filtration rate	Size of particle removed	Average pore size (mm)
54	1 (fast)	Coarse	3.4–5.0
1	4 (medium fast)	Medium	2.1–2.8
50	23 (slow)	Fine	0.4–1.1

Filters

There are occasions when clarification of a liquid is required. Pouring the liquid through muslin can carry out coarse filtration, or 'straining'. Where a finer degree of filtration is required, filter paper, sintered glass filters or membrane filters should be used. Filter paper and membrane filters come in different grades and selection of the correct grade is determined by the size of the particles to be removed. Details of grades of filter paper are found in Table 25.1. Filter paper has the disadvantages of introducing fibres into the filtrate and may also absorb significant amounts of active ingredient. This is less likely with membrane filters.

Heat sources

In the dispensing process it may be necessary to heat ingredients, e.g. melt semi-solids in the preparation of ointments/creams, warm liquids to aid dissolution of solids.

Bunsen (gas) burners

Bunsen burners are useful for small-scale heating if a gas supply is available. They should always be placed on a heat-resistant mat and care taken by the operator to avoid burns. When heating with a Bunsen burner, a blue flame should be used.

Water baths

These are used to provide gentle heat, for example when melting ointment bases or preparing suppositories. Normally the materials to be heated are placed in a porcelain evaporating basin and placed over the hot water in the water bath. There is no necessity to have the water boiling vigorously – this does not increase the heat but does increase the risk of scalding.

Electric hot plates

Electrically heated hot plates can be used for melting and heating and have the advantage of thermostatic controls.

Manipulative techniques

Selection of the correct equipment and using it appropriately is fundamental to good compounding. Several basic manipulative techniques may require practice.

Mixing

The goal of any mixing operation should be to ensure that even distribution of all the ingredients has occurred. If a sample is removed from any part of the final preparation, it should be identical to a sample taken from any other part of the container (Aulton 2007).

Mixing of liquids

Simple stirring or shaking is usually all that is required to mix two or more liquids. The degree of stirring or shaking will be dependent on the viscosities of the liquids. Thus mixing liquids of low viscosities will require only minimal stirring, while mixing two liquids with high viscosities will need more vigorous agitation.

Mixing solids with liquids

Particle size reduction should always be considered. This will either speed up the dissolution process or improve the uniform distribution of the solid throughout the liquid. When a solution is being made, a stirring rod will be adequate. However, a suspension will require a pestle and mortar.

Mixing solids with solids

As well as the correct use of a mortar and pestle, the amounts of material being mixed together must be considered. Where the quantity of material to be mixed is small and the proportions are approximately the same, the materials can be added to an appropriately sized mortar and effectively mixed. Where a small quantity of powder has to be mixed with a large quantity, in order to achieve effective mixing it must be done in stages:

- The ingredient with the smallest bulk is placed in the mortar.
- A quantity of the second ingredient, approximately equal in volume to the first, is added and carefully mixed, using the pestle.
- A further quantity of the second ingredient, approximately equal in volume to the mixture in the mortar, is now added.
- This process, known as 'doubling-up', is continued until all the powder has been added (see Ch. 35).

Mixing semi-solids

This usually occurs in the preparation of ointments where two or more ointment bases may be mixed together. If all the ingredients are semi-solids or liquids, they can be mixed together by rubbing them down on an ointment slab, using a spatula. If there is a significant difference in the quantities of the ingredients, a 'doubling-up' process should be used. An alternative method is the fusion method.

The fusion method

- Place the bases in a porcelain evaporating basin and gently heat until they have just melted. Excess heat should not be used as overheating may cause physical or chemical changes in some materials.
- The basin is then removed from the heat and the contents are stirred continuously, but gently, until the mixture has cooled and set. Stirring at this stage is of vital importance as otherwise the components may segregate on cooling. Rapid stirring should be avoided as it will introduce air bubbles into the mixture.

When using the fusion method, do not be tempted to add any solid active ingredients to the basin before the bases have set. Addition of any further ingredients is best done by rubbing down on an ointment slab. Further details of methods used in the preparation of ointments can be found in Chapter 33.

Tared containers

Liquid preparations should as far as possible be made up to volume in a measure. There are, however, instances when accurate transfer of the preparation to the final container is difficult; for example with some suspensions it can be almost impossible to remove all the insoluble ingredients when pouring from one container to another. Emulsions and viscous preparations can also be difficult to transfer accurately. In these cases a tared container should be used.

To tare a bottle

A volume of water identical to the volume of the product being dispensed is accurately measured. This is then poured into the chosen medicine container and the meniscus marked with the upper edge of a small adhesive label, effectively making the bottle into a single-point measure. The container is then emptied and allowed to drain thoroughly. The preparation is then poured into the container and made up to volume, using the tare mark as the guide. Remove the tare label.

This procedure should be used with discretion and only in situations when major inaccuracies would occur in the transfer of liquids. In addition, it should only be used when water is present as one of the ingredients. Putting medicines into a wet bottle is generally considered bad practice.

Ingredients

All ingredients must be sourced and obtained from reputable suppliers and be of a quality suitable for the preparation and dispensing of pharmaceutical products. Additionally, ingredients must be suitably stored to preserve stability and integrity. For example, regular checks on expiry dates of stored products should be made and any ingredient outside its expiry date should be discarded. Hence arrangements should be made for the regular collection and disposal of pharmaceutical waste (see Ch. 43). Some ingredients may require special storage conditions and these should be provided. Many pharmaceutical ingredients and products require storage in a refrigerator, which should be fitted with a maximum/minimum thermometer and regularly checked on a daily basis.

Selection

When dispensing, selection of the correct product is vital. The label on each container must be read carefully and checked to ensure that it contains the required product. There are many examples of drugs and preparations where names may be misread if care is not taken; examples include folic acid and folinic acid, cefuroxime and cefotaxime. Further examples are given in Chapter 23. Extemporaneously dispensed medicines may contain several ingredients, so the potential for error by wrong selection is increased.

Some ingredients of extemporaneously dispensed medicines may occur in a variety of forms or a synonym is used.

Variety of forms

Coal tar, for example, is available as coal tar solution, strong coal tar solution and coal tar. Clearly if all three containers are on the same shelf, the wrong item may be selected by accident. Some other materials where confusion can occur are listed in Table 25.2. This list is not meant to be comprehensive and only contains common exemplars. The only foolproof method of avoiding errors is to read the container label carefully.

Synonyms

Some substances used in dispensing may be known by more than one name. An awareness of this is useful

Table 25.3 Example of substances with synonyms

Substance	Synonym
Wool fat	Anhydrous lanolin
Hydrous wool fat	Lanolin
Hard paraffin	Paraffin wax
Compound benzoic acid ointment	Whitfield's ointment
Macrogol 2000	Polyethylene glycol 2000 or PEG 2000
Theobroma oil	Cocoa butter

when selecting ingredients. Some examples of commonly used materials are given in Table 25.3. This table is not intended to be comprehensive.

Problem solving in extemporaneous dispensing

For extemporaneous dispensing, it is helpful if a method detailing how to prepare the product is available. Methods for 'official' preparations can sometimes be found in reference sources such as the *Pharmaceutical Codex*. However, on many occasions no method is available. In such a situation, it may be helpful to consider similar formulas in reference

Table 25.2 Some substances which occur in a variety of forms

Substance/form	Use
Light magnesium carbonate	Because of its lightness and diffusible properties, it is used in suspensions
Heavy magnesium carbonate	Normally used in bulk or individual powders
Light kaolin	Used in suspensions
Heavy kaolin	Used in the preparation of kaolin poultice
Precipitated sulphur	This has a smaller particle size than sublimed sulphur and is preferred in preparations for external use, e.g. suspensions, creams and ointments
Sublimed sulphur	Slightly gritty powder which does not produce such elegant preparations as precipitated sulphur
Yellow soft paraffin	Used as an ointment base
White soft paraffin	Bleached yellow soft paraffin normally used when the other ingredients are not strongly coloured

Example 25.2

The following prescription is received:
Sodium bicarbonate ear drops BP
Send 10 mL
Formula:

Sodium bicarbonate 500 mg

Glycerol 3 mL

Freshly boiled and cooled water to 10 mL

Points to note:

- Solubility of sodium bicarbonate is 1 in 11 of water
- Glycerol is a viscous liquid
- The quantity of water in the ear drops is approximately 6.5 mL.

Method:

1. The sodium bicarbonate should be size reduced in a mortar and pestle, if necessary.

2. 500 milligrams of sodium bicarbonate is then weighed and put into a 10 mL conical measuring cylinder.

3. The sodium bicarbonate is soluble, requiring a minimum of 5.5 mL in which to dissolve. Add about 6 mL of water, ensuring that the volume of ingredients does not go beyond the 7 mL mark.

4. Stir the contents of the measure until the sodium bicarbonate is dissolved.

5. Make the volume up to 7 mL with water.

6. The glycerol is viscous and trying to pour 3 mL from a measure is inaccurate. The 3 mL of glycerol can now be added by pouring it into the 7 mL of sodium bicarbonate solution and carefully making the volume in the measure up to 10 mL.

sources. Additionally, the application of simple scientific knowledge, especially of physical properties, is often all that is needed. The following gives an example of how this is done.

Putting theory into practice

Solubility

Always check the solubility of any solid materials. If they are soluble in the main vehicles, then a solution is likely to be produced. If solubility is limited to one liquid, this will assist in achieving uniform dose distribution. Solution will be achieved more quickly if the particle size is small and so size reduction should be considered for any soluble ingredients which are presented in a lumpy or granular form. If the substance is not soluble, then a suspension will need to be produced. Whether a suspending agent will be required should be considered (see Ch. 31). Where one material is an oil and another aqueous, it is likely that an emulsifying agent will be required to produce an emulsion (see Ch. 32).

Volatile ingredients

If an ingredient is volatile then it should be added near the end of the dispensing process. If it is added too early, much may be lost due to evaporation.

Viscosity

The viscosity of a liquid will have a bearing on how it is measured, i.e. is a pipette or measure suitable, or should it be measured by difference, and how will it be incorporated? (See Example 25.1.)

Expiry date

All extemporaneously prepared products should be awarded an expiry date. Ideally stability studies should be undertaken in order to predict an accurate shelf life for all products. This is not usually possible for 'one-off' preparations and most hospital pharmacies have guidelines based on previous stability studies. Further information on stability and appropriate expiry dates is found in Chapter 43.

Example 25.2 illustrates how some very simple facts can be applied to develop an accurate method of preparation.

Counting devices

Tablets and capsules form a large proportion of the medicines which are dispensed today. Most are presented in patient packs or original packs, but occasionally tablets/capsules are supplied in bulk packs and the prescribed amount is counted from them.

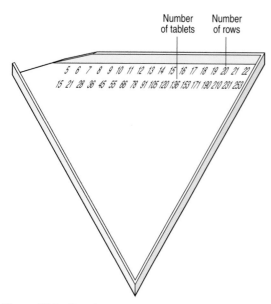

Number of tablets   Number of rows

5 6 7 8 9 10 11 12 13 14 15 16 17 18 19 20 21 22
15 21 28 36 45 55 66 78 91 105 120 136 153 171 190 210 231 253

Figure 25.3 • Counting triangle.

Various methods can be used for this counting:
- The manual method
- A counting triangle or capsule counter
- A counting tray
- An electronic counter.

These methods all have their advantages and disadvantages and it is up to each pharmacist to select the most appropriate for the task, depending on the equipment available. Whichever method is selected it must be noted that the medicines must not be touched by hand (wear disposable gloves to avoid touching the formulation). The equipment should also be carefully cleaned before use (again wear gloves), as powder left from one product could cause contamination of the next one.

The manual method

This consists of pouring the product on to a piece of clean white paper which overlaps another piece. The products are then counted off in tens, using a spatula, on to the second piece of paper. This is formed into a small funnel and the tablets or capsules poured into the appropriate container.

Concentration must be maintained or the wrong quantity may be counted. Remember to wear gloves.

Counting triangles and capsule counters

Counting triangles

This is a fast, accurate and simple way to count tablets. The triangles are made of either metal or plastic. Two rows of figures are printed or etched along the edge. The top row of figures refers to the number of rows and the numbers below refer to the number of tablets contained in that number of rows. This is illustrated in Figure 25.3. Tablets are poured into the triangle and rows completed using a spatula. Any excess of tablets is returned using the spatula and the correct number poured into a tablet bottle.

Capsule counters

Because of their shape, capsules cannot be counted on triangles. A capsule counter, illustrated in Figure 25.4, is a metal tray which consists of 10 rows of grooves. The capsules are poured on to the tray and, using a spatula, lined up in the grooves. Each complete row will contain 10 capsules so the number of complete rows multiplied by 10 gives the number of capsules.

Capsule counters are not as easy to manipulate as triangles but are an efficient method for counting capsules. Studies testing the accuracy of the various counting methods have shown these two devices to be the best.

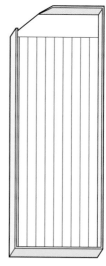

Figure 25.4 • Capsule counter.

Perforated counting trays

These are normally made of clear perspex. They consist of a rectangular box with a sliding lid, on top of which is placed a perforated tray. Each box is supplied with several trays with different sized perforations to accommodate different sizes and types of products (Fig. 25.5). These trays can be used to count tablets or capsules.

The main disadvantage is the necessity to change the trays for different products.

Electronic counters

There are two types of electronic counter, those which use the weight of the product to count and those which count using a photoelectric cell.

Electronic balances

Between 5 and 20 of the required dosage form is put on a balance pan or scoop. From the weight of this reference sample, a microprocessor within the device calculates the total number of dosage forms, as they are added. The main problem with this type of device is that for accurate counting, it requires consistent uniformity of the weight of the tablets or capsules. There can be problems with accuracy when counting sugar-coated or very small tablets.

Photoelectric cell counters

The product to be counted is poured through a hopper on the top of the machine. The tablets or capsules are then channelled into a straight line and counted as they interrupt the beam of light to the photoelectric cell. This is an efficient method of counting and these

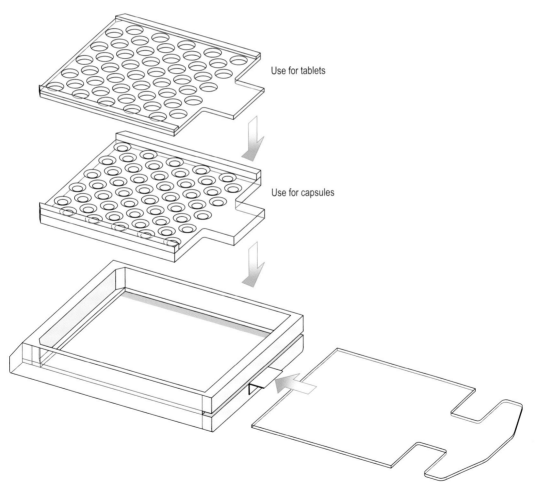

Use for tablets

Use for capsules

Figure 25.5 • Perforated counting tray.

devices are widely used. They are not without their problems, however:

- They do not discriminate between whole and broken tablets
- As the beam of light from the photoelectric cell must be interrupted for counting to occur, these devices cannot count clear capsules
- The speed at which the dosage forms are poured through the hopper must be controlled – if pouring becomes too fast the system will not cope
- They are difficult to clean.

Because of this last point, the Council of the Royal Pharmaceutical Society of Great Britain issued the following advice concerning the use of electronic counters:

Severe allergic reactions can be initiated in previously sensitized persons by very small amounts of certain drugs and of excipients and other materials used in the manufacture of tablets and capsules. In order to minimize that risk, counting devices should be carefully cleaned after each dispensing operation involving any uncoated tablet, or any coated tablet or capsule from a bulk container holding damaged contents. As cross-contamination with the penicillins is particularly serious, special care should be taken when dispensing products containing those drugs.

This type of device should therefore be reserved for counting only coated tablets or capsules or for prepacking operations.

Automated dispensing systems

There are a number of automated dispensing systems available of varying degrees of sophistication. They are linked to a computer, which is used for label production and creation of the patient medication record. The computer 'orders' counting of loose tablets or capsules (using a photoelectric cell counter) into a suitable container, or retrieval of a prepackaged medicine. Some incorporate barcoding technology to improve speed and accuracy.

Tests indicate that these machines are less prone to error than human dispensing.

Conclusion

Developing good practice takes time and requires attention to detail.

KEY POINTS

- Extemporaneous dispensing should only be used when manufactured medicines are not available
- Accurate dispensing requires clean, neat methodical work
- Always comply with SOPs
- Comprehensive records of extemporaneous dispensing are required to be kept for at least 2 years
- Do not use a balance to weigh less than its minimum weighable quantity
- Ensure that liquid measures comply with the weights and measures regulations
- Always use the bottom of the meniscus when measuring liquids
- Viscous liquids should be measured 'by difference'
- Pipettes are used to measure volumes between 0.1 mL and 5 mL
- Select the smallest measure for the volume of liquid to be measured
- A glass mortar and pestle can be used for size reduction of friable materials and mixing small quantities of fine powder
- A porcelain mortar and pestle is used for larger quantities, for mixing solids and liquids, making emulsions, and for size reduction
- 'Doubling-up' is used for mixing a small quantity of powder with a larger quantity
- Confusion can arise with different forms of the same material and the use of synonyms
- Simple problem-solving techniques can produce a satisfactory method of dispensing a product
- Tablets and capsules can be counted manually, or by using a triangle, capsule counter, counting tray or electronic counter
- Tablets and capsules should not be counted in the hand unless wearing gloves

26

Pharmaceutical calculations

Ivan O. Edafiogho and Arthur J. Winfield

STUDY POINTS

- Expressions of concentration
- Calculating quantities from master formulae
- Changing concentrations
- Small quantities (trituration)
- Solubility
- Calculations related to doses
- Reconstitution and rates of infusion

There are examples and self-assessment questions and answers provided to help you assess your progress.

Introduction

Many pharmacy students approach the calculations involved in dispensing and manufacturing with trepidation. There is no need. Most calculations are simple arithmetic. It is true that there are many steps in the dispensing process where things can go wrong and calculating quantities is one of them. However, careful, methodical working will minimize the risk of errors. Always try to relate the calculation to practice, visualize what you are doing and double-check everything.

How to minimize errors

As in all dispensing procedures, an organized, methodical approach is essential:

- Write out the calculation clearly – it is all too easy to end up reading from the wrong line
- If you are transferring data from a reference source, double-check what you have written down is correct
- Write down every step
- Do not take short cuts – you are more likely to make a mistake
- Try not to be totally dependent on your calculator – have an approximate idea of what the answer should be and then if you happen to hit the wrong button on the calculator you are more likely to be aware that an error has been made
- Finally, always double-check your calculation. There is frequently more than one way of doing a calculation, so if you get the same answer by two different methods the chances are that your answer will be correct. Alternatively, try working it in reverse and see if you get the starting numbers.

Expressions of concentration

The metric system is the International System of Units (SI Units) for weight, volume and length. The basic unit for weight is the kilogram (kg) while the basic unit for volume is the litre (L) and the basic unit of length is the metre (m). Appendix 3 gives information about the weights and measures commonly used in pharmacy. The prefix 'milli' indicates one-thousandth (10^{-3}) and 'micro' one-millionth (10^{-6}).

In some countries, the avoirdupois (or imperial) system (pounds and ounces) is still used in commerce and daily life. The imperial system of volume (pints and gallons) is still a common system for commerce and household measurement. Pharmacists need to know about these systems in order to avoid serious errors in interpretation of prescriptions. It is important to be able to change between the systems. Some conversion factors for the metric, avoirdupois

Box 26.1

Weights and measures

- 1000 millilitres (mL) = 1 litre (L)
- 1000 micrograms = 1 milligram (mg)
- 1000 milligrams (mg) = 1 gram (g)
- 1000 grams (g) = 1 kilogram (kg)
- 1 kilogram (kg) = 2.2 pounds (lb)
- 1 teaspoonful (tsp) = 5 mL
- 1 tablespoonful = 15 mL (3 teaspoonfuls)
- 1 grain (Avoir. or Apoth.) = 64.8 mg
- 1 pint (pt) = 473 mL
- 1 gallon (gal) = 3785 mL
- 1 fluid ounce (oz) = 29.57 mL (30 mL)
- 1 fluid ounce (oz) = 480 minims

and apothecary systems are shown in Box 26.1 (Examples 26.1–26.3).

Expressions of strength

Ratio is the relative magnitude of two like quantities. Thus:

$$1 : 10 = 1 \text{ part in } 10 \text{ parts or } 1\,g \text{ in } 10\,g$$

If 1 g of sucrose is in 10 g of solution, the ratio is 1 : 10. Therefore, 10 g of sucrose is in 100 g of solution. This can be expressed as a percentage, so it is equivalent to a 10% w/w (weight in weight) solution.

Ratio strength is the expression of a concentration by means of a ratio, e.g. 1 : 10. Percentage strength is a ratio of parts per hundred, e.g. 10% (Examples 26.4–26.6).

Example 26.1

A prescription is received for a dose of 30 grains of a drug. How many grams is the dose?

1 grain = 64.8 mg. Therefore:
30 grains = 30 × 64.8 mg = 1944 mg = 1.94 g
   (to 2 decimal places)

Example 26.4

Express 0.1% w/w as a ratio strength.

0.1 g/100 g = 1 part/y parts.
y = 100 × 1/0.1
y = 1000

Therefore, the ratio strength = 1 : 1000

Example 26.2

If 60 minims make 1 fluid drachm, and 8 fluid drachms make 1 fluid ounce, what is the volume of 1 minim in the metric system?

60 minims = 1 fluid drachm; and
8 fluid drachms = 1 fluid ounce (30 mL)
60 × 8 minims = 30 mL; 480 minims = 30 mL;
1 minim = 30/480 mL
Therefore 1 minim = 0.06 mL

Example 26.5

Express 1 : 2500 as a percentage strength.

1 part/2500 parts = y parts/100 parts.

Thus, y = 1 × 100/2500 = 0.04%

Example 26.6

Express 1 p.p.m. as a percentage strength.

1 p.p.m. = 1 part per million = 1:1 000 000

Let y be the percentage strength:

Thus, 1 part/1 000 000 = y parts/100 parts
y = 1 × 100/1 000 000 = 0.0001% = 1×10^{-4}%

Example 26.3

Sulfacetamide eye drops contain 200 drops in a 10 mL bottle. Calculate the volume of 1 drop.

200 drops = 10 mL. Therefore:
1 drop = 10/200 mL = 0.05 mL

Percentage weight in weight (w/w)

Percentage weight in weight (w/w) is the number of grams of an active ingredient in 100 grams (solid or liquid) (Example 26.7).

Example 26.7

How many grams of a drug should be used to prepare 240 grams of a 5% w/w solution?
Let y be the weight of the drug needed:

Thus, $y/240 = 5\text{ g}/100\text{ g}$
$y = 5 \times 240/100 = 12\text{ g}$

Percentage weight in volume (w/v)

Percentage weight in volume (w/v) is the number of grams of an active ingredient in 100 mL of liquid (Example 26.8).

Example 26.8

If 5 g of iodine is in 250 mL of iodine tincture, calculate the percentage of iodine in the tincture.
Let y be the percentage of iodine in the tincture:

$y/100\text{ mL} = 5\text{ g}/250\text{ mL}$
$y = 5 \times 100/250 = 2\%\text{ w/v}$

Percentage volume in volume (v/v)

Percentage volume in volume (v/v) indicates the number of millilitres (mL) of an active ingredient in 100 mL of liquid (Example 26.9).

Example 26.9

If 15 mL of ethanol is mixed with water to make 60 mL of solution, what is the percentage of ethanol in the solution?
Let y be the percentage of ethanol in the solution:

$y/100\text{ mL} = 15\text{ mL}/60\text{ mL}$
$y = 15 \times 100/60 = 25\%\text{ v/v}$

Miscellaneous examples

(Examples 26.10–26.13)

Example 26.10

Express 30 g of dextrose in 600 mL of solution as a percentage, indicating w/w, w/v or v/v.
Let y grams be the weight of dextrose in 100 mL:

$y/100\text{ mL} = 30\text{ g}/600\text{ mL}$
$y = 30 \times 100/600\text{ mL} = 5\%\text{ w/v}$

Example 26.11

What is the percentage of magnesium carbonate in the following syrup?

Magnesium carbonate	15 g
Sucrose	820 g
Water, q.s.	to 1000 mL

Percentage is the number of grams of magnesium carbonate in 100 mL of syrup.

$y/100\text{ mL} = 15\text{ g}/1000\text{ mL}$
$y = 15 \times 100/1000 = 1.5\%\text{ w/v (grams in 100 mL)}$

Example 26.12

Calculate the amount of drug in 5 mL of cough syrup if 100 mL contains 300 mg of drug.

By proportion, $y\text{ mg}/5\text{ mL} = 300\text{ mg}/100\text{ mL}$
$y = 5 \times 300/100 = 15\text{ mg}$

Example 26.13

Compute the percentage of the ingredients in the following ointment (to 2 decimal places):

Liquid paraffin	14 g
Soft paraffin	38 g
Hard paraffin	12 g

Total amount of ingredients

$= 14\text{ g} + 38\text{ g} + 12\text{ g} = 64\text{ g}$

To find the amounts of the ingredients in 100 g of ointment, each figure will be multiplied by 100/64:

Liquid paraffin $= (100/64) \times 14 = 21.88\%\text{ w/w}$
Soft paraffin $= (100/64) \times 38 = 59.38\%\text{ w/w}$
Hard paraffin $= (100/64) \times 12 = 18.75\%\text{ w/w}$

It is useful to double-check that these numbers add up to 100% (allowing for the rounding off to 2 decimal places).

Moles and molarity

Concentrations can also be expressed in moles or millimoles (see also Ch. 38). When a mixture contains the molecular weight of a drug in grams in 1 litre of solution, the concentration is defined as a 1 molar solution (1 mol). It has a molarity of 1. Thus, for example, the molecular weight of potassium hydroxide (KOH) is the sum of the atomic weights of its elements, i.e. KOH = 39 + 16 + 1 = 56. Therefore a 1 molar solution (1 mol) of KOH contains 56 g of KOH in 1 litre of solution.

A 1 millimole (mmol) solution of KOH contains one-thousandth of a mole in 1 litre = 56 mg (Examples 26.14–26.16).

Example 26.14

Calculate the number of moles (molarity) of a solution if it contains 117 g of sodium chloride (NaCl) in 1 L of solution (atomic weights: Na = 23, Cl = 35.5).

Molecular weight of NaCl = 23 + 35.5 = 58.5 g
Therefore, 58.5 g of NaCl in 1 litre is equivalent to 1 mole (1 mol) in solution.
Number of moles of NaCl = 117 g/58.5 g = 2 mol

Example 26.15

Calculate the number of milligrams of sodium hydroxide (NaOH) to be dissolved in 1 L of water to give a concentration of 10 mmol (atomic weights: H = 1, O = 16, Na = 23).

Molecular weight of NaOH = 23 + 16 + 1 = 40
1 mmol = 40 mg in 1 L
Therefore, 10 mmol = 400 mg in 1 L

Example 26.16

Express 111 mg of calcium chloride ($CaCl_2$) in 1 L of solution as millimoles (atomic weights: Ca = 40, Cl = 35.5).

Molecular weight of $CaCl_2$ = Ca + (2 × Cl)
= 40 + (2 × 35.5) = 40 + 71 = 111 g
Therefore, 111 mg of $CaCl_2$ = 1 mmol in 1 L

Calculating quantities from a master formula

In extemporaneous dispensing, a list of the ingredients is provided on the prescription or is obtained from a recognized reference source where the quantities of each ingredient are indicated. It may be that this 'formula' is for the quantity requested, but more often the quantities provided by the master formula have to be scaled up or down, depending on the quantity of the product required. This can be achieved using proportion or by deriving a 'multiplying factor'. The latter is the ratio of the required quantity divided by the formula quantity. The following examples illustrate this process (Examples 26.17 and 26.18).

In most formulae where a combination of weights and volumes is required, the formula will indicate that the preparation is to be made up to the required weight or volume with the designated vehicle. However, occasionally, as can be seen in the next example, a combination of stated weights and volumes is used and it is not possible to indicate what the exact final weight or volume of the preparation will be. In these instances an excess quantity is normally calculated for and the required amount measured (Example 26.19).

Example 26.17

Calculate the quantities to prepare the following prescription:

50 g Compound Benzoic Acid Ointment BPC.

The master formula is for 100 g, the prescription is for 50 g, therefore the multiplying factor is 50/100, i.e. each quantity in the master formula is multiplied by 50/100 = 0.5 to give the scaled quantity.

Ingredient	Master formula	Multiplying factor	Scaled quantity
Benzoic acid	6 g	0.5	3 g
Salicylic acid	3 g	0.5	1.5 g
Emulsifying ointment	91 g	0.5	45.5 g

Double-check: the quantities for the master formula add up to 100 g and the scaled quantities add up to 50 g.

Example 26.18

You are requested to dispense 200 mL of Ammonium Chloride Mixture BPC. The formula can be found in a variety of reference books such as *Martindale*. In this example the master formula gives quantities sufficient for 10 mL. As the prescription is for 200 mL, the multiplying factor is 200/10. Thus the quantity of each ingredient in the master formula has to be multiplied by 20 to provide the required amount.

Ingredient	Master formula	Scaled quantity
Ammonium chloride	1 g	20 g
Aromatic solution of ammonia	0.5 mL	10 mL
Liquorice liquid extract	1 mL	20 mL
Water	to 10 mL	to 200 mL

Because this formula contains a mixture of volumes and weights it is not possible to calculate the exact quantity of water which is required. However, it is always good practice to have an idea of what the approximate quantity will be. The liquid ingredients of the preparation, other than the water, add up to 30 mL and there is 20 g of ammonium chloride. The volume of water required will therefore be between 150 mL and 170 mL.

Example 26.19

Calculate the quantities required to produce 300 mL Turpentine Liniment BP 1988.

Ingredient	Master formula
Soft soap	75 g
Camphor	50 g
Turpentine oil	650 mL
Water	225 mL

When the total number of units is added up for this formula it comes to 1000. However, because it is a combination of solids and liquids, it will not produce 1000 mL. The prescription is for 300 mL and experience shows that calculating for 340 units will provide slightly more than 300 mL. The required amount can then be measured.

Ingredient	Master formula	Scaled quantity for 340 units
Soft soap	75 g	25.5 g
Camphor	50 g	17 g
Turpentine oil	650 mL	221 mL
Water	225 mL	76.5 mL

Calculations involving parts

In the following example the quantities are expressed as parts of the whole. The number of parts is added up and the quantity of each ingredient calculated by proportion or multiplying factor, to provide the correct amounts (Example 26.20).

There are some situations when extra care is necessary in reading the prescription (Example 26.21).

Example 26.20

The quantity which is to be prepared of the following formula is 60 g.

Ingredient	Master formula	Quantity for 60 g
Zinc oxide	12.5 parts	7.5 g
Calamine	15 parts	9 g
Hydrous wool fat	25 parts	15 g
White soft paraffin	47.5 parts	28.5 g

The total number of parts adds up to 100 so the proportions of each ingredient will be 12.5/100 of zinc oxide, 15/100 of calamine and so on. The required quantity of each ingredient can then be calculated. Zinc oxide 12.5/100 of 60 g, calamine 15/100 of 60 g, etc. as indicated above.

Example 26.21

Two products are to be dispensed:

Betnovate® cream	1 part
Aqueous cream	to 4 parts

Prepare 50 g

Haelan® ointment	1 part
White soft paraffin	4 parts

Prepare 50 g

At first glance these calculations look similar but the quantities required for each are different. In the Betnovate prescription the total number of parts is 4, i.e. 1 part of Betnovate and 3 parts of aqueous cream to produce a total of 4 parts. However, in the Haelan prescription the total number of parts is 5, i.e. 1 part of Haelan ointment and 4 parts of white soft paraffin.

The quantities required for the prescriptions are as follows:

Betnovate® cream	12.5 g
Aqueous cream	37.5 g
Haelan® ointment	10 g
White soft paraffin	40 g

Calculations involving percentages

There are conventions which apply when dealing with formulae which include percentages:

- A solid in a formula where the final quantity is stated as a weight is calculated as weight in weight (w/w)
- A solid in a formula where the final quantity is stated as a volume is calculated as weight in volume (w/v)
- A liquid in a formula where the final quantity is stated as a volume is calculated as volume in volume (v/v)
- A liquid in a formula where the final quantity is stated as a weight is calculated as weight in weight (w/w) (Example 26.22).

When dealing with preparations where ingredients are expressed as a percentage concentration it is important to check that the standard conventions apply because there are some situations where they do not apply. Two examples are given below:

1. Syrup BP is a liquid – a solution of sucrose and water. If the normal convention applied it would be w/v, i.e. a certain weight of sucrose in a final volume of syrup. However, in the BP formula the concentration of sucrose is quoted as w/w. Therefore Syrup BP is:

   Sucrose 66.7% w/w

   Water to 100%

This means that when preparing Syrup BP the appropriate weight of sucrose is weighed out and water is added to the required weight, not volume.

2. A gas in a solution is always calculated as w/w, unless specified otherwise. Formaldehyde Solution BP is a solution of 34–38% w/w formaldehyde in water.

Changing concentrations

Sometimes it is necessary to increase or decrease the concentration of a medicine by the addition of more drug or a diluent. On other occasions, instructions have to be provided to prepare a dilution for use. These problems can be solved by the dilution equation:

$$C_1V_1 = C_2V_2$$

where C_1 and V_1 are the initial concentration and initial volume respectively; and C_2 and V_2 are the final concentration and final quantity of the mixture respectively.

When three terms of the equation are known, the fourth term can be made the subject of the formula, and solved (Examples 26.24–26.27).

Example 26.22

Prepare 500 g of the following ointment

Ingredient	Master formula	Quantity for 500 g
Sulphur 2%	0.2 g	10 g
Salicylic acid 1%	0.1 g	5 g
White soft paraffin to 10 g	to 10 g	485 g (to 500 g)

The master formula is for a total of 10 g. To calculate the quantities required for 500 g the multiplying factor for each ingredient is 500/10 = 50. Remember do not multiply the percentage figure. This always remains the same no matter how much is being prepared.

In the following example a liquid ingredient, the coal tar solution, is stated as a percentage and a weight in grams of final product is requested. The convention of % w/w is applied (Example 26.23).

Example 26.23

The quantity to be made is 30 g.

Ingredient	Master formula	Quantity for 30 g
Coal tar solution 3%	3 g	0.9 g
Zinc oxide 5 g	5 g	1.5 g
Yellow soft paraffin to 100 g	92 g	27.6 g

Example 26.24

What is the final concentration if 60 mL of a 12% w/v chlorhexidine solution is diluted to 120 mL with water?

$C_1 = 12\%$, $V_1 = 60$ mL, $C_2 = y\%$, $V_2 = 120$ mL

$12 \times 60 = 120 \times y$, therefore

$y = 12 \times 60/120 = 6\%$ w/v

Example 26.25

What concentration is produced when 400 mL of a 2.5% w/v solution is diluted to 1500 mL (answer to 2 decimal places)?

$C_1 = 2.5\%$, $V_1 = 400$ mL, $C_2 = y$, $V_2 = 1500$ mL
$2.5\% \times 400$ mL $= y \times 1500$ mL, therefore
$y = 2.5 \times 400/1500 = 0.67\%$ w/v

Example 26.26

What volume of 1% w/v solution can be made from 75 mL of 5% w/v solution?

$1\% \times V_1 = 5\% \times 75$ mL
$V_1 = 5/1 \times 75 = 375$ mL

Example 26.27

What percentage of atropine is produced when 200 mg of atropine powder is made up to 50 g with lactose as a diluent?
The atropine powder is a pure drug, so its concentration (C_1) is 100% w/w. The initial weight of the atropine powder (W_1) = 200 mg = 0.2 g. Therefore, we can modify the dilution equation to read:

Alligation

Alligation is a method for solving the number of parts of two or more components of known concentration to be mixed when the final desired concentration is known. When the relative amounts of components must be calculated for making a mixture of a desired concentration, the problem is most easily solved by alligation (Examples 26.28 and 26.29).

Calculations where quantity of ingredients is too small to weigh or measure accurately

When preparing medicines by extemporaneous dispensing, the quantity of active ingredient required may be too small to weigh or measure with the equipment available. In these situations a measurable

$$C_1 W_1 = C_2 W_2$$

where C_2 and W_2 are the final concentration and final weight respectively, of the diluted drug. The diluting medium is the lactose.

Thus, $100\% \times 0.2$ g $= C_2 \times 50$ g
Therefore $C_2 = 100 \times 0.2/50 = 0.4\%$ w/w

Example 26.28

Calculate the amounts of a 2% w/w metronidazole cream and of metronidazole powder required to produce 150 g of 6% w/w metronidazole cream (to 2 decimal places).
In alligation, the two starting material concentrations are placed above each other on the left hand side of the calculation. The target concentration is placed in the centre. The arithmetic difference between the starting material and the target is calculated and the answer recorded on the right hand end of the diagonal. The proportions of the two starting materials are then given by reading horizontally across the diagram.

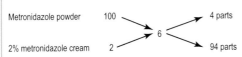

Metronidazole powder   100   4 parts
                              6
2% metronidazole cream   2   94 parts

As shown above, the difference between the concentration

of the pure drug powder (100%, recorded top left) and the desired concentration (6%) is 94 (recorded bottom right). This is equivalent to the number of parts of 2% cream required (read horizontally across the bottom). Similarly, the difference between the concentration of 2% cream (recorded bottom left) and the desired concentration (6%) is 4 (recorded top right). This is equivalent to the number of parts of 100% drug (metronidazole powder) needed for the mixture (read horizontally across the top).

The total amount (4 parts + 94 parts = 98 parts) is 150 g.
Thus, 1 part = 150/98 g.
Therefore, the amount of 2% cream required
= 94 parts $\times$ 150/98 g = 143.88 g.
The amount of pure metronidazole (100%) required
= 4 parts $\times$ 150/98 = 6.12 g.

Example 26.29

Promazine oral syrup is available as 25 mg/5 mL and 50 mg/5 mL. Calculate the quantities to use to prepare 150 mL of 40 mg/5 mL of the oral syrup.

Convert all the concentrations to percentages. Therefore, 25 mg/5 mL is equivalent to 0.025 g in 5 mL = 0.500 g in 100 mL = 0.5% w/v. Similarly, 50 mg/5 mL = 1% w/v; and 40 mg/5 mL = 0.8% w/v.

Using the alligation method:

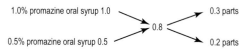

1.0% promazine oral syrup 1.0 → 0.3 parts
0.8
0.5% promazine oral syrup 0.5 → 0.2 parts

Total number of parts

= 0.3 part + 0.2 parts = 0.5 parts = 150 mL.

Amount of 50 mg/5 mL (1.0% w/v) oral syrup needed

= 0.3/0.5 × 150 mL = 90 mL.

Amount of 25 mg/5 mL (0.5% w/v) oral syrup needed

= 0.2/0.5 × 150 mL = 60 mL.

---

quantity has to be diluted with an inert diluent. The process is called 'trituration' (see Ch. 35).

Small quantities in powders

The method for preparing divided powders is described in Chapter 35 (Example 26.30).

Small quantities in liquids

If the quantity of a solid to be incorporated into a solution is too small to weigh, again dilutions are used. In this case a solution is prepared, so the solubility of the substance needs to be considered. Normally a 1 in 10 or 1 in 100 dilution is used (Example 26.31).

Example 26.30

Calculate the quantities required to make 10 powders each containing 200 micrograms of digoxin.
Assume that the balance available has a minimum weighable quantity of 100 mg. An inert diluent, in this case lactose, will be used for the trituration. The convenient weight of each divided powder is 120 mg.
The total weight of powder mixture required will be 10 × 120 = 1200 milligrams = 1.2 g.
Quantities for 10 powders:

Digoxin	2 mg
Lactose	1198 mg
Total	1200 mg

The weight of digoxin is too small to weigh. The minimum weighable quantity of 100 mg is weighed and used in the triturate. A 1 in 10 dilution is produced.

Trituration A

Digoxin	100 mg
Lactose	900 mg
Total	1000 mg

Each 100 mg of this mixture (A) contains 10 mg of digoxin.

Trituration B

Mixture A	100 mg (= 10 mg digoxin)
Lactose	900 mg
Total	1000 mg

Each 100 mg of this mixture (B) contains 1 mg of digoxin. This amount of digoxin is less than the required amount, so mixture B can be used to give the required quantity.

200 mg of mixture B provides the 2 mg digoxin required.

Final trituration (C)

Mixture B	200 mg (= 2 mg digoxin)
Lactose	(1200–200) = 1000 mg
Total	1200 mg

Each 120 mg of this mixture (C) will contain 200 micrograms (0.2 mg) of digoxin.

Example 26.31

Calculate the quantities required to prepare 100 mL of a solution containing 2.5 mg morphine hydrochloride/5 mL. Quantities for 100 mL:

Morphine hydrochloride   50 mg
Chloroform water   to 100 mL
The solubility of morphine hydrochloride is 1 in 24 of water.

The minimum quantity of 100 mg of morphine hydrochloride is weighed and made up to 10 mL with chloroform water (this weight of morphine hydrochloride will dissolve in 2.4 mL).
5 mL of this solution (A) provides the 50 mg of morphine hydrochloride required. Take 5 mL of solution A and make up to 100 mL with chloroform water.

Solubilities

When preparing pharmaceutical products, the solubility of any solid ingredients should be checked. This will give useful information on how the product should be prepared. Examples of the calculations are given in Chapters 25 and 30. The objective of this section is to clarify the terminology used when solubilities are stated.

The solubility of a drug can be found in reference sources such as the drug monograph in *Martindale*. The method of stating solubilities is as follows:

Sodium chloride is soluble 1 in 2.8 of water,

1 in 250 of alcohol and 1 in 10 of glycerol

This means that 1 g of sodium chloride requires 2.8 mL of water, 250 mL of alcohol or 10 mL of glycerol to dissolve it. An example of how knowledge of a substance's solubility can help in extemporaneous dispensing can be found in Chapter 25. Some examples of calculating quantities of liquids required to dissolve solids are found in the self-assessment section (questions 6.1–6.4) at the end of this chapter.

Calculations involving doses

A simple calculation which pharmacists sometimes have to make while dispensing is to calculate the number of tablets or capsules or volume of a liquid medicine to be dispensed (Examples 26.32 and 26.33).

Calculating doses

An overdose of a drug, if given to a patient, can have very serious consequences and may be fatal. It is the responsibility of everyone involved in supplying or administering drugs to ensure that the accuracy and suitability of the dose are checked. The following are some examples of areas where errors can occur.

The standard way to check whether a drug dose is appropriate is to consult a recognized reference book. One of the commonest used for this purpose is the *British National Formulary* (BNF). When first using any reference source it is important to be aware of the terminology used, to avoid misinterpreting the entries, especially where doses are quoted as 'x milligrams daily, in divided doses'. An explanation of the terminology will usually be given in the introduction to the book (Example 26.34).

Example 26.32

The doctor prescribes orphenadrine tablets, 100 mg to be taken every 8 hours for 28 days. Orphenadrine is available as 50 mg tablets. How many tablets should be supplied?
For each dose, 2 tablets are required. Every eight hours means 3 doses per day.
Therefore, the total number of tablets required is
$2 \times 3 \times 28 = 168$ tablets.

Example 26.33

The following prescription is received:

Sodium valproate oral solution:
    100 mg to be given twice daily for 2 weeks.
Sodium valproate oral solution contains sodium valproate 200 mg/5 mL.

This prescription is therefore translated as:
2.5 mL to be given twice daily for 2 weeks.
The quantity to be dispensed will be:
$2.5 \times 2 \times 14 = 70$ mL.

Example 26.34

The following prescription is received:

Verapamil tablets 160 milligrams

Send 56

Take two tablets twice daily

There are a variety of doses quoted for verapamil in the BNF depending on the condition being treated. They are as follows for oral administration:

Supraventricular arrhythmias, 40–120 mg three times daily

Angina, 80–120 mg three times daily

Hypertension, 240–480 mg daily in 2–3 divided doses.

The dose given for hypertension is stated in a significantly different way. Whereas the other doses can be given three times daily, indicating a maximum of 360 mg in any one day, the hypertension dose is the total to be given in any one day and is divided up and given at the stated frequencies, i.e. a maximum of 240 mg, given twice daily or a maximum of 160 mg, given three times daily.

The prescription is for a dose higher than recommended, so consultation with the prescriber would be required. Be alert – variation in terminology and a lack of awareness could have very serious consequences.

Calculations of children's doses

Children often require different doses from those of adults. Ideally these should be arrived at as a result of extensive clinical studies, although this is often not possible. When this is the case an estimate of the dose has to be made. This is best carried out using body weight (see next section), but where this is not available, there are three formulas which relate the child's dose to the adult dose.

Fried's rule for infants

Age (month) $\times$ adult dose/150 = dose for infant

Clark's rule

Weight (in kg) $\times$ adult dose/75 = dose for child

Body surface area (BSA) method

BSA of child $(m^2) \times$ adult dose/1.73 m^2

(average adult BSA) = approximate child's dose

Calculation of doses by weight and surface area

For some drugs the amount of drug has to be calculated accurately for the particular patient. This is normally carried out using either body weight or body surface area. When body weight is being used, the dose will be expressed as mg/kg. In countries which still use pounds, it will be necessary to convert the patient's weight in pounds into kilograms by dividing by 2.2. The total dose required is then obtained by multiplying the weight of the patient by the dose per kilogram.

Body surface area is a more accurate method for calculating doses and is used where extreme accuracy is required. This is necessary where there is a very narrow range of plasma concentration between the desired therapeutic effect and severe toxicity, such as with the drugs used to treat cancer. The body surface area can be calculated from body weight and height using the equation given below, but it is more usual to use a nomogram for its determination. The actual nomogram is published in many reference sources.

$$\text{Body surface area } (m^2) = \text{weight } (kg)^{0.5378}$$
$$\times \text{ height } (cm)^{0.37} \times 0.024265$$

Reconstitution and infusion

Some drugs are not chemically stable in solution and so are supplied as dry powders for reconstitution just before use. Many of these are antibiotics, but there is also a range of chemotherapeutic agents used in cancer treatment. The antibiotics may be for oral use or for injection. An oral antibiotic for reconstitution comes as a powder in a bottle with sufficient space to add the water. The powder itself will remain stable for up to 2 years when dry. When reconstituted, a shelf life of 10–14 days is normal, depending on whether it is refrigerated or not. Those for injection are equally stable when dry, but are intended to be used within hours of reconstitution. Because they are for injection they are sterile powders and are dissolved in sterile water aseptically (see Ch. 29). There are a number of calculations which may be required around the reconstitution processes (Example 26.35).

Example 26.35

What dose of antibiotic will be contained in a 5 mL spoonful when a bottle containing 5 g of penicillin V is reconstituted to give 200 mL of syrup?

For this type of calculation, the simple proportion equation can be used:

$Wt_1/Wt_2 = Vol_1/Vol_2$
5 g = 5000 mg.
Substituting we get:
5000 mg/y mg = 200 mL/5 mL
y = 125 mg.

Example 26.37

The label on an ampicillin bottle indicates that 78 mL of water must be added to produce 100 mL of final syrup. How much water must be added to give the 125 mL final volume?

Thus, the volume of powder in the final syrup is:

100 mL − 78 mL = 22 mL.

Therefore, the volume to add to give 125 mL is:

125 mL − 22 mL = 103 mL.

Example 26.36

We have an ampicillin product for reconstitution. It contains 2.5 g of ampicillin to be made up to 100 mL. To what volume should it be made to give 100 mg per 5 mL dose?

The normal mixture will give a dose of:

2500 mg/y mg = 100 mL/5 mL
y = 125 mg per 5 mL

To calculate the amount of water to add, the same equation is used:

2500 mg/100 mg = y mL/5 mL
y = 125 mL.

Sometimes, the doctor may request a more or less concentrated syrup to be produced which requires altering the amount of water added from that indicated by the manufacturer (Example 26.36).

However, this type of oral mixture is likely to have other ingredients – thickeners, colours, flavours, etc. – which will occupy some of the final volume. So this may not be correct and we need to be able to calculate exactly how much water to add (Examples 26.37 and 26.38).

Drugs for injection solutions do not normally contain ingredients other than the drug (or they make an insignificant contribution to the final volume). However, they are usually packed as a quantity of drug with the final volume left to be calculated by the pharmacist (Example 26.39).

Calculation of infusion rates

Drugs may be given to patients intravenously by adding them to an intravenous (IV) infusion (see Ch. 38). Calculations involve working out how much drug solution should be added, working out how fast, in terms of mL/min, the infusion should be administered, and calculating what this means in terms of 'drops per minute' through the giving set. When an infusion pump is used, this can be set to deliver a specified number of mL/min. The final stage of drops/min is only required for traditional IV 'drips' (see Ch. 38) (Example 26.40).

Example 26.38

A child weighing 60 lb requires a dose of 8 mg/kg of ampicillin. Given that a 5 mL dose is to be given, what volume of water must be added when the powder is reconstituted? Instructions on the label indicate that dilution to 150 mL (by adding 111 mL) gives 250 mg ampicillin per 5 mL.

Conversion of weight to kg: 60/2.2 = 27.27 kg
Calculation of amount of ampicillin required:
27.27 × 8 = 218 mg.

Calculation of amount of ampicillin in container:
250 mg/y mg = 5 mL/150 mL, therefore
y = 7500 mg = 7.5 g
Calculation of amount of water (a) to add to give 218 mg per 5 mL: 218 mg/7500 mg = 5 mL/a mL, therefore
a = 172 mL
Volume occupied by powder: 150 mL − 111 mL = 39 mL
Therefore, volume to be added:
172 mL − 39 mL = 133 mL.

Example 26.39

Calculate the amount of sterile water to be added to a vial containing 200 000 units of penicillin G in order to produce a solution containing 40 000 units per millilitre. Again, simple proportion is used:

40 000 units/200 000 units = 1 mL/y mL, therefore
  y = 5 mL.

Example 26.40

An ampoule of flucloxacillin contains 250 mg of powder with instructions to dissolve it in 5 mL of water for injections. What volume of this solution should be added to 500 mL of saline infusion to provide a dose of 175 mg?

250 mg in 5 mL = 50 mg per mL

Therefore, we require: 175 mg/50 mg/mL = 3.5 mL.

When administering intravenous infusions, the rate of addition is first calculated in terms of millilitres per minute (Example 26.41).

Example 26.41

100 mg of phenylephrine hydrochloride are added to 500 mL of saline infusion. What should be the rate of infusion to give a dose of 1 mg per minute? How long will the infusion take?

Using simple proportion: 100 mg/1 mg = 500 mL/y mL
y = 5 mL and contains the required amount of drug

The infusion rate should be 5 mL per minute.
The total volume is 500 mL, therefore the time taken at 5 mL/min is:

500 mL/5 mL/min = 100 min.

Most infusions are administered using a giving set with a dropping device on the tube (called venoclysis set; see Ch. 38). Partial clamping of the tube can be used to adjust the rate of dropping. Depending on the drop size – that is the number of drops per millilitre – it is then possible to convert a rate of millilitres per minute into drops per minute which the nurse can adjust (Example 26.42).

A variation on this is when the doctor wishes a drug solution to be added to the infusion (Example 26.43).

Example 26.42

A doctor requires an infusion of 1000 mL of 5% dextrose to be administered over an 8 hour period. Using an IV giving set which delivers 10 drops/mL, how many drops per minute should be delivered to the patient?
First convert the time into minutes:

8 hour = 8 × 60 min = 480 min

Next calculate how many mL/min are required:
1000 mL/480 min = 2.1 mL/min

Then calculate the number of drops this requires:

2.1 mL/min × 10 drops/min = 21 drops/min.

Example 26.43

20 mL of a drug solution is added to a 500 mL infusion solution. It has to be administered to the patient over a 5 hour period. Using a set giving 15 drops per millilitre, how many drops per minute are required?
The total volume of infusion is:

20 mL + 500 mL = 520 mL

Then calculate the number of drops which will be administered in total:

520 mL × 15 drops = 7800 drops

The duration of the infusion is to be:

5 (hours) × 60 = 300 min

Calculate how many drops are required per minute:

7800 drops/300 min = 26 drops per min.

KEY POINTS

- Always work methodically and write down calculations clearly
- Check calculations, using a different method where possible
- Estimate the answer before you start
- Try to visualize the quantities you are using in the calculation
- Look carefully to see if a formula gives the quantities of all ingredients or uses 'to' for the vehicle
- Equations can be a useful way of carrying out calculations, but care is required to ensure that the correct figures are being used
- Always check the units being used and be careful not to mix them during a calculation
- Be very careful to read the wording; small changes in terminology can alter the calculation
- Triturates with solids and liquids normally use a 1 in 10 dilution per step
- Be very careful in checking doses, particularly with 'in divided doses' and 'mg/kg' statements in the reference books
- On completion of a calculation, ask yourself whether the answer is 'reasonable' given the numbers you are using

Self-assessment questions

(Express answers to 2 decimal places where appropriate.)

1.1 Express 20 grains in grams.

1.2 Express 300 p.p.m. as a percentage strength.

1.3 Express 324 mg in grains.

1.4 What is the total volume to be dispensed when the prescription states:
5 mL three times daily for 2/52?

1.5 Calculate the number of tablets to be dispensed when the prescription states:
2 tablets four times daily for 2/52.

1.6 Calculate the volume of and total quantity to be dispensed for a prescription for a drug which is available as a 250 mg/5 mL syrup:
100 mg twice daily for 3/52.

2.1 Express the following as percentages (indicating w/w, w/v, v/v, where appropriate):
a 1 g in 220 mL of solution
b 110 mg of sodium chloride in 100 mL of solution
c 0.3 mL in 2.5 mL of solution

d 2 g in 630 g of solution
e 50 mg of sodium chloride in 120 mL
f 2 L of drug in 5000 mL of solution
g 3600 parts per million
h 1 in 4000 solution
i 170 mg of potassium chloride in 90 mL
j 0.15 mL in 13 mL
k 2 g in 630 mL
l 100 microgram/5 mL
m 1.2 mg/mL.

2.2 Express 0.025% w/w as 1 part in ...

2.3 The following are examples of concentrations expressed as percentages. Indicate the amount of drug present in:
a 90 mL of 1.3% w/v solution
b 15 mL of 4.2% w/v preparation
c 2 L of a 0.05% v/v preparation
d 50 mL of 3.2% w/v preparation
e 75 g of a 0.6% w/w mixture
f 150 mL of a 0.002% w/v preparation.

2.4 What weight of lactose is required to make 80 mL of 3.0% w/v solution?

2.5 How much drug is required to prepare 50 g of a 0.3% w/w mixture?

2.6 Express 0.4% w/v as mg/mL.

2.7 How many milligrams of drug are there in 5 mL of 2% w/v solution?

2.8 Calculate the number of milligrams of the following compounds to be dissolved in 1 L of aqueous solution to give a concentration of 10 mmol:
(Atomic weights: $H = 1$, $C = 12$, $N = 14$, $O = 16$, $S = 32$, $Cl = 35.5$, $K = 39$)
a Hydrochloric acid (HCl)
b Sulphuric acid (H_2SO_4)
c Potassium chloride (KCl)
d A drug with the molecular formula $C_{12}H_{12}ONCl$.

2.9 Express 222 mg of calcium chloride ($CaCl_2$) in 2 L of solution as millimoles.
(Atomic weights: $Ca = 40$, $Cl = 35.5$)

2.10 How many grams of aspirin ($C_9H_8O_4$) are contained in 1 millimole?

2.11 How many mmol are there in 15 g of tetracycline hydrochloride ($C_{22}H_{24}N_2O_8HCl$)?

3.1 What weight of each ingredient is required for the extemporaneous preparation if 50 g of the following preparation is to be made?

Hydrocortisone	10 g
Oxytetracycline	30 g
Wool fat	100 g
White soft paraffin	860 g

3.2 Calculate the quantities for the following prescriptions:

a
White beeswax	20 g
Hard paraffin	30 g
Cetostearyl alcohol	50 g
Soft paraffin	900 g
Prepare	150 g

b
Light magnesium carbonate	3 g
Sodium bicarbonate	5 g
Aromatic cardamom tincture	3 mL
Chloroform water, double strength	50 mL
Water	to 100 mL
Send	120 mL

3.3 Calculate the quantities required for the following extemporaneous preparations:

a
Ichthammol	5 parts
Cetostearyl alcohol	3 parts
Wool fat	10 parts
Zinc cream	to 100 parts
Send	120 g

b
Chlorhexidine gluconate 20% solution	5 parts
Cetomacrogol emulsifying wax	25 parts
Liquid paraffin	10 parts
Water	to 100 parts
Send	30 g

c
Zinc oxide	6 parts
Arachis oil	7 parts
Wool fat	2 parts
Water	to 20 parts
Send	60 g

d
Wool alcohols	6%
Soft paraffin	10%
Hard paraffin	24%
Liquid paraffin	60%
Send	30 g

e
Menthol	2%
Eucalyptus oil	10%
Light magnesium carbonate	7%
Water	to 100%
Send	150 mL

f
Cetrimide	3%
Cetostearyl alcohol	13.5 g
White soft paraffin	25 g

| Liquid paraffin | to 50 g |
| Send | 150 g |

g
Starch	7 parts
Zinc oxide	8 parts
Olive oil	2 parts
Wool fat	3 parts
Send	30 g

h
Cetomacrogol emulsifying wax	60 g
Benzyl alcohol	3 g
Methyl paraben	2.3%
Water	to 200 g
Send	40 g

i
Cetrimide	3%
Cetostearyl alcohol	13.5 g
White soft paraffin	25 g
Liquid paraffin	to 50 g
Send	40 g

4.1 How much cetrimide is required to make 30 mL of a solution which, when 1 mL is diluted to 100 mL, produces a 100 parts per million solution?

4.2 What percentage is produced when 200 mg of powder is made up to 40 g with a diluent?

4.3 What concentration is produced when 75 mL of an 8% solution is diluted to 3 L?

4.4 What concentration is produced when 200 mL of a 1 in 40 solution is diluted to 1000 mL?

4.5 What concentration is produced when 75 mL of a 1 in 12.5 solution is diluted to 500 mL?

4.6 What weight of drug must be added to 100 g of 2% ointment to produce a 3.5% ointment?

4.7 Sulphur ointment is available as 5% w/w and 8% w/w. Calculate the quantities needed to prepare 60 g of 6% w/w ointment.

4.8 Orphenadrine syrup is available as 25 mg/ 5 mL and 50 mg/5 mL. Calculate the quantities to use to prepare 1000 mL of 45 mg/5 mL syrup.

4.9 What weight of drug must be added to 50 g of 2% ointment to produce a 3% ointment?

4.10 Calculate the amount of drug and 2.5% w/w ointment to make 60 g of 3.5% ointment.

4.11 How much of a 0.5% solution is required so that when diluted to 600 mL it produces a 1 in 8000 solution?

4.12 What volume of normal saline (0.9% w/v NaCl) can be made from 1.5 g NaCl?

4.13 What volume of 0.8% solution can be made from 300 mL of 2.5% solution?

4.14 What volume of 2% solution can be made from 225 mL of 5% solution?

4.15 What volume of 0.5% solution can be made from 300 mL of 1 in 40 solution?

4.16 How many grams of ichthammol must be added to an ointment base to produce 150 g of a 0.13% w/w ichthammol?

4.17 Calculate the weight of drug which must be added to 1 litre of a 17% w/v solution (density 1.2 g/mL) to make a 20% w/w solution.

4.18 Calculate the volume of 4% solution of cetrimide to prepare 600 mL of a 1 in 1000 solution.

4.19 Calculate the volume of 2% of potassium permanganate required to prepare 1 L of a 0.01% solution.

4.20 Calculate the volume of 1 in 20 solution of chlorhexidine to prepare 250 mL of a 0.2% solution.

5.1 Calculate how to make 30×120 mg powders, each containing 0.5 mg of colchicine.

5.2 Calculate how to make 10×120 mg powders, each containing 2 mg of carbachol.

5.3 Calculate how to make 20×120 mg powders, each containing 0.4 mg of atropine sulphate.

5.4 Calculate how to make 20×120 mg capsules, each containing 0.6 mg of hyoscine hydrobromide.

6.1 How much water is required to dissolve:
  a 5 g of aspirin (solubility 1 in 300)?
  b 50 mg of morphine sulphate (solubility 1 in 21)?
  c 40 mg of hydralazine hydrochloride (solubility 1 in 25)?

6.2 How much lithium carbonate will dissolve in 20 mL of water (solubility 1 in 100)? If 300 mg is to be dispensed, will it dissolve in 20 mL of water?

6.3 300 mg quinine hydrobromide (solubility 1 in 55) is to be dispensed; will it dissolve in 30 mL of water?

6.4 A drug has a solubility 1 in 50 of water and 1 in 14 of alcohol.
  a Will 250 milligrams dissolve in 4 mL of water?
  b Will 4 g dissolve in 60 mL of alcohol?
  c Will 10 micrograms dissolve in 0.002 mL of water?
  d Will 1 kg dissolve in 3 L of alcohol?

  e Will 0.05 g dissolve in 0.2 mL of alcohol?

7.1 For the following prescriptions calculate the dose of active ingredient which the patient will be taking on each occasion and each day.
  a Sudafed elixir
     Mitte 150 mL
     Sig. 3 mL t.i.d.
     (Sudafed elixir contains pseudoephedrine 30 milligrams/5 mL.)
  b Codeine linctus half strength
     Mitte 200 mL
     Sig. 2.5 mL t.i.d.
     (Codeine linctus contains codeine phosphate 15 milligrams/5 mL.)
  c Ketotifen elixir
     Mitte 300 mL
     Sig. 7.5 mL b.i.d.
     (Ketotifen elixir contains ketotifen 1 milligram/5 mL.
  d Alimemazine syrup forte
     Mitte 150 mL
     Sig. 10 mL b.i.d.
     (Alimemazine syrup forte contains alimemazine tartrate 30 milligrams/ 5 mL.)

7.2 For the following prescriptions calculate the volume of liquid which the patient will take on each occasion.
  a Loratadine syrup
     Mitte 500 mL
     Sig. 8 milligrams daily
     (Loratadine syrup contains loratadine 5 milligrams/5 mL.)
  b Methadone oral concentrate is available as 20 mg/mL. What volume is required to provide 2 mg, 17 mg, 43 mg?
  c Promethazine elixir
     Mitte 100 mL
     Sig. 12 milligrams daily
     (Promethazine elixir contains promethazine hydrochloride 5 mg/5 mL.)

7.3 What dose of atenolol should be given to a patient weighing 75 kg to provide a dose of 150 micrograms/kg?

7.4 Calculate the dose of cisplatin to provide 60 mg/m^2 for a patient of estimated surface area 1.57 m^2.

8.1   What is the weight of antibiotic in a 5 mL dose when a bottle containing 15 g antibiotic is made up with water to give 150 mL of syrup?

8.2   What is the total volume, after adding water to 15 g of antibiotic, to provide a 250 mg dose per 5 mL dose?

8.3   The label on a bottle of ampicillin syrup indicates that 92 mL of water should be added to make 100 mL of syrup. How much water should be added to produce 130 mL of syrup?

8.4   An injection of amphotericin B contains 50 mg/10 mL. What volume must be added to 500 mL of normal saline infusion to produce a 1200 microgram/mL solution?

9.1   An infusion solution contains 5 g in 500 mL. What rate of infusion should be used to give 16 mg/min? How long will a 500 mL infusion last?

9.2   In preparing an IV infusion, you have a solution containing 2 g/mL furosemide (molecular weight 330.7). What volume must be added to a 500 mL infusion to provide a 12 mmol total dose?

10.1 Paregoric is 4% v/v tincture of opium which is 10% w/v opium. If opium contains 10% w/w morphine what weight of morphine is contained in a 30 mL bottle of Paregoric?

Self-assessment answers

1.1	1.30 g
1.2	0.03%
1.3	5 grains
1.4	210 mL
1.5	112 tablets
1.6	A 2 mL dose and a total of 84 mL to be dispensed
2.1a	0.45% w/v
2.1b	0.11% w/v
2.1c	12% v/v
2.1d	0.32% w/w
2.1e	0.04% w/v
2.1f	40% v/v
2.1g	0.36%
2.1h	0.03%
2.1i	0.19% w/v
2.1j	1.15% v/v
2.1k	0.32% w/v
2.1l	0.0020% w/v
2.1m	0.12% w/v
2.2	1 in 4000
2.3a	1.17 g
2.3b	0.63 g
2.3c	1 mL
2.3d	1.6 g
2.3e	0.45 g or 450 mg
2.3f	0.003 g or 3 mg
2.4	2.40 g
2.5	0.15 g or 150 mg
2.6	4 mg/mL
2.7	100 mg
2.8a	365 mg
2.8b	980 mg
2.8c	745 mg
2.8d	2215 mg
2.9	1 mmol
2.10	0.18 g or 180 mg
2.11	31.22 mmol

3.1	Hydrocortisone	0.5 g
	Oxytetracycline	1.5 g
	Wool fat	5 g
	White soft paraffin	43 g
3.2a	White beeswax	3 g
	Hard paraffin	4.5 g
	Cetostearyl alcohol	7.5 g
	Soft paraffin	135 g
3.2b	Light magnesium carbonate	3.6 g
	Sodium bicarbonate	6.0 g
	Aromatic cardamom tincture	3.6 mL
	Chloroform water, double strength	60 mL
	Water	to 120 mL
3.3a	Ichthammol	6 g
	Cetostearyl alcohol	3.6 g
	Wool fat	12 g
	Zinc cream	to 120 g
3.3b	Chlorhexidine gluconate 20% solution	1.5 g
	Cetomacrogol emulsifying wax	7.5 g
	Liquid paraffin	3 g
	Water	to 30 g

3.3c	Zinc oxide	18 g
	Arachis oil	21 g
	Wool fat	6 g
	Water	to 60 g
3.3d	Wool alcohols	1.8 g
	Soft paraffin	3 g
	Hard paraffin	7.2 g
	Liquid paraffin	18 g
3.3e	Menthol	3 g
	Eucalyptus oil	15 mL
	Light magnesium carbonate	10.5 g
	Water	to 150 mL
3.3f	Cetrimide	4.5 g
	Cetostearyl alcohol	40.5 g
	White soft paraffin	75 g
	Liquid paraffin	30 g
3.3g	Starch	10.5 g
	Zinc oxide	12 g
	Olive oil	3 g
	Wool fat	4.5 g
3.3h	Cetomacrogol emulsifying wax	12 g
	Benzyl alcohol	0.6 g
	Methyl paraben	0.92 g
	Water	26.48 g
3.3i	Cetrimide	1.2 g
	Cetostearyl alcohol	10.8 g
	White soft paraffin	20 g
	Liquid paraffin	8 g

4.1 0.3 g

4.2 0.5% w/w

4.3 0.2%

4.4 0.5%

4.5 1.2%

4.6 1.55 g

4.7 5% ointment 40 g, 8% ointment 20 g

4.8 25 mg/5 mL 200 mL, 50 mg/5 mL 800 mL

4.9 0.52 g

4.10 Drug 0.62 g, Ointment 59.38 g

4.11 15 mL

4.12 166.67 mL

4.13 937.5 mL

4.14 562.5 mL

4.15 1500 mL

4.16 195 mg or 0.2 g

4.17 The weight of drug to be added = 87.50 g
17% w/v solution = 14.167% w/w
Weight of 1 litre of 17% w/v solution is 1200 g

4.18 15 mL

4.19 5 mL

4.20 10 mL

5.1 Weigh 100 mg drug, dilute with 900 mg lactose, take 150 mg of mixture and mix with 3.450 g of lactose to give 3.6 g total and divide into 30 × 120 mg separately wrapped powders.

5.2 Weigh 100 mg drug, dilute with 900 mg lactose, take 200 mg of mixture and mix with 1.000 g of lactose to give 1.2 g total and divide into 10 × 120 mg separately wrapped powders.

5.3 Weigh 100 mg drug, dilute with 900 mg lactose, take 100 mg of mixture, dilute with 900 mg lactose, take 800 mg of second mixture and mix with 1.600 g of lactose to give 2.4 g total and divide into 20 × 120 mg separately wrapped powders.

5.4 Weigh 100 mg drug, dilute with 900 mg lactose, take 120 mg of mixture and mix with 2.280 g of lactose to give 2.4 g total and divide into 20 × 120 mg separately wrapped powders.

6.1a 1.5 L or 1500 mL

6.1b 1.05 mL

6.1c 1 mL

6.2 0.2 g or 200 mg. No, because 300 mg of lithium carbonate requires 30 mL of water in which to dissolve.

6.3 Yes

6.4a No, because 250 milligrams of drug requires 12.5 mL of water in which to dissolve.

6.4b Yes, because 4 g of drug requires 56 mL of alcohol in which to dissolve.

6.4c Yes, because 10 micrograms of drug requires 0.0005 mL of water in which to dissolve.

6.4d No, because 1 kg of drug requires 14 L of alcohol in which to dissolve.

6.4e No, because 50 milligrams of drug requires 0.7 mL of alcohol in which to dissolve.

7.1a 18 mg per dose, 54 mg per day

7.1b 3.75 mg per dose, 11.25 mg per day

7.1c 1.5 mg per dose, 3 mg per day

7.1d 60 mg per dose, 120 mg per day

7.2a 8 mL of the syrup

7.2b 2 mg in 0.1 mL, 17 mg in 0.85 mL, 43 mg in 2.15 mL

7.2c	12 mL of the elixir		8.3	122 mL
7.3	11.25 mg		8.4	120 mL
7.4	94.2 mg		9.1	1.6 mL/min, 313 min (5 h 13 min)
8.1	0.5 g or 500 mg		9.2	1.98 mL
8.2	300 mL		10.1	12 mg

Packaging

Derek G. Chapman

- Definition of a container
- Considerations made in selecting a container
- The difference between primary and secondary packaging
- The materials used for packaging, including glass, plastics, metal and paper
- Types of container in common use
- Child-resistant closures and tamper-evident seals
- Patient pack dispensing

Introduction

Pharmaceutical formulations must be suitably contained, protected and labelled from the time of manufacture until the patient uses them. Throughout this period the container must maintain the quality, safety and stability of the medicine and protect the product against physical, climatic, chemical and biological hazards. The *British Pharmacopoeia* identifies the closure as part of the container.

To promote good patient compliance the container must be user friendly. This is particularly significant for the elderly who have to take more medicines than the general population and have a greater need for improved compliance (see Ch. 46). Thus containers should be easy to open and reclose, most notably for elderly or arthritic patients. However, other factors must also be considered in the selection of the container used to package a pharmaceutical formulation, including the cost and the need for both child-resistant closures and tamper-evident seals.

Repackaging is performed in the community pharmacy for dispensing purposes (see Chs 25 and 36), in hospital pharmacy and in specialized production facilities. Bulk medicines are repackaged into smaller quantities in dispensing containers for distribution to hospital wards, clinics and general practitioners for direct supply to patients. This is mostly carried out with tablets and capsules that are transferred from bulk quantities into smaller amounts that are more suitable for patient use. In the UK this process is performed in the hospital pharmacy where the Medicines and Healthcare products Regulatory Agency (MHRA) allows the repackaging of small batches of up to 25 containers. Larger batches must be packed in licensed manufacturing premises. The facilities used for these repackaging operations are designed to maintain the quality of the medicine and avoid product contamination and mix up.

Medicines originally contained in patient packs are subdivided into small amounts by transferring small quantities of the medicine in strip or blister packs into secondary cardboard containers. The composition of containers and closures used for the repackaging of bulk medicines must be carefully selected and must be of a quality as good as the original container. Both glass and plastic containers are used for repackaging but glass containers are often preferred due to the more inert qualities of glass.

Primary containers used for repackaging must not:
- Allow product leakage
- Chemically react with the product
- Release components
- Uptake product components.

The container used in the repackaging process must protect the product from:

- Physical damage
- Chemical and microbial contamination
- Light, moisture and oxygen as appropriate.

As the medicine has been transferred into a new container, the expiry date of the repackaged medicine must not exceed 12 months unless the stability of the repackaged product justifies a longer shelf life. The details of these repackaging processes must be recorded.

Each container of the repackaged batch is labelled with the:

- Identity and quantity of the medicine
- Batch number
- Appropriate storage instructions
- Product expiry date
- Requirements for handling and storage.

There are some situations where the repackaging is limited, such as with glyceryl trinitrate tablets, owing to the potential loss of the volatile drug (see Ch. 36). Sterile products cannot easily be repackaged and require effective closure systems to minimize the risk of microbial contamination of the contents within the container. In addition, the pack itself must withstand sterilization procedures. Consequently, care must be applied to the selection of the container and its closure for the packaging of sterile products (see also Chs 38, 39, 40 and 41).

Primary and secondary packaging

Primary packaging materials are in direct contact with the product. This also applies to the closure, which is also part of the primary pack. It is important that this container must not interact with the medicine. It must protect the medicine from damage and from extraneous chemical and microbial contamination. In addition, the primary packaging should support use of the product by the patient. Secondary packages are additional packaging materials that improve the appearance of the product and include outer wrappers or labels that do not make direct contact with the product (Table 27.1). Secondary packages can also supply information about the product and its use. They should provide evidence of tampering with the medicine.

The following terms are used to describe containers:

Single-dose containers hold the medicine that is intended for single use. An example of such a container is the glass ampoule.

Multidose containers hold a quantity of the material that will be used as two or more doses. An example of this system is the multiple dose vial or the plastic tablet bottle.

Well-closed containers protect the product from contamination with unwanted foreign materials and from loss of contents during use.

Airtight containers are impermeable to solids, liquids and gases during normal storage and use. If the container is to be opened on more than one occasion it must remain airtight after reclosure.

Sealed containers such as glass ampoules are closed by fusion of the container material.

Tamper-evident containers are closed containers fitted with a device that irreversibly indicates if the container has been opened.

Light-resistant containers protect the contents from the effect of radiation at a wavelength between 290 nm and 450 nm.

Child-resistant containers, commonly referred to as CRCs, are designed to prevent children accessing the potentially hazardous product.

Table 27.1 Types of primary and secondary packaging materials and their use

Material	Type	Examples of use
Glass	Primary	Metric medical bottle, ampoule, vial
Plastic	Primary	Ampoule, vial, container, infusion fluid dropper bottle
Plastic	Secondary	Wrapper to contain primary pack
Board	Secondary	Box to contain primary pack
Paper	Secondary	Labels, patient information leaflet

Strip packs have at least one sealed pocket of material with each pocket containing a single dose of the product. The pack is made of two layers of film or laminate material. The nature and the level of protection that is required by the contained product will affect the composition of these layers.

Blister packs are composed of a base layer, with cavities that contain the pharmaceutical product, and a lid. This lid is sealed to the base layer by heat, pressure or both. They are more rigid than strip packs and are not used for powders or semi-solids. Blister packs can be printed with day and week identifiers to produce calendar packs. These identifiers will support patient compliance.

Tropicalized packs are blister packs with an additional aluminium membrane to provide greater protection against high humidity.

Pressurized packs expel the product through a valve. The pressure for the expulsion of the product is provided by the positive pressure of the propellant that is often a compressed or liquefied gas (see Ch. 37).

Original packs are pharmaceutical packs that are commercially produced and intended for finite treatment periods. These packs are dispensed directly to the patient in their original form. Manufacturer's information is contained on the pack but the pharmacist must attach a dispensary label.

An important consideration when selecting the packaging for any product is that its main objective is that the package must contribute to delivering a drug to a specific site of effective activity in the patient.

The selection of packaging for a pharmaceutical product is dependent on the following factors:

- The nature of the product itself: its chemical activity, sensitivity to moisture and oxygen, compatibility with packaging materials
- The type of patient: is it to be used by an elderly or arthritic patient or by a child?
- The dosage form
- Method of administering the medication
- Required shelf life
- Product use, such as for dispensing or for an over the counter product.

See also Chapter 36 in *Pharmaceutics: the Science of Dosage Form Design*.

Packaging materials

Glass

Historically, glass has been widely used as a drug packaging material. It continues to be the preferred packaging material for many pharmaceutical products.

Glass does have several advantages:

- It is inert to most medicinal products
- It is impervious to air and moisture
- It allows easy inspection of the container contents
- It can be coloured to protect contents from harmful wavelengths of light
- It is easy to clean and sterilize by heat
- It is available in variously shaped containers.

The disadvantages of glass include:

- It is fragile: glass fragments can be released into the product during transport or contaminants can penetrate the product by way of cracks in the container
- Certain types of glass release alkali into the container contents
- It is expensive when compared to the price of plastic
- It is heavy resulting in increased transport costs.

The chemical stability of glass for pharmaceutical use is given by the resistance of the glass to the release of soluble minerals into water contacting the glass. This is known as the hydrolytic resistance. Details are given in the British Pharmacopoeia (2007) for three types of glass.

Type I glass

This is also known as neutral glass or borosilicate glass. It possesses a high hydrolytic resistance due to the chemical composition of the glass. It is the most inert type of pharmaceutical glass with the lowest coefficient of thermal expansion. As a result, it is unlikely to crack on exposure to rapid temperature changes. Type I glass is suitable for packing all pharmaceutical preparations. However, it is expensive and this restricts its applications. It is widely used as glass ampoules and vials to package fluids for injection. In addition, it is used to package solutions that could dissolve basic oxides in the glass. This would increase the pH of the formulation and could affect the drug stability and potency.

Type II glass

This is made of soda-lime-silica glass with a high hydrolytic resistance due to surface treatment of the glass. Type II glass is used to package aqueous preparations. In general, it is not used by manufacturers to package parenteral formulations with a pH less than 7. This glass has a lower melting point than Type I glass. It is thus easier to produce and consequently cheaper. It is the glass used to produce containers for eye preparations and other dropper bottles.

Type III glass

This is made of a soda-lime-silica glass. It has a similar composition to Type II glass but contains more leachable oxides. Type III glass offers only moderate resistance to leaching and is commonly used to produce dispensary metric medical bottles. It is also suitable for packaging non-aqueous parenteral products and powders for injection.

Types of glass containers

Bottles

These are commonly used in the dispensary as either amber metric medical bottles or ribbed (fluted) oval bottles. Both types of bottle are available in sizes from 50 mL to 500 mL and are supplied with a screw closure.

Amber metric medical bottles have a smooth curved side and a flat side (Fig. 27.1). The bottle was designed to permit the curved side of the bottle to fit into the palm of the hand when pouring from

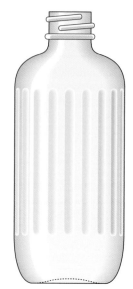

Figure 27.2 • Ribbed oval bottle.

the bottle. The flat side was intended to permit the attachment of a label. In practice, however, the label is commonly attached to the curved surface of the bottle. Amber metric medical bottles are used for packaging a wide range of oral medicines.

Ribbed oval bottles have flutes down one side of the container (Fig. 27.2). The characteristic feel of the flutes warns the user that the contents are not to be taken. A label is attached to the plain front of the bottle. Ribbed oval bottles are used to package various products that should not be taken orally; this includes liniments, lotions, inhalations and antiseptic solutions.

Dropper bottles

Eye drop and dropper bottles for ear and nasal use are hexagonal-shaped amber glass containers fluted on three sides. They are fitted with a cap, rubber teat and dropper as the closure. The bottles are used at a capacity of 10 mL or 20 mL. The label is attached to the plain sides of the bottle.

Jars

Powders and semi-solid preparations are generally packed in wide-mouthed cylindrical jars made of clear or amber glass. The capacity of these jars varies from 15 mL to 500 mL. Ointment jars are used for packing extemporaneously prepared ointments and pastes. They are also used to repackage commercial products where microbial contamination by the patient's fingers is not detrimental to the product.

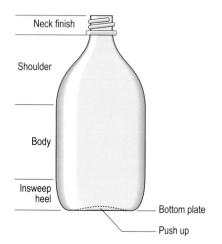

Figure 27.1 • Metric medicine bottle.

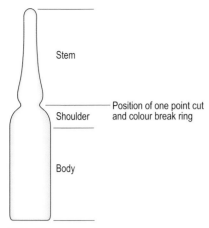

Figure 27.3 • Glass ampoule.

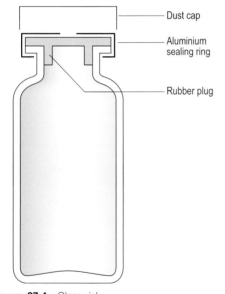

Figure 27.4 • Glass vial.

Containers for parenteral products

Small-volume parenteral products, such as subcutaneous injections, are typically packaged in various containers made of Type I glass. Glass ampoules (Fig. 27.3) are used to package parenteral solutions intended for single use.

Multiple-dose vials (Fig. 27.4) are used to package parenteral formulations that will be used on more than one occasion. Large-volume parenteral fluids have been packaged in 500 mL glass containers but these have been largely superseded by plastic bags.

Plastics

Plastics have been widely used for several years as containers for the product and as secondary packaging in the form of a carton. In more recent times, plastic has been developed for the packaging of parenteral products including infusion fluids and small-volume injections.

Two classes of plastics are used in the packaging of pharmaceutical products. These are known as thermosets and thermoplastics. The thermosets are used for making screw caps for glass and metal containers. Thermoplastic polymers are used in the manufacture of a wide variety of pharmaceutical packages as detailed in Table 27.2.

The advantages of plastics for packaging are that they:

- Release few particles into the product
- Are flexible and not easily broken
- Are of low density and thus light in weight
- Can be heat sealed
- Are easily moulded into various shapes

Table 27.2 The application of thermoplastic polymers for the packaging of pharmaceutical products

Polymer	Examples of application
High-density polyethylene	Solid dosage form containers
Low-density polyethylene	Flexible eye drop bottles
Linear low-density polyethylene	Heat-sealable containers
Polypropylene	Container closures, intravenous solution bottles
Polyvinyl chloride	Laminate for blister packs, intravenous bags
Polystyrene	Containers for oils and creams and solid dosage forms

- Are suitable for use as container, closure and as secondary packaging
- Are cheap.

The disadvantages of plastics are that:

- They are not as chemically inert as Type I glass
- Some plastics undergo stress cracking and distortion from contact with some chemicals
- Some plastics are very heat sensitive
- They are not as impermeable to gas and vapour as glass
- They may possess an electrostatic charge which will attract particles
- Additives in the plastic are easily leached into the product
- Substances such as the active drug and preservatives may be taken up from the product.

Plastic pharmaceutical containers are made of at least one polymer together with additives. The additives used will depend on the composition of the polymer and the production methods used.

Additives used in plastic containers include:

- Plasticizers
- Resins
- Stabilizers
- Lubricants
- Antistatic agents
- Mould-release agents.

Plastic containers

These are used for many types of pack including rigid bottles for tablets and capsules, squeezable bottles for eye drops and nasal sprays, jars, flexible tubes, strip and blister packs. The composition and the physical shape of the containers vary widely to suit the application.

The principal plastic materials used in pharmaceutical packaging

Polyethylene

This is used as high- and low-density polyethylene, both of which are compatible with a wide range of drugs and are extensively used for the packaging of various pharmacy products. Of these two forms of polyethylene, low-density polyethylene (LDPE) is softer, more flexible and more easily stretched than high-density polyethylene (HDPE). Consequently, LDPE is usually the preferred plastic for squeeze bottles. By contrast, HDPE is stronger, stiffer, less clear, less permeable to gases and more resistant to oils,

chemicals and solvents. It is commonly pigmented or printed white to block light transmission and improve label clarity. HDPE is widely used in bottles for solid dosage forms.

Disadvantages of LDPE and HDPE for packaging are that they:

- Are softened by flavouring and aromatic oils
- Are unsuitable for packing oxygen-sensitive products owing to high gas permeability
- Adsorb antimicrobial preservative agents
- Crack on contact with organic solvents.

Polyvinyl chloride (PVC)

This is extensively used as rigid packaging material and as the main component of intravenous bags.

Polypropylene

This is a strong, stiff plastic polymer with good resistance to cracking when flexed. As a result it is particularly suitable for use in closures with hinges which must resist repeated flexing. In addition, polypropylene has been used as tablet containers and intravenous bottles.

Polystyrene

This is a clear, hard, brittle material with low impact resistance. Its use in drug packaging is limited due to its high permeability to water vapour. However, it has been used for tubes and amber-tinted bottles where clarity and stiffness are important and high gas permeability is not a drawback. It is also used for jars for ointments and creams with low water content.

Closures

Any closure system should provide an effective seal to retain the container contents and exclude external contaminants. Child-resistant containers (CRCs) commonly consist of a glass or plastic vial or bottle with a specially designed closure. These CRCs are a professional requirement for dispensing of solid and liquid dosage forms in the UK and are ultimately a compromise between child resistance and ease of opening. They are not an absolute barrier to children accessing medicine containers, therefore the containers should be stored in a safe place. Several designs of child-resistant closures are currently used for pharmaceutical packaging, including cap–bottle alignment systems, push down and turn caps and, less commonly, squeeze and turn caps.

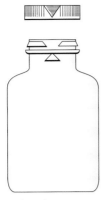

Figure 27.5 • Snap-safe® closure.

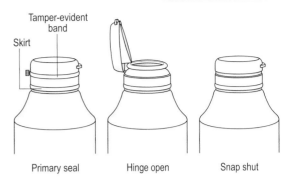

Figure 27.7 • Tamper-evident closure.

The closures in common use with dispensed medicines are the Snap-safe® alignment closure (Fig. 27.5) and the push down and turn Clic-loc® closure (Fig. 27.6). The Clic-loc® child-resistant closures are based on the assumption that young children are unable to coordinate two separate and dissimilar actions; that is, applying pressure and rotating the closure top. The Clic-loc® closure has a two-piece mechanism with springs between the inner and the outer parts. As a result of this design, the closure produces an audible clicking noise when the cap is turned without first being depressed. The inner cap is composed of polypropylene while the outer overcap is made of HDPE.

Contamination of the screw thread with crystallized sugar arising from syrups can increase the torque necessary to open these Clic-loc® closures. This type of problem can restrict their suitability for use. Owing to opening difficulties experienced by some adults,

these closures should not be used on containers supplied to elderly or handicapped patients with poor manual dexterity. They should not be used when a request is made that the product is not dispensed with a child-resistant closure fitted. A Clic-loc® closure must only be dispensed on one occasion as continued use increases the penetration of moisture vapour into the container and decreases the child-resistant properties of the closure.

In recent years greater awareness of the vulnerability of products has led to the development of tamper-evident closures. The closures indicate if unlawful access to the container contents has occurred and are currently available in various designs suitable for different containers and closures. Dispensary stock containers are frequently fitted with a Jaycap® type of tamper-evident closure. These closures are made of either white polypropylene or LDPE. With this closure design the tamper-evident closures snap over a security bead on the neck of the container. The closures cannot be opened until the tamper-evident band connecting the cap to the skirt is torn away (Fig. 27.7). Clic-loc® closures are available with this design whereby an external tamper-evident coloured band must be removed before the closure can be turned. Tamper-evident inner seals are positioned within the closure and are attached to the rim of the opening to the container isolating its contents. The seal must be torn or removed from the container to gain access to the packaged product. These seals are commonly made of a combination of paper, plastic and foil.

Collapsible tubes

These are flexible containers for the storage and dispensing of creams and ointments. Tubes made of tin are used to package certain sterile formulations.

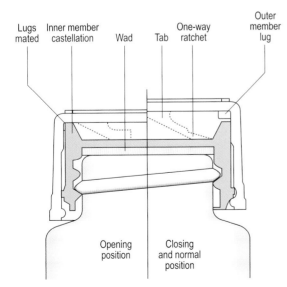

Figure 27.6 • Clic-loc® closure.

Typically the formulation is aseptically filled into the pre-sterilized tubes. However, the most common metal tubes in current use are made of aluminium with an internal lacquered surface. With this package the tube remains collapsed as the product is removed. These tubes are frequently sealed at both ends and the nozzle must be punctured to access the product. An alternative seal that can be used with these packages is a heat seal band between the closure and the container. This band must be torn to gain access to the container contents.

Plastic tubes made from a variety of materials are superseding metal tubes. For example, the tube sleeve may be made of LDPE with either a LDPE or HDPE head or the entire tube may be made of polypropylene.

Unit-dose packaging

This term usually means that a single item such as a tablet or capsule or a specific dose is enclosed within its own disposable packaging. The most commonly used methods for unit-dose packaging are blister packs and strip packs.

Blister packs

These are used for packaging unit doses of tablets and capsules and can act as an aid for patient compliance. The medication is placed in a compartment in a base material made of paper, board, plastic or metal foil or a combination of these. The blister is generally composed of a thermoformed plastic sheet such as PVC. The protection given by the plastic blister depends on its composition, design and the method used to form it. Perforations in the base material allow individual sections of the package to be broken off. Blister packages are rigid, unlike strip packs that are flexible.

Strip packaging

With strip packaging, two webs of material sandwich various types of medicine such as tablets, capsules, suppositories or pessaries. Each of these dosage forms is contained within its own compartment. The composition of the two webs can be selected to meet the necessary protective requirements for the medicine. Aluminium foil is commonly used to manufacture strip packs and provides a good barrier against moisture penetration. The foil is used as a laminate in which the other components add strength to the frag-

ile aluminium foil. They also block small holes which can occur in the thinner foil layer.

Paper

Paper is used more than any other material in packaging. Although it has an insignificant role in primary packaging it remains the predominant secondary and tertiary packaging material. In this role it is used as the carton which contains the primary package and, in the form of board, is the corrugated shipping container which contains both.

Patient pack dispensing

A patient pack consists of a course of medication together with a patient information leaflet in a ready to dispense pack. Liquid formulations are supplied in a standard pack. Solid dose forms are supplied as a strip or blister pack. The size of the sealed patient pack is based on a 28, 30 or 56 dose unit appropriate to the medicine. It is supplied in this amount unless a doctor prescribes that a different quantity of medicine is to be dispensed. The patient pack contains an information leaflet as an aid to improving patient compliance and to supply information to patients about their medication. Pharmacists should be prepared to respond to enquiries after the patient has read the leaflet. The patient pack is designed as a balance between the need for child resistance and the need for ease of opening by the elderly. If requested by the patient, the pack contents can be repackaged in a more suitable container.

Advantages of patient packs

- They contain product information such as product and manufacturer identification and the batch number
- More efficient dispensing results in greater opportunity for patient counselling
- More information is supplied to the patient about the product.

Disadvantages of patient packs

- Increased storage space is required
- Elderly and debilitated patients may experience difficulty in opening the pack.

KEY POINTS

- Containers should preserve the quality of a medicine for its stated shelf life
- Glass has both advantages and disadvantages in use, but remains the preferred material in many situations
- The types of glass have different uses:
  o Type I for ampoules and vials
  o Type II for eye preparations and dropper bottles
  o Type III for metric medical bottles
- Fluted bottles are used for preparations not intended to be swallowed
- Plastics may be thermosets or thermoplastics
- A variety of additives to plastics may enter medicines with which they are in contact
- Child-resistant containers (CRCs) may have alignment closures (Snap-safe®) or push and turn (Clic-loc®)
- Use of CRCs is a professional requirement for dispensed medicines unless requested otherwise
- Tamper-evident closures indicate that there has been no unlawful access to the medicine
- Aluminium is being replaced by plastics for collapsible tubes
- Unit dosage packaging may be either blister or strip packaging
- The main use for paper is for cartons and boxes
- A patient pack consists of the medicine and patient information leaflet in a ready to dispense outer pack

28

Labelling of dispensed medicines

Judith A. Rees

STUDY POINTS

- The reasons for having labels on dispensed products
- Requirements for labels
- Standard details required on labels
- Additional labels
- Specific UK legal requirements
- Patient-specific labels

Introduction

All dispensed medicines should be individually labelled by the dispenser. The label on a dispensed medicine has several main functions:

- To uniquely identify the contents of the container
- To ensure that patients have clear and concise information which will enable them to take or use their medicine in the most effective and appropriate way
- To clearly identify the patient for whom the medicine is dispensed
- To satisfy legal requirements.

In the UK there are both legal (UK and EU) and professional requirements which must be complied with when labelling a dispensed medicine. It is the pharmacist's responsibility to ensure that these requirements are satisfied and that all labelling is accurate and comprehensible. The regulations indicate standard details which must appear on every label. In certain circumstances additional details are also required. Useful sources of information are *Medicines, Ethics and Practice* and the *British National Formulary* (BNF). In this chapter only the requirements for

the labelling of dispensed medicines in the UK are dealt with. However, similar requirements will be in place in other countries. It should also be noted that provision of an adequate label does not remove the need to give advice and counselling to the patient (see Ch. 44).

Standard requirements for labelling dispensed medicines

All labels must be in printed form, either typewritten or computer generated. This should mean that the information on the label is legible; however, there have been reports of labels which were unreadable because the printer was not working properly or the ink or toner cartridges were low or empty. Hence there is a need for pharmacists or dispensers to check each label for legibility before handing the item to the patient. It is also important that the font size of the print is suitable for the patient (see later).

In summary, the details which must appear on the label of a dispensed medicine are:

- The name of the preparation, strength and form (if more than one available)
- The quantity
- Instructions for use
- Precautions relating to the use of the product
- The patient's name
- The date of dispensing
- The name and address of the pharmacy
- 'Keep out of the reach and sight of children'
- The phrase 'For external use' for certain formulations.

Additional labelling requirements

- Warning or advisory labels should be attached to the container, where appropriate
- A batch number should be indicated if the preparation has been prepared extemporaneously
- An expiry date should be indicated if the preparation has been prepared extemporaneously or the shelf life has been shortened, e.g. a diluted preparation
- Additional legal requirements, e.g. 'For animal treatment only' on veterinary prescriptions
- Storage conditions.

The name of the preparation, strength and form

The name which appears on the label must be the same as the one which appears on the prescription. The preparation may be prescribed generically but only be available as a proprietary or branded product; however, the prescribed name must be used. The reason for this is to avoid the patient becoming confused with a variety of names.

The letters NP on a prescription stand for 'nomen proprium' – the proper name of the medicine. Occasionally a prescriber may not wish the name of the preparation to appear on the container. To indicate this they will delete the NP instruction on the prescription. In these cases the type of medicine (e.g. 'the tablets', 'the mixture') should replace the name of the product.

Another occasion when the name may be omitted is when the product contains several active ingredients and has no official or proprietary name and it would be extremely difficult to list all the ingredients on the label. In these instances the pharmaceutical form is used, e.g. 'the ointment', 'the mixture'.

If the preparation is available in more than one strength, the strength must be included on the label, for example, amoxicillin 250 mg capsules and amoxicillin 500 mg capsules. Such information clearly identifies the medicine.

Similarly, the form of the medicines should be included on the label. This is especially important if the product is available in more than one form (e.g. amoxicillin capsules, syrup, suspension, sachets, injection). The inclusion of the form identifies the medicine and may give an indication of how it is to be used/taken (e.g. forms such as suppositories, inhalations, enemas).

Quantity and multiple packs

Normally the quantity which appears on the label will be the quantity which has been prescribed. Nowadays, many medicines are supplied in the manufacturer's patient packs, which will be labelled according to the legal requirements. If the quantity on the prescription requires more than one of these patient packs to be dispensed, for example two patient packs each containing 28 tablets of the same medicinal product (a total of 56 tablets), then the quantity on the label should be the amount in each container. In other words each container should be labelled.

Where several containers (manufacturer's patient packs) of the same medicinal product are required to supply the quantity stated on the prescription (multiple packs), then the name of the product, directions for use and precautions relating to the use of the product need only appear on the package containing the individual packs or on one of the individual packs. All the individual packs must be labelled with the name of the patient, the name and address of the pharmacy, the date of dispensing and the words 'keep out of the reach of children'.

Instructions for use

No patient should leave a pharmacy without knowing how much, how often and how to use/take his or her medication. Although the label should be seen as a back-up to the verbal counselling and advice given by the pharmacist, it is still essential to ensure that the wording on the label is clear, concise and comprehensible to the patient. The prescriber's instructions should therefore be translated into an appropriate form. If instructions are missing or incomplete it is the pharmacist's professional duty to obtain instructions from the prescriber or use professional discretion to interpret BNF statements.

The way in which instructions are worded is very important and will greatly influence how easily a patient understands the message. Pharmacists should therefore give serious consideration to the wording on medicine labels.

The Royal Pharmaceutical Society working party report (1990) on 'The Labelling of Dispensed Medicines' made several recommendations. The use of active verbs is preferred, e.g. 'take' instead of 'to be taken', 'apply' instead of 'to be applied'. The reason is that research has shown that active verbs are more easily understood and remembered than passive verbs. It is

Table 28.1 Recommended wording for directions

Recommended wording	Wording to be replaced
Do not swallow	Not to be taken
Take 'x' times a day, spaced evenly through the day (This wording was considered preferable for antibiotics)	Take every 'y' hours (For analgesics this remains the desirable wording)
Put two drops in the affected eye	Instil two drops in the affected eye
For creams or ointments: Spread thinly	Use sparingly
For pessaries or suppositories: Gently put one into the vagina/rectum	Insert one into the vagina/rectum

bad practice to have two numbers appearing together in instructions, e.g. 'take two three times daily'. It is easy for a patient to mentally transpose the position of the numbers so that the previous instruction becomes 'three twice daily' in the patient's mind. To avoid this, the numbers should always be separated by using the formulation name, e.g. 'take two tablets', 'two capsules', 'two powders three times daily'. Other recommendations in the report can be seen in Table 28.1.

Numbers which are part of an instruction must always be written as words except in the case of 5 mL, when referring to a 5 mL spoonful, or oral syringe quantities, e.g. a 2.5 mL dose using the oral syringe provided.

Many manufacturers' packs of medicines contain a patient information leaflet. These normally give detailed instructions (with illustrations) of how to use a medicine, along with other details about the medicine. Patients should be told to read the patient information leaflet before using the medicine. This is a back-up to the labelling.

Precautions relating to use of the product

Labelling the product with precautions relating to use is for safety reasons. Such labelling will be specific to the product and includes 'Caution flammable: keep away from fire or flames' and 'Not to be consumed by mouth'.

The patient's name

It is a legal requirement that the name of the patient for whom the medication has been prescribed must appear on the label of all dispensed medicines. If possible, the status of the patient, i.e. Mr, Mrs, Miss, Master, Child or Baby, should be included in order to clearly differentiate from other members of a household, where there may be other persons with the same name. For the same reason a full first name should also be included if possible, rather than an initial, e.g. Mr James Burnett instead of J. Burnett.

The date and name and address of the pharmacy

The majority of pharmacies use computer systems for prescription labelling and this information will normally appear automatically, with the date being reset daily. This information is a legal requirement, but enables the source of the medicine to be traced and date of dispensing, if necessary. For example, in the case of possible overdose or poisoning, the label would assist any investigation.

'Keep out of the reach of children'

In order to prevent accidental ingestion of medicines by children, all dispensed medicines are required to carry the label 'Keep out of the reach of children'. Any pharmacist in the UK who issues a dispensed medicine without this warning on the label is guilty of contravening the Medicines Act. Nowadays it is recommended that the wording 'Keep out of the reach and sight of children' is used for consistency because this wording is used on all labels of manufactured patient packs of medicines.

Additional labelling requirements

In addition to the standard details required on all dispensed medicines there are several extra details which are required in certain circumstances. Some information may be specific to a particular type of formulation.

Storage

General information for different types of preparation can be found in the relevant chapters in this book. Some formulations require special storage and this information should be attached to the label, e.g. transdermal patches should be stored in a cool place. Other labels relating to storage include 'protect from light' and 'store in a fridge'. Any specific pharmaceutical precautions relating to storage should always be indicated, for example glyceryl trinitrate tablets should be labelled 'discard after 8 weeks of use'.

The British Pharmacopoeia (and other pharmacopoeias) use the terms 'freshly prepared' and 'recently prepared' for extemporaneously prepared products with a short keeping time. 'Freshly prepared' is defined as having been made no more than 24 hours before issue for use, but there is no indication of when it should be discarded. In this case, it is usual to give a 1 week discard date. The term 'recently prepared' is used for products which should be discarded 4 weeks after issue when stored at 15–25°C.

Information on proprietary medicines can be accessed in the Association of British Pharmaceutical Industries (ABPI) *Medicines Compendium*.

Warnings for patients

Ideally, any liquid preparation should state 'Shake the bottle', and 'For external use only' is a legal requirement on external liquid and gel preparations.

Many drugs cause side-effects about which the patient should be informed. Information on these can be found in Appendix 9 of the BNF (BNF no. 56, September 2008; note that the appendix number may be different in later editions). It is a professional requirement, subject to the pharmacist's discretion, that if indicated, these special warnings should be affixed to the container. Nowadays most computer systems will automatically print these warnings when a label for a particular drug is being produced. However, there are instances when use of this information is inappropriate and professional discretion should be used. For example, the antihistamine chlorphenamine requires the warning: 'Warning. May cause drowsiness. If affected do not drive or operate machinery. Avoid alcoholic drink'. Young children may be prescribed a drug such as this but this warning would be inappropriate. Obviously it is important to draw attention to the problem of sedation and in this case the more suitable warning 'Warning. May cause drowsiness' could be used. If a doctor does not wish the warning labels to appear, the prescription should be endorsed 'NCL' (no cautionary labels).

Some of the BNF warning labels have been known to cause confusion, such as numbers 5, 6, 7, 11 and 14. All of these may require additional explanation to be given to the patient.

- Label number 5: 'Do not take indigestion remedies at the same time of day as this medicine'.
- Label number 6: 'Do not take indigestion remedies or medicines containing iron or zinc at the same time of day as this medicine'.
- Label number 7: 'Do not take milk, indigestion remedies or medicines containing iron or zinc at the same time of day as this medicine'.

Some patients misunderstand the information on these three labels and think that milk, iron preparations and indigestion remedies must not be taken at all. It should be explained to the patient that as long as there is an interval of approximately 2 hours between taking the medicine and any of the remedies, there is not a problem.

- Label number 11: 'Avoid exposure of skin to direct sunlight or sun lamps'.

There have been reports of patients who were frightened to venture outside when taking medication which carried this warning. Again an explanation that as long as exposed areas of skin are adequately covered, e.g. a long-sleeved shirt or a sunhat to shade the face, the patient should not suffer any ill effects.

- Label number 14: 'This medicine may colour the urine'.

It is useful to give the patient an indication of the colour, e.g. phenolphthalein (pink), levodopa (dark reddish) or rifampicin (red).

A batch number

When a product has been prepared extemporaneously it is good practice to award it a batch number and incorporate this onto the label. This is standard practice in hospital pharmacy. When preparing an extemporaneous product, details of the ingredients used should be recorded (see Ch. 25). The batch number allows referral back to this information.

Expiry date

It is not normally necessary to put an expiry date on the label of a dispensed medicine, although with the increasing dispensing of manufacturers' original packs this information will be part of the pack labelling. Manufacturers' expiry dates relate to ideal storage conditions but, unfortunately, when a product has been dispensed and given to the patient there is no longer any control over how it is stored. For this reason, under current legislation, when a product is repackaged for dispensing, no expiry date is stated. Patients should be encouraged to complete the course of medication or, if for any reason a supply is not finished and is no longer required, to bring any remainder back to the pharmacy.

There are, however, specific occasions when an expiry date must be added to the label.

- An expiry date should always be put onto any extemporaneously prepared item.
- An expiry date should always be used when a product has been diluted, thereby affecting its stability and shelf life.
- An expiry date should always be indicated when the preparation is sterile, e.g. eye drops. Once opened the product is no longer sterile and if used beyond a certain timescale there is a serious risk of infection. It is therefore recommended that eye drops and eye ointment, unless otherwise specified by the manufacturer, should be discarded 4 weeks after opening. This instruction should be indicated on the label (see Ch. 39 for further details).

Although the majority of patients will understand what 'expiry date' means, it is important to express the information in a clear and unambiguous way. 'Any unused to be discarded on . . . (date)' or 'Do not use after . . . (date)' are preferred methods of expressing expiry dates.

Legal requirements in certain circumstances

Veterinary dispensed products

The words 'For animal use only' or similar must always be added to the label of a dispensed veterinary product. Instead of the patient's name, the name of the animal's owner should appear, along with the owner's address or address where the animal lives.

Emergency supply

When a preparation is dispensed using the emergency supply procedures, the words 'Emergency supply' must appear on the label.

Private prescriptions

A label for a medicine dispensed from a private prescription must bear a reference number. This reference number will relate to the entry in the private prescription register and will also be endorsed on the private prescription.

Labels for vulnerable patients

Some patients may have difficulty in reading the normal print size of a label due to partial or complete blindness. In such cases consideration should be given to providing additional support to these patients, in the form of large print size on labels or the provision of large print size copies of the labels. In all cases the medicinal products should be labelled. Additionally, consideration should be given to providing Braille labels for those patients able to read Braille.

Some patients may not be able to read the language on the label due to either illiteracy or being a non-native language reader. It may be possible to provide such a patient with a picture or series of pictures to illustrate the instructions. Many pictograms (a symbol representing a concept, object, activity, place or event by an illustration) have been developed for labelling medicines with instructions on how often and how to take medicines. Similarly many toxic chemicals are labelled with pictograms to avoid harm to the public. The Risk-benefit Assessment of Drugs-Analysis and Response (RAD-AR) Council of Japan has recently released a series of new pictograms for use on pharmaceutical packaging. These may be viewed on www.pinktentacle. com/images/pictograms.jpg.

Clearly any patient with difficulty reading or understanding a label on a dispensed medicine should be given advice and counselling by the pharmacist before leaving the pharmacy.

Errors in labelling

The potential for making errors when producing a label is considerable and it is important that constant checking is carried out. Practice procedures should be such that the chances of errors occurring are minimized (see Ch. 24). Dispensing is usually carried out in a busy environment with many distractions and it takes considerable effort to maintain the 100% concentration required to ensure that errors do not occur.

Apart from errors in interpreting prescribers' instructions or missing off any of the details already mentioned, the advent of computerized labelling has brought its own problems, two of which will be mentioned.

Patient's name errors

When using a computer system, if a patient presents a prescription for several items, the patient's name is typed in once and the number of items to be dispensed bearing that patient's name is entered. Occasionally an item may not be dispensed or the number of items may be entered incorrectly. This means that when the next prescription for a different patient is to be dispensed, the name of the first patient will occur on the label even if all the other information is correct.

Transposition of labels

It is not uncommon that two labels have been produced on the pharmacy computer and two medicines have been prepared. At this point the labels could be applied to the incorrect container unless care is taken.

An awareness of how easily these errors can occur is at least one step to ensuring that they do not happen.

KEY POINTS

- A label is used to identify and instruct on the use of a medicine, so simple language should be used
- All labels must be typewritten or computer generated
- All labels must state the name and quantity of the preparation, patient's name and instructions, name and address of pharmacy, date of dispensing and 'Keep out of the reach of children'
- Warning labels may also be required
- Active verbs should be used on the label
- Adjacent numbers should be separated by the formulation name (e.g. 'take two tablets three … ') on a label
- As full a name of the patient as possible should be included on the label
- The BNF contains details of side-effect warnings which should be used unless there is a good reason not to do so
- Some warning labels may require verbal explanation
- It is good practice to give an extemporaneous preparation a batch number
- Expiry dates are required on the label when dispensing diluted, sterile and extemporaneous preparations
- Computer labelling systems can increase the risk of some types of error

Self-assessment questions

1. The following NHS prescription was received:
   Tabs Ibuprofen 400 mg
   Mitte 60
   one t.i.d.

   The name of the patient was Mrs Marjory Nicol. Comment on the accuracy of the following labels produced for this prescription. (Assume that the name and address of the pharmacy and 'Keep out of the reach and sight of children' are included.)
   a 60 Tabs Ibuprofen
      Take one tablet three times daily with or after food
      Mrs Marjory Nicol [12/5/08]
   b 60 Tabs Ibuprofen 400 mg
      Take one three times daily with or after food
      Mrs Marjory Nicol [12/5/08]
   c 60 Tabs Ibuprofen 400 mg
      Take one tablet three times daily with or after food
      M Nicol [12/5/08]

d 60 Tabs Ibuprofen 400 mg

One to be taken three times daily with or after food

Mrs Marjory Nicol [12/5/08]

e 60 Tabs Ibuprofen 400 mg

Take three tablets daily with or after food

Mrs Marjory Nicol [12/5/08]

2. The following NHS prescription is received:
Betnovate® Ointment half Strength

Mitte 50 g

Sig. apply to affected area m. et n.

Mr James Hill

Comment on the following label:

50 g Betnovate® Ointment Half strength

Apply to affected area morning and night

Mr James Hill [12/5/08]

3. You will need to consult Appendix 9 in the BNF to complete this exercise. Using the BNF, indicate the cautionary and advisory labels which should appear on the following products. Are there products where you consider additional information may need to be given?

a Tildiem Retard® tablets

b Ledermycin® capsules

c Solpadol® caplets

d Madopar® capsules

Self-assessment answers

1. a The strength of the drug has been omitted from the label. This will cause problems of identification.

b The instructions have been written with the number of tablets and the dose frequency together, i.e. 'Take one three times . . .' This is bad practice and may lead to errors in dosing.

c The status of the patient and first name have not been included, i.e. M Nicol instead of Mrs Marjory Nicol.

d The passive form of the verb has been used, i.e. 'to be taken'. The active form 'take' is the preferred form.

e The instructions are not clear. Although the patient has been told the correct number of tablets to take in a 24-hour period, information about frequency is missing. This will lead to loss of efficacy and a possible increase in the incidence of adverse effects.

2. This preparation has been diluted, i.e. Betnovate® ointment, 25 g and 25 g of recommended diluent. This has affected the stability and consequently the shelf life so an expiry date should have been indicated on the label. The manufacturer's recommendation is a shelf life of 14 days. This preparation is for external use and the label should have indicated this.

3. a Tildiem Retard® tablets require:

Label 25: 'Swallowed whole, not chewed'.

This is a reasonably simple instruction but the patient's attention should be drawn to it and an explanation of why it is necessary given. The modified release of the preparation will be destroyed if the tablets are crushed or chewed.

b Ledermycin® capsules require:

Label 7: 'Do not take milk, iron preparations or indigestion remedies at the same time of day as this medicine'.

Label 9: 'Take at regular intervals. Complete the prescribed course unless otherwise directed'.

Label 11: 'Avoid exposure of skin to direct sunlight or sun lamps'.

Label 23: 'Take an hour before food or on an empty stomach'.

The main problem here is the considerable amount of information. The patient's understanding of the information should be checked and further explanation given if necessary.

c Solpadol® caplets require:

Label 2: 'Warning. May cause drowsiness. If affected do not drive or operate machinery'.

Label 29: 'Do not take more than 2 at any one time. Do not take more than 8 in 24 hours'.

Label 30: 'Contains paracetamol'.

Again there is a considerable amount of information given, all of which is important. The pharmacist should alert the patient to the paracetamol warning and explain that other paracetamol-containing preparations should not be taken.

d Madopar® capsules require:

Label 14: 'This medicine may colour the urine'.

Label 21: 'Take with or after food'.

Reinforcement of dosing in relation to food intake should be given if the pharmacist considers it necessary. If the patient has not received the medication before, an indication that the urine colour will be reddish should be given.

29

Production of sterile products

Derek G. Chapman

STUDY POINTS

- The requirements for sterile production
- Grades of clean areas
- Design and operation of clean areas
- Isolators
- Environmental monitoring
- Preparation of aseptic products

Introduction

The production of sterile medicinal products has special requirements. These products must be produced in conditions that ensure that they are pure. They must also be free from viable organisms and pyrogens with limited, or ideally no, particulate contamination. It is thus important that only carefully regulated and tested procedures are used to manufacture sterile products.

Owing to their special manufacturing requirements, sterile medicinal products are prepared in special facilities known as clean rooms. These rooms are designed to reduce the risk of microbial and particulate contamination at all stages of the manufacturing process.

The clean area used to produce sterile products is commonly designed as a suite of clean rooms. With this system, the operators enter the clean rooms by way of a changing room. Within this area the operators put on clean room clothing before entering into the clean rooms. The changing room has a lower standard of environmental quality. A clean room with a lower environmental standard is also used to prepare solutions. These solutions are then sterilized by filtration before being transferred into the filling room. The clean room used to fill and seal the product containers is the highest quality of clean room. This will reduce the risk of product contamination.

Sterile products that are marketed in the European Union must be produced in conditions which conform with the conditions given in the revised Annex 1 of Good Manufacturing Practices (Volume IV) of 'The Rules Governing Medicinal Products in the European Union'. This guidance on the procedures for manufacturing sterile products describes the cleanliness of the clean room environment and recommends how pharmaceutical clean rooms should be built and used.

Sterile product production

Production of sterile products should be carried out in a clean environment with a limit for the environmental quality of particulate and microbial contamination. This limit for contamination is necessary to reduce the risk of product contamination. In addition, however, the temperature, humidity and air pressure of the environment should be regulated to suit the clean room processes and the comfort of the operators.

Clean areas for the production of sterile products are classified into grades A, B, C and D. These grades are categorized by the particulate quality of the environmental air when the clean area is operating in both a 'manned' and 'unmanned' state. In addition, these areas are graded by the microbial monitoring of the environmental air, surfaces and operators when the area is functioning. The standards are shown in Tables 29.1 and 29.2.

Table 29.1 Airborne particle contamination for manned and unmanned clean rooms

Grade	Maximum number of particles per cubic metre equal to or above the size indicated			
	Clean room at rest		Clean room operating	
	0.5 μm	5 μm	0.5 μm	5 μm
A	3500	1	3500	1
B	3500	1	350 000	2000
C	350 000	2000	3 500 000	20 000
D	3 500 000	20 000	Varies with procedure	Varies with procedure

Table 29.2 Limits for microbial contamination of an operating clean room

Grade	Viable organisms per cubic metre of air	90 mm settle plate per 4 hours	55 mm contact plate	Glove print (5 fingers)
A	<1	<1	<1	<1
B	10	5	5	5
C	100	50	25	N/A
D	200	100	50	N/A

There are two common procedures used to manufacture sterile products. The first method involves the preparation of products that will be terminally sterilized. The second method involves the aseptic filling of containers that are not exposed to terminal sterilization. Aseptic filling requires a higher environmental quality for the preparation of solutions and the filling of containers. The qualities of the clean rooms used for these production procedures are detailed in Tables 29.3 and 29.4.

Premises

High standards are necessary for the manufacture of sterile medicinal products. The sterile production unit must be separated from the general manufacturing area within the hospital pharmacy or factory. This sterile production unit must not be accessible to unauthorized personnel.

The unit is designed to allow each stage of production to be segregated. It should also ensure a safe

Table 29.3 Conditions for preparing terminally sterilized products

Procedure	Required standard before terminal sterilization
Preparation of solutions for filtration and sterilization	Grade C is used for products which support microbial growth Grade D acceptable if solutions subsequently filtered
Filling small and large volume parenterals	Grade C. For products with a high risk of contamination such as wide-necked containers, a Grade A laminar airflow workstation with Grade C background
Preparation and filling of ointments, creams, suspensions and emulsions	Grade C

Table 29.4 Conditions for the production of aseptically prepared products

Procedure	Required standard
Handling of sterile starting materials	Grade A with Grade B background or Grade C if solution filtered later in production process
Preparation of production solutions	Grade A with Grade B background or Grade C if sterile during filtered production
Filling of aseptically prepared products such as small and large volume parenterals	Grade A with Grade B background
Preparation and filling of ointments, creams, suspensions and emulsions	Grade A with Grade B background

and organized workflow and reduce the need for personnel to move around the clean rooms. The unit is built and the equipment positioned to protect the product from contamination. The layout must allow efficient cleaning of the area and avoid the build up of dust. Premises are also arranged to decrease the risk of mix up or contamination of one product or material by another.

The filling room is typically serviced from an adjacent preparation room. This allows supporting personnel to assemble and prepare materials. Staff within the filling room area then use these materials. Figure 29.1 shows the layout of rooms for the production of terminally sterilized medicines such as small or large volume injections.

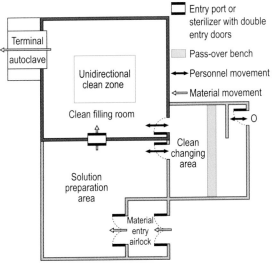

Figure 29.1 • Rooms for the production of terminally sterilized medicines.

Design and construction

Access to clean and aseptic filling areas is limited to authorized personnel. Operators enter clean rooms by way of changing rooms. Within the changing room the operators can don and remove their clean room garments.

A low physical barrier, commonly known as a pass-over (or cross-over) bench, extends across the changing room. It forms a physical barrier that separates the different areas for changing by the operators.

Special precautions are needed to avoid contamination of clean and aseptic filling areas when materials are passed through airlocks or hatchways. Thus, sterilizers and entry ports are fitted with double-sided doors. The doors are interlocked to prevent both doors being opened simultaneously.

Surfacing materials

All clean room surfaces, including the floors, walls and ceilings, should be smooth, impervious and unbroken. This will decrease the release and build-up of contaminating particles and organisms. The surfaces are made of materials that allow the use of cleaning agents and disinfectants. The ceilings are sealed to prevent the entry of contaminants from the space above them. Uncleanable recesses within the clean room should be avoided. This will reduce the collection of contaminating particles. Thus, the junction between the wall and the floor is commonly coved. The presence of shelves, ledges, cupboards and equipment is minimized. Windows should be non-opening and sealed. This will prevent the ingress of contaminants.

Services

Piped liquids and gases should be filtered before entering the clean room. This will ensure that the liquid or gas at the work position will be as clean as the clean room air. The pipes and ducts must be positioned for easy cleaning. All other fittings such as fuse boxes and switch panels should be positioned outside the clean rooms.

Sinks and drains must be excluded from areas where aseptic procedures are performed in clean room areas. They should be avoided in the whole unit wherever possible. In areas where sinks and drains are installed they must be designed, positioned and maintained to decrease the risk of microbial contamination. They are thus often fitted with easily cleanable traps. The traps may contain electrically heated devices for disinfection.

There should be a limited number of entry doors for personnel and ports for materials. Entry doors should be self-closing and allow the easy movement of personnel.

Airlock doors, wall ports, through-the-wall autoclaves and dry heat sterilizers should be fitted with interlocked doors. This will prevent both doors being opened simultaneously. An alarm system should be fitted to all the doors to prevent the opening of more than one door.

Lights in clean rooms are fitted flush with the ceiling to reduce the collection of dust and avoid disturbing the airflow pattern within the room. Similarly, equipment should be positioned in clean rooms to avoid the distribution and the collection of particles and microbial contaminants.

Environmental control

Potential sources of particles and microbial contaminants occurring within the clean room are:

- The air supply of the room
- Inflow of external air
- Production of contaminants within the room.

Each of these possible sources can be minimized as described below.

Air supply

The air supply to a Grade A, B or C clean room must be filtered to ensure the removal of particulate and microbial contamination. This is carried out by filtering the air with high-efficiency particulate air (HEPA) filters. The HEPA filter should be positioned at the inlet to the clean room or close to it. A prefilter may be fitted upstream of the HEPA filter. This will prolong the life of the final filter. A fan is required to pump the air through the filter.

The HEPA filters use pleated fibreglass paper as the filter medium. Parallel pleats of this filter material increase the surface area of the filter and increase the airflow through the filter. This structure allows the filter to retain a compact volume. Aluminium foil is used to form spacers in the traditional type of HEPA filter. Spacers are not used in the more modern 'mini-pleat' type of filter design. These mini-pleat filters are now widely used. They have a shallower depth in construction than the traditional HEPA filter. Within the structure of the filter, the filter material is sealed to an aluminium frame (Fig. 29.2). At least one side of the filter is protected with a coated mild steel mesh. HEPA filters exhibit:

- A high flow rate
- High particulate holding capacity
- Low-pressure drop across the filter.

HEPA filters remove larger particles from the air by inertial impaction, the medium-sized particles by direct interception and the small particles by Brownian diffusion. The HEPA filters are least efficient at removing particles of about 0.3 μm. However, the efficiency of removing particles is affected by the air velocity and the filter packing. Larger and smaller particles will be removed more efficiently.

With a new HEPA filter fitted in a clean room, the air exits from the filter face at a rate of about 0.45 m/s

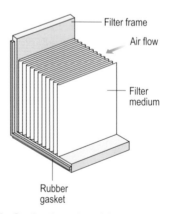

Figure 29.2 • Section through a mini-pleat high-efficiency filter, showing its construction.

and has a 99.997% efficiency at removing 0.3 μm particles. The initial pressure difference across the depth of the filter is about 130 pascal (Pa). At the end of the effective life of the filter the pressure drop across the filter will increase to about 490 Pa. To retain the operating efficiency of the filter, the fan forcing air through the filter must be able to maintain this pressure difference. Sensors are fitted upstream and downstream of the filters to indicate the pressure differential across the filter. An automatic alarm system should be fitted to indicate failure in the air supply or filter blockage.

The HEPA filters for clean room use must conform with the British Standard 5295 (1989) aerosol test. The filters may have faulty seals and can be damaged during delivery or installation. It is thus important that they are tested in situ before use.

The filter material possesses a uniform resistance and is constructed with a large number of parallel pleats. This results in the air downstream of the filter face flowing uniformly with a unidirectional configuration.

The number of air changes in clean rooms is affected by:

- The room size
- The equipment in use
- The number of operators in the area.

In practice 25–35 air changes per hour are common. The airflow pattern within the clean room must be carefully regulated to avoid generating particles from the clean room floor and from the operators. Various options for ventilating clean rooms may be categorized by the airflow pattern within the room. These are:

- Unidirectional airflow systems
- Non-unidirectional airflow systems
- Combination airflow systems.

Unidirectional airflow systems

Air enters the room through a complete wall or ceiling of high-efficiency filters. This air will sweep contamination in a single direction to the exhaust system on the opposing wall or floor (Fig. 29.3). In the interests of economy, the exhaust grill may be fitted low down on the wall. The velocity of the air is about 0.3 m/s in downflow air from ceiling filters and 0.45 m/s in crossflow air. These are highly efficient airflow systems. However, one major disadvantage of these rooms for pharmaceutical use is that they are expensive to construct. They also use much more condi-

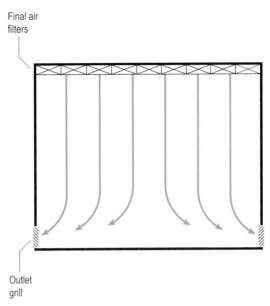

Figure 29.3 • Airflow pattern in a unidirectional airflow clean room.

tioned air than rooms with non-unidirectional airflow. This greatly increases their operating costs. Owing to these factors, unidirectional airflow clean rooms are not often used for pharmaceutical purposes.

Non-unidirectional airflow systems

Air enters the clean rooms through filters and diffusers that are usually located in the ceiling. It exits through outlet ducts positioned low down on the wall or in the floor at sites remote from the air inlet (Fig. 29.4). With the use of this system, the filtered inlet air mixes with and dilutes the contaminated air within the room. As the clean room air has been previously heated and cleaned it can be recirculated to save energy, a little fresh air being introduced with each air change cycle.

Various designs of diffuser are used with this ventilation system. These affect the air movement and the cleanliness of the rooms. The perforated plate diffuser produces a jet flow of air directly beneath it. This jet of air will carry contamination at its edges. However, it does produce high-quality air directly under the diffuser. It is thus important that production procedures are located directly below the diffuser. By contrast, the air released from the bladed diffuser will mix with the clean room air. This diffuser thus produces a reasonably constant quality of air throughout the room.

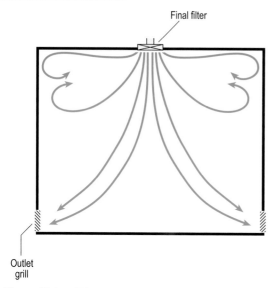

Final filter

Outlet
grill

Figure 29.4 • Airflow pattern in a non-unidirectional airflow clean room.

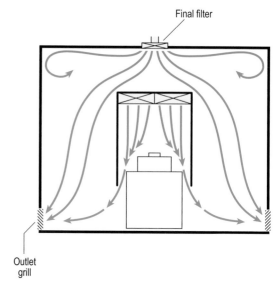

Final filter

Outlet
grill

Figure 29.5 • Airflow patterns in a mixed-flow clean room with non-unidirectional airflow background environment and unidirectional airflow protection for a critical area.

Combination systems

In many pharmaceutical clean rooms it is common to find that the background area is ventilated by a non-unidirectional airflow system. Meanwhile, the critical areas are supplied with high-quality air from unidirectional airflow units.

The combination airflow system is often selected for pharmaceutical clean room applications as it:

- Produces controlled room pressure
- Separates the manufacturing process from the general clean room
- Is cheaper to use.

Several types of unidirectional flow workstations or benches are used in this combination-type room. Various vertical unidirectional airflow systems are used in combination clean rooms. With one system, the critical area is surrounded by a plastic curtain with vertical unidirectional downflow air 'washing' over the manufacturing process and exiting under the plastic curtains into the general clean room area (Fig. 29.5). An alternative system is often used with the small-scale combination-type clean room in hospital pharmacies. With this system, a horizontal airflow cabinet (Fig. 29.6) is used as the workstation. With these cabinets, a fan forces air through a HEPA filter located at the rear wall of the workstation. The air that exits from the filter first washes over the critical work area before washing over the arms and upper body areas of the

operator. Contamination arising from the operator is thus kept downstream of the critical procedures. Grade A environmental conditions are achieved at the critical work area. A similar workstation known as a vertical laminar airflow cabinet (Fig. 29.7) could also be used in the combination room. This cabinet passes air vertically downwards from the ceiling of the cabinet over the critical working area. It produces a

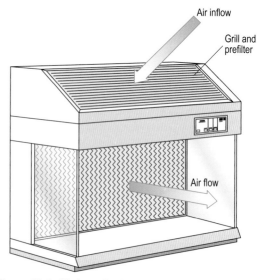

Air inflow

Grill and prefilter

Air flow

Figure 29.6 • Horizontal laminar airflow unit. (Courtesy of John Bass Ltd.)

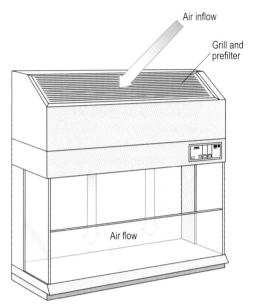

Air inflow

Grill and prefilter

Air flow

Figure 29.7 • Vertical laminar airflow unit. (Courtesy of John Bass Ltd.)

Grade A environmental quality. The air exits from the front of the workstation.

In recent times, there has been a trend towards protecting the critical procedures within combination clean rooms by using isolator cabinets. The isolator cabinet gives a localized high-quality environment. Isolators give protection from potential contamination in clean rooms as they are positively pressurized with air supplied through HEPA filters. The operator works outside the confines of the isolator using glove ports to perform procedures within the enclosed chamber. The gloved hands of clean room operators can transfer microbial contamination into critical working areas within the clean room. To indicate that the required clean room standards have been achieved (Table 29.2), the fingertips of a gloved hand are depressed onto the surface of a suitable solid growth medium. This medium is incubated to show any contamination.

There is also a need to avoid contaminated external air passing into the clean room environment. Thus, the clean room air pressure must exceed that of the surrounding areas. The pressure differential between different standards of clean room should be 10–15 Pa. This level should be comparatively easy to monitor and will decrease the unregulated outflow of air. Adjusting grills known as pressure stabilizers located in the walls of rooms regulate the outflow of clean room air and the room

pressure. The air moves from an area of high pressure to an area of lower pressure. To maintain the room pressure, it is important that the rooms are airtight. However, a small quantity of air will exit from the rooms by way of door spaces.

Temperature and humidity control

The temperature and the humidity are adjusted to suit the procedures being carried out within the clean room and maintain the comfort of the operators. A target temperature of about 20°C with a relative humidity of about 35–45% is usually preferred.

Personnel

The clean room environment is supplied with high-quality air at positive pressure. The main source of contamination in these areas arises from skin scales that are released by the clean room operators.

To limit clean room contamination by personnel, there is a need to:

- Restrict the number of operators working in the clean room
- Restrict operator conversations
- Instruct operators to move slowly
- Minimize general movement throughout the room
- Avoid operators interrupting the airflow between the inlet filter and the work area.

The clean room operator is constantly shedding dead skin scales from the body surface. Not all of these skin particles are contaminated with bacteria. Males shed more particles that are contaminated with bacteria than females. In addition, individual males and females show variable rates of bacterial dispersal. This dispersal from the individual is affected by:

- Personal characteristics
- General health and skin condition.

Body movements of personnel will increase the number of contaminated particles released from the skin surface. Each individual releases more than 10^6 skin scales per minute during normal walking movements. There is a need to contain the dispersion of skin particles from the operators in clean rooms and protect both the environment and the product. Containment of particles is achieved by the operators wearing clean room clothing. This clothing is made from synthetic fabrics that filter out particulate and microbial contamination from the operators without the fabrics releasing contamination. However, this clothing is not absolute and particles can pass through the garments. Operators wearing clean room undergarments reduce this effect. The outer garments are close fitting at the neck, wrists and ankles, but these sites still provide an exit route for particulate matter.

Clean garments should be used for each work session and must provide operator comfort. Disposable single-use garments are available, although most production units employ reusable garments. The clothing is specially laundered in an area with similar standards to those used in the clean room. Garments are laundered by a wet-wash process using particle-free solutions. This is followed by an antibacterial rinse and hot air drying and then the garments are packaged in sealed bags to avoid particulate contamination. This cleaning process fulfils the needs of most pharmaceutical clean room applications, which are a balance between cost and acceptability. For a higher level of sterility assurance the garments are gamma irradiated using ^{60}Co, each garment receiving an approved dose of 25 kGy. This treatment is expensive and decreases the life of the garments. The donning of clean room clothing without contaminating the outer surface of the garments is a rather difficult procedure that is performed in the changing room.

Changing room

Entry of personnel into clean rooms should be through a changing room fitted with interlocking doors. These doors act as an airlock to prevent the influx of external air. This access route is intended for the entry of personnel only. The changing room is subdivided into three areas. Movement through these areas must comply with a strict protocol. They are often colour coded as black, grey and white, black representing the dirtiest area while white represents the cleanest area.

The black area is where jewellery, cosmetics, factory or hospital protective garments and shoes are removed. Long hair may be contained and a mobcap donned to contain the hair completely. The pass-over bench forms a physical separation between the black and the grey areas in the changing room. The operator sits on the pass-over bench, swings his/her legs over the bench and fits clean room covers over the feet before they are placed on the floor of the grey area.

The operator then stands up in the grey area. Wrappings on the various garments are opened to avoid contacting the outer surface of the packaging following the hand-washing procedure. Then the operator washes hands and forearms using an antiseptic solution. Special attention is paid to cleaning the fingernails. The hands are then dried using an automatic air-blow drier as towels shed particles when used for drying hands.

Clothing garments are donned in sequence from head to foot. Throughout this procedure care must be taken to avoid the hands contacting the outer surface of the clean room clothing. Firstly the head and shoulder hood is fitted, ensuring that all the hair is contained within the head cover. A face mask is fitted to prevent the shedding of droplets. The one-piece coverall (or alternatively two-piece trouser suit) is put on. Care must be taken to avoid these garments contacting the floor surface. The shoulder cover of the head and shoulder hood is tucked into the coverall. Then the zip is closed and the studs fastened. Overboots are then fitted over the clean room shoes. The overboots are kept in position with ties that are suitably fastened for operator comfort. For entry into aseptic filling rooms an antiseptic cream is applied to the hands. The clean room powder-free gloves are then donned. Care is needed to avoid contacting the outer surface of the gloves. The cuffs of the coverall are secured within the gloves and the gloved hands disinfected. The operator now enters into the white clean room area and begins work. During the work procedures the gloved hands of the operators are regularly disinfected. Key features of the clothing are given in Table 29.5.

Table 29.5 Clothing for clean room use

Clean room grade	Description of clothing
A/B	Head cover and face mask Single- or two-piece trouser suit Overboots and sterile powder-free rubber or plastic gloves
C	Hair (and beard) cover Single- or two-piece trouser suit Clean room shoes or overshoes
D	Hair (and beard) cover Protective suit Appropriate shoes or overshoes

Cleaning

A strict cleaning and disinfection policy is essential to minimize particulate and microbial contamination in the clean room. Operators release microbial and particulate contamination within the clean room. These contaminants are mostly deposited onto horizontal surfaces. However, other areas of the clean room can become contaminated due to direct contact with the operators' clothing. It is thus essential that a strict cleaning and disinfection policy is implemented within the clean room to minimize both the particulate and the microbial contamination.

There are two main methods of cleaning. Vacuuming is effective at removing gross particulate contamination of particles greater than 100 µm. However, vacuuming is not very effective at removing smaller particles. Small particles are removed by wet wiping. It is important that the wet wipe is sterile and must not generate particulate contamination. The use of wet wipes involves the use of cleaning agents that will remove particulate contamination and have an antibacterial effect.

The ideal cleaning agent should be:

- Effective in removing undesirable contamination
- Harmless to surfaces
- Fast drying
- Non-flammable
- Non-toxic
- Cost-effective.

Anionic or cationic surfactants are used as cleaning agents within the clean room. The disinfectants of choice for clean room use are generally quaternary ammonium compounds, phenols, alcohols and polymeric biguanides. The disinfectant solutions should be freshly prepared before use. Different types of disinfectants should be used in rotation to prevent the development of resistant microbial strains. Most surfactants or detergents will dissipate surface static electricity but the most effective and widely used antistatic agents used in clean rooms are cationic surfactants.

Trained personnel regularly clean critical production areas of clean rooms. A less stringent cleaning protocol is required in the general clean room areas. This applies to the walls and floors where contamination cannot directly contaminate the product. As part of the cleaning protocol, regular microbiological monitoring should be carried out to determine the effectiveness of the disinfection procedures.

Isolators

Commercial manufacturers are using isolators increasingly for the aseptic filling of products, with combination isolators being used. Isolators are also used for sterility testing of products. Robots have been used in isolators for repetitive processes such as sterility testing but they are expensive. Isolators are used in hospital pharmacy departments as an alternative to clean rooms for the small-scale aseptic processing of sterile products. Aseptic procedures performed in the best isolators cannot reach the same levels of sterility assurance achieved by terminal heat sterilization (see Table 29.6). However, when suitably operated they can produce a sterility assurance level better than the conventional clean room. Isolators are often selected for aseptic manipulations of sterile products as they are:

- Relatively inexpensive
- Easily designed for a specific purpose
- Capable of providing operator protection from the product.

Isolators are composed of a chamber that controls the environment surrounding the work procedure (Fig. 29.8). The inlet and exhaust air passes through HEPA filters. The airflow pattern within the isolator chamber may be either unidirectional, non-unidirectional or a combination of both. Vertical unidirectional airflow has the advantage of rapidly purging particles from the isolator chamber. This is an advantage for aseptic processes. The air within the isolator chamber should be frequently changed to maintain the aseptic chamber environment. Particle and microbial contamination of the environment within the isolator chamber must conform with the Grade A standard as detailed in Tables 29.1 and 29.2.

The operator remains outside the isolator chamber environment. To perform manual manipulations within the chamber, the operator inserts his hands and arms into the chamber. Entry occurs by way of a glove port using either a one-piece full-arm-length glove or a glove and sleeve system. With the glove and sleeve system, the easily changeable glove is attached to a sleeve that is attached to the wall of the chamber through an airtight seal. Using either of these glove systems, the operator is able to perform aseptic manipulations in comfort up to a distance of about 0.5 metres within the chamber. The glove system avoids contamination arising from the operator and maintains the integrity of the isolator chamber environment. As cytotoxic materials can diffuse through

Table 29.6 Microbial contamination of batch-produced sterile products

Place of production	Microbial contamination
Industrial production	
Terminal sterilization by dry or moist heat or irradiation	1 in at least 10^6 containers
Aseptic preparation in sealed gassed isolator using sophisticated transfer system	1 in 10^6
Aseptic preparation in conventional clean room using sophisticated laminar airflow system	1 in 10^5
Aseptic preparation in conventional clean room	1 in 10^4
Aseptic complex preparation of large-volume total parenteral nutrition fluids	1 in 10^3
Production in hospital pharmacy	
Terminal sterilization by dry or moist heat containers	1 in at least 10^6
Aseptic preparation in an isolator with surfaces cleaned and wiped with sterile alcohol. Extensively used in many pharmacies	1 in 10^3
Aseptic preparation in a well-managed clean room	1 in 10^3 (or less)

the gloves it is important that they are changed regularly. To perform the work procedure within the chamber, materials must be introduced and prepared products removed without compromising the chamber environment. This transfer procedure is a critical factor in the operation of the isolator and is carried out using a transfer system. The transfer system separates the external environment from the controlled isolator environment. It restricts airflow between these areas while allowing the transfer of materials between them. The transfer system is fitted with an inter-

locked double door entry system. This will provide an airlock that avoids both doors being opened to the external environment simultaneously. A filtered air inlet and exhaust is fitted to the transfer system. However, a risk of microbial contamination during the transfer does exist. This was recorded at the Manchester Children's Hospital in 1994 and is detailed below. The isolator must be positioned in a suitable background environment of at least a Grade D classification. This is typically achieved by positioning the isolator in a dedicated room that is only used for the isolator and its related activities.

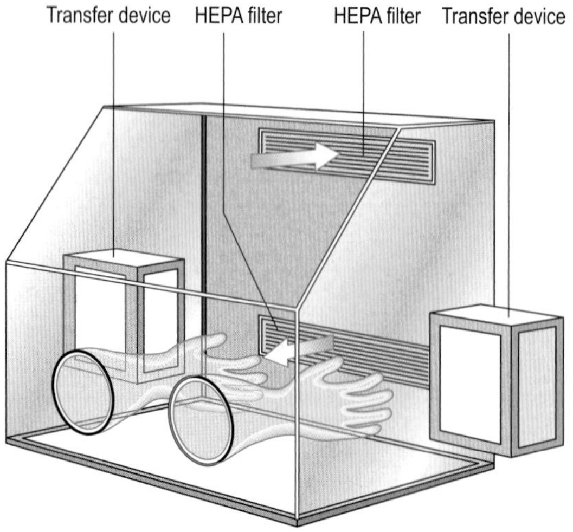

Isolators are divided into positive and negative pressure isolators.

Positive pressure isolator

This isolator operates under positive pressure and protects the product from contamination arising from an external source and from the aseptic process itself. It is used for the aseptic preparation of pharmaceutical products and can be used as a sterility test chamber.

Negative pressure isolator

This isolator will protect the product from contamination arising from an external source and from

Transfer device   HEPA filter   HEPA filter   Transfer device

Figure 29.8 • Isolator cabinet.

the aseptic manipulation. In addition, however, this isolator should protect the operator from hazardous materials such as cytotoxic preparations or radiopharmaceuticals in the isolator chamber. This type of isolator operates under negative pressure. The exhaust air is ducted to the outside through at least one HEPA filter and through an adsorption material such as activated carbon. Rigid negative pressure isolators should be used for radiopharmaceutical manipulations. In this situation, the isolator is frequently used with a lead-free vision panel and a lead glass protector around the product. Alternatively, isolators are available with lead acrylic glass windows.

The chambers of isolators are gas sterilized. The ideal sterilant for use in the isolator chamber should have the following properties:

- Non-corrosive to metals and plastics
- Rapidly lethal to all microorganisms
- Good penetration
- Harmless.

The sterilants in most general use for pharmaceutical applications in isolators do not comply with all of these ideal properties. Those used are peracetic acid vapour and hydrogen peroxide vapour. To reduce the risk of chemical contamination of the sterile product, the sterilant contact time should be carefully regulated. The sterilant must be flushed from the isolator before beginning the aseptic manipulations.

Currently marketed isolators are constructed with either a flexible canopy or a rigid containment medium. The rigid type of isolator is often preferred, owing to the reduced risk of the chamber being punctured. This occurs more readily with the flexible canopy design. Rigid isolators are often constructed from a stainless steel frame with a moulded acrylic window. A further isolator known as a half-suit isolator is currently in use. This is a flexible canopy isolator that is made from material such as nylon-lined polyvinyl chloride. It is designed using a half-suit sealed to a wall of the chamber. This system allows the torso of the operator to be introduced into the suit that is located within the chamber of the isolator. To improve visibility, a transparent helmet is sealed to the neck of the suit that is ventilated by a pressurized air supply. This provides operator comfort over prolonged work sessions. The advantage of the half-suit isolator is that the operator can easily access a large area of the chamber and manoeuvre heavier and larger materials. The half-suit isolator is used as dedicated production equipment for the aseptic compounding of products such as total parenteral nutrition (TPN) fluids.

During a 2-week period in September 1992 eight children died from infection after receiving contaminated TPN fluids at four different hospitals in South Africa. These fluids had been prepared in flexible film isolators. The investigation of this incident revealed that the production equipment was suitable for its purpose but inadequate procedures had allowed contamination and subsequent growth of pathogenic bacteria in the TPN fluids. It should therefore be carefully noted that the use of isolators requires trained staff and good manufacturing practices to maintain product quality.

Isolator tests

Isolators must be frequently tested to ensure that they operate as a sealed chamber and conform with the required level of air quality and surface contamination. They are thus subjected to both physical and microbial tests.

Physical tests include:

- *Integrity tests*. These tests will detect leaks that compromise the integrity of the isolator chamber. The procedure is routinely carried out by sealing the chamber and recording changes in the chamber pressure over time.
- *Glove inspection*. The glove and sleeve are visually inspected and leak tested for pin holes.
- *HEPA filter test*. The integrity of the HEPA filter should be tested with an aerosol generator and a detector.
- *Airborne particle count*. This is carried out in the isolator chamber and the transfer device using a particle counter.

Microbial tests use microbial growth media suitable for the growth of potential contaminants. The tests include:

- *Active air sampling*. This test determines the number of organisms in the air of the isolator chamber. The procedure uses impact and agar impingement samplers.
- *Settle plates*. Settle plates containing growth media are exposed in the chamber for 2–4 hours. Particles and organisms settle by gravity onto the agar surface. The plates are then incubated.
- *Surface tests*. Surfaces are sampled using direct contact plates that are then incubated. Following sampling, it is important to remove materials deposited onto the sampled surfaces

during the test. Alternatively, surfaces are sampled using sterile moistened swabs. The swabs are then streaked onto solid growth media and incubated. Soluble swabs may be dissolved in sterile diluent and the viable count determined.

- *Finger dabs*. The fingertips of the gloved hand are pressed onto the surface of solid growth medium. The medium is then incubated.
- *Broth fill test*. This test challenges both the manipulative procedure of the operator and the facilities. The test simulates routine aseptic procedures by using nutrient medium in place of a product to produce broth-filled units. These units are incubated to indicate microbial contamination.

Environmental monitoring

Following construction of a clean room, it must be tested to ensure that it is providing the required quality of environment. These verification tests are rigorously performed and are similar to the tests that are used to monitor the clean room. The monitoring tests ensure that the clean room continues to provide satisfactory operation.

To ensure that the pharmaceutical clean room is providing the required environmental standards, the following are determined.

Air quality

The air supplied to the clean room must not contribute to particulate or microbial contamination within the room. The HEPA filters for the inlet air must be tested to ensure that neither the filter fabric nor the filter seals are leaking. This is done by introducing a smoke with a known particle size upstream of the filter. The clean room surface of the filter is then scanned for smoke penetration using a photometer or a particle counter.

Air movement

Adequate ventilation throughout the clean room can be determined by air movement tests. These are carried out at the time of clean room validation. Air movement within the clean room is determined by measuring the decay profile of smoke particles released into the clean room. Smoke particle release is

also used to ensure that a clean area within a unidirectional workstation is not being contaminated with air from the clean room environment.

The outflow of air from a clean room with a higher standard of cleanliness to an area with a lower standard is indicated by the pressure differential between the rooms. This is determined using a manometer or magnahelic gauge.

Air velocity

The velocity of the air at several points in a clean room area of critical importance should be determined. This is done both at validation of the clean room and at timed intervals. The procedure involves the use of an anemometer.

Airborne particulate and microbial contamination

The particle count and the microbial bioburden of the clean room provide the basis for the air classification system for grading a clean room as detailed in Table 29.1. The points for sampling and the number of samples taken at each position are determined by the size and the grade of the clean room. Airborne particles are normally sized and counted by optical particle counters.

Microbial monitoring

There should be very few viable organisms present in the clean room air. However, operators within the clean room disperse large numbers of skin particles. Many of these particles are contaminated with bacteria. The dispersal of contaminated particles by the clean room operator is greatly decreased by the wearing of occlusive clothing together with appropriate air ventilation. Sampling for microbial contamination is necessary when people are present in the clean room during production. Monitoring of the microbial contamination during production will ensure that both the use of clean room clothing by the operators and the air ventilation system are producing the required environmental standards. Air sampling is carried out by volumetric sampling or by the use of settle plates. With volumetric sampling, a measured volume of air is drawn from the environment and contaminants are impinged onto a suitable microbial growth medium.

The medium is then incubated and the colonies of microbial growth counted. Settle plates rely on bacteria-carrying particles being deposited onto the exposed solid surface of sterile microbial growth media contained in a 90 or 140 mm diameter Petri dish. When positioning the plates, care is needed to avoid accidental contamination. Owing to the small number of microbial contaminants in the clean room, the settle plates are preferably exposed for about 4 hours.

The surfaces of the clean room should also be tested for microbial contamination, notably in areas that may be contacted by the clothing of the operators. This is achieved by using contact plates or by using sterile moistened swabs. The contact plates allow a sterile agar surface to be pressed onto the clean room surface. These plates are then incubated to reveal microbial growth. Swabbing procedures are carried out as previously detailed in isolator tests.

Aseptic preparation

Parenteral products such as injections, infusions and eye products must be sterile for administration to the patient (see Chs 38 and 39). The preferred method of manufacturing parenteral medicines is to place the product in its final container and then seal this package. The product is then protected from further contamination and is terminally sterilized (see Aulton). At worst this achieves the risk of one product in a million being contaminated following terminal sterilization by dry or moist heat or by irradiation. Some products cannot withstand this sterilization process. An alternative approach known as aseptic preparation must then be used to prepare these medicines. This procedure is carried out in industry with selected products but is extensively used in hospital pharmacy where products are specially compounded to meet the specific needs of patients (see Chs 40 and 41).

As shown in Table 29.6, aseptic preparation of parenteral products provides the lowest level of assurance of sterility of all the methods currently used to produce these formulations. In the pharmaceutical industry, pre-sterilized medicines are aseptically filled into sterile containers. The filling process must avoid recontamination of the sterile medicine and its container during this process. A sterility assurance level of 10^{-6} is achieved, but to achieve this requires highly sophisticated industrial production procedures. In hospital pharmacy, pre-sterilized product components are aseptically compounded using sterile apparatus and then aseptically added to appropriate packaging

for subsequent patient administration. It is critical that the sterile product components and the packaging are not recontaminated with organisms or particulate matter during these aseptic procedures. In order to achieve this, the sterile product components and the sterile package must be manipulated in a high-quality environment. The aseptic preparation and filling of products is performed in a localized Grade A zone that is achieved by a laminar airflow cabinet with a Grade B background. The Grade A environment within an isolator cabinet is also suitable for the compounding of aseptic preparations. It is important that this quality environment is continuous throughout the aseptic preparation process. Great reliance is not only placed on the facility and equipment used to produce the product, but also on the ability of the trained operators to avoid product contamination. It achieves a sterility assurance level of about one in a thousand. The manufacture of aseptic products also needs a stringent quality assurance system to ensure production of a quality product that is fit for its intended purpose. The quality assurance system should have documented, validated and audited procedures with in-process monitoring and standard operating procedures defining each step of the production process.

There is a need for awareness of the potential risk of infection that can occur during the aseptic preparation of pharmacy products. This has been shown by the tragic outcome of the supply of contaminated parenteral nutrition fluids to children at the Royal Manchester Children's Hospital in 1994. These fluids were aseptically compounded in an isolator. Microorganisms were unknowingly transferred from a sink into the isolator chamber on components used to prepare the feeds. The contaminating organisms grew in fluid remaining in assembled tubing used to prepare the feeds in the isolator. Reuse of this tubing resulted in contamination of the feeds that infected the patients. During these events it was shown that the equipment was not faulty, only the manner in which it had been used. This demonstrates the importance of adequately disinfecting the components being transferred into the isolator and for a total quality system for the manufacture of aseptic products.

Chapters 40 and 41 deal with the aseptic preparation of a range of commonly used sterile products.

In order to aseptically prepare a parenteral medicine, it is critical that validated procedures are stringently followed. This must go hand in hand with the other components of the quality assurance system for the preparation of aseptically prepared products of quality that are right first time and every time.

Testing for sterility

Sterility testing is the final method of assuring sterility of the manufactured product. The test is required in most countries for assuring the sterility of aseptically prepared sterile products. Aseptic manufacturing units in hospital pharmacy often perform the test retrospectively following patient administration. A few commercial manufacturers are exempt from performing the sterility test on products that have been terminally sterilized and prepared using highly developed quality assurance procedures incorporating validated and controlled sterilization procedures. This has been referred to as parametric release.

Sterility testing attempts to indicate the presence or absence of viable microorganisms in containers selected from a batch of product. A decision is made as to the sterility of the entire batch from the results obtained by testing the sample. The test has both technical and numerical limitations and thus only provides a partial indication to the state of sterility of each product within a manufactured batch. The numerical limitation arises as only 10% of a batch of parenteral product is sampled, but the probability of accidental contamination in an aseptically manufactured batch can be as high as one in a thousand (10^{-3}) while the probability of contamination of a terminally sterilized batch is at worst only one in a million (10^{-6}).

The details of the test for sterility are provided in the *British Pharmacopoeia* (BP 2007) and this test conforms with the standards of the *European Pharmacopoeia* (EP 2007). These are also very similar to the test in the *Japanese Pharmacopoeia* (2007) and *United States Pharmacopoeia 30* (USP 2007).

KEY POINTS

- Particulate and microbial contamination of sterile products is minimized by preparation in a clean environment
- Quality of clean areas is graded A, B, C, D in decreasing stringency for particulate and microbial content
- Premises must allow segregation of stages of production and protect products from contamination by all possible means of design and operation
- Access to clean areas is restricted and special clothing must be worn
- Environmental control, particularly of the air supply to the room, is required to ensure a minimal contamination hazard
- HEPA filters have a 99.997% efficiency at removing 0.3 μm particles, the size at which their efficiency is lowest
- Airflow may be designed as unidirectional, non-unidirectional or as a combination system
- In addition to general air quality, localized areas of higher quality can be produced either by airflow design in enclosed areas, or by isolator cabinets
- The main source of contamination in clean rooms is the skin scales from operators
- Clean room clothing, made from synthetic fabrics, is designed to minimize release of operator contaminants
- Changing areas are designed and used to minimize the entry of contamination on personnel
- During cleaning, vacuuming and wet wiping are used to remove large and small particles respectively
- Isolators give protection to both the product and the operator at relatively low cost
- Type II isolators protect the operator from hazardous materials in addition to providing the Type I facilities of protection of the product from contamination
- Isolator interiors are sterilized using a gas sterilant
- Isolator integrity is tested using physical and microbial tests
- A range of environmental tests is used in clean rooms to monitor air quality, movement and velocity, airborne particles and microbial contamination
- Aseptic preparation is involved with repackaging sterile products for patient use without terminal sterilization
- Aseptic preparation is performed in laminar airflow cabinets in clean rooms or in isolator cabinets to avoid product contamination
- A stringent quality assurance system is required for aseptic production to ensure a quality product is prepared
- The test for sterility has numerical limitations due to the sample size – cannot guarantee to detect small levels of product contamination

30

Solutions

Arthur J. Winfield

STUDY POINTS

- Definitions of solutions and expressions of solubility
- Advantages and disadvantages of using solutions
- Methods of controlling solubility
- Selection of vehicles
- Use of preservatives and other ingredients in solutions
- Principles of dispensing:
  o Solutions for oral use
  o Diluents
  o Mouthwashes
  o Nasal, oral and aural solutions
  o Enemas
- Use of oral syringes

Introduction

Solutions are homogeneous mixtures of two or more components. They contain one or more solutes dissolved in one or more solvents, usually solids dissolved in liquids. The solvent is often aqueous but can be oily, alcoholic or some other solvent.

There are many types of pharmaceutical solutions, based on their composition or medical use. Solutions may be used as oral dosage forms, mouthwashes, gargles, nasal drops and ear drops and externally as lotions, liniments, paints, etc. Solutions may also be used in injections and ophthalmic preparations, which are discussed in Chapters 38 and 39 respectively.

Solutions for oral dosage

Oral solutions are usually formulated so that the patient receives the usual dose of the medicament in a conveniently administered volume, 5 mL or a multiple thereof, given to the patient using a 5 mL medicine spoon. The term 'teaspoon' and 'tablespoon' should not be used as expressions of a dose for an oral liquid because they are not accurate measures.

Advantages of solutions for oral use over a solid dosage form are that liquids are much easier to swallow than tablets or capsules and the medicament is readily absorbed from the gastrointestinal tract. Ease of taking is especially useful for children, elderly patients or those with chronic conditions such as Parkinson's disease, who may have difficulty swallowing a solid oral dosage form. An advantage of solutions over suspensions is that the medicament is dispersed homogeneously throughout the preparation, without the need to shake the bottle. This makes the preparation easier for the patient to use and should ensure consistent dosage. Sometimes substances with a low aqueous solubility may be made into solution by the addition of another solvent rather than formulate the medicine as a suspension.

Disadvantages of solutions are that they are bulky and not as convenient to carry around as a solid dosage form. They are also less microbiologically and chemically stable than their solid counterparts. Drugs that have an unpleasant taste may not be suitable for administration as an oral solution. The accuracy of oral dosage is dependent on the patient measuring the dose carefully.

The different forms of oral solutions are:

- *Syrups*, which are aqueous solutions that contain sugar. An example is Epilim® syrup (sodium valproate).
- *Elixirs*, which are clear, flavoured liquids containing a high proportion of sucrose or a suitable polyhydric alcohol and sometimes ethanol. Examples are phenobarbital elixir and chloral elixir (see Example 30.5).
- *Linctuses*, which are viscous liquids used in the treatment of cough. They usually contain a high proportion of sucrose, other sugars or a suitable polyhydric alcohol or alcohols. Examples are Simple Linctus BP and diamorphine linctus (see Example 30.4).
- *Mixtures* is a term often used to describe pharmaceutical oral solutions and suspensions. Examples are chloral hydrate mixture and ammonium and ipecacuanha mixture BP (see Example 30.3).
- *Oral drops* are oral solutions or suspensions which are administered in small volumes, using a suitable measuring device. A proprietary example is Abidec® vitamin drops.

Containers for dispensed solutions for oral use

Plain, amber medicine bottles should be used, with a reclosable child-resistant closure. Exceptions to this are if the medicine is in an original pack or patient pack, if there are no suitable child-resistant containers for a particular liquid preparation or if the patient requests it, e.g. if they have severe arthritis in their hands. Advice to store away from children should then be given. A 5 mL medicine spoon or an appropriate oral syringe should be supplied to the patient.

Special labels and advice for dispensed oral solutions

An expiry date should appear on the label for extemporaneously prepared solutions. Most 'official' mixtures and some oral solutions are freshly or recently prepared (see Ch. 43). 'Official' elixirs and linctuses and manufactured products are generally more stable, unless diluted. Diluted products generally have a shorter shelf life than the undiluted preparation. Linc-tuses should be sipped and swallowed slowly, without the addition of water.

Solutions for other pharmaceutical uses

Topical solutions for external use are considered in Chapter 33. Some topical solutions are designed for use in body cavities, such as the nose, mouth and ear.

Mouthwashes and gargles

Gargles are used to relieve or treat sore throats and mouthwashes are used on the mucous membranes of the oral cavity, rather than the throat, to refresh and mechanically clean the mouth. Both are concentrated solutions, although gargles tend to contain higher concentrations of active ingredients than mouthwashes. Both are usually diluted with warm water before use. They may contain antiseptics, analgesics or weak astringents. The liquid is usually not intended for swallowing. Examples are Phenol Gargle BPC and Compound Sodium Chloride Mouthwash BP (see Example 30.7). Proprietary examples are chlorhexidine (Corsodyl®) mouthwash and povidone-iodine (Betadine®) mouthwash.

Containers for mouthwashes and gargles

An amber, ribbed bottle should be used for these extemporaneously prepared solutions. Medicine bottles may be used for products which are intended to be swallowed. Manufactured mouthwashes and gargles are usually packed in plain bottles.

Special labels and advice for mouthwashes and gargles

Directions for diluting the preparations should be given to the patient. If the preparation is not intended for swallowing, the following label is appropriate: 'Not to be swallowed in large amounts'.

Nasal solutions

Most nasal preparations are solutions, administered as nose drops or sprays. They are usually formulated to be isotonic to nasal secretions (equivalent to 0.9% normal saline) and buffered to the normal pH range of nasal fluids (pH 5.5–6.5) to prevent damage to ciliary transport in the nose. The most frequent use of nose drops is as a decongestant for the common cold or to administer local steroids for the treatment of allergic rhinitis. Examples are normal saline nose drops and ephedrine nose drops, 0.5% or 1%. Overuse of topical decongestants can lead to oedema of the nasal mucosa and they should only be used for short periods of time (about 4 days) to avoid rebound congestion, called rhinitis medicamentosa. The nasal route may also be useful for new biologically active peptides and polypeptides which need to avoid the first pass metabolism and destruction by the gastrointestinal fluids. The nasal mucosa rapidly absorbs medicaments applied there to give a systemic effect. There are some products utilizing nasal delivery currently available on the market, e.g. insulin (Exubera®) and desmopressin (e.g. Desmospray®, DDAVP®), used in the treatment of pituitary diabetes insipidus. Accurate dosage is achieved using metered spray devices.

Ear drops

Ear drops are solutions of one or more active ingredient which exert a local effect in the ear, e.g. by softening earwax or treating infection or inflammation. They may also be referred to as otic or aural preparations. Propylene glycol, oils, glycerol (to increase viscosity) and water may be used as vehicles. Examples are aluminium acetate ear drops, almond oil ear drops and Sodium Bicarbonate Ear Drops BP (see Example 30.8).

Containers for nasal and aural preparations

Nose and ear drops that are prepared extemporaneously should be packed in an amber, ribbed hexagonal glass bottle which is fitted with a teat and dropper. Manufactured nasal solutions may be packed in flexible plastic bottles which deliver a fine spray to the nose when squeezed, or in a plain glass bottle with a pump spray or dropper. Manufactured ear drops are usually packed in small glass or plastic containers with a dropper.

Special labels and advice for nasal and aural preparations

Patients should be advised not to share nasal sprays or nose and ear drops in order to minimize contamination and infection. Manufactured nasal sprays and nose and ear drops will usually contain instructions for administration. Patients should be given advice on how to administer extemporaneously prepared nose and ear drops, accompanied by written information if possible (Fig. 30.1). For nose drops, it may be easier if the patient is lying flat with the head tilted back as far as comfortable, preferably over the edge of a bed. The patient should remain in this position for a few minutes after the drops have been administered to allow the medication to spread in the nose.

For ear drops, it may be easier for someone other than the patient to administer the drops. If desired, the drops can be warmed by holding the bottle in the hands before putting them in, but they must not be overheated. The ear lobe should be held up and back in adults, down and back in children, to allow the medication to run in deeper. They may cause some transient stinging. If the drops are intended to soften earwax, then the ears should be syringed after several days of use.

Extemporaneous preparations should be labelled with the appropriate expiry date following the official monographs. 'For external use' is not an appropriate label and so 'Not to be taken' is advised.

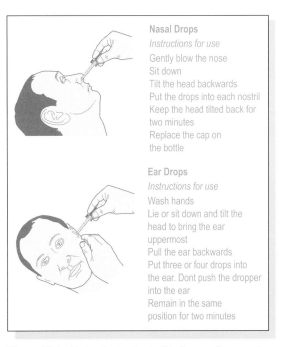

Figure 30.1 • Patient instruction leaflets for use of nose and ear drops.

Nasal Drops
Instructions for use
Gently blow the nose
Sit down
Tilt the head backwards
Put the drops into each nostril
Keep the head tilted back for
two minutes
Replace the cap on
the bottle

Ear Drops
Instructions for use
Wash hands
Lie or sit down and tilt the
head to bring the ear
uppermost
Pull the ear backwards
Put three or four drops into
the ear. Dont push the dropper
into the ear
Remain in the same
position for two minutes

Enemas

Enemas are oily or aqueous solutions that are administered rectally. They are usually anti-inflammatory, purgative, sedative or given to allow X-ray examination of the lower bowel. Examples are arachis oil enema and magnesium sulphate enema. Retention enemas are administered to give either a local action of the drug, e.g. prednisolone, or for systemic absorption, e.g. diazepam. They are used after defecation. The patient lies on one side during administration and remains there for 30 minutes to allow distribution of the medicament. Microenemas are single-dose, small-volume solutions. Examples are solutions of sodium phosphate, sodium citrate or docusate sodium. They are packaged in plastic containers with a nozzle for insertion into the rectum. Large-volume (0.5–1 litre) enemas should be warmed to body temperature before administration.

Containers for enemas

If extemporaneously produced, enemas are packed in amber, fluted glass bottles. Manufactured enemas will usually be packed in disposable polythene or polyvinyl chloride bags sealed to a rectal nozzle.

Special labels and advice for enemas

Patients should be advised on how to use the enema if they are self-administering and the time that the product will take to work. The label 'For rectal use only' should be used.

Expression of concentration

Strengths of pharmaceutical solutions can be expressed in a number of ways. The two most commonly used are in terms of amount of drug contained in 5 mL of vehicle or percentage strength. Thus, for example, a 100 mg/5 mL solution contains 100 mg of drug in each 5 mL. The volume 5 mL is used because it is the commonest oral dose administered. A percent weight in volume (% w/v) describes the number of grams of a constituent in 100 mL of preparation. For example, a 2% w/v preparation contains 2 g of a constituent in 100 mL of preparation. A percent volume in volume (% v/v) describes the number of millilitres of a constituent in 100 mL of preparation. For example, a 1% v/v preparation contains 1 mL of a constituent in 100 mL of preparation (see also Ch. 26).

Formulation of solutions

Solutions comprise the medicinal agent in a solvent as well as any additional agents. These additional agents are usually included to provide colour, flavour, sweetness or stability to the formulation. Most solutions are now manufactured on a large scale although it may be occasionally required to make up a solution extemporaneously. When compounding a solution, information on solubility and stability of each of the solutes must be taken into account.

Chemical and physical interactions that may take place between constituents must also be taken into account, as these will affect the preparation's stability or potency. For example, esters of *p*-hydroxybenzoic acid, which can be used as preservatives in oral solutions, have a tendency to partition into certain flavouring oils. This could reduce the effective concentration of the preservative agent in the aqueous vehicle of the preparation to a level lower than that required for preservative action.

Solubility

The saturation solubility of a chemical in a solvent is the maximum concentration of a solution which may be prepared at a given temperature. For convenience, this is usually simply called solubility. Solubilities for medicinal agents in a given solvent are given in the *British Pharmacopoeia* (BP) and Martindale and other reference sources. Solubilities are usually stated as the number of parts of solvent (by volume) that will dissolve one part (by weight or volume) of the substance. In other situations, words are used to describe the solubility (see Example 30.2). Using this information it is often possible to calculate whether a solution can be prepared. Most solutions for pharmaceutical use are not saturated with solute.

Example 30.1

Potassium chloride is soluble in 2.8–3 parts of water. This means that 1 g of potassium chloride will dissolve in 2.8–3 mL of water at a temperature of 20°C (taken as normal room temperature).

Example 30.2

Diazepam is described as being 'very slightly soluble' in water (which means 1 in 1000 to 1 in 10 000), 'soluble' in alcohol (which means 1 in 10 to 1 in 30) and 'freely soluble' in chloroform (which means 1 in 1 to 1 in 10).

This means that 1 g of diazepam will dissolve in between 10 and 30 mL of alcohol, but would need 1000–10 000 mL of water to dissolve, at a temperature of 20°C.

Vehicles

In pharmacy, the medium which contains the ingredients of a medicine is called the vehicle. In solutions, this is the solvent. The choice of a vehicle depends on the intended use of the preparation and on the nature and physicochemical properties of the active ingredients.

Water as a vehicle

Water is the vehicle used for most pharmaceutical preparations. It is widely available, relatively inexpensive, palatable and non-toxic for oral use and non-irritant for external use. It is also a good solvent for many ionizable drugs. Different types of water are available as outlined below:

- *Potable water* is drinking water, drawn freshly from a mains supply. It should be palatable and safe for drinking. Its chemical composition may include mineral impurities which could react with drugs, e.g. the presence of calcium carbonate in hard water.
- *Purified water* is prepared from suitable potable water by distillation, by treatment with ion-exchange materials or by any other suitable treatment method such as reverse osmosis. Distilled water is purified water that has been prepared by distillation.
- *Water for preparations* is potable or freshly boiled and cooled purified water, which can be used in oral or external preparations which are not intended to be sterile. The boiling removes dissolved oxygen and carbon dioxide from solution in the water. Any stored water, for example drawn from a local storage tank, should

not be used because of the risk of contamination with microorganisms.

- *Water for injections* is pyrogen-free distilled water, sterilized immediately after collection and used for parenteral products (for further details see Ch. 38).
- *Aromatic waters* are near-saturated aqueous solutions of volatile oils or other aromatic or volatile substances, and are often used as a vehicle in oral solutions. Some have a mild carminative action, e.g. dill. Aromatic waters are usually prepared from a concentrated ethanolic solution, in a dilution of 1 part of concentrated water with 39 parts of water. Chloroform water is used as an antimicrobial preservative and also adds sweetness to preparations (see also p. 440).

Other vehicles used in pharmaceutical solutions

- *Syrup BP* is a solution of 66.7% sucrose in water. It will promote dental decay and is unsuitable for diabetic patients. Hydrogenated glucose syrup, mannitol, sorbitol, xylitol, etc. can replace the sucrose to give 'sugar-free' solvents.
- *Alcohol (ethyl alcohol, ethanol)*. This is rarely used for internal preparations but is a useful solvent for external preparations.
- *Glycerol (glycerin)* may be used alone as a vehicle in some external preparations. It is viscous and miscible both with water and alcohol. It may be added as a stabilizer and sweetener in internal preparations. In concentrations above 20% v/v it acts as a preservative.
- *Propylene glycol* is a less viscous liquid and a better solvent than glycerol.
- *Oils*. Bland oils such as fractionated coconut oil and arachis oil may be used for fat-soluble compounds, e.g. Calciferol Oral Solution BP. Care is required when using nut oils due to hypersensitivity reactions.
- *Acetone* is used as a cosolvent in external preparations.
- *Solvent ether* can be used as a cosolvent in external preparations for preoperative skin preparation. The extreme volatility of ether and risk of fire and explosion limit its usefulness.

Factors affecting solubility

Compounds that are predominantly non-polar tend to be more soluble in non-polar solvents, such as chloroform or a vegetable oil. Polar compounds tend to be more soluble in polar solvents, such as water and ethanol. The pH will also affect solubility, as many drugs are weak acids or bases. The ionized form of a compound will be the most water soluble, therefore a weakly basic drug will be most soluble in an aqueous solution that is acidic. Acid or alkali may therefore be added to manipulate solubility. Most compounds are more soluble at higher temperatures. Particle size reduction will increase the rate of solution.

Increasing the solution of compounds with low solubility

Cosolvency

The addition of cosolvents, such as ethanol, glycerol, propylene glycol or sorbitol, can increase the solubility of weak electrolytes and non-polar molecules in water. They are discussed in more detail in Aulton (2007).

Solubilization

Surfactants may be used as solubilizing agents. Above the critical micelle concentration (CMC), they form micelles which are used to help dissolve poorly soluble compounds. The dissolved compound may be in the centre of the micelle, adsorbed onto the micelle surface, or sit at some intermediate point, depending on the polarity of the compound. Examples of surfactants used in oral solutions are polysorbates, while soaps are used to solubilize phenolic disinfectants for external use.

Preservation of solutions

Most water-containing pharmaceutical solutions will support microbial growth unless this is prevented. Contamination may come from raw materials or be introduced during extemporaneous dispensing.

Preservatives may be added to the formulation to reduce or prevent microbial growth. Chloroform is the most widely used in oral extemporaneous pre-

parations although there are disadvantages to its use, including its high volatility and reported carcinogenicity in animals. Use in the UK is limited to a chloroform content of 0.5% (w/w or w/v). For oral solutions, chloroform at a strength of 0.25% v/v will usually be incorporated as Chloroform Water BP. Alternatively, double strength chloroform water may be included in pharmaceutical formulae as half the total volume of the solution, to effectively give single strength chloroform water in the finished medicine (see Example 30.3). Benzoic acid at a strength of 0.1% w/v is also suitable for oral administration, as are ethanol, sorbic acid, the hydroxybenzoate esters and syrup. Some of the alternative preservatives have pH-dependent activity.

Syrups can be preserved by the maintenance of a high concentration of sucrose as part of the formulation. Concentrations of sucrose greater than 65% w/w will usually protect an oral liquid from growth of most microorganisms by its osmotic effects. A problem with their use occurs when other ingredients are added to the syrup, as this decreases the sucrose concentration. This may cause a loss in the preservative action of the sucrose. Accidental dilution by, for example, using a damp bottle, may have a similar effect.

Preservatives used in external solutions include chlorocresol (0.1% w/v), chlorbutanol (0.5% w/v) and the parahydroxybenzoates (parabens).

Additional ingredients

Solutions that are intended for oral use may contain excipients such as flavouring, sweetening and, sometimes, colouring agents. These are added to improve the palatability and appearance of a solution for the patient. Stabilizing and viscosity enhancing agents may also be used.

Flavouring agents

Flavours added to solutions can make a medicine more acceptable to take, especially if the drug has an unpleasant taste. Selection of flavours is a complex process in the pharmaceutical industry. Flavours should be chosen to mask particular taste types, e.g. a fruit flavour helps to disguise an acid taste. The age of the patient should be taken into account when selecting a flavour, as children will tend to enjoy fruit or sweet flavours. Some flavours are associated with particular uses, e.g. peppermint is associated with antacid preparations. The flavour and colour should also complement each other. Extemporaneous medicines tend to use natural flavours added as juices (raspberry), extracts (liquorice), spirits (lemon and orange), syrups (blackcurrant), tinctures (ginger) and aromatic waters (anise and cinnamon). Some synthetic flavours are used in manufactured medicines.

Sweetening agents

Many oral solutions are sweetened with sugars, including glucose and sucrose. Sucrose enhances the viscosity of liquids and also gives a pleasant texture in the mouth. Prolonged use of liquid medicines containing sugar will lead to an increased incidence of dental caries, particularly in children. Attempts should be made to formulate oral solutions without sugar as a sweetening agent, using sorbitol, mannitol, xylitol, saccharin and aspartame as alternatives. Oral liquid preparations that do not contain fructose, glucose or sucrose are labelled 'sugar free' in the *British National Formulary* (BNF). These alternatives should be used where possible.

Colouring agents

Colouring agents are added to pharmaceutical preparations to enhance the appearance of a preparation or to increase the acceptability of a preparation to the patient. Colours are often matched to the flavour of a preparation, e.g. a yellow colour for a banana-flavoured preparation. Colour is also useful to give a consistent appearance where there is natural variation between batches. Colours can give distinctive appearances to some medicines, e.g. the green colour of the Drug Tariff formula of methadone mixture.

Colouring agents should be non-toxic and free of any therapeutic activity themselves. Natural colourants are most likely to meet this criterion and include materials derived from plants and animals, e.g. carotenoids, chlorophylls, saffron, red beetroot extract, caramel and cochineal. As with all natural agents, the disadvantage is that batches may vary in quality. Mineral pigments such as iron oxides are not often used in solutions because of their low solubility in water. Synthetic organic dyes such as the azo compounds are alternatives for colouring pharmaceutical solutions as they give a wide range of bright, stable colours. Colours appear in pharmaceutical formulae less often now, especially in children's medicines. Some consumers see their use as unnecessary and some colouring agents, e.g. tartrazine, have been implicated in allergic reactions and hyperactivity of chil-

dren. Additionally, coloured dyes in medicines can lead to confusion when diagnosing diseases, e.g. a red dye appearing in vomit could be wrongly assumed to be blood. In the European Union, colours are selected from a list permitted for medicinal products, with designated 'E' numbers between 100 and 180.

Stabilizers

Antioxidants may be used where ingredients are liable to degradation by oxidation, e.g. in oils. Those which are added to oral preparations include ascorbic acid, citric acid, sodium metabisulphite and sodium sulphite. These are odourless, tasteless and non-toxic.

Viscosity-enhancing agents

Syrups may be added to increase the viscosity of an oral liquid. They also improve palatability and ease pourability. Other thickening agents may also be used (see Ch. 31).

Shelf life of solutions

There may be individual variations, but most solutions which are prepared extemporaneously should be freshly or recently prepared. The data sheets should be consulted for information about particular manufactured solutions and for storage conditions.

Oral syringes

If fractional doses are prescribed for oral liquids, they should not be diluted, but an oral syringe should be supplied with the dispensed oral liquid. The standard 5 mL or 10 mL capacity oral syringe is marked in 0.2 mL divisions to measure fractional doses. An adapter fits into the neck of all common sizes of the medicine bottle. Instructions should be supplied with the oral syringe. Shake the bottle and then remove the lid and insert the adapter firmly into the top of the bottle. Push the tip of the oral syringe into the hole in the adapter and turn the bottle upside down. Pull the syringe plunger to draw liquid to the appropriate volume. It may be desirable to indicate this on the syringe. Turn the bottle right way up and carefully remove the syringe, holding the barrel. Gently put the tip into the child's mouth to be inside the cheek. Slowly and gently push the plunger in and allow the child to swallow the medicine before removing the syringe. Do not squirt the liquid or direct it towards the throat. After completing the process, remove the adapter and replace the cap on the bottle. The adapter and syringe should be rinsed and left to dry. Patient information leaflets are available to accompany the oral syringe.

Diluents

If a prescriber insists that a manufactured solution is diluted, then a suitable diluent must be selected. Information sources to obtain this information are the *Medicines Compendium* or the National Pharmaceutical Association (NPA) *Diluent Directory*. An indication of the expiry date for the diluted preparation is also given in these references. The dilution should be freshly prepared.

A short shelf life for a diluted solution may require patients to return to the pharmacy to collect the balance of their medication. This may happen, for instance, where an oral sodium chloride solution has been prescribed for 1 month. The solution has a 2-week expiry, and must therefore be supplied in two instalments. The patient, or their representative, should be issued with an owing slip, or some similar documentation. This should state the name of the patient, the pharmacy, the item and quantity of medicine owed and the date of issue. A record should also be kept in the pharmacy. Most computer labelling systems have the facility to handle 'owings'.

they may be useful as a placebo and they are inexpensive.

Formulation notes. Ammonium bicarbonate, ipecacuanha and camphor water are mild expectorants. Anise water acts as a mild expectorant and a flavouring agent. Liquid liquorice extract is used as a mild expectorant, flavouring and sweetening agent. Chloroform water acts as a sweetener and a preservative. Ammonium bicarbonate is soluble 1 in 5 of water, so will dissolve to give a solution. All other ingredients are liquids.

Method of preparation. Weigh the ammonium bicarbonate on a suitable balance and dissolve in approximately 15 mL water, in a 100 mL conical measure. Add the double strength chloroform water to this solution. Measure the other liquid ingredients and add to the solution. Make up to volume with water in the conical measure. Pack into an amber medicine bottle with a child-resistant closure. Polish the bottle and label, and provide a 5 mL spoon.

Shelf life and storage. Store in a cool, dry place. It is recently prepared, therefore a shelf life of 2–3 weeks is applicable.

Advice and labelling. 'Shake well before use'. While this is not strictly required, it is good practice to include it.

Example 30.3

Rx Ammonium and Ipecacuanha Mixture BP. Mitte 100 mL.

	Master formula	For 100 mL
Ammonium bicarbonate	200 mg	2 g
Liquorice liquid extract	0.5 mL	5 mL
Ipecacuanha tincture	0.3 mL	3 mL
Concentrated camphor water	0.1 mL	1 mL
Concentrated anise water	0.05 mL	0.5 mL
Double strength chloroform water	5 mL	50 mL

Example 30.4

Rx 200 mL of Diamorphine linctus.

	Master formula	For 200 mL
Diamorphine hydrochloride	3 mg	120 mg
Oxymel	1.25 mL	50 mL
Glycerol	1.25 mL	50 mL
Compound tartrazine solution	0.06 mL	2.4 mL
Syrup	to 5 mL	to 200 mL

Action and uses. A cough suppressant in terminal care.

Formulation notes. Oxymel is a solution of acetic acid, water and purified honey, used as a demulcent and sweetening agent in linctuses. Glycerol is also a demulcent and sweetener. Compound tartrazine solution is a colouring agent and syrup is a demulcent vehicle. Diamorphine is soluble 1 in 1.6 of water and 1 in 12 of alcohol, so a solution will be produced.

Method of preparation. Weigh 120 mg diamorphine on an appropriate balance. Transfer to a 200 mL

Action and uses. Expectorant cough preparation. The benefit of expectorant mixtures is doubtful, but

measuring cylinder. Dissolve the diamorphine in the oxymel and glycerol. Add about 50 mL of syrup, then add the compound tartrazine solution. Transfer to a previously tared amber medicine bottle (see Ch. 25). Make up to volume with the syrup in the tared bottle in order to overcome difficulties in draining all the viscous mixture from a measure. Close with a child-resistant closure, polish and label the bottle and give a 5 mL medicine spoon or oral syringe with the medicine (depending on the dosage prescribed).

Shelf life and storage. Store in a cool, dry place. It is recently prepared, therefore a shelf life of 2–3 weeks is applicable.

Advice and labelling. 'Shake well before use'. The linctus should be sipped and swallowed slowly, undiluted. 'Warning. May cause drowsiness. Avoid alcoholic drink' (BNF Label 2). Since this patient is terminally ill, they are unlikely to be driving or operating machinery so this part of the advisory label can be omitted. Alcohol should be avoided as this will increase the sedative effect.

Example 30.5

℞ 50 mL Chloral elixir, paediatric. For an 8-month-old baby.

	Master formula	For 50 mL
Chloral hydrate	200 mg	2 g
Water	0.1 mL	1 mL
Blackcurrant syrup	1 mL	10 mL
Syrup	to 5 mL	to 50 mL

Action and uses. For short-term use in insomnia.

Formulation notes. Chloral hydrate is soluble 1 in 0.3 of water and has an unpleasant taste. Blackcurrant syrup is used as a flavouring agent to mask this.

Method of preparation. Weigh 2 g chloral hydrate on a suitable balance. Transfer it to a 50 mL measuring cylinder and dissolve it in water. Add the blackcurrant syrup. Add some of the syrup (rinsing the measure used for the blackcurrant syrup). Transfer the mixture to a tared, 50 mL amber medicine bottle and make up to volume, to avoid loss of the viscous product in the measures. Polish and label the bottle and give a 5 mL medicine spoon or oral syringe with the medicine.

Shelf life and storage. Store in a cool, dry place. Chloral hydrate is volatile and sensitive to light. It is

recently prepared and a shelf life of 2–3 weeks is appropriate.

Advice and labelling. 'Shake well before use' and BNF Labels 1 and 27. An appropriate dose for a child up to 1 year is one 5 mL spoonful to be given, well diluted with water, at bedtime. The parent should be advised that this might make the child drowsy.

Example 30.6

℞ 200 mL Potassium Citrate Mixture BP.

	Master formula	For 200 mL
Potassium citrate	3 g	60 g
Citric acid monohydrate	500 mg	10 g
Syrup	2.5 mL	50 mL
Quillaia tincture	0.1 mL	2 mL
Lemon spirit	0.05 mL	1 mL
Double strength chloroform water	3 mL	60 mL
Water	to 10 mL	to 200 mL

Action and uses. Alkalinization of urine to relieve discomfort in mild urinary tract infections or cystitis.

Formulation notes. Citric acid and potassium citrate are the active ingredients; both are soluble 1 in 1 of water. Lemon spirit, which is lemon oil in alcoholic solution, is a flavouring agent. The oil tends to be displaced from solution in an aqueous medium, especially in the presence of a high concentration of salts. The quillaia tincture is a surfactant used to emulsify any displaced lemon oil. Syrup is a sweetening agent.

Method of preparation. The solids should be size reduced, weighed and dissolved in the double strength chloroform water and syrup. The quillaia tincture should be added before the lemon spirit is added with stirring, so that immediate emulsification of the oil will be achieved if required. Make up to volume with water. Pack in an amber medicine bottle with a child-resistant closure. Polish and label the bottle and give a 5 mL medicine spoon with the medicine.

Shelf life and storage. Store in a cool, dry place. It is recently prepared, therefore a shelf life of 2–3 weeks is applicable.

Advice and labelling. 'Shake well before use'. The medicine should be diluted with plenty of water (BNF Label 27).

Example 30.7

Rx Compound Sodium Chloride Mouthwash BP. Mitte 500 mL.

	Master formula	For 500 mL
Sodium chloride	1.5 g	7.5 g
Sodium bicarbonate	1 g	5 g
Concentrated peppermint emulsion	2.5 mL	12.5 mL
Double strength chloroform water	50 mL	250 mL
Water	to 100 mL	to 500 mL

Action and uses. Mechanically cleans and freshens the mouth.

Formulation notes. Concentrated peppermint emulsion is used as a flavouring and the chloroform water is a sweetener and preservative. Sodium chloride is soluble 1 in 3 of water and sodium bicarbonate is soluble 1 in 11 of water.

Method of preparation. The solids are weighed on a suitable balance and dissolved in a 500 mL conical measure in approximately 100 mL of water. Add the double strength chloroform water and the concentrated peppermint emulsion. Make up to volume with water. Pack in an amber ribbed bottle with a child-resistant closure. Polish and label the bottle.

Shelf life and storage. Store in a cool, dry place. It is recently prepared, therefore a shelf life of 2–3 weeks is applicable.

Advice and labelling. 'Shake well before use'. The patient should be directed to use about 15 mL diluted in an equal volume of warm water, usually morning and night, unless otherwise directed. The solution should be used as a mouthwash and should not be swallowed, although reassure the patient that it is not harmful to swallow small amounts of the mouthwash.

Example 30.8

Rx 10 mL Sodium Bicarbonate Ear Drops BP.

	Master formula	For 10 mL
Sodium bicarbonate	5 g	500 mg
Glycerol	30 mL	3 mL
Water	to 100 mL	to 10 mL

Action and uses. For the softening and removal of earwax (usually prior to syringing with warm water).

Formulation notes. Sodium bicarbonate is soluble 1 in 11 of water. Glycerol is a viscous liquid used to thicken the drops, but presents problems in measuring the volume accurately.

Method of preparation. Weigh 500 mg sodium bicarbonate and dissolve in 6 mL of water, using a 10 mL conical measure. Carefully make up to 7 mL using water. Carefully add glycerol up to the 10 mL mark (this will result in 3 mL of glycerol being added to the solution). Pack in a 10 mL hexagonal, amber, ribbed bottle with a dropper. Polish and label the bottle on the three smooth sides.

Shelf life and storage. Store in a cool, dry place. The drops are recently prepared, therefore a shelf life of 2–3 weeks is applicable.

Advice and labelling. 'Shake well before use' and 'Not to be taken'. The bottle may be warmed in the hands before placing drops in the ears. A patient information leaflet should be used to describe how to use the drops (see Fig. 30.1).

KEY POINTS

- Pharmaceutical solutions are given different names depending on their nature and use
- There are both advantages and disadvantages in the use of oral solutions
- Most oral solutions should be freshly or recently prepared
- Solutions may also be used for mouthwashes, gargles, nasal drops and sprays, ear drops and enemas
- Many different vehicles may be used in pharmaceutical solutions, but water is the most common
- Water is available in different forms for different uses
- Saturation solubility of a drug in a solvent is affected by polarity of both drug and solvent
- Saturation solubility can be increased by techniques such as cosolvency and solubilization
- Antimicrobial preservation is required for most aqueous solutions
- Various additives such as flavours, sweeteners and colours may be added to improve the palatability of oral solutions
- Oral syringes will be required for doses of less than 5 mL and its use explained

Suspensions

Arthur J. Winfield

Introduction

Suspensions contain one or more insoluble medicaments in a vehicle, with other additives such as preservatives, flavours, colours, buffers and stabilizers. Most pharmaceutical suspensions are aqueous, but an oily vehicle is sometimes used. Suspensions may be used for oral administration, inhalation, topical application, as ophthalmic preparations, for parenteral administration and as aerosols.

A pharmaceutical suspension may be defined as a disperse system in which one substance (the disperse phase) is distributed in particulate form throughout another (the continuous phase). Most are classified as a coarse suspension which is a dispersion of particles with a mean diameter greater than 1 μm. A colloidal suspension is a dispersion of particles with a mean diameter less than 1 μm. Suspended solids slowly separate on standing, but redispersion may be difficult if they form a compacted sediment.

Pharmaceutical applications of suspensions

Suspensions may be used pharmaceutically for a number of reasons. Some are given below:

- Drugs that have very low solubility are usefully formulated as suspensions.
- If people have difficulty swallowing solid dosage forms, the drug may need to be dispersed into a liquid form.
- Drugs that have an unpleasant taste in their soluble form can be made into insoluble derivatives, and formulated as a suspension, which will be more palatable; for example chloramphenicol (soluble) and chloramphenicol palmitate (insoluble).
- In oral suspensions the drug is delivered in finely divided form, therefore optimal dissolution occurs immediately in the gastrointestinal (GI) fluids. The rate of absorption of a drug from a suspension is usually faster than when delivered as a solid oral dosage form, but slower than the rate from solution. The rate of availability of drug from a suspension is also dependent on the viscosity; the more viscous the product, the slower the release of drug.
- Insoluble forms of drugs may prolong the action of a drug by preventing rapid degradation of the drug in the presence of water.

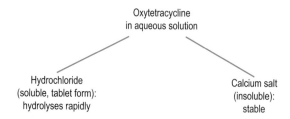

Oxytetracycline
in aqueous solution

Hydrochloride
(soluble, tablet form):
hydrolyses rapidly

Calcium salt
(insoluble):
stable

- After gentle shaking, the medicament stays in suspension long enough for a dose to be accurately measured
- The suspension is pourable
- Particles in suspension are small and relatively uniform in size, so that the product is free from a gritty texture.

- If the drug is unstable when in contact with the vehicle, suspensions should be prepared immediately prior to handing out to the patient in order to reduce the amount of time that the drug particles are in contact with the dispersion medium. For example, with ampicillin suspension, water is added to powder or granules prior to giving out to the patient. A 14-day expiry date is given, if the product is to be kept in the fridge.
- Drugs which degrade in aqueous solution may be suspended in a non-aqueous phase, for example tetracycline hydrochloride is suspended in a fractionated coconut oil for ophthalmic use.
- Bulky, insoluble powders can be formulated as a suspension so that they are easier to take, for example kaolin or chalk (see Example 31.2). Examples of suspensions for oral use are Kaolin Mixture Paediatric BP, kaolin and morphine mixture (see Example 31.1) and antacids such as Magnesium Trisilicate Mixture BP.
- Intramuscular, intra-articular or subcutaneous injections are often formulated as suspensions to prolong the release of the drug.
- Lotions containing insoluble solids are formulated to leave a thin coating of medicament on the skin. As the vehicle evaporates, it gives a cooling effect and leaves the solid behind. Examples are Calamine Lotion BP (see Example 31.5) and Sulphur Lotion Compound BPC (see Ch. 33).

Properties of a good pharmaceutical suspension

In preparing a pharmaceutically elegant product, several desirable properties are sought:
- There is ready redispersion of any sediment which accumulates on storage

Formulation of suspensions

The three steps that can be taken to ensure formulation of an elegant pharmaceutical suspension are:
1. Control particle size. On a small scale, this can be done using a mortar and pestle, to grind down ingredients to a fine powder
2. Use a thickening agent to increase viscosity of the vehicle, by using suspending or viscosity-increasing agents
3. Use a wetting agent.

Some of the theoretical and practical aspects of these will be considered in the context of extemporaneous dispensing. Further details about the industrial aspects are given in Aulton (2007).

The insoluble medicament may be a diffusible solid or an indiffusible solid:

Diffusible solids (dispersible solids). These are insoluble solids that are light and easily wetted by water. They mix readily with water, and stay dispersed long enough for an adequate dose to be measured. After settling they redisperse easily. Examples include magnesium trisilicate, light magnesium carbonate, bismuth carbonate and light kaolin (see Example 31.1).

Indiffusible solids. Most insoluble solids are not easily wetted, and may form large porous clumps in the liquid. These solids will not remain evenly distributed in the vehicle long enough for an adequate dose to be measured. They may not redisperse easily. Examples for internal use include aspirin, phenobarbital, sulfadimidine and chalk (see Example 31.2) and for external use calamine, hydrocortisone, sulphur and zinc oxide.

Problems encountered when formulating insoluble solids into a suspension

Various factors need to be considered when formulating insoluble solids into a suspension.

Sedimentation

The factors affecting the rate of sedimentation of a particle are described in Stokes' equation:

$$y = \frac{2\,gr^2\,(\rho_1 - \rho_2)}{9\eta}$$

where y = velocity of a spherical particle of radius r, and density ρ_1, in a liquid of density ρ_2, and viscosity η, and where g is the acceleration due to gravity.

The basic consequences of this equation are that the rate of fall of a suspended particle in a vehicle of a given density is greater for larger particles than it is for smaller particles. Also, the greater the difference in density between the particles and vehicle, the greater will be the rate of descent. Increasing the viscosity of the dispersion medium, within limits so that the suspension is still pourable, will reduce the rate of sedimentation of a solid drug. Thus a decrease in settling rate in a suspension may be achieved by reducing the size of the particles and by increasing the density and the viscosity of the continuous phase.

Flocculation

The natural tendency of particles towards aggregation will determine the properties of a suspension. In a deflocculated suspension, the dispersed solid particles remain separate and settle slowly. However, the sediment that eventually forms is hard to redisperse and is described as a 'cake' or 'clay'. In a flocculated suspension, individual particles aggregate into clumps or floccules in suspension. Because these flocs are larger than individual particles, sedimentation is more rapid, but the sediment is loose and easily redispersible. Excess flocculation may prevent 'pourability' due to its effect on rheological properties.

The ideal is to use either a deflocculated system with a sufficiently high viscosity to prevent sedimentation, or controlled flocculation with a suitable combination of rate of sedimentation, type of sediment and pourability.

Wetting

Air may be trapped in the particles of poorly wetted solids which causes them to float to the surface of the preparation and prevents them from being readily dispersed throughout the vehicle. Wetting of the particles can be encouraged by reducing the interfacial tension between the solid and the vehicle, so that adsorbed air is displaced from solid surfaces by liquid. Suitable wetting agents have this effect, but decrease interparticular forces thereby affecting flocculation.

Hydrophilic colloids such as acacia and tragacanth can act as wetting agents. However, care should be taken when using these agents as they can promote deflocculation. Intermediate HLB (hydrophilic–lipophilic balance) surfactants (see Ch. 32) such as polysorbates and sorbitan esters are used for internal preparations. Solvents such as ethanol, glycerol and the glycols also facilitate wetting. Sodium lauryl sulphate and quillaia tincture are used in external preparations.

Suspending agents

Suspending agents increase the viscosity of the vehicle, thereby slowing down sedimentation. Most agents can form thixotropic gels which are semi-solid on standing, but flow readily after shaking. Care must be taken when selecting a suspending agent for oral preparations, as the acid environment of the stomach may alter the physical characteristics of the suspension, and therefore the rate of release of the drug from suspension. Some suspending agents may also bind to certain medicaments, making them less bioavailable.

Suspending agents can be divided into five broad categories: natural polysaccharides, semi-synthetic polysaccharides, clays, synthetic thickeners and miscellaneous compounds. Brief information on these classes of suspending agents is given below, with more detailed information available from the *Pharmaceutical Codex* or Aulton (2007).

Natural polysaccharides

The main problem with these agents is their natural variability between batches and microbial contamination. Tragacanth is a widely used suspending agent and is less viscous at pH 4–7.5. As a rule of thumb, 0.2 g Tragacanth Powder is added per 100 mL suspension or 2 g Compound Tragacanth Powder per 100 mL suspension. Tragacanth Powder requires to be dispersed with the insoluble powders before water is added to prevent clumping (see Example 31.2). Compound Tragacanth Powder BP 1980 contains tragacanth, acacia, starch and sucrose and so is easier to use. Other examples include acacia gum, starch, agar, guar gum, carrageenan and sodium alginate. These materials should not be used externally as they leave a sticky feel on the skin.

Semi-synthetic polysaccharides

These are derived from the naturally occurring poly-saccharide cellulose. Examples include methylcellu-lose (Cologel®, Celacol®), hydroxyethylcellulose (Natrosol 250®), sodium carboxymethylcellulose (Carmellose sodium) and microcrystalline cellul-ose (Avicel®).

Clays

These are naturally occurring inorganic materials which are mainly hydrated silicates. Examples include bentonite and magnesium aluminium silicate (Veegum®).

Synthetic thickeners

These were introduced to overcome the variable qual-ity of natural products. Examples include carbomer (Carboxyvinyl polymer, Carbopol®), colloidal silicon dioxide (Aerosil®, Cab-o-sil®) and polyvinyl alcohol.

Miscellaneous compounds

Gelatin is used as a suspending and viscosity-increasing agent.

Preservation of suspensions

Water is the most common source of microbial con-tamination. All pharmaceutical preparations that con-tain water are therefore susceptible to microbial growth. Also the naturally occurring additives such as acacia and tragacanth may be sources of microbes and spores. Preservative action may be diminished because of adsorption of the preservative onto solid particles of drug, or interaction with suspending agents. Useful preservatives in extemporaneous preparations include chloroform water, benzoic acid and hydroxybenzoates.

The dispensing of suspensions

The method of dispensing suspensions is the same for most, with some differences for specific ingredients.

- Crystalline and granular solids are finely powdered in the mortar. The suspending agent should then be added and mixed thoroughly in the mortar. Do not apply too much pressure, otherwise gumming or caking of the suspending agent will occur and heat of friction will make it sticky.
- Add a little of the liquid vehicle to make a paste and mix well until smooth and free of lumps. Continue with gradual additions until the mixture can be poured into a tared bottle. Further liquid is used to rinse all the powder into the bottle, where it is made up to volume.

Variations

- If wetting agents are included in the formulation, add them before forming the paste
- If syrup and/or glycerol are in the formulation, use this rather than water to form the initial paste
- If soluble solids are being used, dissolve them in the vehicle before or after making the paste
- Leave addition of volatile components, colourings or concentrated flavouring tinctures such as chloroform spirit, liquid liquorice extract and compound tartrazine solution until near the end.

Most 'official' suspensions will be prepared from the constituent ingredients. There may be some occasions where an oral solid dosage form, such as a tablet or capsule, will have to be reformulated by the pharmacist into an oral suspension, e.g. where the medicine is for a child (see Example 31.3). It is important to obtain as much information (physical, chemical and microbiological) as possible about the manufactured drug and its excipients. This can usu-ally be obtained from the manufacturer. Typically, the tablet will be crushed or capsule contents emp-tied into the mortar and a suspending agent added. A paste is formed with the vehicle and then diluted to a suitable volume, with the addition of any other desired ingredients such as preservative or flavour. A short expiry of no more than 2 weeks (more likely to be 7 days) should be given owing to the lack of knowledge about the stability of the formulation.

Preparation of suspensions from dry powders and granules for reconstitution

Suspensions may have to be prepared from previously manufactured dry powders or granules if the liquid preparation has a limited shelf life because of chem-ical or physical instability. Powders should firstly be loosened from the bottom of the container by lightly tapping against a hard surface. The specified amount of cold, purified water should then be added, sometimes in two or more portions, with shaking, until all the dry powder is suspended. The container is usually over-sized in order to allow adequate shaking for reconstitution. The patient may prepare some suspensions immediately before taking from individually packed sachets of powder or from bulk solids. This is considered in more detail in Chapter 35.

Containers for suspensions

Suspensions should be packed in amber bottles, plain for internal use and ribbed for external use. There should be adequate air space above the liquid to allow shaking and ease of pouring. A 5 mL medicine spoon or oral syringe should be given when the suspension is for oral use.

Special labels and advice for suspensions

The most important additional label for suspensions is 'Shake well before use', as some sedimentation of medicament would normally be expected. Shaking the bottle will redisperse the medicament and ensure that the patient can measure an accurate dose.

'Store in a cool place'. Stability of suspensions may be adversely affected by both extremes and variations of temperature. Some suspensions, such as those made by reconstituting dry powders, may need to be stored in a refrigerator.

Extemporaneously prepared and reconstituted suspensions will have a relatively short shelf life. They are usually required to be recently or freshly prepared, with a 1–4-week expiry date. Some official formulae state an expiry date, but many do not. The pharmacist may have to make judgments about the expiry date for a particular preparation, based on its constituents and likely storage conditions. The manufacturer's literature for reconstituted products will give recommended storage conditions.

Inhalations

Suspensions are useful formulations for inhalations. The volatile components are adsorbed onto the surface of a diffusible solid to ensure uniform dispersion throughout the liquid. When hot water is added, the oils vaporize. Where quantities are not stated, 1 g of light magnesium carbonate is used for each 2 mL of oil (such as eucalyptus oil) or 2 g of volatile solid (such as menthol). An example of an inhalation is menthol and eucalyptus inhalation (see Example 31.4).

Example 31.1

Rx 150 mL Kaolin and Morphine Mixture BP.

	Master formula	For 150 mL
Light kaolin	2 g	30 g
Sodium bicarbonate	500 mg	7.5 g
Chloroform and morphine tincture	0.4 mL	6 mL
Water	to 10 mL	to 150 mL

Action and uses. As an adjunct to fluid replacement in treatment of acute diarrhoea.

Formulation notes. Light kaolin is a diffusible solid, therefore no suspending agent is required.

Method of preparation. Weigh the light kaolin and place in the mortar. Dissolve the sodium bicarbonate in about 100 mL of water. Gradually add this to the light kaolin in the mortar with mixing to disperse the solid. Add the chloroform and morphine tincture. Wash the mixture into a tared, amber medicine bottle, and make up to volume with water. Seal with a child-resistant closure. Polish and label the bottle and give a 5 mL medicine spoon with the medicine.

Shelf life and storage. Store in a cool, dry place. It is recently prepared (unless the kaolin has been sterilized), therefore a shelf life of 2–3 weeks is applicable.

Advice and labelling. 'Shake well before use'. The usual dose is 10 mL every 4 hours in water. The importance of rehydration therapy should be stressed to the patient.

Example 31.2

Rx Chalk Mixture, Paediatric BP. Mitte 100 mL.

	Master formula	For 100 mL
Chalk	100 mg	2 g
Tragacanth	10 mg	200 mg
Syrup	0.5 mL	10 mL
Concentrated cinnamon water	0.02 mL	0.4 mL
Double strength chloroform water	2.5 mL	50 mL
Water	to 5 mL	to 100 mL

Action and uses. As an antidiarrhoeal mixture for children, in addition to fluid replacement.

Formulation notes. Chalk is practically insoluble in water and is an indiffusible solid which requires a suspending agent. Tragacanth Powder is used in this formulation. The concentrated cinnamon water is a flavouring agent and the syrup increases the viscosity as well as acting as a sweetener. Chloroform water is the preservative.

Method of preparation. The chalk and tragacanth should be weighed and lightly mixed in a mortar and pestle. Add the syrup and mix to make a paste. The double strength chloroform water should be gradually added, with mixing, followed by the concentrated cinnamon water. The mixture should be rinsed into a previously tared 100 mL amber medicine bottle and made up to volume with water. Shake the suspension well and seal with a child-resistant closure. Polish and label the bottle and give a 5 mL medicine spoon with the medicine.

Shelf life and storage. Store in a cool, dry place. It is freshly prepared, therefore a shelf life of 1 week is applicable.

Advice and labelling. 'Shake well before use'. A dose of 5 mL every 4 hours is normally used. Advice on the importance of fluid replacement, using oral rehydration sachets, should be given if necessary.

Example 31.3

Rx Spironolactone suspension 15 mg/5 mL. Sig. 5 mL t.d.s. Mitte 100 mL. For a 4-year-old child.

	Master formula	For 100 mL
Spironolactone	q.s.*	300 mg
Compound orange spirit	0.2%	0.2 mL
Cologel	20%	20 mL
Water	to 100%	100 mL

*q.s. means sufficient (see Appendix 2)

Action and uses. A potassium-sparing diuretic used in oedema of heart failure and nephrotic syndrome.

Formulation notes. Spironolactone is practically insoluble in water. Cologel® (methylcellulose) acts as the suspending agent. Compound orange spirit is a flavouring agent.

Method of preparation. Tablets may be used, and sufficient crushed in a mortar and pestle to give 300 mg spironolactone (e.g. 6 × 50 mg tablets). Alternatively, weigh the powder and transfer to a mortar

and pestle. Add the Cologel® and mix to a paste. Gradually add some of the water. Add the compound orange spirit. Rinse the suspension into a tared, amber medicine bottle and make up to volume with water. Shake the bottle well and seal with a child-resistant closure. Polish and label the bottle and give a 5 mL medicine spoon with the medicine.

Shelf life and storage. It is recently prepared with a shelf life of 4 weeks when stored in a refrigerator. Spironolactone should be protected from light.

Advice and labelling. 'Shake well before use' and 'Give one 5 mL spoonful three times a day'. BNF Label 21 should be used. Reinforce the storage conditions.

Example 31.4

Rx Menthol and Eucalyptus Inhalation BP 1980. Mitte 100 mL.

	Master formula
Menthol	2 g
Eucalyptus oil	10 mL
Light magnesium carbonate	7 g
Water	to 100 mL

Action and uses. For relief of nasal congestion.

Formulation notes. Light magnesium carbonate has a large surface area and is used to adsorb the volatile ingredients which helps to ensure a uniform dispersion. Menthol is freely soluble in fixed and volatile oils, so will dissolve in the eucalyptus oil.

Method of preparation. Grind the menthol to a fine powder in a glass mortar and add the eucalyptus oil, which will dissolve the menthol. Gradually add the light magnesium carbonate to the mortar and mix well. Add the water gradually to produce a pourable suspension; this may take a while to achieve. Rinse into a tared, amber ribbed bottle and make up to volume. Seal with a child-resistant closure.

Shelf life and storage. Store in a cool, dry place. It is recently prepared, therefore a shelf life of 2–3 weeks is applicable.

Advice and labelling. 'Shake well before use' and 'Not to be taken'. The patient should be told to add 1 teaspoonful to 1 pint of hot, not boiling, water. A towel should be placed over the head and bowl and the vapour inhaled for 5–10 minutes. Patients should be made aware of the potential danger of scalding to themselves and others, particularly small children.

Example 31.5

℞ 200 mL Calamine Lotion BP.

	Master formula	For 200 mL
Calamine	15 g	30 g
Zinc oxide	5 g	10 g
Bentonite	3 g	6 g
Sodium citrate	500 mg	1 g
Liquefied phenol	0.5 mL	1 mL
Glycerol	5 mL	10 mL
Water	to 100 mL	to 200 mL

Action and uses. As a cooling lotion for sunburn or skin irritation and pruritis.

Formulation notes. Calamine is a coloured zinc carbonate and is practically insoluble in water, as is zinc oxide. Both are indiffusible solids. Sodium citrate is added to control the flocculation of calamine. Bentonite is a thickening agent and glycerol will thicken the product and help powder adherence to the skin. Liquefied phenol acts as a preservative and antiseptic.

Method of preparation. The dry powders should be weighed and mixed in a mortar so that the bentonite is well distributed. Add the glycerol to the powders and mix. The sodium citrate is dissolved in about 140 mL of water, and gradually added to the mixture in the mortar, so that a smooth paste is produced. Add the liquefied phenol, taking care not to splash, as it is caustic. Transfer the mixture to a tared, amber ribbed glass bottle, adding washings from the mortar, and make up to volume. Seal with a child-resistant closure.

Shelf life and storage. Store in a cool, dry place. It is recently prepared, therefore a shelf life of 2–3 weeks is applicable.

Advice and labelling. 'For external use only', 'Shake well before use' and 'Do not apply to broken skin'. The lotion should be applied to the affected areas when required and allowed to dry.

KEY POINTS

- Suspensions can be used to administer an insoluble solid by the oral route
- Suspensions may be used to replace tablets, to improve dissolution rate, to prolong action and to mask a bad taste
- Solids may be diffusible or indiffusible and require different dispensing techniques
- Stokes' equation can be applied when formulating a suspension to help ensure accurate dosage of the drug
- Flocculated particles settle quickly and redisperse easily, while deflocculated particles settle slowly but tend to cake
- Hydrophobic solids may require wetting agents
- Suspending agents are added to slow down the rate of settling of the solid
- Suspending agents may be natural polysaccharides, semi-synthetic polysaccharides, clays or synthetic polymers
- Some suspensions are made by adding water to reconstitute manufactured powders when stability is a problem
- 'Shake well before use' and 'Store in a cool place' should be part of the labels on a suspension
- Inhalations are suspensions of a volatile material adsorbed onto a diffusible solid

32

Emulsions

Arthur J. Winfield

STUDY POINTS

- The uses of pharmaceutical emulsions
- The different types of emulsion and their identification
- Considerations during the formulation of emulsions
- Selection of emulsifying agents and other ingredients
- The dispensing processes for emulsions

Introduction

An emulsion consists of two immiscible liquids, one of which is uniformly dispersed throughout the other as fine droplets normally of diameter 0.1–100 μm. To prepare a stable emulsion, a third ingredient, an emulsifying agent, is required. Oral emulsions are stabilized oil-in-water dispersions that may contain one or more active ingredients. They are a useful way of presenting oils and fats in a palatable form. Emulsions for external use are known as lotions, applications or liniments if liquid, or creams if semi-solid in nature. Some parenteral products may also be formulated as emulsions. Most important of these is total parenteral nutrition (TPN), which is discussed in detail in Chapter 41. Pharmaceutically, the term 'emulsion', when no other qualification is used, is taken to mean an oil-in-water preparation for internal use. Information about other types of emulsion, together with some of the science of emulsions, can be found in Aulton (2007).

Pharmaceutical applications of emulsions

Emulsions have a wide range of uses, including:

- Oral, rectal and topical administration of oils and oil-soluble drugs
- Formulation of oil- and water-soluble drugs together
- To enhance palatability of oils when given orally by disguising both taste and oiliness
- Increasing absorption of oils and oil-soluble drugs through intestinal walls. An example is griseofulvin suspended in oil in an oil-in-water emulsion
- Intramuscular injections of some water-soluble vaccines: these provide slow release and therefore a greater antibody response and longer-lasting immunity
- Total parenteral nutrition: this makes use of a sterile oil-in-water emulsion to deliver oily nutrients intravenously to patients, using non-toxic emulsifying agents, such as lecithin (see Ch. 41).

Examples of emulsions for oral use are cod liver oil emulsion (see Example 32.3), liquid paraffin oral emulsion (see Example 32.4) and castor oil emulsion. Examples of emulsions for external use are Turpentine Liniment BP (see Example 33.3) and Oily Calamine Lotion BP (see Example 32.5).

Emulsion types

Emulsions may be oil-in-water (o/w) emulsions, where oil is the disperse phase in a continuous phase of water, or water-in-oil (w/o) emulsions, where water is the disperse phase in a continuous phase of oil. It is also possible to form a multiple emulsion, e.g. a water droplet enclosed in an oil droplet, which is itself dispersed in water – a w/o/w emulsion. These may be used for delayed-action drug delivery systems.

If the emulsion is for oral or intravenous administration it will always be oil-in-water. Intramuscular injections may be water-in-oil for depot therapy. When selecting emulsion type for preparations for external use, the therapeutic use, texture and patient acceptability will be taken into account. Oil-in-water emulsions are less greasy, easily washed off the skin and more cosmetically acceptable than water-in-oil emulsions. They have an occlusive effect, which hydrates the upper layers of the skin (called an emollient, see Ch. 33). Water-in-oil emulsions rub in more easily.

Identification of emulsion type

There is a range of tests available to identify the emulsion type. Some of the tests that can be used are outlined below.

Miscibility test. An emulsion will only mix with a liquid that is miscible with its continuous phase. Therefore an o/w emulsion is miscible with water, a w/o emulsion with an oil.

Conductivity measurement. Systems with an aqueous continuous phase will conduct electricity, while systems with an oily continuous phase will not.

Staining test. A dry filter paper impregnated with cobalt chloride turns from blue to pink on exposure to stable o/w emulsions.

Dye test. If an oil-soluble dye is used, o/w emulsions are paler in colour than w/o emulsions. If examined microscopically, an o/w emulsion will appear as coloured globules on a colourless background while a w/o emulsion will appear as colourless globules against a coloured background.

Formulation of emulsions

An ideal emulsion has globules of disperse phase that retain their initial character, that is the mean globule size does not change and the globules remain evenly distributed. The formulation of emulsions involves the prevention of coalescence of the disperse phase (often called 'cracking') and reducing the rate of creaming.

Emulsifying agents

Emulsifying agents help the production of a stable emulsion by reducing interfacial tension and then maintaining the separation of the droplets by forming a barrier at the interface. Most emulsifying agents are surface-active agents. Emulsion type is determined mainly by the solubility of the emulsifying agent. If the emulsifying agent is more soluble in water (i.e. hydrophilic) then water will be the continuous phase and an o/w emulsion will be formed. If the emulsifying agent is more soluble in oil (i.e. lipophilic), oil will be the continuous phase and a w/o emulsion will be formed. If a substance is added which alters the solubility of the emulsifying agent, this balance may be altered and the emulsion may change type. The process is called phase inversion. The ideal emulsifying agent is colourless, odourless, tasteless, non-toxic, non-irritant and able to produce stable emulsions at low concentrations.

Emulsifying agents can be classed into three groups: naturally occurring, synthetic surfactants and finely divided solids.

Naturally occurring emulsifying agents

These agents come from vegetable or animal sources. Therefore the quality may vary from batch to batch and they are susceptible to microbial contamination and degradation.

Polysaccharides. Acacia is the best emulsifying agent for extemporaneously prepared oral emulsions as it forms a thick film at the oil–water interface to act as a barrier to coalescence. It is too sticky for external use. Tragacanth is used to increase the viscosity of an emulsion and prevent creaming. Other polysaccharides, such as starch, pectin and carrageenan, are used to stabilize an emulsion.

Semi-synthetic polysaccharides. Low-viscosity grades of methylcellulose (see Example 32.4) and carboxymethylcellulose will form o/w emulsions.

Sterol-containing substances. These agents act as water-in-oil emulsifying agents. Examples include beeswax, wool fat and wool alcohols (see Ch. 33).

Synthetic surfactants

These agents are classified according to their ionic characteristics as anionic, cationic, non-ionic and ampholytic. The latter are used in detergents and soaps but are not widely used in pharmacy.

Anionic surfactants. These are organic salts which, in water, have a surface-active anion. They are incompatible with some organic and inorganic cations and with large organic cations such as cetrimide. They are widely used in external preparations as o/w emulsifying agents. They must be in their ionized form to be effective and emulsions made with anionic surfactants are generally stable at more alkaline pH.

Many different ones are used pharmaceutically. Some examples include:

- Alkali metal and ammonium soaps such as sodium stearate (o/w)
- Soaps of divalent and trivalent metals such as calcium oleate (w/o) (see Example 32.5)
- Amine soaps such as triethanolamine oleate (o/w)
- Alkyl sulphates such as sodium lauryl sulphate (o/w).

Cationic surfactants. These are usually quaternary ammonium compounds which have a surface-active cation and so are sensitive to anionic surfactants and drugs. They are used in the preparation of o/w emulsions for external use and must be in their ionized form to be effective. Emulsions formed by a cationic surfactant are generally stable at acidic pH. The cationic surfactants also have antimicrobial activity. Examples include cetrimide and benzalkonium chloride.

Non-ionic surfactants. These are synthetic materials and make up the largest group of surfactants. They are used to produce either o/w or w/o emulsions for both external and internal use. The non-ionic surfactants are compatible with both anionic and cationic substances and are highly resistant to pH change. The type of emulsion formed depends on the balance between hydrophilic and lipophilic groups which is expressed as the HLB (hydrophilic–lipophilic balance) number (see below). Examples of the main types include glycol and glycerol esters, macrogol ethers and esters, sorbitan esters and polysorbates.

The HLB (hydrophilic–lipophilic balance) system. An HLB number, usually between 1 and 20, is allocated to an emulsifying agent and represents the relative proportions of the lipophilic and hydrophilic parts of the molecule. The lower the number, the more oil soluble the emulsifying agent. Higher numbers (8–18) indicate a hydrophilic molecule which

Table 32.1 HLB values of emulsifying agents

Emulsifying agent	HLB value
Acacia	8.0
Sorbitan laurate (Span 20®)	8.6
Sorbitan stearate (Span 60®)	4.7
Polysorbate 20 (Tween 20®)	16.7
Polysorbate 80 (Tween 80®)	15.0
Sodium lauryl sulphate	40.0
Sodium oleate	18.0
Tragacanth	13.2
Triethanolamine oleate	12.0

produces an o/w emulsion. Low numbers (3–6) indicate a lipophilic molecule which produces a w/o emulsion. Oils and waxy materials have a 'required HLB number' which helps in the selection of appropriate emulsifying agents when formulating emulsions. Liquid paraffin, for example, has a required HLB value of 4 to obtain a w/o emulsion and 12 for an o/w emulsion. Two or more surfactants can be combined to achieve a suitable HLB value and often give better results than one surfactant alone. (See Aulton (2007) or the *Pharmaceutical Codex* for more details.) HLB values of some commonly used emulsifying agents are given in Table 32.1.

Finely divided solids

Finely divided solids can be adsorbed at the oil–water interface to form a coherent film that prevents coalescence of the dispersed globules. If the solid particles are preferentially wetted by oil, a w/o emulsion is formed. Conversely, if the particles are preferentially wetted by water, an o/w emulsion is formed. They form emulsions with good stability which are less prone to microbial contamination than those formed with other naturally derived agents. Examples are bentonite, aluminium magnesium silicate and colloidal silicon dioxide. Colloidal aluminium and magnesium hydroxides are used for internal preparations. For example liquid paraffin and magnesium hydroxide oral emulsion is stabilized by the magnesium hydroxide.

Choosing an emulsifying agent

The active ingredients that are to be emulsified and the intended use of the product will determine the choice of emulsifying agent. Because they are non-toxic and non-irritant, the natural polysaccharides (acacia) and non-ionic emulsifying agents are useful for internal emulsions. Quillaia can be used in low concentrations, but soap emulsions irritate the gastro-intestinal tract and have a laxative effect. The taste should be bland and palatable, again suggesting the use of natural polysaccharides. Polysorbates have a disagreeable taste, therefore flavouring ingredients are necessary. Only certain non-ionic emulsifying agents are suitable for parenteral use including lecithin, polysorbate 80, methylcellulose, gelatin and serum albumin. A wider range of emulsifying agents can be used externally, although the polysaccharides are normally considered too sticky.

Antioxidants

Some oils are liable to degradation by oxidation and therefore antioxidants may be added to the formulation. They should be preferentially soluble in the oily phase.

Antimicrobial preservatives

Emulsions contain water, which will support microbial growth. Microbes produce unpleasant odours, colour changes and gases. In addition they may affect the emulsifying agent, possibly causing the breakdown of the emulsion. Other ingredients in emulsions can provide a growth medium for microbes. Examples include arachis oil which supports *Aspergillus* species and liquid paraffin which supports *Penicillium* species. Contamination may be introduced from a variety of sources including:

- Natural emulsifying agents, e.g. starch and acacia
- Water, if not properly stored
- Carelessly cleaned equipment
- Poor closures on containers.

Antimicrobial preservative agents should be free from toxic effects, odour, taste (for internal use) and colour. They should be bactericidal rather than bacteriostatic, have a rapid action and wide antibacterial spectrum over a range of temperatures and pH. Additionally emulsion ingredients should not affect their activity and they should be resistant to attack by microorganisms. The effect of the partition coefficient is also important. Microbial growth normally occurs in the aqueous phase of an emulsion, therefore it is important that a sufficient concentration of preservative is present in the aqueous phase. A preservative with a low oil/water partition coefficient will have a higher concentration in the aqueous phase. A combination of preservatives may give the best preservative cover for an emulsion system. The ratio of the disperse phase volume to the total volume is known as the phase volume or phase volume ratio. If, for example, a preservative is soluble in the oil and if the proportion of oil is increased, the concentration of preservative in the aqueous phase decreases. This could reduce the concentration in the aqueous phase below an effective concentration.

Some preservatives in use are listed below:

- Benzoic acid: effective at a concentration of 0.1% at a pH below 5
- Esters of parahydroxybenzoic acid such as methyl paraben (0.01–0.3%)
- Chloroform, as chloroform water (0.25% v/v)
- Chlorocresol (0.05–0.2%)
- Phenoxyethanol (0.5–1.0%)
- Benzyl alcohol (0.1–3%)
- Quaternary ammonium compounds, e.g. cetrimide, which can be used as a primary emulsifying agent but can also be used as a preservative
- Organic mercurial compounds such as phenyl mercuric nitrate and acetate (0.001–0.002%).

Colours and flavourings

Colour is rarely needed in an emulsion, as most have an elegant white colour and thick texture. Emulsions for oral use will usually contain some flavouring agent.

Stability of emulsions

Phase inversion

This is the process in which an emulsion changes from one type to another, say o/w to w/o. The most stable range of disperse phase concentration is 30–60%. As the amount of disperse phase approaches or exceeds a theoretical maximum of 74% of the total volume, so the tendency for phase inversion to occur increases. Addition of substances which alter the solubility of an emulsifying agent may also cause phase inversion. The process is irreversible.

Creaming

The term 'creaming' is used to describe the aggregation of globules of the disperse phase at the top or bottom of the emulsion, similar to cream on milk. The process is reversible and gentle shaking redistributes the droplets throughout the continuous phase. Creaming is undesirable because it is inelegant and inaccurate dosing is possible if shaking is not thorough. Additionally, creaming increases the likelihood of coalescence of globules and therefore the breakdown of the emulsion due to cracking.

Cracking

Cracking is the coalescence of dispersed globules and separation of the disperse phase as a separate layer. It is an irreversible process and redispersion cannot be achieved by shaking.

Causes and prevention of cracking or creaming

- *Globule size*. Stable emulsions require a maximal number of small sized (1–3 μm) globules and as few as possible larger (>15 μm) diameter globules. A homogenizer will efficiently reduce droplet size and may additionally increase the viscosity if more than 30% of disperse phase is present. Homogenizers force the emulsion through a small aperture to reduce the size of the globules.
- *Storage temperature*. Extremes of temperature can lead to an emulsion cracking. When water freezes it expands, so undue pressure is exerted on dispersed globules and especially the emulsifying agent film, which may lead to cracking. Conversely, an increased temperature decreases the viscosity of the continuous phase and disrupts the integrity of the interfacial film. An increasing number of collisions between droplets will also occur, leading to increased creaming and cracking.
- *Potential for globule coalescence*. Increasing the viscosity of the continuous phase will reduce the potential for globule coalescence as this reduces the movement of globules. Emulsion stabilizers, which increase the viscosity of the continuous phase, may be used in o/w emulsions, e.g. tragacanth, sodium alginate and methylcellulose.
- *Changes which affect the interfacial film*. These may be chemical, physical or biological effects: microbiological contamination may destroy the emulsifying agent, especially if a polysaccharide emulsifying agent is being used, addition of a common solvent, addition of an emulsifying agent of opposite charge, for instance cationic to anionic.
- *Incorporation of excess disperse phase*, as discussed above.

Dispensing emulsions

Emulsions can be extemporaneously prepared on a small scale using a mortar and pestle. Electric mixers can also be used, although incorporation of excess air may be a problem. All equipment used must be thoroughly clean and dry. All oil-soluble and water-soluble components of the emulsion are separately dissolved in the appropriate phase. A suitable emulsifying agent must then be used.

Emulsions for oral use

Acacia gum is usually used when making extemporaneous o/w emulsions for oral use, unless otherwise specified. A primary emulsion should be prepared first. This is a thick, stable emulsion prepared using optimal proportions of the ingredients. These vary with the nature of the oil.

Calculating quantities for primary emulsions

Proportions or 'parts' for preparation of primary emulsions are given in Table 32.2. These refer to parts by volume for the different types of oil and water and weight for the acacia gum. If more than one oil is to be incorporated, the quantity of acacia for each is calculated separately and the sum of the quantities used.

Example 32.1

Calculate the quantities for a primary emulsion for the following:

℞
Cod liver oil	30 mL
Water	to 100 mL

Primary emulsion quantities:
Cod liver oil is a fixed oil, therefore the primary emulsion proportions are 4:2:1. Hence:

Cod liver oil	30 mL	4 parts
Water	15 mL	2 parts
Powdered acacia gum	7.5 g	1 part

Table 32.2 Quantities for primary emulsions

Type of oil	Examples	Oil	Water	Gum
Fixed	Almond, arachis, cod liver, castor	4	2	1
Mineral (hydrocarbon)	Liquid paraffin	3	2	1
Volatile	Turpentine, cinnamon, peppermint	2	2	1
Oleo-resin	Male fern extract	1	2	1

Variations to primary emulsion calculations

If the proportion of oil is too small, modifications must be made. Acacia emulsions containing less than 20% oil tend to cream readily. A bland, inert oil, such as arachis, sesame, cottonseed or maize oil, should be added to increase the amount of oil and so prevent this from happening. Care should be taken in selection of the bulking oil because of the increasing incidence of nut allergy. It is often, therefore, advisable to avoid oils such as arachis, especially for children.

Example 32.2

R$_X$ Calciferol solution, 0.15 mL per 5 mL dose.
The percentage of oil in each dose is 3%. The oil content must be made up to at least 20% to produce a stable emulsion.

Since 20% of 5 mL = 1 mL, the volume of bland oil required is 1.0−0.15 = 0.85 mL.

Formula for primary emulsion (for 50 mL):

Calciferol solution	1.5 mL	4 parts
Cottonseed oil	8.5 mL	
Water	5 mL	2 parts
Acacia	2.5 g	1 part

Methods of preparation of extemporaneous emulsions

There are two possible methods, the dry gum method being the more popular.

Dry gum method of preparation

- Measure the oil accurately in a dry measure. It is important that the measure is dry.
- Allow measure to drain into a dry mortar with a large, flat bottom.
- Weigh acacia gum.
- Measure the water for the primary emulsion in a clean measure.
- Add acacia to the oil and mix lightly to disperse lumps. Do not over-mix, and keep the suspension in the bottom of the mortar.
- Immediately add all of the water (aim to do this within 10–15 seconds of adding the acacia to the oil) and stir continuously and vigorously until the mixture thickens and the primary emulsion is formed. The mixture thickening, becoming white and producing a 'clicking' sound, characterizes this.
- Continue mixing for a further 2–3 minutes to produce the white stable emulsion. The whiter the product, the smaller the globules.
- Gradually dilute the primary emulsion with small volumes of the vehicle, ensuring complete mixing between additions.
- Gradually add any other ingredients, transfer to a measure and make up to final volume with the vehicle.

Wet gum method of preparation

Water is added to the acacia gum and quickly triturated until the gum has dissolved to make a mucilage. Oil is added to this mucilage in small portions, triturating the mixture thoroughly after each addition until a thick primary emulsion is obtained. The primary emulsion should be stabilized by mixing for several minutes and then completed in the same way as for the dry gum method.

Problems when producing the primary emulsion

The primary emulsion may not form and a thin oily liquid is formed instead. Possible causes are:

- Phase inversion has occurred
- Incorrect quantities of oil or water were used
- There was cross-contamination of water and oil
- A wet mortar was used
- The mortar was too small and curved, or the pestle head was too round, giving insufficient shear
- Excessive mixing of oil and gum before adding water (dry gum method)
- Diluting the primary emulsion too soon
- Too rapid dilution of primary emulsion
- Poor-quality acacia.

Emulsions for external use

Liquid or semi-liquid emulsions may be used as applications, liniments and lotions (see Ch. 33). The extemporaneous preparation of emulsions for external use does not require the preparation of a primary emulsion. Soaps are commonly used as the emulsifying agent and some are prepared 'in situ' by mixing the oily phase containing a fatty acid and the aqueous phase containing the alkali. Alternatively the emulsifying agent can be dissolved in the oily or aqueous phase and the disperse phase added to the continuous phase, either gradually or in one portion.

Creams are semi-solid emulsions which may be o/w (e.g. aqueous cream) or w/o (e.g. oily cream). These are considered in more detail in Chapter 33.

Shelf life and storage

Emulsions should be stored at room temperature and will either be recently or freshly prepared. Some official preparations will have specific expiry dates. They should not be frozen.

Containers

An amber medicine bottle is used, plain for internal use and ribbed for external use, with an airtight child-resistant closure. Containers with a wide mouth are useful for very viscous preparations.

Special labelling and advice for emulsions

- 'Shake well before use'
- 'Store in a cool place'. This is to protect the emulsion against extremes of temperature which will adversely affect its stability

- Expiry date
- 'For external use only', for external emulsions.

Example 32.3

Rx Prepare 200 mL cod liver oil emulsion to the following formula:

Cod liver oil	60 mL
Chloroform	0.4 mL
Cinnamon water	to 200 mL

Action and uses. A rich source of vitamins A and D.

Formulation notes. Cod liver oil is a fixed oil that requires the addition of acacia gum as an emulsifying agent. The proportions are 4 oil : 2 water : 1 gum. Therefore 60 mL cod liver oil, 30 mL of cinnamon water and 15 g of acacia gum will be used to prepare the primary emulsion. Cinnamon water acts as a flavouring agent and vehicle. It may need to be prepared from concentrated cinnamon water, at a dilution of 1 part to 39 parts of water. Since 60 mL of the emulsion is the cod liver oil, it is not necessary to prepare 200 mL of cinnamon water, so 160 mL is adequate. Therefore, 4 mL of concentrated cinnamon water will be diluted to 160 mL with water. Chloroform is dense and only slowly soluble and acts as a preservative.

Method of preparation. Use the dry gum method. Weigh 15 g of acacia, measure 60 mL of cod liver oil and 30 mL of cinnamon water, which will be used to create the primary emulsion. Place the cod liver oil in a dry, flat-bottomed mortar. Add the acacia and mix very lightly and briefly. Immediately add the cinnamon water, mixing vigorously until a clicking sound is heard and a white primary emulsion is formed. Continue mixing for a few minutes to stabilize the primary emulsion. Scrape the mortar and pestle with a spatula to ensure that all the oil is incorporated. Add the chloroform by pipette and mix thoroughly. Gradually add most of the remainder of the cinnamon water to the emulsion in the mortar, stirring well between additions. Transfer the emulsion to a 200 mL measure, rinsing the mortar with cinnamon water, adding these washings to the measure. Make up to volume with cinnamon water and pack in an amber medicine bottle with a child-resistant closure. Polish and label the bottle and give a 5 mL medicine spoon with the medicine.

Shelf life and storage. Store in a cool, dry place. It is recently prepared, therefore a shelf life of 2–3 weeks is applicable.

Advice and labelling. This is an unofficial formula, and should be labelled 'Cod liver oil 30% v/v emulsion'. 'Shake well before use'. A normal dose is 10 mL three times a day, with or after food.

Example 32.4

Rx 100 mL Liquid Paraffin Oral Emulsion BP 1968.

Liquid paraffin	50 mL
Vanillin	50 mg
Chloroform	0.25 mL
Benzoic acid solution	2 mL
Methylcellulose 20	2 g
Saccharin sodium	5 mg
Water	to 100 mL

Action and uses. A lubricant laxative for chronic constipation.

Formulation notes. Methylcellulose 20 at a concentration of 2% acts as an emulsifying agent for the mineral oil, liquid paraffin. A primary emulsion is not required. Benzoic acid and chloroform act as preservatives and vanillin and saccharin sodium act as flavouring and sweetening agent respectively. The amount of saccharin sodium is not weighable on a dispensing balance and will be obtained by trituration using water as the diluent (since this is the vehicle for the emulsion).

Trituration for saccharin sodium:

Saccharin sodium	100 mg
Water	to 100 mL

5 mL of water will contain 5 mg of saccharin sodium.

Method of preparation. Firstly, prepare a mucilage by mixing the methylcellulose 20 with about six times its weight of boiling water and allow to stand for 30 minutes to hydrate. Add an equal weight (about 15 g) of ice and stir mechanically until the mucilage is homogeneous. Dissolve the vanillin in the benzoic acid solution and chloroform. Add this mixture to the mucilage and stir for 5 minutes. Make up the saccharin sodium trituration and stir in the appropriate volume of solution to the mucilage. Make the volume of the mucilage up to 50 mL, taking care to ensure that there is no entrapped air in the mucilage. Make the emulsion by mixing together 50 mL of liquid paraffin and 50 mL of prepared mucilage with constant stirring. The emulsion is more stable if passed through a hand homogenizer. Pack in an amber medicine bottle with a child-resistant closure. Shake well to ensure that the emulsion is thoroughly mixed. Polish and label the bottle and give a 5 mL medicine spoon with the medicine.

Shelf life and storage. Store in a cool, dry place. This is an official preparation and should remain stable on storage, however a 4-week expiry date is recommended.

Advice and labelling. 'Shake well before use'. The emulsion should not be taken within 30 minutes of meal times and preferably on an empty stomach. It should not be taken at bedtime. The importance of fibre and fluid intake in the diet should be emphasized.

Example 32.5

Rx 100 mL Oily Calamine Lotion BP 1980.

Calamine	5 g
Wool fat	1 g
Oleic acid	0.5 mL
Arachis oil	50 mL
Calcium hydroxide solution	to 100 mL

Action and uses. Soothing lotion for the treatment of eczema, sunburn and other inflammatory conditions.

Formulation notes. The emulsifying agent for the arachis oil is the soap calcium oleate produced from the calcium hydroxide and oleic acid when they are shaken together. Wool fat is included as an emulsion stabilizer. This is a w/o emulsion.

Method of preparation. The wool fat, oleic acid and arachis oil should be warmed gently together in an evaporating basin (using a water bath or heating block) until melted. Mix them thoroughly. The calamine should be sieved and weighed and placed on a warm ointment tile. Add a little of the oily mixture and rub in with a large spatula until smooth. Gradually add more of the oily mixture until it is fluid. Transfer back to the evaporating basin and stir to evenly distribute the calamine powder. Pour into a previously tared, amber ribbed bottle and add the calcium hydroxide solution to the bottle in small amounts, shaking well between additions. Make up to volume and seal with a child-resistant closure. Polish and label the bottle.

Shelf life and storage. Store in a cool, dry place. It is unpreserved, therefore a shelf life of 2–3 weeks is applicable.

Advice and labelling. 'Shake well before use' and 'For external use only'.

KEY POINTS

- Emulsions may be oil-in-water (o/w) or water-in-oil (w/o)
- Emulsions may be used orally, externally or by intramuscular and intravenous injection
- Oral emulsions are always o/w
- The type of emulsion may be determined by miscibility, conductivity, staining and dye tests
- Emulsifying agents are required to reduce the interfacial tension and act as a barrier between the oil and water phases
- Naturally occurring emulsifying agents include polysaccharides (acacia), semi-synthetic polysaccharides (methylcellulose) and sterols (wool fat)
- Synthetic surfactants can be used and are selected using the HLB number
- Care is required to avoid anion–cation incompatibilities
- Some finely divided solids will stabilize emulsions
- Emulsions require antimicrobial preservation
- Phase inversion, creaming and cracking are instabilities of emulsions which must be avoided
- A primary emulsion is prepared when making an emulsion using acacia as the emulsifying agent using either the 'dry gum' or 'wet gum' method
- The ratio of oil : water : acacia used for the primary emulsion will vary with the type of oil in the formulation
- Liquid emulsions should have 'Shake well before use' and 'Store in a cool place' labels and should not be frozen

33

External preparations

Arthur J. Winfield

STUDY POINTS

- Skin structure and sites of action of drugs
- The types and functions of solid, liquid and semi-solid skin preparations
- The ingredients used in skin preparations
- Dispensing preparations for use on the skin
- Transdermal drug delivery for systemic activity

Introduction

Skin is the largest organ in the body and has three distinct regions. The hypodermis is the innermost and is often called subcutaneous fat. The dermis is the bulk of the thickness of the skin and contains blood vessels, nerve fibres, sweat glands and hair follicles. The outermost region is the epidermis, which is made up of several layers. One of these layers is the stratum basale, in which cells divide and as they move towards the surface they change appearance and function. The outermost layer, the stratum corneum, acts as the skin barrier. It is made up of about 20 layers of dead keratinized cells. The hair follicles and sweat ducts pass through the stratum corneum to reach the surface. A simplified diagram showing the main skin structures is given in Figure 33.1.

There are a large number of diseases which may affect different regions of the skin. Any drug used will require to reach the site of the disease in order to act. Unless it is for a surface effect only, the drug must either pass through the stratum corneum or go through hair follicles or sweat ducts. Examples of drugs applied to the skin and their sites of action are shown in Figure 33.1. Once in the skin, a lipid-soluble drug will tend to accumulate in lipid regions, while more water-soluble drugs will tend to enter the blood capillaries and be removed from the skin. There are also many metabolic enzymes in the skin which can deactivate drugs. A more detailed discussion of these factors and the physicochemical principles involved is given in Aulton (2007).

Pharmacokinetics is seldom applied to skin administration and dosage is often imprecise. However, by effective formulation it is possible to achieve adequate and reproducible percutaneous absorption. The main advantage is that close to zero order kinetics can be produced. This also carries an inherent warning because traditionally it has been assumed that absorption from the skin is minimal. As a consequence, the skin is seen as 'safe' even if quite toxic materials are applied. This is not true and great care is required, so that gloves should always be warn when extemporaneously preparing external preparations.

There are an increasing number of drugs that are effective against skin diseases, but drugs are not the only way of treating skin conditions. Creating physiological changes in the skin can also be beneficial. The main change is to control the moisture content of the skin. Normal skin has 10–25% moisture in the stratum corneum. This level may be reduced in, for example, eczema, or increased, as in skin maceration between the toes. By using an occlusive product (that is, an oily product), water leaving the body through the skin will be trapped and moisture content will increase. These products are called emollients. An excess of moisture may be removed using an astringent, a hygroscopic material or, to a lesser extent, a dusting powder. Where an oily vehicle is needed, but moisture must not increase, adding solid particles to the vehicle

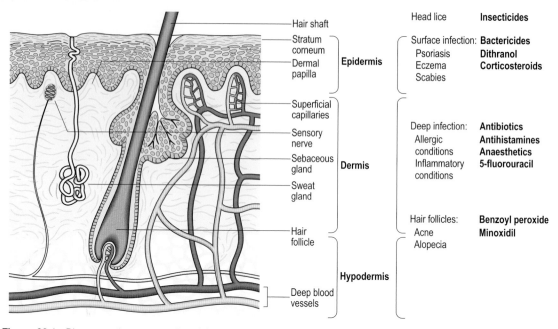

Figure 33.1 • Diagrammatic representation of the skin showing the main structures, location of diseases and the sites of action of drugs.

will allow water to escape. Lubrication of sensitive skin is achieved by using finely divided solids, applied either as a powder or, more efficiently, as a suspension. Cooling the skin relieves inflammation and eases discomfort. It is achieved by evaporating a solvent, usually water or a water and alcohol mixture. Volatile solvents sprayed on the skin give intense cooling.

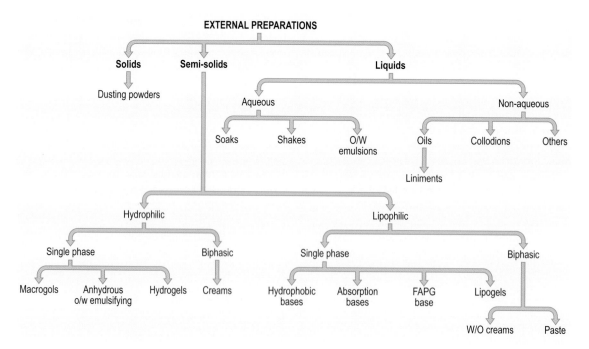

Figure 33.2 • Schematic representation of types of external medicines.

Types of skin preparation

There are a large number of different types of external medicine, ranging from dry powders through semi-solids to liquids. The names are often traditional making classification difficult. Figure 33.2 illustrates the formulation of the main types of preparation used on the skin.

Solids

Dusting powders are applied to the skin for a surface effect such as drying or lubricating, or an antibacterial action. They are made of a fine-particle-size powder which may be a drug alone or together with excipients.

Liquids

Soaks have an active ingredient dissolved in an aqueous solvent and are often used as astringents, for cooling or to leave a film of solid on the skin. Oily vehicles can be used in bath additives to leave an emollient film on the skin surface.

Applications are solutions or emulsions that frequently contain parasiticides (see Example 33.4).

Liniments are alcoholic or oily solutions or emulsions (see Example 33.3) designed to be rubbed into the skin. The medicament is usually a rubefacient.

Lotions are aqueous solutions, suspensions (see Example 33.1) or emulsions that cool inflamed skin and deposit a protective layer of solid.

Paints and *tinctures* are concentrated aqueous or alcoholic antimicrobial solutions.

Collodions are organic solvents containing a polymer and keratolytic agent for treating corns and calluses.

There are also many other liquid products including shampoos, pomades and foot washes.

Semi-solids

Ointments are usually oily vehicles that may contain a surfactant to allow them to be washed off easily (barrier creams). They are used as emollients, or for drug delivery either to the surface or for deeper penetration.

Creams are traditionally oil-in-water (o/w) emulsions while *oily creams* are water-in-oil (w/o) emulsions. However, there are also 'creams' that are not emulsions. Emulsified creams usually give cooling, are less greasy than ointments and can be used for drug delivery onto or into the skin. They require antimicrobial preservatives.

Pastes are vehicles (aqueous or oily) with a high concentration of added solid. This makes them thick so they do not spread and so localizes drug delivery (e.g. Dithranol in Lassar's Paste, see Example 33.11). They can also be used for sun blocks.

Gels (jellies) are usually aqueous gels used for lubrication or applying a drug to the skin. Oily gels are also available where occlusion is required.

Ingredients used in skin preparations

Water-miscible vehicles

These include water, alcohol and the macrogols. Alcohol is often added to water to increase the rate of evaporation and produce a more intense cooling effect. Industrial denatured alcohol (IDA) (formerly known as industrial methylated spirit) is normally used for external preparations because it is exempt from excise duty. The macrogols (polyethylene glycols) are available with a range of molecular weights. As chain length increases, so the properties change from liquid, through semi-solid to waxy solid. They have good solvent properties for a wide range of drugs and can be blended to produce intermediate consistencies. They tend to dry the skin, inactivate some antimicrobials, interact with some plastics and can give poor release of drugs.

Oily vehicles

Oils used in external preparations come from one of three sources.

Mineral oils (paraffins) are the most widely used. They are complex mixtures of mainly saturated hydrocarbons which are available in different fractions. Different names are used in different pharmacopoeias (Table 33.1).

Light liquid paraffin is not normally used in external medicines. Soft paraffin is the main ingredient in many products, with liquid or hard paraffin being used to thin or thicken them respectively. There are two forms of soft paraffin – yellow and white. The latter has been bleached, residues of which may remain. As a general rule, white is used with white or pale coloured

Table 33.1 Paraffins used in external preparations: the names used are different in the UK, USA and European pharmacopoeias

UK	USA	European
Light liquid paraffin	Light mineral oil	Paraffinium perliquidum
Liquid paraffin	Mineral oil	Paraffinium liquidum
Soft paraffin	Petrolatum	Paraffinium molle
Hard paraffin	Paraffin	Paraffinium durum

Table 33.2 Materials based on wool fat: different names are used in the UK, USA and European pharmacopoeias

UK	USA	European
Wool fat	Lanolin	Adeps lanae
Wool alcohols	Lanolin alcohols	Alcoholes adipis lanae
Hydrous wool fat	Hydrous lanolin	Adeps lanae cum aqua

ingredients, while yellow is used for darker ingredients. The paraffins are occlusive and chemically inert, but do not give good skin penetration.

Vegetable oils come from many plant sources such as peanut, castor, olive and coconut. They may be used as a mobile solvent (as in a liniment, see Example 33.2) or as part of an ointment or cream. If they require thickening, a high melting point material such as cetostearyl alcohol can be used. They are occlusive and give good skin penetration, but may go rancid. Sufficient skin penetration may occur to cause severe reactions in patients with nut allergies.

Synthetic oils, such as the silicone oils (Dimeticone BP), are used as water repellents and occlusives because they are very hydrophobic. The semi-synthetic isopropylmyristate is similar to vegetable oil in properties and use.

Emulsifying agents

Liquid and semi-solid emulsions, both o/w and w/o, are used externally and require the addition of emulsifying agents. The latter may also be added to an oil without water as in Emulsifying Ointment BP. The presence of a surfactant usually increases the skin penetration of any drug. A wide range of materials can be used as surfactants, either alone or in combinations. Selection is made in view of the type of emulsion required (o/w or w/o) and the charge on the other ingredients (anionic, cationic or non-ionic).

Emulsifiers – w/o

Wool fat, obtained from sheep wool, is a pale yellow sticky material. It is a complex mixture of fatty acid esters of cholesterol and other sterols and alcohols. While it is similar to human sebum, it has been implicated in sensitization in some people. Where this is a problem there are an increasing number of hypoallergenic commercial products available. Wool alcohol, a solid, is richer in cholesterol and lanesterol and freer from impurities. Both it and wool fat increase the 'water-holding' capacity of greasy bases. Hydrous wool fat is 7 parts wool fat and 3 parts water and is a softer material. Different names are used, as shown in Table 33.2. Beeswax is a traditional w/o emulsifier which is occasionally used.

Emulsifiers – o/w

The main group of materials used extemporaneously are the emulsifying waxes. Each one has two ingredients – cetostearyl alcohol and a surface-active agent, as shown in Table 33.3. All three are waxy solids that mix with oily materials. Addition of water produces an o/w emulsion – a cream. Both the non-aqueous blends and the creams are easily washed off the skin. Varying the amount of bodying agent, usually cetostearyl alcohol, can control consistency. The ratio of oil to water will also alter the consistency of a cream.

Table 33.3 The ingredients used in the emulsifying waxes described in the *British Pharmacopoeia* (BP) and *British Pharmaceutical Codex* (BPC)

Charge	Surfactant	CSA : SAA ratio[*]	Name
Anionic	Sodium lauryl sulphate	9 : 1	Emulsifying Wax BP
Cationic	Cetrimide	9 : 1	Cetrimide Emulsifying Wax BPC
Non-ionic	Cetomacrogol 1000	8 : 2	Cetomacrogol Emulsifying Wax BPC

[*] CSA, cetostearyl alcohol; SAA, surface active agent.

Other emulsifiers

The gums used in oral emulsions (see Ch. 32) are too sticky for external use, but a number of other emulsifying agents are used.

Calcium soaps are produced by mixing a fatty acid with lime water (calcium hydroxide solution) to form a soap in situ (see Example 32.5). They form w/o emulsions. Soft soap is a sticky green material that can be used to make o/w emulsions (see Example 33.3).

Synthetic surface-active agents are used particularly in commercial products. Low HLB (hydrophilic–lipophilic balance) materials will produce w/o emulsions, while higher HLB surfactants give o/w emulsions.

Suspending agents

These materials can be used for suspending solids in shake lotions, or to produce gels, depending on the concentration used. Those used in oral suspensions (see Ch. 31) are too sticky for use in external liquid suspensions. The main group of materials used for this purpose are the clays, of which there are many forms, including bentonite, attapulgite, montmorrilonite and Veegum® (aluminium magnesium silicate). They leave a lubricant layer of powder on the skin. They are unsuitable for use below pH 3.5 and their consistency may be affected by alcohol and electrolytes (see Example 31.5).

Gelling agents can be used to produce a wide range of consistency from slightly thickened (as in artificial tears), through lubricants and semi-solids for the delivery of drugs to very thick bases used to immobilize the skin. For aqueous gels the materials used include tragacanth, alginates, pectin, gelatin, methylcelluloses, carbomer, polyvinyl alcohol and clays. Oils may be thickened using cetostearyl alcohol, hard paraffin, beeswax (see Example 33.7), wool alcohols and poly-valent soaps such as magnesium stearate. The latter, when heated with an oil, produces a clear 'lipogel'.

Other ingredients

Wetting agents are required for hydrophobic solids. Tincture of quillaia is the traditional material (see Example 33.1), but alcohol alone may be effective. Synthetic materials, such as Manoxol OT, can also be used.

Humectants are materials added to reduce the rate of water loss from creams and gels. They are all hygroscopic materials and include glycerol, propylene glycol, PEG 300 and sorbitol syrup, typically used at concentrations of 5–15%.

Solids may be added to semi-solid occlusive bases. They provide channels for the migration of water from the skin surface and so reduce the occlusiveness. Solids used include zinc oxide, talc, starch and Aerosil. Some, such as talc, must be sterilized to kill bacterial spores (see Ch. 35).

Whenever there is a danger of microbial growth, antimicrobial preservation is required.

Dispensing of external preparations

A wide range of dispensing techniques are used in compounding external medicines, some of which have been reviewed in other chapters (see Chs 25, 30, 31, 32 and 35). In the section that follows, only those types of product which require different dispensing techniques are described in detail.

Dusting powders

A simple mixing in a mortar and pestle using 'doubling-up' is used (see Ch. 35). Sieving may be necessary to disperse aggregates of cohesive powders. A 180 μm sieve should be used. Powders such as starch, which contains a lot of moisture, may need drying to ensure optimum flow properties. With coloured materials, considerable working with the pestle is required before proceeding to 'doubling-up' otherwise a speckled product may result. A liquid may be added by pipette to a small quantity of the powder and be worked in before further mixing. A worked example of a dusting powder is given in Example 35.3.

Liquid preparations

These include solutions, suspensions and emulsions. The same basic dispensing techniques employed in making the corresponding oral systems are used (see Chs 30, 31 and 32). Most liquid preparations are used unsterilized, but if they are intended for application to broken skin, eyes or body cavities, they should be sterilized. They should be packed in ribbed bottles, labelled 'For external use only', and carry a 'Shake the bottle' label if they are emulsions or suspensions. Worked examples are given of a lotion in Example 31.5 and of an oily lotion in Example 32.5.

Example 33.1

Rx Compound Sulphur Lotion BPC

Send 100 mL Compound Sulphur Lotion BPC.

	Master formula	For 100 mL
Precipitated sulphur	40 g	4 g
Quillaia tincture	5 mL	0.5 mL
Glycerol	20 mL	2 mL
Industrial methylated spirit (now IDA)	60 mL	6 mL
Calcium hydroxide solution	to 1000 mL	to 100 mL

Action and uses. This is used as a treatment for acne, scabies and as a mild antiseptic.

Formulation notes. This an example of a shake lotion, an aqueous suspension prepared without a suspending agent, but including a wetting agent for the hydrophobic sulphur.

Method of preparation. Sieve the precipitated sulphur. Weigh out 4 g and place in a glass mortar. Using a 1 mL pipette, add 0.5 mL quillaia tincture and work well into the sulphur using a pestle. Add 6 mL of industrial methylated spirits followed by 2 mL glycerol, working in after each addition (thus achieving

maximum wetting before water is added). Add 20–30 mL calcium hydroxide solution to produce a pourable suspension. Transfer to a tared bottle. Rinse the mortar with calcium hydroxide solution, adding it to the bottle, before making up to volume.

Shelf life and storage. There are no special requirements for storage. An expiry date of 4 weeks is suitable.

Example 33.2

Rx Methyl Salicylate Liniment BP

Prepare 100 mL methyl salicylate liniment.

	Master formula	For 100 mL
Methyl salicylate	250 mL	25 mL
Arachis oil	to 1000 mL	to 100 mL

Action and uses. Methyl salicylate is a rubefacient, used to treat muscular aches and pains.

Formulation notes. The methyl salicylate requires to enter the skin. The vegetable oil, arachis oil, is used as the solvent to assist in this process. Other similar fixed oils can be used.

Method of preparation. Measure 25 mL of methyl salicylate in a 100 mL measure and add arachis oil to make up to volume. Transfer to a dry 100 mL amber ribbed bottle.

Shelf life and storage. This liniment should be kept in a well-closed container in a cool place. An expiry date of 4 weeks is appropriate.

Example 33.3

Rx Turpentine Liniment BP

Send 100 mL of turpentine liniment.

	Master formula	To send 100 mL (120 units)
Turpentine oil	650 mL	78 mL
Racemic camphor	50 g	6 g
Soft soap	75 g	9 g
Purified water, freshly boiled and cooled	225 mL	27 mL

Action and uses. Both turpentine oil and camphor are rubefacients which are rubbed into the skin to relieve muscular aches and pains.

Formulation notes. The BP formula adds up to 1000. However, this is a mixture of weights and volumes so the final volume is not known. It is usual to calculate in the ratio 120 'units' per 100 mL.

This is an emulsion made using an alkali soap. When using soft soap, it is usual to use it at 10% by weight of an oil (as in this example), or 20% by weight of a fat.

Method of preparation. Weigh the camphor and place in a porcelain mortar. Grind it to a small particle size. Choose the softer, greener parts of the soap. Weigh (on a piece of paper) and mix thoroughly with the camphor. Measure the turpentine oil and add small aliquots (5–10 mL at first) to the soap and camphor followed by thorough mixing. When an even, pourable dispersion is obtained, transfer this to a 250 mL stoppered measuring cylinder. Use the remaining oil to rinse the mortar and add to the cylinder. Measure the water and add it, as quickly as possible, to the measure, stopper and shake it vigorously until a creamy white emulsion is formed. Allow it to stand for a few minutes (for air bubbles to separate) before transferring 100 mL to a tared bottle. Avoid plastic containers because turpentine reacts with some plastics.

Shelf life and storage. There are no special storage requirements. An expiry date of 4 weeks is appropriate.

Example 33.4

℞ Benzyl Benzoate Application BP
Prepare 100 mL of benzyl benzoate application.

	Master formula	For 100 mL
Benzyl benzoate	250 g	25 g
Emulsifying wax	20 g	2 g
Purified water, freshly boiled and cooled	to 1000 mL	to 100 mL

Action and uses. Benzyl benzoate is a liquid insecticide used for treating scabies and lice. It is usually applied with a brush over the whole body. It should not be applied to broken or inflamed skin.

Formulation notes. Benzyl benzoate is water immiscible and is being emulsified using the anionic Emulsifying Wax BP. The application is an o/w emulsion.

Method of preparation. Weigh the emulsifying wax and place it in an evaporating basin on a water bath or hot plate to melt. Add the benzyl benzoate and mix and warm. Warm about 75 mL of the water to the same temperature. Add about half of this to the evaporating basin and mix very gently. Transfer the mixture, again very gently to avoid frothing, to a tared bottle. Add warmed water to volume. Close the bottle and shake vigorously. Care is required to avoid frothing when water is present, because it will be very difficult to make up to the tare mark when froth has formed. Shake frequently during cooling.

Shelf life and storage. The application should be kept in a cool place, but not be allowed to freeze. An expiry date of 4 weeks is appropriate.

Semi-solid preparations

Mixing by fusion

The compounding of many semi-solid preparations includes the blending together of oily materials, some of which are solids at room temperature. The process called 'mixing by fusion' achieves this. As the name implies, it involves melting the ingredients together (see Example 33.5). The process is carried out in an evaporating basin on a water bath or hot plate. It should be noted that a high temperature is not required so 60–70°C is usually adequate. Waxy solids should be grated before weighing and should be added first, so that melting can start while other ingredients are being measured. When all the ingredients are melted, remove the basin from the water bath and gently stir until cold. Mixing, which should be gentle to avoid air bubbles, is necessary to avoid lumps forming. This could happen because the higher melting point ingredients in the eutectic system may precipitate out. Any medicament may be added at different stages of preparation depending on its properties. If soluble and stable, it can be added when the base is molten. If it is less stable, or insoluble but easy to disperse, it can be added during cooling. However, if it is unstable or if dispersion is difficult, it should be added when cold using mixing by trituration.

When evaporating basins are being used, recovery of all the product is not possible. Thus, in order to be able to pack the prescribed amount, it is necessary to make an excess of about 10%.

Example 33.5

Rx Simple Ointment BP
Send 50 g simple ointment.

	Master formula	For 60 g
Wool fat	50 g	3 g
Hard paraffin	50 g	3 g
Cetostearyl alcohol	50 g	3 g
Yellow or white soft paraffin	850 g	51 g

Action and uses. Simple ointment is used as an emollient, or for making other ointments.

Formulation notes. This is a simple blend of solid and semi-solid oily ingredients made by fusion. Yellow or white soft paraffin is chosen according to the colour of the finished product. In this case, since there is nothing else to be added, white soft paraffin should be used; 60 g is made to allow 50 g to be dispensed.

Method of preparation. Grate the hard paraffin and cetostearyl alcohol. Weigh 3 g of each and place in an evaporating basin on a water bath or hot plate. Weigh the wool fat, using a piece of paper to allow full re-covery of the material, and add it to the evaporating basin, followed by the soft paraffin (also weighed on paper). Stir gently until fully melted. Remove from the heat and continue to stir gently until cold. Weigh 50 g of base into a tared ointment jar or pack into a collapsible tube (see Example 33.10). If an ointment jar is used, a greaseproof paper disc should be placed on the surface of the ointment to protect the liner of the lid from the greasiness.

Shelf life and storage. Store in a cool place. An expiry date of 4 weeks is appropriate.

Mixing by trituration

Insoluble solids or liquids are incorporated into bases using the technique called 'mixing by trituration'. Any powders should be passed through a 180 μm sieve before weighing to avoid grittiness in the fin-ished product. Mixing by trituration is carried out on an ointment slab or tile, which may be made of glass or glazed porcelain. A flexible spatula is used to work the materials together. Powders are placed on the tile and incorporated into the base using 'dou-bling-up' as it is worked in. However, it is usually necessary to have two to three times the volume of base to powder, otherwise it will 'crumble'. Liquids, if present, are usually present in small amounts. To in-corporate a liquid, a portion of the base is placed on the slab and a recess made to hold the liquid which is then worked in gently. Larger quantities of liquid should be added a little at a time using the same method. In theory it is possible to recover all material from the slab, but it is normal to allow up to 10% excess for losses. These processes can be carried out in a mortar with a flat base using a pestle with a flat head. However, because recovery of the product is difficult, this is usually reserved for larger-scale batches.

Example 33.6

Rx Sulphur Ointment BP
Send 50 g sulphur ointment.

	Master formula	For 50 g	For 55 g
Precipitated sulphur, finely sifted	100 g	5 g	5.5 g
Simple ointment	900 g	45 g	49.5 g

Action and uses. The ointment is used to treat acne and scabies.

Formulation notes. The BP directs that the simple ointment be prepared with white soft paraffin. If simple ointment is available, the trituration can be carried out on a slab and all the product recov-ered. However, if simple ointment is also being made, 50 g should be adequate to ensure that 45 g are available. Precipitated sulphur, while of smaller particle size than sublimed sulphur, can give a gritty feel unless it is passed through a 180 μm sieve.

Method of preparation. Sieve and then weigh out the precipitated sulphur and place it on the slab. Weigh out the simple ointment (using a piece of paper to prevent it sticking to the balance), and place it on a different part of the slab. Take a portion of the sulphur and a portion of the base of about three times the volume of the sulphur and work them together vigor-ously until there is no sign of any particles of sulphur. Spreading a thin layer on the slab helps check this. Gradually add the remaining sulphur and base. Col-lect the ointment together on the slab using the spat-ula and pack 50 g.

Shelf life and storage. Store in a cool place. An expiry date of 4 weeks is appropriate.

Example 33.7

Rx Methyl Salicylate Ointment BP
Send 30 g methyl salicylate ointment.

	Master formula	For 35 g
Methyl salicylate	500 g	17.5 g
White beeswax	250 g	8.75 g
Hydrous wool fat	250 g	8.75 g

Action and uses. Methyl salicylate is a volatile material used as a rubefacient.

Formulation notes. Methyl salicylate is a liquid. With the high proportion present, the product would be runny without the addition of the beeswax as a thickening agent. The base ingredients require to be blended by fusion.

Method of preparation. Grate and weigh the beeswax. Melt it with the hydrous wool fat (weighed on a piece of paper) in an evaporating basin on a water bath or hot plate. Remove from the heat and stir until almost cold before adding the methyl salicylate (it is volatile). Continue stirring until cold. Pack 30 g in a glass ointment jar (plastic should be avoided with methyl salicylate).

Shelf life and storage. Store in a cool place. An expiry date of 4 weeks is appropriate.

Creams

Creams are emulsified preparations containing water. They are susceptible to microbial growth which may cause spoilage of the cream or disease in the patient. While preservatives are included, they are usually inadequate to cope with a heavy microbial contamination and so the possibility of microbial contamination during preparation should be minimized. Ideally aseptic techniques should be used, but this is not normally possible in extemporaneous dispensing and so thorough cleanliness is employed. As a minimum, all apparatus and final containers should be thoroughly cleaned and rinsed with freshly boiled and cooled purified water, then dried just prior to use. Swabbing of working surfaces, spatulas and other equipment with ethanol will also reduce the possibility of microbial contamination.

The basic method of making an emulsified cream is to warm both the oily phase and aqueous phase separately to a temperature of about 60°C, mix the phases and stir until cold. It is important that the temperatures of the two phases are within a few degrees of each other and it is advisable to use a thermometer to check this. Rapid cooling will cause the separation of high melting point materials, and excessive aeration as a result of vigorous stirring will produce a granular appearance in the product. Medicaments may, if they are stable, be dissolved in the appropriate phase before emulsification, or can be added by trituration when cold.

Example 33.8

Rx Aqueous Cream BP
Send 50 g aqueous cream.

	Master formula	For 55 g
Emulsifying ointment	300 g	16.5 g
Phenoxyethanol	10 g	0.55 g
Purified water, freshly boiled and cooled	690 g	37.95 g

Action and uses. Aqueous cream is an emollient and can be used as a base for drugs.

Formulation notes. This is an o/w cream made using an anionic emulsifying agent. To reduce the risk of microbial contamination, all equipment should be washed before use. Phenoxyethanol is present as an antimicrobial preservative. It is a liquid, so has to be weighed, or, if its density is obtained, it could be measured by pipette. If the emulsifying ointment has to be made, exactly 16.5 g can be made because the emulsification can be carried out in the same evaporating basin.

Method of preparation. The phenoxyethanol is dissolved in the water warmed to 60°C. Weigh the emulsifying ointment (using a piece of paper to prevent it sticking) and melt it in an evaporating basin on a water bath or hot plate. Ensure that both phases are close to 60°C, then add the aqueous phase to the melted ointment. Remove from the heat and stir continuously until cold, taking care not to incorporate too much air. Weigh 50 g and pack in an ointment jar or collapsible tube.

Shelf life and storage. The preparation should be stored in a cool place, but not allowed to freeze. A shelf life of 2–3 weeks is appropriate because the preparation has not been made in the cleanest conditions.

Example 33.9

℞ Hydrous Ointment BP (also known as Oily Cream)
Send 50 g oily cream.

	Master formula	For 60 g
Wool alcohols ointment	500 g	30 g
Phenoxyethanol	10 g	0.6 g
Dried magnesium sulphate	5 g	0.3 g
Purified water, freshly boiled and cooled	485 g	29.1 g

Actions and uses. Oily cream is used as an emollient in treating dry skin conditions.

Formulation notes. This is a w/o cream prepared using wool alcohols as the emulsifying agent. Phenoxyethanol is present as preservative, but all equipment should be washed before use. Phenoxyethanol is a liquid and so must be weighed, or, if its density is obtained, it can be measured by pipette. Quantities for 55 g produce amounts that cannot be weighed on a dispensing balance, so 60 g is made. If the wool alcohols ointment is also to be made, exactly 30 g is adequate, because it does not have to be removed from the evaporating basin.

Method of preparation. All equipment should be thoroughly cleaned before use. Dissolve the magnesium sulphate and phenoxyethanol in the water and warm to 60°C on a water bath or hot plate. Weigh the wool alcohols ointment, using a piece of paper, and melt it in an evaporating basin at 60°C. Check that the two temperatures are the same. Add the water, little by little, to the ointment, stirring constantly until a smooth creamy mixture is produced, while maintaining the temperature at 60°C. When all the water is added, remove from the heat and stir gently until the cream is at room temperature. Pack 50 g in an ointment jar or collapsible tube.

Shelf life and storage. Store in a cool place but do not allow to freeze. If liquid separates on storage, stirring may reincorporate it. An expiry date of 4 weeks is appropriate.

Dilution of creams

It is sometimes necessary to prepare a dilution of a commercially produced cream, although the practice is undesirable. Choice of diluent is crucial, since the diluent may impair the preservative system in the cream, may affect the bioavailability of the medica-ment, or be incompatible with other ingredients. The process of dilution also increases the risk of microbial contamination. Thus, dilutions should only be made with the diluent(s) specified in the manufacturer's data sheet and heat must be avoided. All diluted creams should be freshly prepared and be given a 2-week shelf life.

Example 33.10

A method for filling a collapsible tube extemporaneously.

1. Cut a piece of greaseproof paper about 5 cm longer than the tube and of a width that will go round the tube about twice. Place this on a clean slab, and fold up about 1 cm on one long edge (Fig. 33.3).
2. Place the cream on the paper, parallel to the fold, so that the length is about the same as that of the tube. Then fold the loose edge of the paper into the fold, so covering the cream. (This stage is rather like wrapping a powder – see Fig. 35.1.) Roll the paper from the fold, so that the cream is held in a cylinder of paper which will slide inside the tube.
3. Push the paper and cream right down the tube. Then, using a spatula or fingers, close the paper at the open end and gently pull it out, leaving the cream behind in the tube.
4. When fully withdrawn, hold a spatula blade firmly down on the open end of the tube, about 2.5 mm in from the end, and raise the cap end to produce a fold. Use the spatula, or a crimping tool if one is available, to complete the fold. Repeat this to produce a second fold.

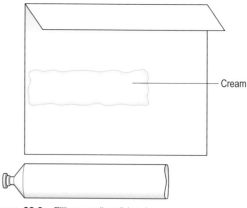

Cream

Figure 33.3 • Filling a collapsible tube.

Pastes

Pastes are dispersions of high concentrations of solid in either an aqueous or oily vehicle. They can be used to treat infections by making use of their high osmotic pressure, or as very thick materials to prevent irritant drugs spreading over the skin surface. Incorporation of the solid is by mixing on an ointment slab.

Example 33.11

℞ Dithranol Paste BP

Send 100 g of weak dithranol paste.

	Master formula	For 100 g
Dithranol	1 g	0.1 g
Lassar's paste	999 g	99.9 g

Lassar's paste:	Master formula	For 110 g
Zinc oxide	240 g	26.4 g
Salicylic acid	20 g	2.2 g
Starch	240 g	26.4 g
White soft paraffin	500 g	55 g

Action and uses. Dithranol is used to treat psoriasis. There are two strengths of dithranol paste, 'weak' is 0.1% and 'strong' is 1%, although a range of intermediate strengths are prescribed by dermatologists.

Formulation notes. The Lassar's paste has to be made first before incorporating the dithranol. Dithranol is prone to oxidation, so contact with metal should be avoided. Gloves should be worn during preparation

Method of preparation. Sieve the zinc oxide and salicylic acid through a 180 μm sieve before weighing. Weigh the soft paraffin (on a piece of paper) and melt in an evaporating basin on a water bath. Take some of the powder and stir into the melted base. Continue until all the powder is added, then stir gently until cold. Weigh out the Lassar's paste (using paper to avoid sticking). Only when the Lassar's paste has been completed, weigh out the dithranol. Care is required because it is very irritant to skin. Place it on a slab and incorporate it in a small portion of the paste using a plastic spatula, ensuring that a smooth, even product is produced. Dilute gradually with the remainder of the paste. Pack in a 120 g (4 ounces) brown ointment jar, with a circle of greaseproof paper and a tight-fitting closure, or a collapsible tube. The label should include the words 'To be spread thinly' (British National Formulary Label 28).

Shelf life and storage. The product should be kept in a cool place, protected from light. An expiry date of 2 weeks is appropriate because of chemical instability.

Transdermal delivery systems

Transdermal drug delivery systems aim to provide continuous drug release over a period of time which can be from a few hours to 7 days.

The principle of this dosage form is that, by optimization of physicochemical factors, the drug is absorbed through the skin into the systemic circulation. Absorption through the skin is variable so the rate of release of the drug must be controlled to a slower rate than the skin can absorb it. This may be achieved either by using a matrix system or a rate-limiting membrane. These devices are commonly known as 'patches'. Further details about the pharmaceutics of the patches are given in Aulton (2007). There is also a glyceryl trinitrate ointment (Percutol) which gives systemic activity.

Drugs available as transdermal therapeutic systems include:

- Glyceryl trinitrate for the treatment of angina. These patches are designed to deliver the drug over a 24-hour period, although it is recommended that a drug-free period is allowed each day to prevent tolerance. These patches are normally applied to the chest area.

- Estradiol for the alleviation of menopausal symptoms and the prevention of osteoporosis. These patches are applied once or twice weekly to skin below the waist (away from the breasts). They can be used alone or in combination with progestogens.

- Nicotine, in the alleviation of withdrawal symptoms in smoking cessation, provides an alternative route of administration to the gums, sprays etc. Patches are used for 16-hour per day periods and are available in a range of 'strengths' – that is rate of delivery of nicotine (e.g. 5 mg/ 16 hours). By providing a steady delivery of nicotine, they avoid the high plasma levels obtained during smoking. They may also have beneficial effects in other disease states. They are applied to the trunk.

- Hyoscine is available for the prevention of symptoms of travel sickness for up to 72 hours. It is applied behind the ear.
- Testosterone is used for hormone replacement and is applied to the trunk.
- Fentanyl patches can treat chronic intractable pain over a 72-hour period. They are applied to the torso.

Advantages

- Continuous drug delivery, producing steady-state plasma levels.
- No drug deactivation in the gastrointestinal tract.
- No first pass effect, as the liver is bypassed (although there is metabolism in the skin).
- Cessation of treatment by removing the patch. (This is not immediate because of a reservoir effect which will continue to deliver drug from the skin for several hours.)

Although these are benefits, various problems are associated with this type of dosage form. For these reasons, few drugs so far have been formulated in this way.

Disadvantages

- Only potent drugs, i.e. those with a small therapeutic dose, are suitable to be incorporated into a patch. Skin permeability is inadequate to allow larger doses from an acceptable size of patch.
- Because the drug is being absorbed through the skin, lipid-soluble drugs are most likely to be effective.
- Drugs with long half-lives are not suitable for this type of formulation.
- There have been reports of local skin reactions due to irritancy by drugs. Clonidine was withdrawn for this reason. To minimize possible skin reactions, new patches should be placed on fresh skin each time, the same site being used for at least 7 days.
- In some instances the steady-state blood levels have produced tolerance, e.g. glyceryl trinitrate. This has led to the practice of patients being given a 'nitrate-free' period which prevents tolerance occurring. A patch is applied and remains in place for 16 hours and is then removed. A period of 8 hours is allowed to elapse before a new patch is applied.

- Steady-state blood levels of nicotine have caused central nervous system disturbance; in particular, patients have reported suffering nightmares. Normally nicotine levels in a smoker will fall during the hours of sleep as no cigarette smoking occurs. No such fall will occur when 24-hour nicotine patches are used. For this reason manufacturers have developed patches which are applied for 16 hours then removed. A new one is applied 8 hours later.

Method of use

It is important that patients are informed how to use patches correctly. All patients who purchase or are prescribed patches should be given the following information about their use:

- To ensure adequate adhesion, the patch must be applied to a clean, dry area of skin.
- The old patch must always be removed before applying a new one.
- When a patch is replaced with a new one it must be applied to a different area of skin. The area of skin from which a patch has just been removed will be soft and possibly moist. This alters the permeability of the skin. In order to maintain the same level of drug absorption, a different, intact area of skin must be used.
- The patch must be disposed of carefully. It should be folded together to prevent it being stuck on to another person's skin. Particular care should be taken to keep patches away from children.

KEY POINTS

- Drugs applied to the skin are usually for a local effect, although systemic action is possible
- Skin preparations may be solids, liquids or semi-solids
- For liquids and semi-solids, the vehicles may be water based, water miscible, oily or emulsified
- A wide range of emulsifying agents may be used to produce either o/w or w/o emulsions
- Suspending agents used on the skin are usually clays
- Other ingredients include wetting agents, humectants and finely divided solids
- Powders should normally be passed through a 180 μm sieve before use
- Containers for liquid preparations should be brown and ribbed

- All skin preparations should carry the label 'For external use only'
- Dusting powders are simple mixtures made by 'doubling-up'
- Lotions are aqueous solutions, suspensions or emulsions
- Liniments are oily solutions or emulsions
- Mixing by fusion is the process of melting together the ingredients of ointment bases followed by stirring until cold

- Mixing by trituration is the incorporation of solids or liquids into semi-solid vehicles on an ointment slab
- Cleanliness is essential when making creams to avoid excessive microbial contamination
- Transdermal delivery systems (skin patches) are used to give prolonged constant plasma concentrations for a number of drugs
- Patients must be carefully counselled on the use of skin patches

Suppositories and pessaries

Arthur J. Winfield

STUDY POINTS

- Ideal suppository bases
- Types of base
- Suppository moulds and mould calibration
- Displacement values
- Methods of preparation of suppositories and pessaries
- Containers, labelling and patient advice for suppositories and pessaries

Introduction

Drug administration by the rectum can be used for local or systemic action. Dosage forms used include suppositories, rectal tablets, capsules, ointments and enemas. Vaginal administration can also be for both local and systemic action, using dosage forms which include pessaries and vaginal formulations of tablets, capsules, solutions, sprays, creams, ointments and foams. This chapter gives details of how suppositories and pessaries are prepared extemporaneously, the substances and equipment used in their preparation, the calculations involved and patient advice. Details about the formulation, manufacture and biopharmacy can be found in Aulton (2007).

Suppositories and pessaries are drug delivery systems where the drug is incorporated into an inert vehicle. The vehicle is referred to as the base. They are formed by melting the base, incorporating the drug and then allowing them to set in a suitable mould (made of metal or plastic).

Suppository bases

A range of materials is available for use as bases. A number of criteria can be identified as desirable in an ideal base, including the following:

- Melt at, or just below, body temperature or dissolve in body fluids
- Solidify quickly after melting
- Be easily moulded and removed from the mould
- Be chemically stable even when molten
- Release the active ingredient readily
- Be easy to handle
- Be bland, i.e. non-toxic and non-irritant.

No base meets all these requirements, so a compromise is usually required. There are two groups of materials, the fatty bases and the water-soluble or water-miscible bases.

The fatty bases

These bases, which melt around body temperature, are the naturally occurring theobroma oil and synthetic fats.

Theobroma oil, which has been used as a suppository base for over 200 years, has a melting point range of 30–36°C and so readily melts in the body.

It liquefies easily on heating but sets rapidly when cooled. It is also bland, therefore no irritation occurs. However, for a number of reasons the newer synthetic bases have now largely superseded it. The main technical difficulty is the ease with which lower melting point polymorphic forms of theobroma oil are formed. The stable β-form has a melting point of 34.5°C and forms after melting at 36°C and slowly cooling. However, if it is overheated, the unstable α-form (melting point 23°C) and γ-form (melting point 19°C) are produced. These forms will eventually return to the stable form but this may take several days. The melting point is also a problem in hot climates and can be reduced further by the addition of a soluble drug. The latter effect can be counteracted by adding beeswax (up to 10%), but care must be taken not to raise the melting point too high, as the suppository would then not melt in the rectum. In addition theobroma oil is prone to oxidation, and in common with many naturally occurring substances, may vary from batch to batch. Theobroma oil shrinks only slightly on cooling and therefore tends to stick to the suppository mould. For this reason the mould must be lubricated before use.

Synthetic fats

These are prepared by hydrogenating suitable vegetable oils. They have many of the advantages of theobroma oil but fewer disadvantages. However, there are a few potential problems:

- The viscosity of the melted fats is lower than that of theobroma oil. As a result there is a greater risk of drug particles sedimenting during preparation leading to a lack of uniform drug distribution which can give localized irritancy. This problem is partly compensated for in that these bases set very quickly.
- These bases become brittle if cooled too rapidly, so should not be refrigerated during preparation.
- Most manufacturers produce a series of grades of synthetic fatty bases, each with different hardness and melting point ranges. These can be used to compensate for melting point reduction by soluble drugs. However, release and absorption of the drug in the body may vary depending on the base being used.

Further information on these bases can be found in the *Pharmaceutical Codex* (1994).

Water-soluble and water-miscible bases

Glycerol-gelatin bases

These bases are a mixture of glycerol and water stiffened with gelatin. The commonest is Glycerol Suppositories Base BP, which has 14% weight in weight (w/w) gelatin, and 70% w/w glycerol. In hot climates the gelatin content can be increased to 18% w/w. Gelatin is a purified protein produced by the hydrolysis of the collagenous tissue, such as skins and bones, of animals. Grades of gelatin for pharmaceutical use must be heat treated during their preparation to ensure that the product is pathogen free. Some people may have ethical problems with the use of material from an animal source.

Two types of gelatin are used for pharmaceutical purposes: Type A, which is prepared by acid hydrolysis and is cationic, and Type B, which is prepared by alkaline hydrolysis and is anionic. Type A is compatible with substances such as boric acid and lactic acid while Type B is compatible with substances like ichthammol and zinc oxide. The 'jelly strength' or 'Bloom strength' of gelatin is important, particularly when it is used in the preparation of suppositories or pessaries.

Glycerol-gelatin bases have a physiological effect which can cause rectal irritation because of the small amount of liquid present. As they dissolve in the mucous secretions of the rectum, osmosis occurs producing a laxative effect. In addition they are also hygroscopic and therefore require careful storage. They are much more difficult to prepare and handle than other bases and the solution time depends on the content and quality of the gelatin and also the age of the suppository. Because of the water content, microbial contamination is more likely than with the fatty bases. Preservatives may be added to the product, but can lead to problems of incompatibilities.

Macrogols

These polyethylene glycols can be blended together to produce suppository bases with varying melting points, dissolution rates and physical characteristics. Drug release depends on the base dissolving rather than melting (the melting point is often around 50°C). Higher proportions of high molecular weight polymers produce preparations which release the drug slowly and are also brittle. Less brittle products which release the drug more readily can be prepared by mixing high polymers with medium and low polymers. Details of combinations which are used are found in the *Pharmaceutical Codex* (1994, p. 172). Macrogols have several properties which make them useful as suppository bases including the absence of a physiological effect, are not prone to microbial contamination and have a high water-absorbing capacity. As they dissolve, a viscous solution is produced which means there is less likelihood of leakage from the body.

There are, however, a number of disadvantages. They are hygroscopic, which means they must be carefully stored, and this could lead to irritation of the rectal mucosa. This latter disadvantage can be alleviated by dipping the suppository in water prior to insertion. They become brittle if cooled too quickly and also may become brittle on storage. Incompatibility with several drugs and packaging materials, e.g. benzocaine, penicillin and plastic, may limit their use. In addition crystal growth occurs, with some drugs causing irritation to the rectal mucosa and, if the crystals are large, prolonged dissolution times.

Preparation of suppositories

Suppositories are made using a suppository mould which may be made of metal or plastic. Traditional metal moulds for extemporaneous dispensing (Fig. 34.1) are in two halves which are clamped together with a screw. The internal surface is normally plated to ensure that the suppositories have a smooth surface.

Before use it is important to ensure that the mould is completely clean and it should be washed carefully in warm, soapy water and thoroughly dried, taking care not to scratch the internal surface. The exact shape can vary slightly from one mould to another.

Preparation of suppositories containing an active ingredient which is insoluble in the base

The bases used most commonly for extemporaneous preparation of suppositories and pessaries are the synthetic fats and glycerol-gelatin base.

1. It is always advisable when calculating the quantity of ingredients to calculate for an excess of 2 to allow for unavoidable wastage, e.g. if required to prepare 12 suppositories, calculate for 14.
2. The mould should be carefully washed and dried.
3. Ensure that the two halves fit together correctly. This is necessary to ensure that there is no leakage of material. They usually have code letters and/or numbers which should match.
4. For some bases the mould will need to be lubricated. The lubricants are given in Table 34.1.
5. If a lubricant is necessary, apply it carefully to the two halves of the mould using gauze or other non-fibrous material. Do not use cotton wool as fibres may be left on the mould surface and become incorporated into the suppositories.
6. Invert the mould to allow any excess lubricant to drain off.
7. Accurately weigh the required amount of base. If large lumps are present the material should be grated.
8. Place in a porcelain basin and warm gently using a water bath or hot plate. Allow approximately two-thirds of the base to melt and remove from the heat. The residual heat will be sufficient to melt the rest of the base.
9. Reduce the particle size of the active ingredient, if necessary. Either grinding in a mortar and pestle or sieving will do this.

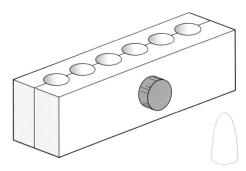

Figure 34.1 • Dispensing suppository mould.

Table 34.1 Lubricants for use with suppository bases

Base	Lubricant
Theobroma oil	Soap spirit
Glycerol-gelatin base	Almond oil, liquid paraffin
Synthetic fats	No lubricant required
Macrogols	No lubricant required

10. Weigh the correct amount of medicament and place on a glass tile (ointment slab).

11. Add about half of the molten base to the powdered drug and rub together with a spatula.

12. Scrape the dispersion off the tile using the spatula and place it back in the basin.

13. If necessary, put the basin back over the water bath to remelt the ingredients.

14. Remove from the heat and stir constantly until almost on the point of setting. If the mixture is not stirred at this stage the active ingredient will sediment and uniform distribution of the drug will not be achieved.

15. Quickly pour into the mould, slightly overfilling each cavity to allow for contraction on cooling. Do not start pouring the suppositories while the mixture is still very molten. If this is done, a suspended drug will sediment to the bottom of the mould and the base shrinks excessively so that the tops become concave.

16. Leave the mould and its contents to cool for about 5 minutes and then, using a spatula, trim the tops of the suppositories. Do not leave the suppositories too long before trimming as they will be too hard and trimming becomes very difficult.

17. Allow cooling for another 10–15 minutes until the suppositories are completely firm and set. Do not try to speed up the cooling process by putting the mould in a refrigerator. Synthetic fats in particular are inclined to become brittle and break if cooled too quickly.

18. Unscrew the mould and remove the suppositories.

19. Each perfect suppository should then be wrapped in greaseproof paper and packed in an appropriate container and labelled.

When preparing suppositories where the active ingredient is a semi-solid, is soluble in the base or is a liquid which is miscible with the base, the melting point of the base will be lowered. In these situations a base with a higher than normal melting point should be used if available. The base is melted as normal and the active ingredient is added directly to the base and incorporated by stirring.

Moulds are made in four sizes: 1 g, 2 g, 4 g and 8 g. Unless otherwise stated, the 1 g size is used for suppositories. The same moulds are used to prepare pessaries, when the two larger sizes are generally used. A suppository mould is filled by volume, but the suppository is formulated by weight. The capacity of a suppository mould is nominal and each mould will have minor variations. Therefore the weight of material contained in different moulds may be different and will also depend on the base being used. It is therefore essential that each mould be calibrated for each different base.

Mould calibration

The capacity of the mould is confirmed by filling the mould with the chosen base. The total weight of the perfect suppositories is taken and a mean weight calculated. This value is the calibration value of the mould for that particular base (see Example 34.1).

Example 34.1

A 1 g suppository mould is to be used to prepare a batch of suppositories. The base to be used is a synthetic fat. Some base is melted in an evaporating basin over a water bath or hot plate. When about two-thirds of the base has melted the basin is removed from the heat. The contents of the basin are stirred and the remaining base melts with the residual heat. Continue stirring the base until it is almost on the point of setting (it starts to thicken, becomes slightly cloudy and small crystals can be seen on the surface). The base is then poured into the mould cavities, slightly overfilling to allow for shrinkage. They are trimmed after about 5 minutes and left to set for a further 10–15 minutes. The mould is then opened and the suppositories removed. Only the perfect products should be weighed. Any which are chipped or damaged should be discarded.

From the above exercise, five perfect suppositories were obtained. The total weight was 5.05 g. The mould calibration figure is therefore 5.05/5 = 1.01 g. This is the value which should be used for that particular combination of mould and base.

Displacement values

The volume of a suppository from a particular mould is uniform but its weight can vary when a drug is present because the density of the drug may be different from that of the base. For example a drug which has twice the density of the base will occupy half the volume which the same weight of base occupies, and a drug whose density is four times that of the base will occupy a quarter the volume which the same weight of base occupies. Allowance must be made for this by using displacement values (DVs).

The displacement value of a drug is the number of parts by weight of drug which displaces 1 part by weight of the base.

Displacement values for a variety of medicaments are given in Table 34.2. Other reference sources such as the *Pharmaceutical Handbook* (Wade 1980) and the *Pharmaceutical Codex* also give information on displacement values. Minor variations may occur in the values quoted so it is always advisable to indicate the source of your information.

Displacement values in the literature normally refer to values for theobroma oil. These values can also be used for other fatty bases. With glycerol-gelatin suppository base, approximately 1.2 g occupies the same volume as 1 g of theobroma oil. Using this information the relevant displacement values can be calculated.

Table 34.2 Displacement values with respect to fatty bases

Medicament	Displacement value
Aspirin	1.1
Bismuth subgallate	2.7
Chloral hydrate	1.4
Cinchocaine hydrochloride	1.0
Codeine phosphate	1.1
Hamamelis dry extract	1.5
Hydrocortisone	1.5
Ichthammol	1.0
Liquids	1.0
Metronidazole	1.7
Morphine hydrochloride	1.6
Paracetamol	1.5
Pethidine hydrochloride	1.6
Phenobarbital	1.1
Zinc oxide	4.7

There may be occasions when information on the DV of a drug is not available. In these situations the DV must be determined.

Example 34.2

Prepare six suppositories each containing 250 mg bismuth subgallate.

Not all material can be removed from the evaporating basin, so quantities are calculated for an excess of two suppositories. Therefore calculate for eight suppositories.
DV of bismuth subgallate = 2.7 (*Pharmaceutical Codex*), i.e. 2.7 g of bismuth subgallate displaces 1 g of base.
A 1 g mould will be used with mould calibration = 0.94.
To calculate the amount of base required, a simple equation is used:

$$\text{Amount of base} = (N \times y) - (N \times D)/DV$$

where N is the number of suppositories to be made, y is the mould calibration, D is the dose in one suppository, DV is the displacement value.
Using the terms in the equation for this example:

$N = 8$
$Y = 0.94$
$D = 250$ mg $= 0.25$ g
DV $= 2.7$

Using the equation:

Amount of base required
$= (8 \times 0.94) - (8 \times 0.25)/2.7 = 7.52 - 0.741$
$= 6.779$ g $= 6.78$ g

Example 34.3

To calculate the DV of a drug:

A batch of unmedicated suppositories is prepared and the products weighed.
A batch of suppositories containing a known concentration of the required drug is prepared and the products are weighed.

Weight of six unmedicated suppositories = 6 g.
Weight of six suppositories containing 40% drug = 8.8 g.
Weight of base is then = 60% = 60/100 × 8.8 = 5.28 g.
Weight of drug in suppositories = 40% = 40/100 × 8.8 = 3.52.
Weight of base displaced by drug = 6 × 5.28 = 0.72g.
If 0.72 g of drug is displaced by 3.52 g of base, then 1 g of base will be displaced by 3.52/0.72 g = 4.88 g.
Therefore displacement value of drug = 4.9 (rounded to one decimal place).

Calculation of quantities when the active ingredient is stated as a percentage

A displacement value is not required when calculating quantities stated as percentages.

Example 34.4

Prepare eight suppositories containing 18% zinc oxide. Calculate for 10 suppositories (2 excess).

Mould calibration = 1
Weight of base required to fill mould = 10 × 1 = 10 g.
Zinc oxide is 18% of total = 1.8 g.
Weight of base required = 10 − 1.8 = 8.2 g.

When there is more than one active ingredient present the quantity of each medicament is calculated and the amount of base is calculated using the displacement value for each ingredient.

Example 34.5

Calculate the quantities required to make 15 suppositories each containing 150 mg hamamelis dry extract and 560 mg of zinc oxide.
A 2 g mould, with mould calibration of 2.04, will be used. Calculate for 17 suppositories (2 excess).
DV of hamamelis dry extract = 1.5 (*Pharmaceutical Codex*).
DV of zinc oxide = 4.7 (*Pharmaceutical Codex*).
Weight of hamamelis dry extract = 17 × 0.15 = 2.55 g.
Weight of zinc oxide = 17 × 0.56 = 9.52 g.
Weight of base = 17 × 2.04 − (2.55/1.5 + 9.52/4.7) = 34.68 − (1.7 + 2.03) = 30.95 g.

Preparation of suppositories using a glycerol-gelatin base

The formula for Glycerol Suppository Base BP is:

Gelatin	14%
Glycerol	70%
Water	to 100%

1. The gelatin strip is cut into small pieces, approximately 1 cm square, trimming off any hard outer edges.

2. The required amount of gelatin is weighed and placed in a previously weighed porcelain evaporating basin.
3. Sufficient water to just cover the gelatin is added and the contents left for about 5 minutes.
4. When the gelatin has softened (hydrated), any excess water is drained off. This step is not necessary if powdered gelatin is being used.
5. The exact amount of glycerol is then weighed into the basin.
6. The basin is heated gently on a water bath or hot plate and the mixture gently stirred until the gelatin has dissolved. Do not stir vigorously as this will create air bubbles which are very difficult to remove. At this stage the base may need to be heat treated as noted below.
7. When the gelatin is dissolved, the basin is removed from the heat and weighed. If the weight is less than the required total (basin plus ingredients), water is added to give the correct weight. If the contents of the basin are too heavy, it must be heated further to evaporate the excess water.
8. When the correct weight is achieved, the active ingredient is added, with careful stirring.
9. The mixture is then poured into the prepared mould and lubricated with an oil such as almond oil or liquid paraffin. The mould must not be overfilled because glycerol-gelatin base cannot be trimmed.
10. The preparation is left to set. After removing from the mould, each suppository should be smeared with liquid paraffin before being wrapped in greaseproof paper.

Note: Gelatin which is of a grade suitable for pharmaceutical use should not contain any pathogens, but as a precaution, the base may be heat treated. This is done by heating the base for 1 hour at 100°C in an electric steamer. This should be done before the base is adjusted to weight (at Stage 7 above).

This base is commonly used for the preparation of pessaries, as described in the following example.

Containers for suppositories

Glass or plastic screw-topped jars are possibly the best choice of container for extemporaneously prepared suppositories and pessaries. Cardboard cartons may

Example 34.6

Prepare 12 pessaries containing 10% ichthammol. A 4 g mould (calibration value 4.0) is used.

Calculate for 14 pessaries to allow for wastage. Additional base is required because it is more dense than the oily bases. The density factor is 1.2.
Mould calibration for glycerol-gelatin base is 4.0 × 1.2 = 4.8 g.
A displacement value is not required because the ichthammol is expressed as a percentage.

Formula for the base:

Gelatin	14 g
Glycerol	70 g
Water	to 100 g

Formula for the pessaries:

Ichthammol	10% w/w
Glycerol-gelatin base	90% w/w

The total weight required to prepare the pessaries is 14 × 4.8 g = 67.2 g. For ease of calculation prepare 70 g. Quantities are therefore:

Ichthammol	7 g
Base	63 g

It is advisable to make a small excess of base, taking care to choose quantities which give easily weighable amounts, i.e. do not try to weigh to several decimal points. In this case 65 g can be prepared.

Using the method described above, prepare 65 g of the base, taking care that the correct type of gelatin is chosen. Because the active ingredient is ichthammol, Type B should be used. When the 65 g of base has been prepared, 2 g should be removed from the basin, leaving the required 63 g. The base is removed from the heat, allowed to cool a little before 7 g of ichthammol is added with careful stirring. The mixture is then poured into the lubricated mould and left to set.

be used but these offer little protection from moisture or heat. They are therefore not suitable for hygroscopic materials.

Shelf life

Provided they are well packaged and the storage temperature is low, suppositories and pessaries are relatively stable preparations. Unless other information is available, an expiry date of 1 month is appropriate.

Labelling for suppositories

Adequate information should appear on the label so that the patient knows how to use the product. In addition the following information should appear: 'Store in a cool place' and 'For rectal use only' or 'For vaginal use only', whichever is appropriate.

'Do not swallow' can be put on the label but do not use 'For external use only' – the preparation is being inserted into a body cavity and this instruction is therefore incorrect.

Patient advice

In addition to what appears on the label, patients should be told to unwrap the suppository or pessary (this may appear to be unnecessary advice but there is sufficient evidence to show that it is not always done) and insert it as high as possible into the rectum or vagina. It may be helpful to provide the patient with a diagram and instruction leaflet, such as that produced by the National Pharmaceutical Association. When suppositories are for children it is likely that an adult will have to carry out the insertion.

KEY POINTS

- Both rectal and vaginal administration can be used for local or systemic drug action
- Bases may be fatty or water miscible
- Synthetic bases, made from hydrogenated vegetable oils, are easier to use than theobroma oil
- Glycerol-gelatin base produces a laxative effect
- Type A (anionic) or Type B (cationic) gelatin can be used to avoid incompatibilities
- Macrogol bases are blends of high and low molecular weight polymers which dissolve in rectal contents
- Suppository moulds have nominal capacities of 1, 2, 4 and 8 g and must be calibrated with the base to be used
- When using theobroma oil and glycerol-gelatin base, the mould has to be lubricated
- To allow for contraction on cooling, overfilling with oily bases is required
- Each mould should be calibrated for each base

- Because glycerol-gelatin base has a higher density than fatty bases, moulds hold approximately 1.2 times the nominal weight
- The displacement value is the number of parts by weight of drug which displaces one part by weight of base

- Unless the density of the drug and base are the same, a displacement value is required to calculate the amount of base displaced by the drug
- Labels should include either 'For rectal use only' or 'For vaginal use only', and 'Store in a cool place'

35

Powders and granules

Arthur J. Winfield

STUDY POINTS

- The pharmaceutical uses of powders
- Bulk and divided powders
- The mixing of powders
- Diluents used with powders
- Calculations required when preparing powders
- How to dispense powders
- The folding of powders

Introduction

A powder may be defined as a solid material in a finely divided state. Granules are powders agglomerated to produce larger free-flowing particles. Powders and granules can be used to prepare other formulations, such as solutions, suspensions and tablets. A powdered drug on its own can be a dosage form for taking orally (called a simple powder), when they are usually mixed with water first, or for external application as a dusting powder. Alternatively the drug may be blended with other ingredients (called a compound powder).

Powders for internal use

Powders for oral administration will comprise the active ingredients with excipients such as diluents, sweeteners and dispersing agents. These may be presented as undivided powders (bulk powders) or divided powders (individually wrapped doses).

Magnesium Trisilicate Powder Compound BP (see Example 35.4) and Compound Kaolin Powder BP are examples of bulk powders for internal use. Proprie-

tary powders and granules include Dioralyte®, Electrolade® (both oral rehydration salts), Normacol® (sterculia) and Fybogel® (ispaghula husk). Individually wrapped powders tend not to be official formulae (see Examples 35.1 and 35.2).

Bulk powders

Supplying as an undivided powder is useful for non-potent, bulky drugs with a large dose, e.g. antacids, or when the dry powder is more stable than its liquid-containing counterpart. A bulk powder can be supplied to the patient although this is rarely seen nowadays because the dosage form is inconvenient to carry and there are possible inaccuracies in measuring the dose. Some liquid mixtures may be prepared in the pharmacy from a bulk powder by the addition of a specific volume of water, e.g. Magnesium Trisilicate Mixture BP. This reduces transport and packaging costs.

Individually wrapped powders

Individually wrapped powders are used to supply some potent drugs, where accuracy of dose is important. Extemporaneously produced powders are wrapped separately in paper. They are convenient dosage forms for children's doses of drugs which are not commercially available at the strength required, such as levothyroxine (thyroxine) or ibuprofen (see Example 35.2). Sealed sachets of powders are available commercially, e.g. Paramax (paracetamol and metoclopramide) and oral rehydration salts. They are mixed with water prior to taking and are useful for patients who have difficulty swallowing or where rapid absorption of the drug is required.

Granules for internal use

Some preparations are supplied to the pharmacy as granules, for reconstitution immediately before dispensing, e.g. antibiotic suspensions. This protects drugs which are susceptible to hydrolysis or other degradation in the presence of water until the time of dispensing in order to give an adequate shelf life (see Ch. 31).

Particle size

The particle size of a powder is described using standard descriptions given in the *British Pharmacopoeia* (BP). These refer to either the standardized sieve size that they are capable of passing through in a specified time under shaking, or to the microscopically determined particle size. Thus powders for oral use would normally be a 'moderately fine' or a 'fine' powder. The former is able to pass through a sieve of nominal mesh aperture 355 μm and the latter one of 180 μm. Comminution is the process of particle size reduction. On a small scale, this can be achieved using a mortar and pestle when it is usually called trituration. This is a common first step in extemporaneous dispensing,

after which the powder should be passed through the appropriate sieve before weighing.

Mixing the powder

Ingredients of powders should be mixed thoroughly, using the technique of 'doubling-up' (sometimes called geometric dilution) to ensure an even distribution. This process involves starting with the ingredient which has the smallest bulk. In Example 35.1 this is hyoscine hydrobromide. The other ingredient(s) are added progressively in approximately equal parts by volume. In this way the amount in the mortar is approximately doubled at each addition. Mixing in between additions continues until all the ingredients are incorporated. The powder can then be packed.

Preparing individually wrapped powders

The minimum weight of an individually wrapped powder is 120 mg. Dilution of a drug with a diluent, usually lactose, is often necessary to produce this weight.

Occasionally manufactured tablets or capsules may be used to prepare oral powders (see Example 35.2). This involves either crushing the tablet in a

---

Example 35.1

Hyoscine hydrobromide 300 micrograms. Mitte 4 powders.
Label 'One to be given 30 minutes before the journey'.

Action and uses. Antimuscarinic drug used in the prevention of motion sickness.
Calculation and method of preparation. Calculate for five powders. Use lactose as the diluent, each powder to weigh 120 mg.

Hyoscine hydrobromide (5 × 300)
= 1500 micrograms = 1.5 mg
Lactose (5 × 120 mg) to 600 mg

The minimum weighable quantity (using a Class B balance) is 100 mg.

Step A

Make a 1 in 10 dilution of hyoscine hydrobromide with lactose:
Hyoscine hydrobromide 100 mg
Lactose 900 mg

Mix by doubling-up and remove 100 mg (triturate A).
100 mg of triturate A contains 100/1000 × 100 = 10 mg hyoscine hydrobromide.

Step B

Make a 1 in 10 dilution of triturate A with lactose:

Triturate A	100 mg
Lactose	900 mg

Mix by doubling-up and remove 150 mg (triturate B).
150 mg of triturate B contains 10/1000 × 150 = 1.5 mg hyoscine hydrobromide.

Step C

Triturate B	150 mg
Lactose ((5 × 120 mg) − 150 mg) = 450 mg	

Mix by doubling-up. 120 mg portions of this final powder will contain 300 micrograms of hyoscine hydrobromide. Weigh 120 mg aliquots and wrap in a powder paper.

mortar and pestle, or emptying the contents of the capsule and adding a suitable diluent. Lactose is the most commonly used diluent because it is colourless, odourless, soluble, is generally harmless and has good flow properties. Some patients may be unable to tolerate lactose and a suitable inert alternative diluent, for instance light kaolin, would then be used.

Powder calculations

Quantities should be calculated to allow for loss of powder during manipulation. It is usual to allow for at least one extra powder. If the total amount of active ingredient required is less than the minimum weighable quantity, dilutions will be necessary. In this process, also called trituration, the minimum quantity of the active ingredient(s) is weighed and diluted, over several steps if necessary, in order to obtain the dose(s) required. Example 35.1 illustrates the process where two dilution steps are required (see also Ch. 26).

Folding papers

White glazed paper, called demy paper, is used for wrapping powders. A suitable size is 120 mm × 100 mm. The wrapping should be carried out on a clean tile or larger sheet of demy to protect the product. The papers should be folded with their long edges parallel to the front of the bench. Follow the steps illustrated in Figure 35.1 in order to fold the paper:

- The long edge, furthest away from the dispenser, should be turned over to about one-seventh of the paper width (step A).
- The powder should be weighed accurately and placed on the paper towards the folded edge of the centre of the paper (step B).
- The unfolded long edge (nearest the dispenser) should then be brought over the powder to meet the crease of the folded edge and the flap closed over it (step C).
- The folded edge should then be folded over (towards the dispenser) so that it covers about half the powder packet (step D).
- The short edges of the powder packet should be folded over, using a powder cradle if available, so that the flaps are of equal lengths and the folded powder fits neatly into a box or jar (steps E and F). Before making these folds, ensure that there is no powder in the ends to be folded, otherwise it may fall out and be lost.

The creases can be sharpened with a spatula, taking care not to tear the paper or use excessive pressure which would compress the powder inside the pack.

The powders can be packed in pairs, back to back, or in one bundle, with the final powder placed back to back. They should be held together with an elastic band. In a well-wrapped product, there will be no powder in the fold or flaps, so that all the powder is available for easy administration when unwrapped.

Manufactured powders are subject to a uniformity of weight test, or uniformity of content test if each dose contains less than 2 mg of active ingredient or the content of active ingredient represents less than 2% of the total weight.

Shelf life and storage of internal powders

Extemporaneously prepared powders should have an expiry of between 2 and 4 weeks. Proprietary powders often have a longer shelf life because of the protective packaging. Some powders may be hygroscopic, deliquescent or volatile and will need to be protected from decomposition. Storage for these powders should be moisture proof and airtight.

Containers for internal powders

Extemporaneously prepared individually wrapped powders are often dispensed in a paperboard box. However, it is preferable to use a screw-top glass or plastic container which provides an airtight seal and protection against moisture. Proprietary powders in individual sachets which are moisture proof may be dispensed in a paperboard box. Bulk powders are packed in an airtight glass or plastic jar. A 5 mL spoon should also be supplied with bulk powders.

Special labels and advice for internal powders

Powders are usually mixed with water or another suitable liquid before taking, depending on their solubility. Powders for babies or young children can be placed directly into the mouth on the back of the tongue, followed by a drink to wash down the powder. Bulk powders should be shaken and measured carefully before dissolving or dispersing in a little water and taking.

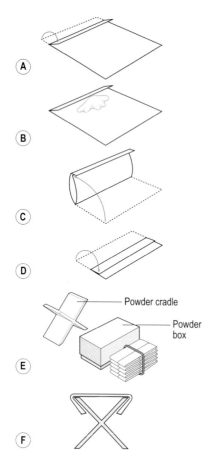

Figure 35.1 • Steps for the folding of individually wrapped powders.

Powders for external use

Powders, with or without medicament, are frequently applied to the skin. Dusting powders contain one or more substances in fine powder and may be dispensed as single-dose or multidose preparations (see Example 35.3). They are used to treat a variety of skin conditions or to soothe skin. Examples are antifungal powders for athlete's foot or talc dusting powder for the prevention of chafing and skin irritation. Zinc oxide and starch are added to formulations to absorb moisture and talc is used for lubricant properties. Talc, kaolin and other natural mineral materials are liable to contamination with bacteria such as *Clostridium tetani*, *C. perfringens* and *Bacillus anthracis*. These ingredients should be sterilized by dry heat or the final product should be sterilized. Dusting powders should be sterile if they may be applied to large areas of open skin or wounds. They should not be used where there

is a likelihood of large volumes of exudate, as hard crusts will form.

Preparing powders for external use

A sieve size of 180 μm should be used to obtain the finely divided powder. The constituents should be mixed using the doubling-up method, as described previously.

Shelf life and storage for powders for external use

Dry powders should remain stable over a long period of time if packaged and protected from the atmosphere. For extemporaneously prepared products, an expiry of 4 weeks is appropriate.

Containers for powders for external use

Powders for external use may be packed in glass, metal or plastic containers with a sifter-type cap. Some are also available commercially in pressurized containers, containing other excipients such as a propellant and lubricants.

Special labels and advice for powders for external use

'For external use only' and 'Store in a cool, dry place'.
    Examples of official powders for external use include Zinc Oxide Dusting Powder Compound BPC, Chlorhexidine Dusting Powder BP and Talc Dusting Powder BP. Proprietary examples of powders for

---

Example 35.2

Send 18 ibuprofen powders for a child of 3 years to provide 20 mg/kg daily. Take 1 twice daily (child's weight is 14 kg).

The dose required = 20 × 14 = 280 mg daily.
Therefore each powder to contain 140 mg.

	For 1 powder	For 20 powders (2 excess)
Ibuprofen	140 mg	2.8 g

---

external use include Daktarin (miconazole), Cicatrin (neomycin sulphate, bacitracin zinc, cysteine, glycine and threonine) and Canesten powder (clotrimazole).

Action and uses. Non-steroidal anti-inflammatory drug, used to treat fever, pain and juvenile arthritis at a dose of up to 40 mg/kg daily.

Formulation notes. A diluent is not required, since the weight of each powder will be above the minimum 120 mg required. Pure ibuprofen powder can be used. However, if it is not available, manufactured 200 mg ibuprofen tablets (not modified release) can be used to prepare these powders.

Method of preparation. Take 14 × 200 mg ibuprofen tablets (contain 2.8 g ibuprofen) and weigh them. This is necessary to allow for the weight of the tablet excipients. Grind to a fine powder in a mortar and pestle. Pass the resulting powder through a 250 µm sieve and lightly remix. Divide the original weight of tablets by 20, and weigh aliquots of the resulting amount of powder. Pack into individual powder papers. Fasten the 18 powders together with an elastic band and pack in an amber glass jar or plastic container with a screw cap.

Shelf life and storage. Store in a cool, dry place. A shelf life of 2–3 weeks is appropriate.

Advice and special labels. The powders should be given after food, in water (or directly into the child's mouth, followed by a drink of water).

Example 35.3

R$_X$ Zinc, Starch and Talc Dusting Powder BPC. Mitte 100 g.

	Master formula	For 100 g
Zinc oxide	25%	25 g
Starch	25%	25 g
Sterilized purified talc 50%	50 g	

Action and uses. A soothing preparation to absorb moisture and act as a lubricant, preventing friction in skin folds.

Method of preparation. Sieve the powders, using a 180 µm sieve, weigh and mix them by doubling-up in a mortar and pestle. Pack in an amber glass jar or plastic container with a screw cap (with a perforated, reclosable lid if possible).

Shelf life and storage. Store in a dry place. An expiry date of 4 weeks is advisable.

Advice and special labels. 'For external use only'. Lightly dust the powder onto the affected area. The area should not be too wet as the powder will cake and abrade the skin. It should not be applied to broken skin or large raw areas.

Example 35.4

R$_X$ Compound Magnesium Trisilicate Oral Powder BP 1988. Mitte 200 g.

	Master formula	For 200 g
Magnesium trisilicate	250 mg	50 g
Chalk	250 mg	50 g
Heavy magnesium carbonate	250 mg	50 g
Sodium bicarbonate	250 mg	50 g

Action and uses. Antacid preparation for dyspepsia.

Method of preparation. Sieve the powders, using a 250 µm sieve, weigh and mix them by doubling-up, using a mortar and pestle. Pack in an amber glass jar or plastic container with a screw cap.

Shelf life and storage. Store in a dry place. A 4-week expiry date is reasonable if kept dry.

Advice and special labels. 'Dissolve or mix with water before taking' (British National Formulary Label 13). A normal dose is 1–5 g of the powder taken in liquid, when required. Antacids are usually taken between meals and at bedtime.

KEY POINTS

- Powders may be prepared as bulk powders, divided powders or granules
- Powders may be used internally or externally
- The particle size of a fine powder should be less than 180 µm
- The minimum weight of a divided powder is 120 mg
- Lactose is a good diluent for internal powders
- Trituration is the process used to obtain small doses which are below the minimum weighable quantity
- Ideally powders should be packed in a glass or plastic container
- A 5 mL spoon should be provided with bulk powders for oral use
- When dispensing divided powders, an excess of one or two should be prepared to allow for losses during processing

36

Oral unit dosage forms

Arthur J. Winfield

STUDY POINTS

- Different types of tablets
- Excipients used in tablets and capsules
- Dispensing commercially produced tablets and capsules
- Extemporaneous dispensing of capsules and cachets

Introduction

Tablets and capsules are the most popular way of delivering a drug for oral use. They are convenient for the patient and are usually easy to handle and identify. They are mass produced on a commercial scale at a relatively low manufacturing cost. Because they are manufactured by the pharmaceutical industry where quality assurance is in place, a high accuracy of dosage is achievable with oral unit dosage forms and they are free from the problems of stability found in aqueous mixtures and suspensions. Packaging in blister packs can also enhance the stability of these dosage forms (see Ch. 27). Their main disadvantages are that there is a slower onset of action relative to liquids and some people have difficulty swallowing solid oral dosage forms, e.g. the very young or very old.

Tablets

Tablets are solid preparations each containing a single dose of one or more active ingredient(s). They are normally prepared by compressing uniform volumes of particles, although some tablets are prepared by moulding. The process of tablet production is outside the scope of this book, but can be found in Aulton (2007) or the *Pharmaceutical Codex*.

Many different types of tablet are available, which may also be in a variety of shapes and sizes. The types include dispersible, effervescent, chewable, sublingual and buccal tablets, lozenges, tablets for rectal or vaginal administration and solution tablets. Some tablets are designed to release the drug after a time lag, or slowly for a prolonged drug release or sustained drug action (see Ch. 21). The design of these modified-release tablets uses formulation techniques to control the biopharmaceutical behaviour of the drug. These issues are discussed in Aulton (2007).

In addition to the drug(s), several excipients must be added. These will aid the process of tableting and ensure that the active ingredient will be released as intended. Excipients include:

- *Diluents*. These add bulk to make the tablet easier to handle. Examples include lactose, mannitol, sorbitol and calcium carbonate.
- *Binders*. These enable granules to be prepared which improves flow properties of the mixture during manufacture. Examples include acacia mucilage, polyvinylpyrrolidone and microcrystalline cellulose.
- *Disintegrants*. These encourage the tablet to break into smaller particles after ingestion. Examples include modified cellulose and modified starch.
- *Lubricants, glidants, antiadherents*. These are essential for flow of the tablet material into the tablet dies and preventing sticking of the compressed tablet in the punch and die. Examples of lubricants are magnesium and calcium stearate,

sodium lauryl sulphate and sodium stearyl fumarate. Colloidal silica is usually the glidant of choice. Talc and magnesium stearate are effective antiadherents.

- *Miscellaneous agents* may be added, such as colours and flavours in chewable tablets.

Some tablets have coatings, such as sugar coating or film coating. Coatings can protect the tablet from environmental damage, mask an unpleasant taste, aid identification of the tablet and enhance its appearance. Enteric coatings on tablets resist dissolution or disruption of the tablet in the stomach, but not in the intestine. This is useful when a drug is destroyed by gastric acid, is irritating to the gastric mucosa, or when bypassing the stomach aids drug absorption. See Aulton (2007) for details about coatings and other specialized formulation and manufacturing techniques.

Dispensing of tablets

Many tablets in the UK and other countries are packaged by the manufacturer into patient packs suitable for issue to the patient without repacking by the pharmacist. Patient information leaflets are also contained in these patient packs. When dispensing these packs to patients, the pharmacist must ensure that they are labelled correctly, according to the prescriber's instructions (see Ch. 28), and that the patient is counselled on the use of the medication (see Ch. 44). Further supplies of patient information leaflets are available from the manufacturer when required. For some controlled-release tablets, variations in bioavailability may occur with different brands. It is important that patients are given the brand that they are stabilized on in order to maintain therapeutic outcome. Examples where this is important include theophylline, lithium and phenytoin.

Tablets may also be supplied in a bulk container. The required number of tablets needs to be counted out (see Ch. 25) and placed in a suitable container for dispensing to the patient (see Ch. 27). It is important to minimize errors by ensuring that the correct bulk container has been selected and the correct drug dispensed. The pharmacist should verify this by checking the label of the bulk container and by examining the shape, size and markings on the dispensed tablets where appropriate, with the prescription. A copy of the patient information leaflet should be included.

Some tablets are supplied in a strip-packed form where each tablet has its own blister. A development

of this is the calendar pack where the day or date on which the tablet is to be taken is indicated on the pack.

Shelf life and storage of tablets

Most tablets should be stored in airtight packaging, protected from light and extremes of temperature. When stored properly they generally have a long shelf life. The expiry date will be printed on the package or the individual strip packs. Some tablets need to be stored in a cool place, e.g. Ketovite® and Leukeran® (chlorambucil) (both stored between 2 and 8°C). Some tablets contain volatile drugs, e.g. glyceryl trinitrate, and must be packed in glass containers with tightly fitting metal screw caps (see Ch. 27). An additional warning must be placed on these tablets, when dispensed to patients, to advise them to throw away the tablets 8 weeks after opening, as they lose potency.

Containers for tablets

Strip or blister packs are dispensed in a paperboard box and tablets counted from bulk containers are placed in amber glass or plastic containers with airtight, child-resistant closures.

Special labels and advice on tablets

Most tablets should be swallowed with a glass, or 'draught', of water. A draught of water refers to a volume of water of about 50 mL. This prevents the dosage form becoming lodged in the oesophagus, which can cause problems such as ulceration. Tablets may be coated and shaped to aid swallowing.

Some tablets should be dissolved or dispersed in water before taking, e.g. effervescent analgesic tablets. Other tablets, particularly those with coatings or modified-release properties, should be swallowed whole. There are also some tablets which should be chewed or sucked before swallowing, e.g. antacid tablets. Appropriate labels should be placed on the container (see Ch. 28).

Coated tablets, e.g. enteric coatings, require specific advice on avoiding indigestion remedies at the same time of day, as these will affect the pH of the stomach, and therefore cause premature breakdown of the enteric coating on the tablet.

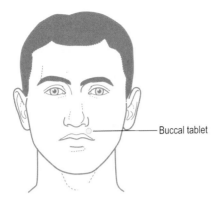

Figure 36.1 • Positioning of a buccal tablet.

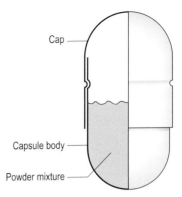

Figure 36.2 • Hard gelatin capsule shell: body and cap.

Buccal and sublingual tablets are not swallowed whole and it is important that patients know how to use them. If these formulations are swallowed then they will not have their intended therapeutic effect. Figure 36.1 illustrates the positioning for buccal tablets. Sublingual tablets are placed under the tongue.

Capsules

Capsules are solid preparations intended for oral administration made with a hard or soft gelatin shell. One (or more) medicament is enclosed within this gelatin container. Most capsules are swallowed whole, but some contain granules which provide a useful premeasured dose for administering in a similar way to a powder, e.g. formulations of pancreatin. Some capsules enclose enteric-coated pellets, e.g. Erymax (erythromycin). Capsules are elegant, easy to swallow and can be useful in masking unpleasant tastes. Capsules may also be used to hold powder or oils for inhalation, e.g. Intal® capsules (sodium cromoglicate) or Karvol®, or for rectal and vaginal administration, e.g. Gyno-Daktarin® (miconazole nitrate) (see Ch. 34).

Soft shell capsules

A soft gelatin capsule consists of a flexible solid shell containing powders, non-aqueous liquids, solutions, emulsions, suspensions or pastes. Such capsules allow liquids to be given as solid dosage forms, e.g. cod liver oil. They also offer accurate dosage, improved stability and overcome some of the problems of dealing with powders. They are formed, filled and sealed in one manufacturing process.

Hard shell capsules

Empty capsule shells are made from gelatin and are clear, colourless and essentially tasteless. Colourings and markings can be easily added for light protection and to ease identification. The shells are used in the preparation of most manufactured capsules and for the extemporaneous compounding of capsules. The shell comprises two sections, the body and the cap, both being cylindrical and sealed at one end. Powder or particulate solid, such as granules and pellets, can be placed in the body and the capsule closed by bringing the body and cap together (Fig. 36.2). Some capsules have small indentations on the body and cap which 'lock' together. If not, they must be sealed by moistening the outside top of the body before putting the top in place. Technical aspects of capsule manufacture are given in Aulton (2007).

Compounding of capsules

Occasionally hand filling of capsules may be required, particularly in a hospital pharmacy or when preparing materials for clinical trials. A suitable size of capsule shell should be selected so that the finished capsule looks reasonably full. Hard shell capsules are available in eight sizes. These are listed in Table 36.1, with the corresponding approximate capacity (based on lactose). The bulk density of a powder mixture will also affect the choice of capsule size.

Calculations for compounding capsules

The recommended minimum weight for filling a capsule is 100 mg. If the required weight of the drug is smaller than this, a diluent should be added by

Table 36.1 Sizes of hard gelatin capsules and their approximate capacities

Capsule no.	000	00	0	1	2	3	4	5
Content (mg)	950	650	450	300	250	200	150	100

trituration (see Ch. 35). If the quantity of the drug for a batch of capsules is smaller than the minimum weighable amount, 100 mg on a Class B balance, then trituration will also be required. Lactose, magnesium carbonate, starch, kaolin and calcium phosphate are commonly used diluents. To allow for small losses of powder, an excess should be calculated, e.g. two extra capsules. Example 36.1 gives a worked example.

Filling capsules

The number of capsules to be filled should be taken first and set to one side. This avoids the danger of contaminating empty capsules. The powder to be encapsulated should be finely sifted (180 μm sieve) and prepared. Magnesium stearate (up to 1% weight in weight (w/w)) and silica may be added as a lubricant and glidant respectively, to aid filling of the capsule. Various methods of filling capsules on a small scale are possible.

Filling from a powder mass

The prepared powder can be placed on a clean tile or piece of demy paper and powder pushed into the capsule body with the aid of a spatula until the required weight has been enclosed. The empty capsule body could also be 'punched' into a heap of powder

until filled. Alternatively create a small funnel from demy paper and fill the capsule body with the required weight. Gloves or rubber finger cots should be worn to protect the capsules from handling with bare fingers.

Filling with weighed aliquots

Weighed aliquots of powder may be placed on paper and channelled into the empty capsule shell. A sharp fold in the paper helps direct the powder. Alternatively, simple apparatus is available for small-scale manufacture of larger numbers of capsules. A plastic plate with rows of cavities to hold the empty capsule bodies is used, different rows holding different sizes of capsules. A plastic bridge containing a row of holes corresponding to the position of the capsule cavities can then be used to support a long-stemmed funnel. The end of the funnel passes into the mouth of the capsule below. The stem of the funnel should be as wide as possible for the size of the capsule to assist with powder flow. A weighed aliquot of powder can then be poured into the capsule via the funnel. A thin glass or plastic rod or wire may be used to 'tamp' the powder to break blockages or to lightly compress the material inside the capsule. After filling the capsule, the top can be fitted loosely and the weight checked before sealing.

Capsules are subject to tests for uniformity of weight and content of active ingredient, and uniformity

---

Example 36.1

℞ Caps atropine sulphate 600 micrograms. Mitte 4. Calculate for six capsules.

Atropine sulphate (6 × 600) = 3600 micrograms = 3.6 mg. Lactose (6 × 100 mg) to 600 mg.

Step A

Atropine sulphate	100 mg
Lactose	900 mg

Mix by doubling-up in a small mortar and pestle. Weigh 100 mg of this mixture (triturate A). Triturate A contains 10 mg of atropine sulphate.

Step B

Triturate A	100 mg
Lactose	900 mg

Mix by doubling-up in a small mortar and pestle. Weigh 360 mg of this mixture (triturate B) which contains 3.6 mg of atropine sulphate.

Step C

Add sufficient lactose to triturate B to make the final weight up to 600 mg.
The powder mixture is now ready to be placed into capsules.

of content where the content of active ingredient, is less than 2 mg or less than 2% by weight of the total capsule fill.

Shelf life and storage of capsules

If stability data are not available for extemporaneously filled capsules, then a short expiry date (up to 4 weeks) should be given. Manufactured capsules will generally be very stable and will be assigned expiry dates on the container or on the packed strips or blister packs. Most capsules need to be stored in a cool, dry place. Some capsules need to be stored in a cool place, e.g. Restandol (testosterone), which needs to be stored in the refrigerator at 2–8°C until it is dispensed to the patient, when it can be stored at room temperature for 3 months.

Containers for capsules

Containers used are similar to those for tablets. Some capsules are susceptible to moisture absorption, and desiccants may be included in the packaging, either integrally (e.g. in the cap of the container for Losec capsules) or as separate sachets. These capsules have a limited shelf life once dispensed to a patient. Desiccant sachets should not be dispensed to patients, in case they are mistaken for a capsule and ingested.

Special labels and advice on capsules

Capsules should be swallowed whole with a glass of water or other liquid. Advice may be sought from the pharmacist about whether it is acceptable to empty the contents of a capsule onto food or into water for ease of swallowing. In giving this advice, the release characteristics of the dosage form should be considered; for instance, whether it is an enteric-coated or prolonged-release formulation. Additional labels and advice may be required for capsules, depending on the drug contained.

Other oral unit dosage forms

Pastilles

These contain a glycerol and gelatin base. They are sweetened, flavoured and medicated and are popular over the counter remedies for soothing coughs and sore throats.

Cachets

These are very rarely used in practice today. They are made from rice flour and each cachet comes in two halves ready to be filled with powder. They are available as dry seal or wet seal. They are dipped in water then swallowed whole with water and prevent the patient from tasting the powder. Filled cachets are packed in cardboard boxes.

Example 36.2

R_X Haloperidol 10 mg capsules, with 1% w/w magnesium stearate. Mitte 8 caps.

	For 1 capsule	For 10 capsules
Haloperidol	10 mg	100 mg
Magnesium stearate	1 mg	10 mg
Lactose	89 mg	890 mg

Action and uses. Used in managing acute and chronic psychosis.

Formulation notes. Magnesium stearate is added to act as a lubricant to aid flow of the powder into the capsule. 10 mg is not weighable, so a trituration must be carried out. Lactose acts as a diluent to bring the weight of each capsule fill to 100 mg.

Trituration for magnesium stearate

Magnesium stearate	100 mg
Lactose	900 mg

Take a 100 mg portion of this mixture, which will contain 10 mg of magnesium stearate and 90 mg of lactose.

Method of preparation. Sieve the powders using a 180 μm sieve. Prepare the magnesium stearate triturate. Weigh 100 mg of haloperidol, and mix this with the magnesium stearate triturate in a mortar and pestle. Gradually add 800 mg of lactose to this mixture, by doubling-up. This gives a total powder quantity of 1000 mg (equivalent to 10 × 100 mg capsules). Fill the capsule shells (size 4 or 5) with 100 mg aliquots, checking the weight of each capsule before sealing. Pack eight capsules in an amber glass or plastic tablet container with a child-resistant closure.

Storage and shelf life. Store in a cool, dry place and protect from light. Expiry date of 2 weeks, since stability in capsule form is unknown.

Advice and labelling. 'Warning. May cause drowsiness. If affected do not drive or operate machinery. Avoid alcoholic drink' (*British National Formulary* Label 2).

KEY POINTS

- Tablets and capsules are the most common dosage forms
- Excipients are added to improve manufacture, handling and release of the drug
- Bioavailability of some tablets may vary between manufacturers
- Checking of labels and contents of bulk containers is essential in minimizing errors
- Tablets should be swallowed normally with about 50 ml of water

- Some tablets are designed to be chewed, dissolved, swallowed whole or delivered by the buccal or sublingual route. Ensure the patient understands the route of delivery
- Indigestion remedies should be avoided with enteric-coated tablets and capsules
- Tablets cannot be made extemporaneously, but capsules are filled, especially in hospitals and when preparing for clinical trials
- Capsule size is selected so that they look reasonably full
- The minimum weight of contents in an extemporaneous capsule is 100 mg
- Manufactured tablets and capsules are subject to uniformity of weight and drug content tests
- Medicated glycerol-gelatin-based pastilles are popular for coughs and sore throats
- Rice flour cachets are little used today

37

Inhaled route

Peter M. Richards

STUDY POINTS

- The rationale for using the inhaled route
- The appropriate use of the most widely prescribed inhaled medicines
- The role of the peak flow meter
- The different types of inhaler, and inhaler technique
- Nebulized therapy

The role of the pharmacist

Inhaled products are specialized dosage forms, which are designed to deliver medicines directly to the lung. A variety of inhaler devices are in use, all of which require the user of the inhaler to adopt an appropriate inhaler technique. Failure to use the correct inhaler technique will result in treatment failure. The pharmacist, who is usually the person who gives (dispenses) the inhaler to the patient, is ideally placed to demonstrate the appropriate inhalation technique for that inhaler. Using an inhaler is a skill subject to the development of 'bad habits' which can lead to poor technique. Inhaler technique should therefore be regularly checked to ensure that the technique is optimal; again the pharmacist is ideally placed to perform this function.

Pharmacists can also provide education to patients beyond a discussion of a patient's inhalers and other medicines, to include education about the patient's disease (e.g. asthma) and its management. Pharmacists also run asthma clinics and may do so as supplementary or independent prescribers. A few pharmacists have specialist respiratory consultant posts in secondary care. A pharmacist wishing to undertake a specialist role in respiratory medicine will need to gain appropriate experience and undertake further training such as that offered by the National Respiratory Training Centre, Warwick.

This chapter describes the most frequently prescribed inhaled therapies in the context of asthma and chronic obstructive pulmonary disease (COPD). The most widely prescribed inhaler devices are outlined along with instructions in their use.

Introduction

Many patients on inhaled therapy will be using more than one inhaler and may also have been prescribed a peak flow meter (PFM) to aid in monitoring their condition. In order for pharmacists to be able to provide useful education and advice to these patients, pharmacists will need to understand the condition being treated and the role of the medicines and devices prescribed. This chapter will provide that understanding in the context of the two most common airways diseases treated with inhaled medicines, namely asthma and COPD. It is beyond the scope of the chapter to discuss the diseases themselves, or the role of oral therapy and non-drug management of these conditions (see *Clinical Pharmacy and Therapeutics*, Walker & Whittlesea 2007). It should be remembered that the most important intervention in COPD is smoking cessation, and that oral steroids can be life-saving in acute severe asthma.

There are significant differences in the way that inhalers are prescribed for asthma and COPD. In

COPD the emphasis of treatment is on the use of bronchodilators, and it may be appropriate for a COPD patient to have a long-acting inhaled beta-agonist without an inhaled steroid. This is different from asthma treatment where a long-acting beta-agonist should always be prescribed with an inhaled steroid. The scope of this chapter is limited to commonly used inhaled treatments and devices used for these inhaled treatments. By being familiar with national treatment guidelines for asthma and COPD, pharmacists can be assured that the advice that they give patients is likely to be consistent with that given by other healthcare professionals. These guidelines are widely available, e.g. in the *British National Formulary* (BNF) or at http://www.sign.ac.uk/guidelines/ and click on 'By subject' then 'Respiratory Medicine' for asthma guidelines, and http://guidance.nice.org.uk/cg12 for COPD guidelines.

Asthma is a very common condition in the UK, affecting at least 5% of adults and up to 20% of children. It is therefore likely that 1 in 5 of the population will experience symptoms attributable to asthma at some time in their life.

COPD has been an under-publicized condition. Prevalence in 40–70-year-olds in the USA is estimated at around 10% and prevalence is likely to be similar in the UK. The decline in lung function leading to COPD is age related but this decline can be rapidly accelerated in some smokers. COPD is thus an increasing problem in an ageing population.

Asthma and COPD are not mutually exclusive and some patients will have features of both diseases; this is often referred to as 'mixed disease'.

The prevalence of asthma, COPD and related conditions means that pharmacists will not only frequently be encountering patients on inhaled therapy during dispensing, but will also encounter patients on inhaled therapy when giving advice on the sale of over the counter medicines. This chapter not only provides pharmacists with the knowledge to confidently discuss with patients their use of inhaled therapy but also to be aware of some signs and symptoms that may be associated with poor disease control.

The inhaled route

The inhaled route delivers medicines to the lungs. Inhaled medicines may have a local effect on the lungs, or may be absorbed to give a systemic effect. The inhaled route is generally used when the lung is the target organ, e.g.:

- The antibiotic colistin is nebulized to treat lung infections associated with cystic fibrosis
- The antiviral zanamivir is presented as a dry-powder inhaler for treating influenza.

Using the inhaled route when the lung is the target organ has a number of advantages:

- A smaller dose can be used. The normal adult oral dose of salbutamol is 4 mg, but the normal inhaled dose of salbutamol is 200 micrograms (0.2 mg)
- The risk of unwanted systemic effects is reduced
- A faster onset of action may be achieved with some drugs, e.g. salbutamol
- Topically active drugs with poor oral bioavailability can be used.

The main disadvantage of the inhaled route is that inhaling a drug is more difficult than swallowing a tablet. Some drugs are ineffective by the inhaled route, e.g. theophylline.

Using the inhaled route does not result in the entire quantity of drug in the inhaler device reaching the lung. Even if an inhaler device is used perfectly, it

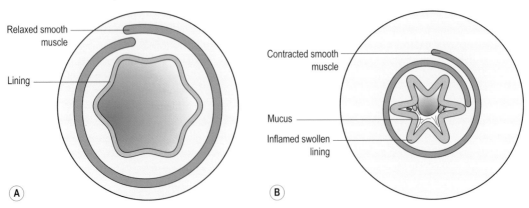

Figure 37.1 • Airways obstruction in asthma. (A) Unobstructed airway. (B) Obstructed airway.

is unlikely that any more than 20% of the drug reaches the lung. The majority of the rest of the drug remains in the oropharynx and is normally swallowed.

The lungs are designed to prevent the inhalation of anything other than gas. However, particles with a diameter of approximately 5 μm can be inhaled and have sufficient mass to settle in the lung. Particles larger than 10 μm remain in the oropharynx. Particles smaller than 1 μm are inhaled, but are then exhaled. Decreasing particle size increases the chance of penetration further down the tracheobronchial tree. It may be that a particle needs to be less than 3 μm to reach the 8th to 23rd branch generation. These particle sizes apply to the adult lung, and a smaller particle size of the order of 2.5 μm may be optimal in infant lungs.

The specific target in the lung for medicines used in asthma and COPD is the bronchiole. Branching from bronchi, bronchioles are the first airways in the lung not to contain cartilage and are less than 1 mm in diameter. The absence of cartilage means that smooth muscle contraction reduces the size of the airway. Inflammation also results in reduction in size of the airway (Fig. 37.1).

Inhaled medicines used for asthma and COPD

Short-acting beta$_2$ agonists

Salbutamol and terbutaline are short-acting beta$_2$ agonists and are the most widely used inhaled bronchodilators. They act on beta$_2$ receptors in the smooth muscle of bronchioles to reverse bronchospasm. The latter can cause symptoms including wheeze, coughing, breathlessness and a feeling of tightness of the chest. For this reason, short-acting beta$_2$ agonists are often referred to as 'relievers' and should be used 'as required' to relieve symptoms. If a reliever inhaler is required for asthma more than three times a week most weeks, the addition of a 'preventer' (usually a steroid) inhaler should be considered.

Points to note

- The inhaler itself is not dangerous – but asthma is potentially life-threatening
- Appropriate, 'as required' use of a reliever inhaler provides a useful marker of the severity of the condition

- Frequent usage of a reliever inhaler may indicate severe uncontrolled asthma
- There is no risk that using the reliever inhaler whenever needed will result in a diminishing response, but worsening asthma will not respond to a reliever inhaler alone – additional treatment is required
- If the reliever inhaler is not relieving symptoms, urgent medical attention is required
- If reliever inhaler usage has increased, or is being used more than three times a week most weeks, review of treatment is required
- The reliever inhaler can be used 15–20 minutes before sport/exercise to prevent exercise-induced asthma in susceptible individuals
- A reliever inhaler is normally blue.

For COPD, a short-acting beta$_2$ agonist may be prescribed for regular four times a day use as well as for symptom relief. In COPD, if a short-acting beta$_2$ agonist is not sufficient, the next step may be to add a short-acting beta$_2$ agonist/anticholinergic bronchodilator.

Unwanted effects of inhaled beta$_2$ agonists are rare but tremor can occur.

Short-acting anticholinergics (antimuscarinics)

The most commonly prescribed short-acting anticholinergic bronchodilator is ipratropium. Smooth muscle relaxation is achieved by opposing the parasympathetic nervous system. Ipratropium requires four times daily inhalation, and is more commonly used in patients with COPD than in asthmatics.

Long-acting beta$_2$ agonists

Salmeterol and formoterol are inhaled long-acting beta$_2$ agonist bronchodilators. They are normally used twice daily, and are indicated for people with asthma who are symptomatic despite adequate doses of inhaled steroids. Formoterol is also licensed for once-daily use. These inhalers are sometimes referred to as 'protectors'.

Points to note

- Protector inhalers should be used regularly and not on an 'as required' basis

- A reliever inhaler (short-acting beta$_2$ agonist) should be used to relieve breakthrough symptoms
- Inhaled steroids (preventer inhalers) should be continued.

For COPD, a long-acting bronchodilator (beta$_2$ agonist or anticholinergic) is the next step to short-acting bronchodilators (beta$_2$ agonist and anticholinergic). A short-acting beta$_2$ agonist will also be required to relieve breakthrough symptoms.

Long-acting anticholinergics

Tiotropium is a once-a-day inhaled anticholinergic indicated as regular preventative therapy for COPD.

Inhaled steroids

The powerful anti-inflammatory actions of steroids ideally suit them to control the inflammatory processes in asthma.

The inhaled route allows small doses of steroid to be used, minimizing the risk of systemic effects. The ideal inhaled steroid's properties would include:

- Poor absorption from the gastrointestinal tract to minimize systemic effects due to the swallowed portion
- Almost complete metabolism in the 'first pass' through the liver
- High topical activity
- Metabolism in the lung to inactive metabolites (absorption from the lung circumvents the 'first pass' through the liver).

Using a spacer device with the steroid inhaler, and/or rinsing the mouth with water and spitting immediately after using the inhaled steroid may further reduce systemic effects.

Beclometasone, budesonide and fluticasone are examples of inhaled steroids. They are normally used twice daily. Budesonide is also licensed for once-daily use. Ciclesonide is a recently introduced inhaled steroid licensed for once-a-day use. Inhaled steroids are often referred to as 'preventers'.

Inhaled steroids should normally be introduced:

- After a severe exacerbation of asthma
- If an asthmatic is using his short-acting beta$_2$ agonist more than three times a week
- If asthma is causing waking one night a week or more.

The above measures form the basis for assessing control of asthma; in addition, limitation of exercise due to asthma and measures of lung function can be considered.

Points to note

- Inhaled steroids should be used regularly, not on an 'as required' basis
- Inhaled steroids have no immediate effect
- Improved asthma control will take a minimum of 1–3 days, and it may be 14–28 days before maximum improvement is seen after starting or increasing the dose of inhaled steroid
- Steroid inhalers are normally brown, orange or maroon.

Unwanted systemic effects of inhaled steroids are extremely rare provided that the total daily dose is less than the equivalent of 800–1000 micrograms beclometasone diproprionate.

Unwanted local effects of inhaled steroids are:

- Oral candidiasis (thrush)
- Dysphonia.

Combination long-acting beta$_2$ agonist/steroid inhalers

Salmeterol is combined with fluticasone in three different strength combinations as an aerosol metered dose inhaler (MDI) and in three different strength combinations as a dry powder inhaler (DPI). Formoterol and budesonide are combined in three different strength combinations as a dry powder inhaler. These inhalers are convenient for patients who require both an inhaled steroid and a long-acting beta$_2$ agonist.

In general these combination inhalers are used as regular preventative therapy with the dose adjusted to achieve long-term control of asthma; a short-acting beta agonist inhaler being used for control of breakthrough symptoms. However, a budesonide 200 microgram/formoterol 6 microgram dry powder inhaler has recently been granted a license for preventer (maintenance) and reliever use for asthma. Thus some asthmatics who are using a budesonide 200 microgram/formoterol 6 microgram inhaler may only need to have one inhaler. A budesonide 200 microgram/formoterol 6 microgram inhaler can only be used for relief of symptoms if also being used as a regular preventer. It is not licensed for use before exercise to prevent exercise-induced asthma; an additional short-acting beta$_2$ agonist should be used for this purpose.

Fluticasone 500 microgram/salmeterol 50 microgram dry powder inhaler and budesonide 400 microgram/formoterol 12 microgram dry powder inhaler, twice daily, are licensed for certain patients with COPD. That is for those whose forced expiratory volume in 1 second (FEV$_1$) is less than 50% predicted and who are frequent exacerbators (two or more exacerbations per year).

The peak flow meter

The peak flow meter (PFM) is a simple inexpensive device, prescribable on the NHS, which gives a useful objective measure of airways obstruction. A peak flow meter and its correct use is illustrated in Figure 37.2. The PFM measures peak expiratory flow rate (PEFR). PEFR is expressed in litres per minute (L/min). Flow rate of gas through a tube is proportional to the diameter of the tube when the pressure exerted on the gas is constant. Thus the maximum rate at which individuals can expel air from their lungs is proportional to the patency of the tubes in their lungs. A reduced PEFR indicates that there is obstruction to airflow in the lungs.

Asthmatics will obtain useful information about their condition by using the PFM twice daily and charting their results for 2–4 weeks in the following situations:

- To confirm a diagnosis of asthma (a diurnal variation of PEFR of more than 20% is characteristic of asthma)

1 Set marker to zero
2 Stand up, hold PFM horizontally, avoiding touching or blocking the movement of the marker
3 Breathe in deeply then blow into the PFM as fast and hard as possible
4 Note reading, reset marker and repeat twice
5 The peak flow is the highest of the three readings

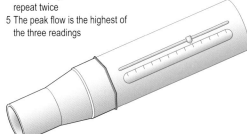

Figure 37.2 • The correct use of a peak flow meter (PFM).

- To establish the level of control of asthma on current therapy
- To track improvement of control of asthma following the introduction of a new treatment
- To ensure asthma control is maintained when treatment is stepped down
- As an aid to self-management of asthma.

Normal values are available for PEFR in graph or chart form or on 'wheels'. In adults, normal values for PEFR vary by age, sex and height; for children, PEFR varies just by height. Normal or average values of PEFR are just that and values of 50–100 L/min above or below a predicted value fall within the normal range. An increase of at least 20% in PEFR following the use of an inhaled short-acting beta$_2$ agonist such as salbutamol is diagnostic of asthma. This is known as a reversibility test.

The PFM is of less value in COPD as the airways obstruction tends to be fixed rather than variable, and lung volumes may be more important. Spirometry, which measures FEV$_1$ and forced vital capacity (FVC) is a more useful test of lung function in COPD.

Types of inhaler device

Aerosol inhalers

Metered dose inhaler (MDI)

An MDI (Fig. 37.3) delivers an aerosol of drug dissolved or suspended in a propellant. Immediately an MDI is actuated, some of the propellant rapidly evaporates to produce droplets of appropriate size to be inhaled into the lung. Further evaporation of propellant may occur in the mouth and the so-called

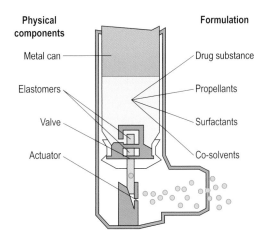

Physical components

Metal can
Elastomers
Valve
Actuator

Formulation

Drug substance
Propellants
Surfactants
Co-solvents

Figure 37.3 • The main elements of a metered dose inhaler.

'cold-freon effect' occurs if there is further evaporation of propellant (freon) when the aerosol impacts on the back of the throat. The sensation produced by the cold-freon effect can be sufficient in a minority of individuals to stop the inhalation and means that these individuals cannot use MDIs. The propellants currently used are generally hydrofluoro-alkanes (HFAs). Chlorofluoroalkanes, also known as chlorofluorocarbons (CFCs), were formerly used as propellants, but are now banned by international treaty because of their ozone-depleting properties. Medical aerosols were given exemption from the ban on CFCs, until alternatives were found and tested. Currently the change from CFCs to HFAs is not complete. It should perhaps be noted that while HFAs do not have the ozone-depleting effects of CFCs, both CFCs and HFAs are 'greenhouse' gases.

Patients who have previously had CFC-containing MDIs may be concerned when they start using a CFC-free MDI, because the taste and 'feel' of the aerosol is different. These differences are largely due to the fact that most CFC-containing MDIs are suspensions of drug in propellant, whereas most CFC-free MDIs are solutions of drug in propellant. Suspensions of drug in propellant result in nearly all the propellant evaporating after actuation and this can cause the cold-freon effect (see above). For many people this cooling sensation provides feedback that they are inhaling the drug. Solutions of drug in propellant result in only a fraction of the propellant evaporating after actuation, resulting in a reduced potential for the cold-freon effect but also a different 'feel' for the patient.

Surfactants such as oleic acid and cosolvents such as ethanol may be used to facilitate the production of an appropriate suspension or solution of drug in propellant.

The propellants, which are gases at room temperature, are maintained as liquids by filling under pressure into the metal aerosol canister.

A metered dose is achieved by having an appropriate size reservoir in the valve, which fills by gravity as the valve re-seats after each actuation.

The correct method of using an MDI is shown in Figure 37.4.

Common errors in using an MDI include:

- Inability to coordinate actuation of the inhaler with inspiration
- Taking a short, sharp inspiration, instead of a long, steady inspiration (this is often at least in part due to not exhaling before using the inhaler)

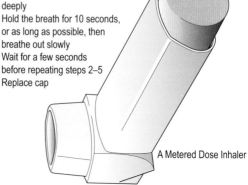

**HOW TO USE A
METERED DOSE INHALER**

1 Remove the cap
2 Shake the inhaler
3 Breathe out gently
4 Put the mouthpiece in the mouth and at the start of inspiration, which should be slow and deep, press the canister down and continue to inhale deeply
5 Hold the breath for 10 seconds, or as long as possible, then breathe out slowly
6 Wait for a few seconds before repeating steps 2–5
7 Replace cap

A Metered Dose Inhaler

**ALWAYS DEMONSTRATE TO THE PATIENT HOW TO USE THE
METERED DOSE INHALER**

Figure 37.4 • How to use a metered dose inhaler. (Source: National Respiratory Training Centre.)

- Actuating the inhaler twice (or more) on one inspiration.

Breath-actuated MDI

Inhaling through a breath-actuated MDI triggers a mechanism that 'fires' (actuates) the aerosol. These inhalers are particularly useful for those patients who have difficulty coordinating inspiration with actuation of the MDI.

Easi-Breathe® is a type of breath-actuated MDI; its correct use is shown in Figure 37.5.

Autohaler® is another breath-actuated MDI. Using an Autohaler® is essentially the same as using an Easi-Breathe® except that the Autohaler® is primed by raising a lever on the top of the inhaler, whereas the Easi-Breathe® is primed by opening the mouthpiece cover.

Common errors when using a breath-actuated MDI include:

- Not achieving a sufficiently high inspiratory flow rate to actuate the device
- Stopping inhaling immediately the inhaler actuates.

HOW TO USE THE EASI-BREATHE®

1 Shake the inhaler
2 Hold the inhaler upright. Open the cap
3 Breathe out gently. Keep the inhaler upright, put the mouthpiece in the mouth and close lips and teeth around it (the airholes on the top must not be blocked by the hand)
4 Breathe in steadily through the mouthpiece. DON'T stop breathing when the inhaler 'puffs' and continue taking a really deep breath
5 Hold the breath for 10 seconds
6 After use, hold the inhaler upright and immediately close the cap
7 For a second dose, wait a few seconds before repeating steps 1–6

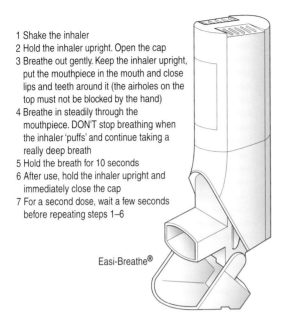

Easi-Breathe®

ALWAYS DEMONSTRATE TO THE PATIENT HOW TO USE THE EASI-BREATHE®

Figure 37.5 • How to use the Easi-Breathe®. (Source: National Respiratory Training Centre.)

**HOW TO USE A SPACER DEVICE
e.g. VOLUMATIC®**

Single breath technique

1 Remove the cap
2 Shake the inhaler and insert into the device
3 Place the mouthpiece in the mouth
4 Press the canister once to release a dose of the drug
5 Take a deep, slow breath in
6 Hold the breath for about 10 seconds, then breathe out through the mouthpiece
7 Breathe in again but do not press the canister
8 Remove the device from the mouth
9 Wait about 30 seconds before repeating steps 2–8

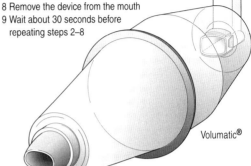

Volumatic®

ALWAYS DEMONSTRATE TO THE PATIENT HOW TO USE THE SPACER DEVICE

Figure 37.6 • How to use a spacer device, e.g. Volumatic®. Method for patients who can use the device without help. (Source: National Respiratory Training Centre.)

MDI + spacer

A chamber device (spacer) may be attached to an MDI (Fig. 37.6).

A spacer consists of a plastic chamber with a port at one end for the MDI and in most cases a one-way valve and mouthpiece at the other end.

An MDI + spacer is best used by firing a single dose from the MDI; inhalation should then start as soon as possible.

A spacer may be used with an MDI for the following reasons:

• To overcome difficulty in coordinating inspiration with actuation of the MDI, as the inspirable particles remain available for inhalation for some seconds after actuation

• To decrease deposition of non-respirable particles in the oropharynx. The larger particles are deposited in the spacer, rather than the oropharynx. This may be particularly important for high-dose inhaled steroids

• To allow those unable to distinguish between inspiration and expiration (e.g. young children) to benefit from inhaled therapy by simply inhaling and exhaling across the one-way valve

• To deliver a large dose of bronchodilator in an acute attack. The MDI is 'fired' a number of times into the spacer and the asthmatic inhales the drug by breathing through the one-way valve.

A mask may be attached or be integral to a spacer. The mask can then be placed over the mouth and nose of babies or infants to enable them to benefit from inhaled therapy. The correct use of a spacer and facemask is shown in Figure 37.7.

Examples of spacers are Volumatic®, Nebuhaler® and Aerochamber®.

Dry powder inhaler (DPI)

Medicines for inhalation can be presented as a micronized powder. The powder may be pure drug as in the Turbohaler®, or be drug and a carrier powder such as lactose, as in Rotacaps®, Diskhaler® and Accuhaler®.

When a carrier powder is used, the drug particles are adhered by weak electrostatic forces to the much larger carrier particles. As the drug/carrier powder is

HOW TO USE A LARGE VOLUME SPACER AND MASK

1 Remove the mouthpiece cover from the inhaler
2 Attach the mask to the spacer mouthpiece. The Laerdal® mask attaches to the Volumatic® and the new 'McCarthy' mask to the Nebuhaler®
3 Shake the inhaler and insert into the spacer device
4 Tip the spacer to an angle of 45° or more to enable the valve to remain open
5 Apply the mask to the child's face covering nose and mouth with as tight a seal as possible
6 Press the inhaler canister once to release a dose of the medication, keep the mask on the child's face to allow 5 or 6 breaths
7 Wait for 30 seconds before repeating steps 3–6
8 When using this method to administer inhaled steroids, remember to wash the child's face after each treatment

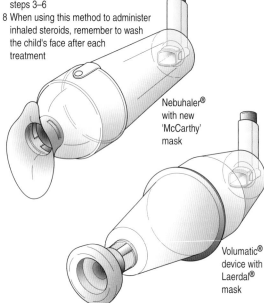

Nebuhaler® with new 'McCarthy' mask

Volumatic® device with Laerdal® mask

ALWAYS DEMONSTRATE TO THE PATIENT HOW TO USE THE LARGE VOLUME SPACER AND MASK

Figure 37.7 • How to use a large-volume spacer and face mask. (Source: National Respiratory Training Centre.)

inhaled from the inhaler, the small respirable drug particles fly off the larger non-respirable carrier particles. The lactose carrier thus remains in the mouth. Patients using DPIs that employ a carrier powder should be reassured that even when using the inhaler correctly they will have carrier powder left in the mouth.

Patients inhaling pure drug from a Turbohaler® may experience little or no taste.

The correct method of using the Turbohaler® is shown in Figure 37.8 and the Accuhaler® in Figure 37.9.

All inhalers are boxed with instruction leaflets. However, the best way to learn how to use an inhaler is to have the technique demonstrated, then to

HOW TO USE THE TURBOHALER®

1 Unscrew and lift off the white cover
2 Hold Turbohaler® upright and twist the grip then twist it back again as far as it will go. You should hear a click
3 Breathe out gently, put the mouthpiece between the lips and teeth and breathe in as deeply as possible. Even when a full dose is taken there may be no taste. (Do not breathe out into Turbohaler®)
4 Remove the Turbohaler® from the mouth and hold breath about 10 seconds
5 For a second dose repeat steps 2-4
6 Replace white cover
7 A red line appears in the window on the side of the Turbohaler® when there are 20 doses left. When the whole window is red the inhaler is empty

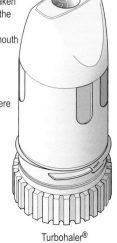

Turbohaler®

ALWAYS DEMONSTRATE TO THE PATIENT HOW TO USE THE TURBOHALER®

Figure 37.8 • How to use the Turbohaler®. (Source: National Respiratory Training Centre.)

HOW TO USE THE ACCUHALER®

1 Open the Accuhaler® by holding outer casing of the Accuhaler® in one hand whilst pushing the thumb grip away until a click is heard
2 Hold the Accuhaler® with the mouthpiece towards you, slide the lever away until it clicks. This makes the dose available for inhalation and moves the dose counter on
3 Holding the Accuhaler® level, breath out gently away from the device, put mouthpiece in mouth and take a breath in steadily and deeply
4 Remove the Accuhaler® from the mouth and hold breath for about 10 seconds
5 To close, slide the thumb grip back towards you as far as it will go until it clicks
6 For a second dose repeat steps 1–5
7 The dose counter counts down from 60 to 0. The last 5 numbers are red

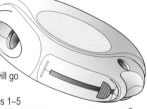

Accuhaler®

ALWAYS DEMONSTRATE TO THE PATIENT HOW TO USE THE ACCUHALER®

Figure 37.9 • How to use the Accuhaler®. (Source: National Respiratory Training Centre.)

Table 37.1 Differences in the use and care of metered dose inhalers and dry powder inhalers

MDI	DPI
Coordination of actuation and inhalation required	No coordination required as the release of powder and inhalation is a two-step process
Long, slow inhalation is the ideal to allow vaporization of propellants	Inhalation should be vigorous to disperse drug particles
Should be washed at least once a week to prevent blockage of actuator	Inhalers containing drug, e.g. Turbohaler®, must never be washed. Inhalers that do not contain drug, e.g. Rotahaler®, may be washed but must be completely dry before use
Exhalation prior to inhalation can be into the inhaler	Exhalation must never be into the inhaler

attempt to use the inhaler under supervision so that any errors can be corrected. Many patients will benefit from pharmacists providing this service. Similarly, for pharmacists to best learn how to provide this service, they too should be shown how to use the inhaler and how to spot common errors. Medical representatives from companies that market inhalers are usually more than happy to train pharmacists how to use, demonstrate and check inhaler technique. As part of this service, the medical representative will provide placebo inhalers, to allow the pharmacist to demonstrate the correct inhaler technique, instruction leaflets and other patient education material.

The use and care of a DPI differs from that of an MDI, as shown in Table 37.1.

Nebulizers

Medicines for inhalation can be presented as solutions or suspensions for nebulization. A nebulizing system (Fig. 37.10) usually consists of a compressor supplying compressed air to a nebulizing chamber, which delivers the nebulized drug to the patient via a mouthpiece or face mask. The face mask is most commonly used but when deposition of the nebulized drug on the face is undesirable (e.g. a steroid), then a mouthpiece is preferable, or the face under the mask should be protected with petroleum jelly.

The principle of jet nebulization is shown in Figure 37.11. The gas used to drive the nebulization process may be oxygen or air, but in either case a minimum flow rate of 8 L/min at a pressure of at least 69 kPa (10 psi) is required.

Patients using more than one nebulized medicine may have two different solutions mixed in the nebulizing chamber to be nebulized together. The Summary of Product Characteristics (SPC) may give advice on other solutions and diluents that may be appropriately mixed with a given medicine for nebulization. It is possible that one solution will precipitate the other; this can normally be detected by the mixed solutions in the nebulizer changing from clear to cloudy. Such a change means that the mixed solutions are not compatible and should not be nebulized together. Consideration should also be given to the total volume of the mixed solutions, as the larger the volume, the longer it will take to be nebulized.

Nebulizers are used when high doses of drug are required and/or when the patient is unable to use any form of inhaler. Nebulizers do not require the patient to learn any technique and are effective on normal or shallow breathing.

Nebulizers are used in the treatment of severe acute asthma and this is best done under medical supervision:

- To ensure that an adequate objective and maintained response to treatment is achieved (e.g. by measuring PEFR before and after nebulization)
- To assess if other treatment is indicated, e.g. oral or parenteral steroids
- To plan follow-up and possible review of chronic medication.

Nebulized treatment may also be used in the latter stages of COPD often in conjunction with domiciliary oxygen therapy. Domiciliary oxygen cylinders do not provide sufficient flow rates to produce adequate nebulization, so a compressor unit should be used.

Drugs for nebulization are normally presented as unit dose vials; examples of these are Nebules® and Respules®.

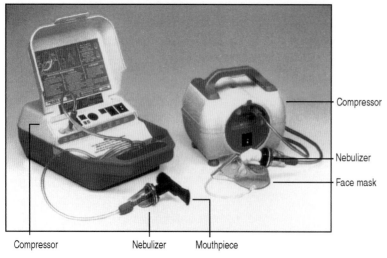

Figure 37.10 • Nebulization equipment.

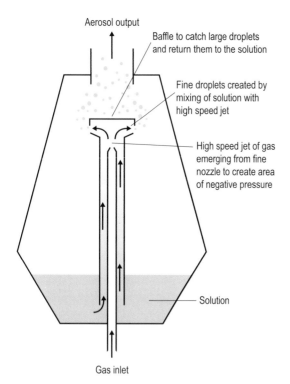

Figure 37.11 • The principle of jet nebulization.

KEY POINTS

- Asthma and COPD are common conditions, treatment of which is largely dependent on the inhaled route
- The vast majority of inhaled treatments for asthma and COPD can be divided into two pharmacological classes of drugs: inhaled bronchodilators and inhaled steroids
- Inhaled bronchodilators can be further subdivided into beta$_2$ agonists and anticholinergics (antimuscarinics). Each of these classes can be further subdivided into short acting and long acting
- National and international management guidelines are available for asthma and COPD and treatment is based on a step-wise approach
- A range of inhalation devices is available to deliver drugs directly to the lungs. This has clear advantages including using much lower doses compared to oral therapy
- The use of inhalers is technique dependent and patients require training in their use
- Medicines to be inhaled are presented as aerosol inhalers, dry powder inhalers or liquids to be nebulized
- The most widely prescribed inhaler device is the aerosol metered dose inhaler (MDI). The MDI may be used in conjunction with a spacing device (a 'spacer'). A modified form of the MDI, triggered to actuate by inhalation, is a breath-actuated MDI. Both the 'spacer' and the breath-actuated MDI overcome the main difficulty of using an MDI, the need to coordinate inhalation with actuation of the MDI, and allow a wider range of individuals to successfully use an MDI
- Dry powder inhalers (DPIs) were originally developed to overcome the difficulty some patients have coordinating inhalation with actuation of an MDI
- DPIs vary widely in appearance and the method by which the powder is made available for inhalation, but all rely on inhalation to mobilize the powder from the inhaler and through the mouthpiece

- Liquids for nebulization are either solutions or permanent suspensions. It may be that solutions are more reliably nebulized and inhaled than permanent suspensions
- Caution should be exercised when mixing two liquids for nebulization in the nebulizer as one liquid can cause precipitation in the other
- The peak flow meter is a simple prescribable device which gives an objective measurement of lung function, and can be useful from time to time for asthmatics, e.g. when commencing a new treatment. It may also be used to aid self-management of asthma

- Many asthmatic and COPD patients will have at least two or three different inhalers. They will obtain greatest benefit from their inhalers if they understand something about their condition, the rationale for the different inhalers and how and when to use them
- Pharmacists with an understanding of asthma and COPD treatment and the correct use of inhalers can provide advice, education and training for patients on inhaled therapy which can markedly improve patients' quality of life

Parenteral products

Derek G. Chapman

STUDY POINTS

- The reasons for parenteral administration
- The routes available for parenteral administration
- The various forms and types of parenteral product
- The design of containers and methods of administration of parenteral products
- The formulation and uses of parenteral products
- Pyrogens
- Tonicity adjustment
- Large-volume sterile products

Introduction

Parenteral products are dosage forms that are delivered to the patient by a route outwith the alimentary canal. The parenteral route of administration is often used for drugs that cannot be given orally. This may be because of patient intolerance, the instability of the drug, or poor absorption of the drug if given by the oral route. In practice, parenteral products are often regarded as dosage forms that are implanted, injected or infused directly into vessels, tissues, tissue spaces or body compartments. From the site of administration the drug is then transported to the site of action. With developing technology, parenteral therapy is being used outside the hospital or clinic environment. Patients are increasingly using it at home and in the workplace, allowing them to administer their own medication.

Parenteral therapy is used to:

- Produce a localized effect
- Administer drugs if the oral route cannot be used
- Deliver drugs to the unconscious patient
- Rapidly correct fluid and electrolyte imbalances
- Ensure delivery of the drug to the target tissues.

Parenteral injections are either administered directly into blood for a fast and controlled effect or into tissues outside the blood vessels for a local or systemic effect. An injection can be administered intravenously to rapidly increase the concentration of drug in the blood plasma, but the concentration soon falls due to the reversible transfer of the drug from blood plasma into body tissues, a process known as distribution. The drug concentration remaining in the blood plasma is affected both by the administered dose and by the quantity of drug transferred into body tissues. Thereafter, there is a slower decrease in the drug concentration due to irreversible excretion and metabolism. An intravenous infusion administers a large volume of fluid at a slow rate and ensures that the drug enters the general circulation at a constant rate. In this procedure, the drug concentration in the blood plasma rises soon after the start of the infusion and achieves a steady state when the rate of drug addition equals the rate of drug loss. When infusion is stopped, elimination of the drug from the body by metabolism and/or excretion generally follows first-order kinetics.

Following subcutaneous and intramuscular injection there is a delay in the systemic effects of the drug. The delay is due to the time for the drug to first pass through the epithelial cells and basement membrane that forms the walls of the capillaries before entering into the blood. This occurs by passive diffusion that is promoted by the concentration gradient across the capillary wall. Other factors are also important, including the permeability characteristics and the number of capillaries in the area. Most plasma solutes pass freely across the capillary walls, while water-soluble substances such as glucose and amino acids pass through intercellular aqueous spaces of the capillary wall. After passing through the capillary wall the drug concentration in the blood plasma rises to a peak level and then falls due to distribution to the tissues followed by metabolism and excretion.

Administration procedures

Intravenous injections and infusions

Administration by this route provides strict control of the drug concentration in the circulating blood. The vein that is selected for administering the formulation depends on several factors. These include the size of the delivery needle or catheter, the type and volume of fluid to be administered and the rate of administering the fluid. The fluids are administered into a superficial vein, commonly on the back of the hand or in the internal flexure of the elbow (see Fig. 21.1). The intravenous route is widely used to administer parenteral products, but it must not be used to administer water-in-oil emulsions or suspensions.

Subcutaneous injections

These are injected into the loose connective and adipose tissue immediately beneath the skin (Fig. 38.1). Typically, the volume injected does not exceed 1 mL. Injection sites include the abdomen, the upper back,

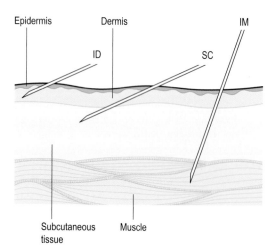

Figure 38.1 • Injection routes. ID, intradermal; SC, subcutaneous; IM, intramuscular.

the upper arms and the lateral upper hips. This route is used if the medicine cannot be administered orally. The drugs are more rapidly and predictably absorbed than when administered by the oral route. Following administration, the site of the injection, the body temperature, age of the patient and the degree of massaging of the injection site affect drug distribution. However, absorption of the drug after subcutaneous injection is slower and less predictable than when administered by the intramuscular route.

Intramuscular injections

Small-volume aqueous solutions, solutions in oil and suspensions are administered directly into the body of a relaxed muscle (see Fig. 38.1). Several muscle sites are used for these injections, including the gluteal muscle in the buttock, the deltoid muscle in the shoulder and the vastus lateralis of the thigh. In adults, the gluteal muscle is often used as larger volumes can be tolerated. In infants and small children, the vastus lateralis of the thigh is usually more developed than other muscle groups and is thus used. For rapid absorption of the medicament, the deltoid muscle in the shoulder is often used.

Other routes of parenteral administration are described below.

Intradermal injections

A volume of about 0.1 mL is injected into the skin between the epidermis and the dermis. Absorption from intradermal injections is slow. This route is often used for diagnostic tests for allergy or immunity. It is also used to administer some vaccines.

Intra-arterial injections

The drug is administered directly into an artery. Owing to the fast flow of blood in the artery it is likely that the drug will be rapidly dispersed throughout the blood system. However, manipulative difficulties restrict the use of intra-arterial injections but drugs can be administered by this route to target a specific organ or tissue that is served by the artery.

Intracardiac injections

These are aqueous solutions that are administered in emergency directly into a ventricle or the cardiac muscle for a local effect.

Intraspinal injections

These are aqueous solutions that are injected in volumes less than 20 mL into particular areas of the spinal column. They are categorized as intrathecal, subarachnoid, intracisternal, epidural and peridural injections. The specific gravity of these injections may be adjusted to localize the site of action of the drug.

Intra-articular injections

These are administered as an aqueous solution or suspension into the synovial fluid in a joint cavity. They are often used for the local administration of anti-inflammatory agents.

Products for parenteral use

Parenteral products are sterile formulations that are administered into the body by various routes including injection, infusion and implantation.

Injections

These are subdivided into small- and large-volume parenteral fluids. Small-volume parenterals are sterile, pyrogen-free injectable products. They are packaged in volumes up to 100 mL. Small-volume parenteral fluids are packed as:

- Single-dose ampoules
- Multiple-dose vials
- Prefilled syringes.

Single-dose ampoules

Most small-volume parenterals are currently packaged as either ampoules or vials. Glass ampoules are thin-walled containers made of Type I borosilicate glass (see Fig. 27.3). Injections packaged in glass ampoules are manufactured by filling the product into the ampoules, which are then heat sealed. To achieve the quality required of these products, the packaged solution must be sterile and practically free of particles. These products are typically prepared in clean room conditions (see Ch. 29). However, the great concern with using glass ampoules relates to the hazards of opening them because the product may become contaminated with glass particles. Opening

is easier with glass ampoules with a weakened neck. This is achieved by applying a ceramic paint ring to the ampoule neck. The paint, after a process of heat baking, has the effect of weakening the neck. Even though the subsequent opening of the ampoules is physically easier, a large number of glass particles still contaminate the product. Another ampoule design has a score on the glass at the ampoule neck with a painted dot marker on the opposing side. These are known as one-point cut ampoules. They are easier to open, but glass particles continue to be released when they are opened.

Plastic ampoules are prepared, filled and sealed by a procedure known as blow–fill–seal. This is a four-step continuous procedure in which granules of plastic are heated to a semi-solid state. The plastic is then blow moulded and formed into ampoules. These containers are filled with the product and immediately sealed. This system is only used to package simple solutions. The plastic may take up drug components from the product. When the ampoule is opened by rotating the integral plastic closure, few particles are released into the solution.

Ampoules should have a reliable seal that can be readily leak tested. A good seal will not deteriorate during the lifetime of the product. Medicines packaged in ampoules are intended for single use only. As a result, these products do not contain chemical antimicrobial preservatives. The ampoule must also contain a slight excess volume of product. This is necessary to allow the nominal injection volume to be drawn into a syringe.

Multiple-dose vials

These are composed of a thick-walled glass container that is sealed with a rubber closure. The closure is kept in position by an aluminium seal that is crimped to the neck of the glass vial (see Fig. 27.4). These closures are then covered with a plastic cap. The cap is removed before a needle, attached to a syringe, is inserted through the rubber closure to withdraw a dose of product. The contents of the vial may be removed in several portions.

The glass vial packaging system has the advantage of increased dose flexibility and decreased costs per unit dose. There are also certain disadvantages with the use of glass vials. Fragments of the closure may be released into the product when the needle is inserted through the closure. There is also the risk of interaction between the product and the closure. Repeated withdrawal of injection solution from these containers increases the risk of microbial contamination of the product. These products must, therefore, contain an antimicrobial preservative unless the medicine itself has antimicrobial activity. An example of such a multidose product is insulin. Each dose is withdrawn from the vial when required and administered by the patient.

Prefilled syringes

With these devices, the injection solution is aseptically filled into sterile syringes. The packed solution has a high level of sterility assurance and does not contain an antimicrobial preservative. The final product is available for immediate use. Prefilled syringes are expensive and so only limited products are packaged in this way.

Administration of small-volume parenteral products

Hypodermic syringes and needles are extensively used for administering small volumes of parenteral formulations to the patient. These syringes have been sterilized by ethylene oxide gas or, occasionally, by gamma irradiation following packaging. Various sizes of hypodermic syringes are available. They are composed of a barrel, having a graduated scale, together with a plunger and a headpiece, known as a piston (Fig. 38.2). These components are often made of polypropylene, although the piston could be made of medical grade rubber.

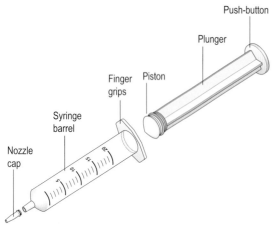

Figure 38.2 • Hypodermic syringe for single use.

Formulation of parenteral products

Vehicles for injections

The drug is generally present in an injection in low concentration. The vehicle provides the highest proportion of the formulation and should not be toxic nor have any therapeutic activity.

Mains water often contains a wide variety of contaminants such as electrolytes, organisms and particulate matter, and dissolved gases, such as carbon dioxide and chlorine. The wide variety of these contaminants causes a problem in the preparation of water for use in injections. This is called 'water for injections' and must be used as the vehicle for parenteral products. It is often used to prepare ophthalmic products but these could be made using purified water.

Water for injections

Water for injections is the most extensively used vehicle in parenteral formulations. Water for injections is well tolerated by the body and ionizable electrolytes readily dissolve in water. Water for injections must be free of pyrogens. It must also have a high level of chemical purity. The *British Pharmacopoeia* (BP; 2007) considers that water for injections can only be prepared by distillation in order to produce a consistent supply of the required quality of water.

Preparation of water for injections

The usual method of preparing water for injections in Europe and North America is distillation. While other processes can achieve a similar quality of product, these alternative systems cannot produce a consistent water quality. The source water used in the preparation of water for injections by distillation is usually potable water. This water varies in quality and may be contaminated with dissolved gases, suspended minerals and organic substances, mineral salts, chemicals, endotoxins and microorganisms. The high standard required of water for injections is only achieved if the quality of the source water is improved by suitable pretreatment before it is supplied as feed water for final processing. The pretreatment of the source water usually involves:

- Chemical softening
- Filtration
- De-ionization
- pH adjustment.

The water is then treated by reverse osmosis to yield purified water. This water is often used as the feed water for distillation and has a low silica content and a low total organic carbon content. A wide variety of designs of still are used in the production of water for injections. These stills are typically made of stainless steel, although chemically resistant glass could be used.

The single effect still is used to produce volumes less than 90 L/h. This usually fulfils the demands of small-scale production as required by a hospital pharmacy. The single effect still requires de-ionized feed water and has three main structural components:

- An evaporator containing the heater
- A vapour-liquid disengaging section
- A condenser.

When this still is functioning, the feed water in the horizontal evaporator is heated. Steam is produced at atmospheric pressure and at slow velocity. Some steam will condense before it enters a vertical vapour-liquid disengaging unit that is attached to the horizontal evaporator. Baffle plates at the base of the vapour-liquid unit reduce the risk of water droplets being carried in the steam into this unit. The water droplets and the non-volatile impurities are returned to the water in the evaporator. The vapour-liquid disengaging unit often contains a centrifugal device that spins the steam as it rises in this unit. This has the effect of throwing entrapped water droplets in the steam onto the wall of this vertical cylindrical section where it condenses and returns to the evaporator. Only pure steam exits from this unit into the condenser where the heat of vaporization is removed and converts the water vapour to the liquid distillate. Only stills designed to produce high purity water may be used in the production of water for injections.

In operation, the first portion of the distillate must be discarded. The remainder is collected in a suitable storage vessel. Freshly collected distillate is usually free of microbial contaminants and should contain not more than 0.25 international units of endotoxin per mL as determined by the bacterial endotoxin test (see later). However, the distillate is regularly sampled and tested for microbial contamination. It is acceptable if there are fewer than 10 organisms per 100 mL present at any instance; no *Pseudomonas* bacteria should be present. To ensure that the distillate is of a suitable purity, the electrical conductivity of the distillate is measured. This measurement is used as an indicator of the quality of ionizable materials in the collected water. The electrical conductance should be less than 1.1 mS/cm when measured at 20°C. However, the measurement of electrical conductivity alone as an indicator of water quality can be misleading, as it does not detect silica in the distillate. To conform with the quality standards of the BP (2007) and the *European Pharmacopoeia* (EP; 2007), the distillate will also have the following quality limits:

Total organic carbon	Not more than 0.5 mg per litre
Chlorides	Not more than 0.5 parts per million (p.p.m.)
Ammonium	Not more than 0.2 p.p.m.
Nitrates	Not more than 0.2 p.p.m.
Heavy metals	Not more than 0.1 p.p.m.
Oxidizable substances	Not more than 5 p.p.m.
pH	5.0–7.0

Care is required in handling the freshly collected distillate as it is subject to microbial contamination during storage and distribution. Two systems are commonly used for the storage of water for injections: batch storage and dynamic storage.

Batch storage

With this system the water for injections is stored as a batch of discrete unit volumes which may be sterilized. Quality control tests are performed on this batch. Only after the batch is identified as being of suitable quality is it released for use. This system provides maximum product accountability before use. It is, however, an expensive storage system.

Dynamic storage

With this system the storage tank is a surge tank, usually made of quality polished stainless steel. As the level of water for injections in the tank falls then more water for injections is produced and filled into the tank. The fresh water for injections mixes with water remaining in the tank. This system is cheaper and simpler to operate than batch storage. However, it does lack batch accountability and the water may become contaminated through corrosion of the steel tank. Owing to the potential problem with Gram-negative bacterial contamination, it is important that the distillate is stored at 80°C to prevent bacterial growth. Heating the water in the tank is achieved with a steam-heated jacket around the tank.

Surge tanks require sterilization at timed intervals. They are fitted with a filter vent used to equilibrate the tank pressure during filling and emptying the tank. The filter prevents airborne bacterial contamination of the water for injections within the tank.

Distribution

A loop distribution system may be used to deliver the water for injections to the point of use. The water in the distribution system can become contaminated with organisms. As a result, the water in the stainless steel pipes is constantly circulated from the tank to avoid stagnation and to maintain the temperature. This distribution system has one major disadvantage in that the point of use may not require high-temperature water. Thus a cooling system may be fitted close to the point of use. Microbial growth may then occur in the cooled water.

Sterilized water for injections

This is prepared by packing a volume of water for injections in sealed containers. These containers are then moist-heat sterilized which yields a sterile product that remains free of pyrogens. Sterilized water for injections is used to dissolve or dilute parenteral preparations before administration to the patient.

Pyrogens

Water is potentially the greatest source of pyrogens in parenteral products. Untreated pyrogenic water is contaminated with pyrogens and these must be removed before the water can be used in parenteral products. This is achieved in the preparation of water as a vehicle for injections by distillation in the UK. Pyrogens are fever-producing substances. The injection of distilled water may produce a rise in body temperature if it contains pyrogens, while water that is free of this effect is described as apyrogenic.

Microbial pyrogens arise from components of Gram-negative and Gram-positive bacteria, fungi and viruses. Non-microbial pyrogens, such as some steroids and plasma components, also produce a pyrogenic response if injected. The most important pyrogens in pharmacy products are high molecular weight endotoxins that are found in the outer membrane of Gram-negative bacteria. Therefore endotoxins potentially exist in all situations harbouring bacteria.

Freshly prepared parenteral products must not be contaminated with organisms that could produce pyrogens. They must be prepared in conditions that reduce microbial contamination because bacteria contaminating aqueous solutions can release endotoxins. Contaminated solutions will become more pyrogenic with the passage of time. Therefore, these products must be sterilized shortly after preparation.

Endotoxins produce significant physiological changes when injected. Their detection and elimination is very important for manufacturers of parenteral products.

Nature of endotoxins

Endotoxins isolated from the outer membrane of Gram-negative bacteria are composed of three areas. The inner region is composed of lipid A that is linked to a central polysaccharide core. This polysaccharide core is joined to long projections known as the O-antigenic side chains. Lipid A is responsible for most of the biological activity of endotoxin. By itself it is not very soluble in water. However, it is joined to a core polysaccharide by an eight-carbon sugar that acts as a solute carrier for the lipid A in aqueous solutions.

The molecular weight of endotoxin is important in determining its biological activity. In a pure aqueous environment, endotoxin has a relative molecular mass of about 10^6. This is equivalent to the relative molecular mass of a virus particle and is the most common size of endotoxin found in large-volume parenteral formulations. In the presence of magnesium and calcium, the endotoxin forms bilayer sheets or vesicles with a diameter of about 0.1 μm. These small structures can easily pass through a 0.22 μm membrane filter. This size of filter is commonly used in the production of pharmacy products.

Biological activity of pyrogens

The injection of endotoxins and other pyrogens can produce many physiological effects. The most important arising from the use of pharmacy products is the pyrogenic effect, where the lipid A directly affects the thermoregulatory centres in the brain. At high dose levels, endotoxin will also:

- Activate the coagulation system
- Alter carbohydrate and lipid metabolism
- Produce platelet aggregation
- Produce shock and ultimately death.

As pyrogens can produce these toxic effects, they should never be knowingly injected. Their detection and elimination is very important for the production of parenteral products. The contamination of large-volume parenteral solutions with pyrogens is especially serious, owing to the large volumes that are administered to seriously ill patients.

Although endotoxins are the predominant pyrogen in parenteral formulations, other pyrogenic substances also exist. These agents include peptidoglycan, from Gram-positive bacteria, and bacterial exotoxins, as evidenced by the erythrogenic response produced by *Streptococcus* group A organisms which cause the skin to turn red. Viruses induce a pyrogenic response that often appears like the fever induced by the common cold virus. Moulds and yeasts also produce a pyrogenic effect following intravenous injection.

Tests for pyrogens

The rabbit test included in the BP (2007) and in the EP (2007) is very similar to the original rabbit test included in the 1948 edition of the BP. However, in recent times, alternative tests for bacterial endotoxins have been extensively used. The rabbit test that is used to identify the presence of a wide range of pyrogens does have problems for testing pharmacy products. It is an expensive and slow test that is difficult to perform even in specialized test centres. The bacterial endotoxin test is a specific test for endotoxins of bacterial origin. Bacterial endotoxin is the main pyrogen found in parenteral products and the test is carried out on both the components and the final parenteral products.

Bacterial endotoxin tests

This test, as detailed in Appendix XIV of the BP (2007), is commonly referred to as the limulus amoebocyte lysate (LAL) test. It detects or quantifies endotoxins from Gram-negative bacteria. The BP test allows the use of a lysate of amoebocytes from either the American or Japanese horseshoe crab. Not surprisingly, however, in practice the lysate used in tests in Europe and North America is obtained from amoebocytes of the American horseshoe crab *Limulus polyphemus*, while the lysate of the Japanese crab (*Tachypleus tridentatus*) is used in tests carried out in Asia. Although six tests are detailed in the BP (2007), these tests can be grouped into one of three types, known as: the gel clot end point, the turbidimetric test and the kinetic chromogenic test. The gel clot end point is based on the formation of a solid gel clot. It is an in vitro test for bacterial endotoxins that does have some advantages, as it is cheap, rapid, simple to perform and sensitive to low endotoxin concentrations. This test is often used by hospital and small-scale manufacturers and is used as a definitive test if doubt exists regarding results obtained by the other test methods.

With the gel clot procedure, a solution containing the endotoxin is added to a solution of the lysate. The reaction requires a proclotting enzyme system and a clottable protein coagulogen that are provided by the lysate. The reaction that takes place is shown in Figure 38.3. The rate of this reaction is affected by several factors, including the concentration of endotoxin, the pH and the temperature. In the test procedure, the lysate is mixed with an equal volume of the test solution in a depyrogenated container, such as a glass tube. The tube is then incubated undisturbed at 37°C for a period of about 60 minutes. The test is a pass or fail test. The end point is identified by gently inverting the glass tube. A positive result is indicated by the formation of a solid clot of coagulin. This clot does not disintegrate when the tube is inverted. A negative result is indicated if no gel clot has been formed. This test needs appropriate positive and negative controls. For a positive control, a known concentration of endotoxin is added to the lysate alone and then repeated with a product sample. As a negative control, water that is free of endotoxin is added to the lysate. All the controls must produce appropriate results for the test to be valid. The sensitivity of the assay is limited by the sensitivity of the lysate used in the test. The gel clot test will detect between 0.02 and 1.0

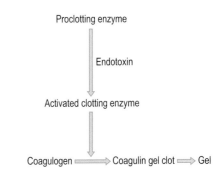

Figure 38.3 • The lysate clotting mechanism.

endotoxin units per millilitre. Some recently developed biopharmaceuticals have shown similar activity to endotoxin in this and the other endotoxin tests. Before this test is carried out, it is necessary to determine that:

- The test equipment does not adsorb endotoxins
- The lysate is of suitable sensitivity
- No interfering agents are present.

The turbidimetric test is used in the testing of water systems and for testing simple pharmacy products. The test measures the opacity change in the LAL test due to the formation of insoluble coagulin. An increase in the endotoxin concentration produces a proportional increase in opacity due to the precipitation of the clottable protein coagulin.

The kinetic chromogenic test is an automated test used by commercial parenteral manufacturers to test large numbers of complex products. The test gives an accurate result over a wide range of endotoxin concentrations. The test measures the colour change induced by the release of the chromogenic chemical *para*-nitroanilide. This is released as a by-product of the clotting reaction during the LAL test. The quantity of *para*-nitroanilide produced is directly proportional to the endotoxin concentration.

Pyrogen testing

The BP pyrogen test involves measuring the rise in body temperature of healthy mature rabbits. This temperature rise is recorded after the rabbits have been intravenously injected with a sterile solution of the test substance. The environment and the equipment used in the test are detailed in the BP (2007). This test can only be carried out where the rabbits can tolerate the test product.

The test itself is preceded by a preliminary test to identify and exclude any animal with an unusual response to the trauma of the injection. With the preliminary test, a warmed pyrogen-free saline solution is injected into the rabbits. The temperature of the rabbits is recorded from 90 minutes before the test to 3 hours after the injection, as specified in the BP (2007). The fever response in the rabbits after the injection with pyrogens follows a biphasic response. After the injection, there is a lag time of about 15–18 minutes, which is followed by a rapid temperature rise to a peak within 2 hours. The temperature then falls and is followed by a second rise in temperature. This returns to normal after 6–9 hours. False-positive

temperature increases occur with rabbits as a result of:

- Injury
- Badly positioned recording devices
- Distress.

The rabbits may develop a resistance to pyrogens. As a result, they are tested at specified time intervals.

Depyrogenation

Depyrogenation is the elimination of all pyrogens from the production materials, solutions and equipment. It is achieved by either removal or inactivation of the pyrogens. The main method of preventing pyrogens contaminating parenteral products is strict control of the ingredients used. That is solvents, raw materials, packaging materials and equipment should not be contaminated with pyrogens.

A simple method of removing small amounts of pyrogens from surfaces such as packaging components is by rinsing the surfaces with non-pyrogenic water. As pyrogens are non-volatile, distillation is the principal method of avoiding contamination of water used in parenteral products. This is achieved by positioning a trap, fitted with baffles, in the still. The trap removes the droplets of water by impingement and prevents pyrogens being carried over into the distillate. However, the freshly collected distillate that is initially pyrogen-free water can become contaminated with organisms and pyrogens if stored for more than 4 hours at 22°C. To avoid microbial growth in this water, it must be sterilized soon after collection or stored at high temperatures to suppress microbial growth. Pyrogens can be removed from solutions by ultrafiltration that separates pyrogens by a process based on their relative molecular mass. This specialized system has been used to depyrogenate antibiotic products during their commercial production. These filters are different from the 0.22 µm filters often used in pharmacy production.

Various methods are used to inactivate pyrogens including heat treatment, acid–base hydrolysis and oxidation. High temperature is widely used to incinerate pyrogens especially for glassware, thermostable equipment and formulation components. Dry heat at 250°C for 30 minutes is normally used. The commonly used dry or moist heat sterilization cycles (see Aulton 2007) will not greatly reduce the pyrogen burden of parenteral products.

Non-aqueous solvents

Water-miscible cosolvents, such as glycerin and pro-pylene glycol, are used as vehicles in small-volume parenteral fluids. They are used to increase the solu-bility of drugs and to stabilize drugs degraded by hydrolysis.

Metabolizable oils are used to dissolve drugs that are insoluble in water. For example steroids, hor-mones and vitamins are dissolved in vegetable oils. These formulations are administered by intramuscu-lar injection.

Additives

Various additives, such as antimicrobial agents, anti-oxidants, buffers, chelating agents and tonicity-adjusting agents, are included in injection formula-tions. Their purpose is to produce a safe and elegant product. Both the types and amounts of additives to be included in formulations are given in the appropri-ate monograph in the BP (2007).

Antimicrobial agents

These are added to products that are packaged in multiple-dose vials. They are not used in large-volume injections or if the drug formulation itself has sufficient antimicrobial activity (such as Meth-ohexital Sodium Injection). Antimicrobial agents are added to inhibit the growth of microbial organ-isms that may accidentally contaminate the product during use. The antimicrobial agents must be stable and effective in the parenteral formulation. Because they are effective in the free form, their activity can be greatly reduced by interaction with components of the injection. Rubber closures have been shown to take up antimicrobial preservatives from the in-jection solution. Preservative uptake is more signif-icant with natural and neoprene rubber and much less with butyl rubber closures.

There is concern about the toxic effects of injec-tions containing preservatives. As a result, a low but effective antimicrobial concentration is used in injections. Challenging the product with selected organisms can test the effectiveness of antimicrobi-al agents. The test procedure will evaluate the an-timicrobial activity of the preservative in the packaged product. The test procedure is detailed in BP 2007. Table 38.1 gives details for some com-monly used preservatives.

Table 38.1 Examples of antimicrobial preservatives used in aqueous multiple dose injections

Antimicrobial preservative	Concentration (% w/v)
Benzyl alcohol	1–2
Chlorocresol	0.1–0.3
Cresol	0.25–0.5
Methyl hydroxybenzoate	0.1
Phenol	0.25–0.6
Thiomersal	0.01

Antioxidants

Many drugs in aqueous solutions are easily degraded by oxidation. Small-volume parenteral products of these drugs often contain an antioxidant. Bisulphites and meta-bisulphites are commonly used antioxidants in aqueous injections. Antioxidants must be carefully selected for use in injections to avoid interaction with the drug. Anti-oxidants have a lower oxidation potential than the drug and so are either preferentially oxidized or block oxida-tive chain reactions. Injection formulations may, in addi-tion to antioxidants, also contain chelating agents. Chelating agents such as EDTA or citric acid remove trace elements which catalyse oxidative degradation.

Buffers

The ideal pH of parenteral products is pH 7.4. If the pH is above pH 9, tissue necrosis may result, while below pH 3, pain and phlebitis in tissues can occur.

Buffers are included in injections to maintain the pH of the packaged product. Changes in pH can arise through interaction between the product and the con-tainer. However, the buffer used in the injection must allow the body fluids to change the product pH after injection. Acetate, citrate and phosphate buffers are commonly used in parenteral products.

Tonicity-adjusting agents

Isotonic solutions have the same osmotic pressure as blood plasma and do not damage the membrane of red blood cells. Hypotonic solutions have a lower osmotic pressure than blood plasma and cause blood cells to swell and burst because of fluids passing into the cells by osmosis. Hypertonic solutions have a higher os-motic pressure than plasma; as a result the red blood cells lose fluids and shrink. Following the administra-tion of an injection it is important that tissue damage and irritation are minimized and haemolysis of red blood cells is minimized. Thus, the BP (2007) states that aqueous solutions for large-volume infusion fluids, together with aqueous fluids for subcutaneous, intradermal and intramuscular administration, should be made isotonic. Intrathecal injections must also be isotonic to avoid serious changes in the osmotic pressure of the cerebrospinal fluid. Aqueous hypotonic solutions are made isotonic by adding either sodium chloride, glucose or, occasionally, mannitol. The latter two agents are incompatible with some drugs. If the solution is hypertonic, it is made isotonic by dilution.

Some components of injections, such as buffers and antioxidants, affect the tonicity. Other components, such as preservatives, which are present in low concentration, have little effect on the tonicity.

Injection solutions are often made isotonic with 0.9% sodium chloride solution. The amount of solute, or the required dilution necessary to make a solution isotonic, can be determined from the freezing point depression. The freezing point depression of blood plasma and tears is $-0.52°C$. Thus solutions that freeze at $-0.52°C$ have the same osmotic pressure as body fluids. Hypotonic solutions have a smaller freezing point depression and require the addition of a solute to depress the freezing point to $-0.52°C$.

The amount of adjusting substance added to these solutions may be calculated from the equation:

$$W = (0.52 - a)/b$$

where W = percentage concentration of adjusting substance in the final solution, a = freezing point depression of the unadjusted hypotonic solution, b = freezing point depression of a 1% weight in volume (w/v) concentration of the adjusting substance.

An extensive list of freezing point depression values is detailed in Table 6 (pp 53–64) in the chapter 'Solution properties' in the 12th edition of the *Pharmaceutical Codex* (1994) (Example 38.1).

Other methods that are used to estimate the amount of adjusting substances required to make a solution isotonic include:

- Sodium chloride equivalents
- Molar concentrations
- Serum osmolarity.

Details of these methods are given in the chapter 'Solution properties' (pp 64–67) in the 12th edition of the *Pharmaceutical Codex* (1994).

Units of concentration

The concentration of the components in parenteral products may be expressed in various ways (see also Ch. 26):

- *Percentage weight/volume*. Examples include: magnesium sulphate injection 50%, sodium chloride intravenous infusion 0.9%.
- *Weight per unit volume*. Examples include: atropine sulphate 600 micrograms/mL or ephedrine hydrochloride injection 30 mg/mL.
- *Millimoles per unit volume*. Examples include: potassium chloride solution, strong (sterile) contains 2 mmol each of K^+ and Cl^- per mL; Calcium Chloride Injection BP contains 2.5 mmol of Ca^{2+} and 10 mmol of Cl^- in 5 mL.

During the formulation of injections and infusions, the units of interest are the ions of electrolytes and the molecules of non-electrolytes. For molecules, 1 millimole (mmol) is the weight in milligrams corresponding to its relative molecular mass. A mole of an ion is its relative atomic mass weighed in grams. The number of moles of each of the ions of a salt in solution depends on the number of each ion in the molecule of the salt (Example 38.2).

Example 38.1

A 100 mL volume of a 2% w/v solution of glucose for intravenous injection is to be made isotonic by the addition of sodium chloride.

A 1% w/v solution of glucose depresses the freezing point of water by 0.1°C and a 1% solution of sodium chloride depresses the freezing point of water by 0.576°C.
The depression of freezing point of the unadjusted solution of glucose (a) will therefore be:

$$(a) = 2 \times 0.1 = 0.2$$

A 1% w/v solution of sodium chloride depresses the freezing point of water by 0.576°C (b).
Substituting these values for a and b in the above equation:

$$W = (0.52 - 0.2)/0.576 = 0.32/0.576 = 0.555$$

The intravenous solution thus requires the addition of 0.555 g of sodium chloride per 100 mL volume to make it isotonic with blood plasma.

Example 38.2

Sodium chloride has one sodium and one chloride ion. Thus, 1 mole of sodium chloride provides 1 mole of both sodium and chloride ions. The weight of sodium chloride which provides a 1 mmol quantity is 58.5 mg. This weight corresponds to its relative molecular mass and provides 1 mmol of both sodium and chloride ions.

Magnesium chloride has one magnesium and two chloride ions. The weight in milligrams that provides 1 mmol of magnesium and 2 mmol of chloride ions is 203 mg. This weight corresponds to the relative molecular mass of this salt. The quantity of salt in milligrams containing 1 mmol of a particular ion can be determined by dividing the relative molecular mass of the salt by the number of the particular ions that it contains. Weights of common salts that provide 1 mmol are given in Table 4 in the chapter 'Solution properties' (pp 49–50) in the 12th edition of the *Pharmaceutical Codex* (1994).

Example 38.3

Calculate the quantities of salts required for the following electrolyte solution:

Sodium	12 mmol
Potassium	4 mmol
Magnesium	6 mmol
Calcium	6 mmol
Chloride	40 mmol
Water for injections	to 1 L

From Table 4 in the *Pharmaceutical Codex* (1994), 4 mmol of potassium ion is provided by 4 × 74.5 mg of potassium chloride, which also yields 4 mmol of chloride ions.

6 mmol of magnesium ions is provided by 6 × 203 mg of magnesium chloride, which also yields 2 × 6 = 12 mmol of chloride ions as there are two chloride ions in the molecule. 6 mmol of calcium ions is provided by 6 × 147 mg of calcium chloride, which also yields 12 mmol of chloride ions as there are two chloride ions in the molecule. 12 mmol of sodium ions is provided by 12 × 58.5 mg of sodium chloride that also yields 12 mmol of chloride. The formula can, therefore, be shown as in Table 38.2. It should be noted that the charges on the anions and cations are equally balanced.

Table 38.2 The formula for Example 38.3

		Na$^+$	K$^+$	Millimoles of Mg^{2+}	Ca^{2+}	Cl$^-$
Sodium chloride	12 × 58.5 = 0.702 g	12				12
Potassium chloride	4 × 74.5 = 0.298 g		4			4
Magnesium chloride	6 × 203 = 1.218 g			6		12
Calcium chloride	6 × 147 = 0.882 g				6	12
Water for injections to 1 L Total (mmol/L)		12	4	6	6	40

Conversion equations

Useful conversion equations include the following:

mg per litre $= W \times M$
grams per litre $= (W \times M)/1000$
% w/v $= (W \times M)/10\,000$

where W = the number of milligrams of salt containing 1 mmol of the required ion, M = the number of millimoles per litre (Examples 38.3–38.5).

Special injections

These are more complex formulations than solutions for injection.

Example 38.4

Calculate the number of millimoles of dextrose and sodium ions in 1 litre of sodium chloride and dextrose injection containing 5% anhydrous dextrose and 0.9% w/v of sodium chloride.

Use the conversion equation for % w/v calculations:

$$\%w/v = (W/M)10\,000$$

From this equation:

$$M = \%\,w/v \times 10\,000/W$$

For dextrose

As dextrose is a non-electrolyte, $W = 180.2$. Thus:

$$M = 5.0 \times 10\,000/180.2 = 277\ \text{mmol}$$

The 1 litre of solution contains 277 mmol.

For sodium chloride

$$M = 0.09 \times 10\,000/58.5 = 15.4\ \text{mmol}$$

As 1 mmol of sodium chloride provides 1 mmol of both sodium and chloride ions, 1 litre of the solution will contain 15.4 mmol of both sodium and chloride ions.

Example 38.5

Calculate the number of millimoles of magnesium and chloride ions in 1 litre of a 2% solution of magnesium chloride.

$$M = 0.2 \times 10\,000/203 = 9.85$$

Each mole of magnesium chloride provides 1 mole of magnesium ions and 2 moles of chloride ions. Thus, 1 litre of the solution contains 9.85 mmol of magnesium ions and 19.7 mmol of chloride ions.

Suspensions

Commonly, suspensions for injection contain less than 5% of drug solids with a mean particle diameter within the range 5–10 μm. Owing to the presence of particles in these formulations, these injections are more difficult to process and sterilize than solutions for injection. During the manufacture of suspensions for injection, the components are prepared and sterilized separately. They are then aseptically combined (see Ch. 29). The final product cannot be filter sterilized owing to the presence of particles in the formulation. Powders for use in sterile suspensions can be sterilized by gas, but gas residues must be avoided.

Dried injections

With these products the dry sterile powder is aseptically added to a sterile vial. Alternatively, a sterile filtered solution can be freeze dried in a vial. The dry drug powder is reconstituted with a sterile vehicle before use.

Non-aqueous injections

Drugs that are insoluble in an aqueous vehicle can be formulated in solution using an oil as the vehicle. These formulations are less common than aqueous suspensions. Several oils are used in these formulations, including arachis oil and sesame oil, which are easily metabolized. These viscous injections give a depot effect with slow release of the drug and are administered by intramuscular injection.

Large-volume parenteral products

These are parenteral products that are packed and administered in large volumes. They are formulated as single-dose injections that are administered by intravenous infusion. They are sterile aqueous solutions or emulsions with water for injections as the main component. It is important that they are free of particles. During the administration of these fluids, additional drugs are often added to the fluids (see Ch. 40). This may be carried out by the injection of small-volume parenteral products to the administration set of the fluid, or by the 'piggyback' method. In this procedure a second, but smaller, volume infusion of an additional drug is added to the intravenous delivery system.

Large-volume parenteral products include:

- Infusion fluids
- Total parenteral nutrition (TPN) solutions
- Intravenous antibiotics
- Patient-controlled analgesia
- Dialysis fluids
- Irrigation solutions.

All of these products have direct contact with blood or are introduced into a body cavity. Large-volume parenterals are variously formulated and packaged and have been used to:

- Restore fluid and electrolyte imbalance in patients suffering from dehydration, shock or injury
- Provide nutrition in circumstances where patients are malnourished, e.g. TPN
- Act as a vehicle for administration of medicines
- Perform dialysis
- Allow irrigation of body parts.

Large-volume parenterals must be terminally heat sterilized. While water for injections is the main component of these products, they also incorporate other ingredients including:

- Carbohydrates, e.g. dextrose, sucrose and dextran
- Amino acids
- Lipid emulsions which contain vegetable or semisynthetic oil
- Electrolytes such as sodium chloride
- Polyols, including glycerol, sorbitol and mannitol.

Most large-volume parenteral fluids are clear aqueous solutions, except for the oil-in-water emulsions. The production of emulsions for infusion is highly specialized as they are destabilized by heat. This results in production difficulties, particularly because the size of the oil droplets must be carefully controlled during the heat sterilization.

Production of large-volume parenteral products

The fluids are produced and filled into containers in a high-standard clean room environment (see Ch. 29). The high standards are required to limit the contamination of these products with organisms, pyrogens and particulate matter. Use of stringent quality assurance procedures is essential to ensure the quality of the products.

In commercial manufacturing facilities, large volumes of fluids are used in the production of a batch of product. The fluids are packaged from a bulk container into the product container in highly mechanized operations using high-speed filling machines. Just before the fluid enters the container, particulate matter is removed from the fluid by passing it through an in-line membrane filter. Immediately after filling, the neck of each glass bottle is sealed with a tight-fitting rubber closure that is kept in place with a crimped aluminium cap. The outer cap is also aluminium and an outer tamper-evident closure is used.

When using plastic bags, the preformed plastic bag is aseptically filled and immediately heat sealed. As an alternative, a blow–fill–seal system can be used. This integrated system involves melting the plastic, forming the bag, filling and sealing in a high-quality clean room environment. Blow–fill–seal production decreases the problems with product handling, cleaning and particulate contamination. Following filling of the product into containers, the fluids are examined for particulate matter and the integrity of container closures established.

Moist heat should be used to sterilize parenteral products, irrigation solutions and dialysis fluids wherever possible. This should be carried out as soon as possible after the containers have been filled. Plastic containers must be sterilized with an over-pressure during the sterilization cycle to avoid the containers bursting.

Containers and closures

Large-volume parenteral fluids are packaged into:

- Glass bottles
- Polyvinyl chloride (PVC) collapsible bags
- Semi-rigid polythene containers.

The containers and closures that are used for packaging parenteral products must:

- Maintain the sterility of the packed fluids
- Withstand sterilization
- Be compatible with the packed fluid
- Allow withdrawal of the contents.

Glass bottles are normally made of Type II glass (Fig. 38.4), but Type I glass is used for products that have a high pH, despite the increased costs. Glass bottles have advantages for packaging these fluids as

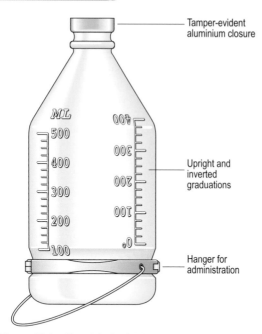

Figure 38.4 • Glass infusion fluid container.

- They permit a high moisture penetration
- They adsorb some drugs
- They require an extended sterilization time due to the heat resistance of the PVC
- Moist heat sterilization requires air ballasting to avoid pouch explosion.

Semi-rigid plastic containers are used for volumes of 100 mL for electrolyte solutions, 3 L for TPN solutions and up to 5 L for dialysis solutions.

Semi-rigid containers:

- Are more drug compatible than PVC containers
- Are difficult to break
- Do not fully collapse
- Need extended heat sterilization times
- Need air equilibration.

Semi-rigid bags are designed with two ports. One port allows the attachment of the administration set. The other port permits the addition of small-volume parenteral products or small-volume infusion fluids. These containers are intended for single use. They have a graduated scale that can be read either in an inverted or upright position (Fig. 38.5). To enable containers of large-volume parenterals to be

they are transparent and chemically inert. They may be used for products that are incompatible with plastic containers. Glass bottles also have some disadvantages. They are much heavier than plastic and therefore less transportable. Although they are strong, they are also brittle, and subject to damage during transport and storage. During use they require the use of an air inlet filter device for pressure equilibration within the container. Particles of glass can be released into the injection fluids. Damage to the neck of the bottles may result in contamination of the container contents from the external environment. A further problem with glass containers may occur during moist heat sterilization. This results in contamination of the fluid due to a pressure imbalance between the internal and external environment. Owing to these difficulties with glass containers, plastic containers have become widely used.

PVC collapsible bags are used to package most infusion fluids. They are designed with a port for the attachment of the administration set and an additive port for the addition of small-volume parenteral fluids.

PVC collapsible bags are:

- Resistant to impact
- Flexible and collapse during fluid administration and so do not require an air inlet system.

The disadvantages of plastic bags are:

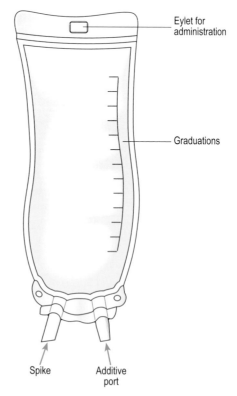

Figure 38.5 • Semi-rigid infusion bag.

suspended from a drip stand for administration, bags are made with an eyelet opening that can be pierced to suspend the bag. Glass bottles are supplied with a plastic band that fits around the container to allow the bottle to be suspended during fluid administration.

Administration of large-volume parenteral fluids

All large-volume parenterals are administered to the patient by a parenteral route using a wide variety of administration sets. Most infusion fluids are administered using the standard infusion set specified in British Standard 2463 (Part 2, 1989). These sets are packaged as sterile units intended for single use (Fig. 38.6). Fluid moves through them by gravity, at a rate that is affected by the physical characteristics of the fluid and the fluid pressure, determined by the height of the infusion above the patient. The administration set is made up of a rigid plastic spike that is inserted into the rubber septum of an infusion container. A filter that removes any particles from the fluid is positioned above a clear drip-control chamber,

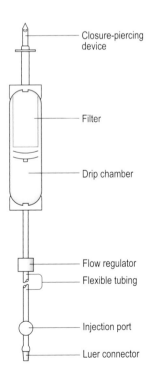

Closure-piercing device

Filter

Drip chamber

Flow regulator

Flexible tubing

Injection port

Luer connector

Figure 38.6 • Diagram of a typical administration set. (From BS 2463: Part 2, 1989, reproduced with permission.)

which aids monitoring the fluid flow rate. These components are connected by at least a 150 cm length of clear flexible tubing. The tubing has a flow regulator and a rubber injection port. The tubing is fitted with a Luer connector for attachment to a needle or catheter that is inserted into the vein of a patient.

Labelling

Batch-produced products have identical labels attached to both the product and the outer packaging carton that is used for transport. With flexible plastic containers, the labelling requirements are commonly printed directly on to the container prior to filling. With bags containing TPN fluids, a label is placed on the bag itself and an identical label is attached to the outer plastic cover on the bag. Labels are attached to infusion fluid containers. The labels on parenteral fluids should include the following details:

- Product identity and details of the contained volume
- Solution strength in terms of the amount of active ingredient in a suitable dose-volume
- Batch number and product expiry date
- Storage requirements
- For TPN solutions, the name of the patient, the unit number, ward and infusion rate.

Containers often carry a warning label to discard the remaining product when treatment is completed.

Aseptic dispensing

Most parenteral fluids are terminally moist heat sterilized. However, some products are aseptically compounded from sterile ingredients in the hospital pharmacy. These products are prepared and dispensed for individual patients. Examples of aseptically prepared products are TPN fluids and the aseptic reconstitution of freeze-dried formulations. These freeze-dried products are often reconstituted using either water for injections or 0.9% sodium chloride injection. Aseptic dispensing is performed in a Grade A clean room environment or a Grade A isolator chamber (see Ch. 40). The dispensing of these products relies on good aseptic procedures to ensure the sterility of the product. Owing to the absence of terminal sterilization, it is important that manufacture is performed using rigorous quality assurance procedures. Aseptically dispensed products are given a very limited expiry time.

Infusion fluids used for nutrition

Nutrients can be delivered to patients by intravenous administration. This is known as total parenteral nutrition and should allow for both tissue synthesis and anabolism. Some patients require TPN for prolonged periods. Initially patients are provided with their TPN in hospital. They may then undergo training to allow self-administration at home. This is known as home parenteral nutrition. Information on total and home parenteral nutrition is given in Chapter 41.

Admixtures

These are prepared by adding at least one sterile injection to an intravenous infusion fluid for administration. The injections to be added are packed in an ampoule or vial, or may be reconstituted from a solid. These additions should be carried out using aseptic procedures in a Grade A environment within an isolator cabinet or clean room facility. This environment is required to maintain the sterility of the product and avoid contamination of the product with particulate matter, microorganisms and pyrogens. Following the additions, a sealing cap may be placed over the additive port of the infusion bag to prevent further, potentially incompatible, additions at ward level. Hospital pharmacies often have a centralized intravenous additive service (CIVAS) as detailed in Chapter 40. These facilities ensure that additions to infusion fluids are carried out in a suitable environment.

Novel delivery systems

Special delivery systems are used to facilitate self-medication by patients in a home environment. Some of these delivery systems are described below.

Infusion devices

There are situations that require strict control of the volume of fluids that are infused into a patient. Accurate flow control with infusion devices is vital for patient safety and for optimum efficacy of the infusion. A range of delivery systems are available that regulate the volume of fluid administered to the patient.

These systems are used both in the hospital and for the self-administration of fluids by patients at home. The selection of an infusion device for the self-administration of medicines by patients requires careful consideration of several factors including:

- Delivery volume and control of flow rate
- Complexity of the administration procedure
- Type of therapy being administered
- Frequency of dosing
- Reservoir volume available in the infusion device.

Infusion devices available include:

- Infusion pumps and controllers
- Elastomeric infusers
- Electromechanical syringe pumps.

All these devices should be:

- Mechanically reliable with accurate flow rates
- Able to provide an output pressure which will not damage the injection site
- Supported with a back-up power supply if electrically operated
- Compact and portable
- Simple to operate for hospital staff and home care patients.

Infusion pumps

These devices use pressure as the driving force to allow administration of fluids into the patient. Infusion pumps, which can be divided into those that move fluid by a piston and valve mechanism and those that move the fluid by peristalsis, are widely used. Infusion pumps are expensive to purchase and operate but allow fluids to be accurately infused into the patient at a slow rate. These devices are becoming more sophisticated with greater electronic controls.

Infusion controller

This is a simple device that can accurately deliver the required fluid volume, although difficulties occur with the administration of viscous solutions. The device relies on gravity moving the infusion fluid down the intravenous administration set. The drop rate in the administration set drop chamber is monitored by a photoelectric mechanism. The device then applies a constriction on the tube of the administration set to give a preselected flow rate.

Elastomeric infusers

These devices are made of a rigid or flexible outer shell with an inner flexible reservoir (Fig. 38.7). The reservoir inside the device is aseptically filled with the fluid. The elasticity of the filled reservoir exerts a constant pressure. This forces the fluid through an

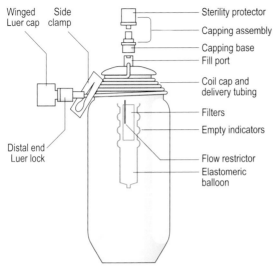

Winged Side
Luer cap clamp

Distal end
Luer lock

Sterility protector
Capping assembly
Capping base
Fill port
Coil cap and
delivery tubing
Filters
Empty indicators
Flow restrictor
Elastomeric
balloon

Figure 38.7 • Elastomeric infuser. (Courtesy of Baxter Health-care Ltd.)

integrated flow restriction device that controls the rate of fluid outflow. The tube from the infuser can be connected to an indwelling cannula in a central vein of the patient. These devices are expensive but they are simple to operate and allow easy home care use.

Syringe infusers

These devices are used for controlling the delivery of small volumes of intravenous infusions over a predetermined period of time. The syringe driver is widely used as an infusion controller for the administration of intravenous antibiotics and patient-controlled analgesia. They are often powered by mains electricity, or may be battery operated, although clockwork syringe infusers have limited low-risk applications. Syringe infusers move the syringe plunger by a motor-driven screw forcing the fluid into tubing for delivery to the patient. These small, lightweight devices allow the administration of precise volumes of fluids. Syringe devices provide good patient home care for patient-controlled analgesia where the drug is often infused over long periods. Patient-controlled analgesia is used by patients to self-regulate the intravenous administration of pain-relieving drugs at controlled intervals. Parenteral administration gives a rapid onset of drug action.

Irrigation solutions

These solutions are applied topically to bathe open wounds and body cavities. They are sterile solutions for single use only. Examples of irrigation fluids are 0.9% w/v sodium chloride solution or sterile water for irrigation. Most irrigation fluids are now available in rigid plastic bottles. Urological irrigation solutions are used for surgical procedures; they are usually sterile water or sterile glycine solutions and are used to remove blood and maintain tissue integrity during an operation.

Water for irrigation is sterilized distilled water that is free of pyrogens. The water is packed in containers and is intended for use on one occasion only. The containers are sealed and sterilized by moist heat.

Peritoneal dialysis fluids

Peritoneal dialysis involves the administration of dialysis solutions directly into the peritoneum by way of an indwelling catheter. The fluid is then drained after a 'dwell-time' to remove toxic waste products from the body. Peritoneal dialysis solutions are sterile solutions manufactured to the same standards as parenteral fluids. The composition of peritoneal dialysis fluid simulates potassium-free extracellular fluid. These fluids are packaged in volumes of 3–5 L in plastic containers that are similar to the bags used for TPN (see Ch. 41).

Haemodialysis

In this dialysis procedure, blood is removed and returned to the patient by way of a catheter, or a double needle arrangement, using a fistula where an artery and vein are joined together. The dialysis procedure involves the use of an artificial disposable membrane within a 'dialyser' machine that acts as an artificial kidney. An electrolyte fluid, simulating body fluid, bathes one side of the membrane, with blood from the patient on the other side. There is no direct contact between the blood and the dialyser fluid. Thus fluids for haemodialysis do not require to be sterile or free of pyrogens or particulate matter.

Fluid volumes of 30–50 L are used daily in haemodialysis procedures (see Ch. 41).

Blood products

These products are not usually identified as sterile products although they are commonly packaged as sterile large-volume parenteral fluids. These biological products include albumin, human plasma and blood protein fractions. All these products must be treated to inactivate virus contamination prior to packaging. This is usually achieved by specialized heat treatment or filtration. These products are unstable to heat sterilization. Therefore, they are filter sterilized and then aseptically filled into containers in large-scale production facilities. Most of these products are packed as liquids, although a few blood protein fractions such as factor VIII and factor IX are freeze dried. The collection, management and distribution of these products is carried out by the blood transfusion service.

KEY POINTS

- Convention uses the term 'parenteral' for dosage forms which are placed directly into the body
- The three main routes are subcutaneous, intramuscular and intravenous, but many others are used in particular situations
- Parenteral products are sterile forms used for injection, infusion or implantation
- Glass ampoules are convenient for small volumes, but glass particles can fall into the injection during opening
- Multiple-dose injections must have an antimicrobial preservative
- Water for injections must be used as the aqueous ingredient in all injections
- Water for irrigations is used in large volumes to irrigate body cavities and other areas
- Pyrogens cause fever and must be eliminated from water for injections and water for irrigations

- Endotoxins, from Gram-negative bacteria, are a major type of pyrogen
- Bacterial endotoxin is detected using the LAL tests, while pyrogens in general are detected by the rabbit pyrogen test
- Additives to injections include antimicrobial preservatives, antioxidants, buffers, tonicity adjusters and cosolvents
- Injection solutions for subcutaneous, intradermal, intramuscular, intrathecal and large-volume intravenous use should be made isotonic
- Tonicity calculations are normally based on freezing point depression, but sodium chloride equivalents, molar concentrations and serum osmolarity can be used
- There is a wide range of large-volume parenteral products, including infusion fluids, total parenteral nutrition, dialysis fluids and irrigation solutions
- All large-volume parenteral products must be sterilized after filling into their final containers
- Large-volume parenteral products may be packaged in glass bottles, semi-rigid or collapsible plastic containers
- When aseptic dispensing is required, rigorous quality assurance is essential and a 1-week expiry date is given to the product
- A range of infusion devices is available for hospital use and to assist patients' self-administration of infusions at home
- Sterile solutions have other uses, such as in peritoneal dialysis

Ophthalmic products

R. Michael E. Richards

STUDY POINTS

- Discuss the formulation, preparation and uses of single- and multiple-dose ophthalmic solutions
- Discuss the formulation, preparation and uses of ophthalmic ointments
- Explain the packaging and labelling requirements for ophthalmic preparations
- Advise patients on the use of eye medication and on any adverse effects they experience
- Describe the anatomy and physiology of the eye in relation to the administration of medication and the wearing of contact lenses
- Explain the properties of contact lenses in relation to their physicochemical composition
- Discuss the wearing of and caring for contact lenses and the various products available to facilitate comfort, effectiveness, convenience and safety
- Highlight the role of antimicrobial preservatives in ophthalmic products with particular reference to the high-risk microbial contaminants *Pseudomonas aeruginosa* and *Acanthamoeba*
- Advise patients on the possible adverse effects of concurrent medication and the sensible use of cosmetics when wearing contact lenses

Introduction

The human eye is a remarkable organ and the ability to see is one of our most treasured possessions. Thus the highest standards are necessary in the compounding of ophthalmic preparations and the greatest care is required in their use. It is necessary that all ophthalmic preparations are sterile and essentially free from foreign particles.

These preparations may be categorized as follows:

- Eye drops including solutions, emulsions and suspensions of active medicaments for instillation into the conjunctival sac
- Eye lotions for irrigating and cleansing the eye surface, or for impregnating eye dressings
- Eye ointments, creams and gels containing active ingredient(s) for application to the lid margins and/or conjunctival sac
- Contact lens solutions to facilitate the wearing and care of contact lenses
- Parenteral products for intracorneal, intravitreous or retrobulbar injection
- Ophthalmic inserts placed in the conjunctival sac and designed to release active ingredient over a prolonged period
- Powders for the preparation of eye drops and powders for the preparation of eye lotions.

Medicaments contained in ophthalmic products include:

- Anaesthetics used topically in surgical procedures
- Anti-infectives such as antibacterials, antifungals and antivirals
- Anti-inflammatories such as corticosteroids and antihistamines
- Antiglaucoma agents to reduce intraocular pressure, such as beta-blockers
- Astringents such as zinc sulphate
- Diagnostic agents such as fluorescein which highlight damage to the epithelial tissue
- Miotics such as pilocarpine which constrict the pupil and contract the ciliary muscle, increasing drainage from the anterior chamber

● Mydriatics and cycloplegics such as atropine which dilate the pupil and paralyse the ciliary muscle and thus facilitate the examination of the interior of the eye.

Anatomy and physiology of the eye

Figure 39.1 gives an indication of the relevance of the external structures of the eye and the structure of the eyelids to the application of medication and the wearing of contact lenses.

Formulation of eye drops

The components of an eye drop formulation are given below:
● Active ingredient(s) to produce desired therapeutic effect

● Vehicle, usually aqueous but occasionally may be oil, e.g. tetracycline hydrochloride
● Antimicrobial preservative to eliminate any microbial contamination during use and thus maintain sterility; it should not interact adversely with the active ingredient(s)
● Adjuvants to adjust tonicity, viscosity or pH in order to increase the 'comfort' in use and to increase the stability of the active ingredient(s); they should not interact adversely with other components of the formulation
● Suitable container for administration of eye drops which maintains the preparation in a stable form and protects from contamination during preparation, storage and use.

The single most important requirement of eye drops is that they are sterile. During the 1940s and 1950s there were several instances reported where microbially contaminated eye drops were used and consequently introduced infection into the eyes being treated. The results were particularly damaging when

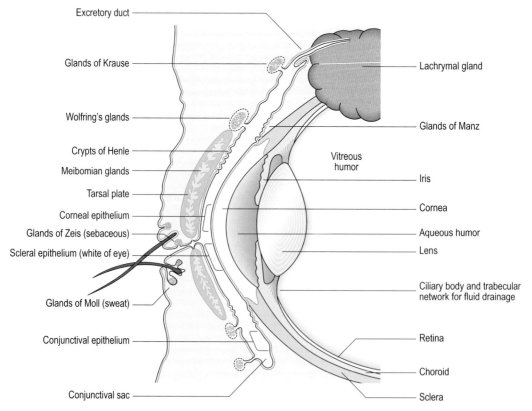

Figure 39.1 ● Section of the eye showing the glands which produce the fluids that form the tears, the epithelial sites of drug action and absorption and the internal sites of pharmacological action.

Box 39.1

Preservatives suitable for specific eye drops

Benzalkonium chloride 0.01% w/v	**Chlorhexidine acetate 0.01% w/v**	**Phenylmercuric nitrate* 0.002% w/v**
Atropine sulphate	Cocaine	Tetracaine
Carbachol	Cocaine and homatropine	Chloramphenicol
Cyclopentolate		Fluorescein[†]
Homatropine		Hydrocortisone and neomycin
Hyoscine		Lachesine
Hypromellose		Neomycin
Phenylephrine		Sulfacetamide
Physostigmine		Zinc sulphate
Pilocarpine		Zinc sulphate and adrenaline
Prednisolone		

[*] The acetate may also be used.
[†] This is preferably used as single dose preparations.

the contaminating organism was *Pseudomonas aeruginosa*, which is difficult to treat successfully and can cause loss of the eye.

Antimicrobial preservatives

It is essential that multiple-dose eye drops contain an effective antimicrobial preservative system which is capable of withstanding the test for efficacy of antimicrobial preservatives of the *British Pharmacopoeia* (BP; 2007). This is to ensure that the eye drops are maintained sterile during use and will not introduce contamination into the eyes being treated. Normal healthy eyes are quite efficient at preventing penetration by microorganisms. Eyes that have damaged epithelia have their defences compromised and may be colonized by microorganisms. This has to be guarded against. The lack of vascularity of the cornea and certain internal structures of the eye make it very susceptible and difficult to treat once infection has been established.

No single substance is entirely satisfactory for use as a preservative for ophthalmic solutions. The systems that have been used, based on work of the author and others in the 1960s, have formed the basis of effective preservation over the subsequent years.

Eye drops specifically formulated for use during intraocular surgery should not contain a preservative because of the risk of damage to the internal surfaces of the eye. Diagnostic dyes should preferably be supplied as single-dose preparations. Preservatives which

are suitable for a selection of eye drops are given in Box 39.1.

Benzalkonium chloride

This quaternary ammonium compound is the preservative of choice. It is in over 70% of commercially produced eye drops and over a third of these also contain disodium edetate, usually at 0.1% weight in volume (w/v).

Rather surprisingly benzalkonium chloride is not a pure material, but is a mixture of alkylbenzyldimethyl ammonium compounds. This permits a mixture of alkyl chain lengths containing even numbers of carbon atoms between 8 and 18 and results in products of different activities. The longer the carbon chain length, the greater the antibacterial activity but the less the solubility. Therefore the manufacturer should seek to maximize the activity within the constraints of solubility. This means maximizing the proportions of C_{12}, C_{14} and C_{16}. It should be noted that Benzalkonium Chloride BP contains 50% w/v benzalkonium chloride.

Benzalkonium chloride is well tolerated on the eye up to concentrations of 0.02% w/v but is usually used at 0.01% w/v. It is stable to sterilization by autoclaving. The compound has a rapid bactericidal action in clean conditions against a wide range of Gram-positive and Gram-negative organisms. It destroys the external structures of the cell (cell envelope). It is active in the controlled aqueous environment and pH values of ophthalmic solutions.

Activity is reduced in the presence of multivalent cations (Mg^{2+}, Ca^{2+}). These compete with the antibacterial for negatively charged sites on the bacterial cell surface. It also has its activity reduced if heated with methylcellulose or formulated with anionic and certain concentrations of non-ionic surfactants. Benzalkonium chloride is incompatible with fluorescein (large anion) and nitrates and is sorbed from solutions through contact with rubber.

The antibacterial activity of benzalkonium is enhanced by aromatic alcohols (benzyl alcohol, 2-phenylethanol and 3-phenylpropanol) and its activity against Gram-negative organisms is greatly enhanced by chelating agents such as disodium edetate. These agents chelate the divalent cations, principally Mg^{2+}, of Gram-negative cells. These ions form bridges and bind the polysaccharide chains which protrude from the outer membrane of these cells. Thus the integrity of the membrane is compromised and the benzalkonium chloride activity enhanced. This is particularly valuable in preserving against contamination with the most feared bacterial contaminant *Pseudomonas aeruginosa*.

The surface activity of benzalkonium chloride may be used to enhance the transcorneal passage of non-lipid-soluble drugs such as carbachol. Care must be taken since the preservative can solubilize the outer oily protective layer of the precorneal film. This film has an internal mucin layer in contact with the corneal and scleral epithelia, a middle aqueous layer and an outer oily layer. The oil prevents excessive aqueous evaporation and protects the inner surface of the lids from constant contact with water. The blink reflex helps maintain the integrity of the precorneal film. For these reasons it is important not to use benzalkonium chloride to preserve local anaesthetic eye drops which abolish the blink reflex. The combined effect of the two agents causes drying of the eye surface and irritation of the cornea.

Chlorhexidine acetate or gluconate

Chlorhexidine is a cationic biguanide bactericide with antibacterial properties in aqueous solution similar to benzalkonium chloride. Its activity is often reduced in the presence of other formulation ingredients. It is used at 0.01% w/v. Its antibacterial activity against Gram-negative bacteria is enhanced by aromatic alcohols and by disodium edetate. Activity is antagonized by multivalent cations. Stability is greatest at pH 5–6 but it is less stable to autoclaving than benzalkonium chloride. Chlorhex-

idine salts are generally well tolerated by the eye although allergic reactions may occur.

Chlorobutanol

This chlorinated alcohol is used at 0.5% w/v and is effective against bacteria and fungi. Chlorobutanol is compatible with most ophthalmic products. The main disadvantages are its volatility, absorption by plastic containers and lack of stability at high temperatures. For example, at autoclaving temperatures it breaks down to produce hydrochloric acid which produces solutions of pH 3–4. Although chlorobutanol is more stable at low pH, such solutions are not desirable for eye drops.

Organic mercurials

Phenylmercuric acetate and nitrate and thiomersal are organic mercurials. They are slowly active, at concentrations of 0.001–0.004% w/v, over a wide pH range against bacteria and fungi. Absorption by rubber is marked.

Opinion is against using heavy metals as preservatives if there are suitable alternatives. The organic mercurials should not be used in eye drops which require prolonged usage because this can lead to intraocular deposition of mercury (mercurialentis). Allergy to thiomersal is also possible.

Tonicity

Where possible, eye drops are made isotonic with lachrymal fluid (approximately equivalent to 0.9% w/v sodium chloride solution). In practice the eye will tolerate small volumes of eye drops having tonicities in the range equivalent to 0.7–1.5% w/v sodium chloride. Nevertheless it is good practice to adjust the tonicity of hypotonic eye drops by the addition of sodium chloride to bring the solution to the tonicity of the lachrymal fluid. Methods for calculating the amount of sodium chloride required are given in Chapter 38. Likewise non-essential increases in the tonicity of hypertonic solutions should be avoided. Some preparations are themselves hypertonic and this cannot be avoided.

If the physiology of the eye is adversely affected, such as when tear film is deficient, or even where hard contact lenses are worn, then the eye surface is more sensitive to variations in tonicity and eye drops should be as near as possible isotonic.

Viscosity enhancers

There is a general assumption that increasing the viscosity of an eye drop increases the residence time of the drop in the eye and results in increased penetration and therapeutic action of the drug. Most commercial preparations have their viscosities adjusted to be within the range 15–25 millipascal seconds (mPas). It should be noted that gently pressing downwards on the inside corner of the closed eye restricts the drainage channel into the nasal cavity and prolongs contact time. This has been recommended to increase the therapeutic index of antiglaucoma medications. Under normal conditions a large proportion of a typical 50 μL drop will have drained from the conjunctival sac (capacity 25 μL) within 30 seconds. There will be no trace of the drop after 20 minutes.

Viscolizing agents include methylcellulose derivatives and polyvinyl alcohol.

Hypromellose

The hydroxypropyl derivative of methylcellulose is the most popular cellulose derivative employed. It has good solubility characteristics (soluble in cold but insoluble in hot water) and good optical clarity. Typical concentrations in eye drop formulations are 0.5–2.0% w/v since higher concentrations tend to form crusts on the eyelids.

Polyvinyl alcohol

This is used at 1.4% w/v. It has a good contact time on the eye surface and good optical qualities. As well as withstanding autoclaving, it can be filtered through a 0.22 μm filter.

Polyvinylpyrrolidone, polyethylene glycol and dextrin have also been used as viscolizing agents.

pH adjustment

The best compromise is required after considering the following factors:

- The pH offering best stability during preparation and storage
- The pH offering the best therapeutic activity
- The comfort of the patient.

Most active ingredients are salts of weak bases and are most stable at an acid pH but most active at a slightly alkaline pH.

The lachrymal fluid has a pH of 7.2–7.4 and also possesses considerable buffering capacity. Thus a 50 μL eye drop which is weakly buffered will be rapidly neutralized by lachrymal fluid. Where it is possible, very acidic solutions, such as adrenaline acid tartrate or pilocarpine hydrochloride, are buffered to reduce a stinging effect on instillation. Suitable buffers are shown in Box 39.2.

Antioxidants

Reducing agents are preferentially oxidized and are added to eye drops in order to protect the active ingredient from oxidation. Active ingredients requiring protection include adrenaline (epinephrine), proxymetacaine, sulfacetamide, tetracaine, phenylephrine and physostigmine. With physostigmine, the antioxidant is purely cosmetic as the initial breakdown product is formed by hydrolysis. The antioxidant only prevents the subsequent discolouration of this product produced by oxidation.

Sodium metabisulphite and sodium sulphite

Both may be used as antioxidants at 0.1% w/v. The former is preferred at acid pH and the latter at alkaline pH. Both are stable in solution when protected from light. Sodium metabisulphite possesses marked antimicrobial properties at acid pH and enhances the activity of phenylmercuric nitrate at acid pH. It is incompatible with prednisolone phosphate, adrenaline (epinephrine), chloramphenicol and phenylephrine.

Chelating agents

Traces of heavy metals can catalyse breakdown of the active ingredient by oxidation and other mechanisms. Therefore chelating agents such as disodium edetate may be included to chelate the metal ions and thus enhance stability. It is seen that disodium edetate is a very useful adjuvant to ophthalmic preparations at concentrations of up to 0.1% w/v to enhance antibacterial activity and chemical stability. It has also been used at higher concentrations as an eye drop for the treatment of lime burns in cattle.

Bioavailability

The effect of pH on the therapeutic activity of weak bases such as atropine sulphate has already been indicated under the section on pH adjustment. At acid pH these bases exist in the ionized hydrophilic form. In order to penetrate the cornea, the bases need to be at alkaline pH so that they are in the unionized lipophilic form. Thus at tear pH (7.4) they are able to penetrate the outer lipid layer of the lipid–water–lipid sandwich which constitutes the physicochemical structure of the cornea. Once inside the epithelium the undissociated free base will partially dissociate. The water-soluble dissociated moiety will then traverse the middle aqueous stromal layer of the cornea. When the dissociated drug reaches the junction of the stroma and the endothelium it will again partially associate, forming the lipid-soluble moiety and thus cross the endothelium. Finally the drug will dissociate into its water-soluble form and enter the aqueous humour. From here it can diffuse to the iris and the ciliary body which are the sites of its pharmacological action (see Fig. 39.1). Thus it is seen that the most effective penetration of the lipophilic–hydrophilic–lipophilic corneal membrane is by active ingredients having both hydrophilic and lipophilic forms. For example, highly water-soluble steroid phosphate esters have poor corneal penetration but the less water-soluble, more lipophilic steroid acetate has much better corneal penetration. This also explains why the more lipophilic dipivalyladrenaline 0.1% w/v is as active as 2% w/v of the more hydrophilic adrenaline.

Storage conditions

To minimize degradation of eye drop ingredients, storage temperature and conditions must be considered at the time of formulation. The stability of several drugs used in eye drops is improved by refrigerated storage (2–8°C) and the following eye drops are recommended for such storage: Chloramphenicol, Eppy, Minims, Mydrilate, Neosporin, Otosporin, Sno-Phenicol and Sno-Pilo.

Containers for eye drops

Containers should be regarded as part of the total formulation. They should protect the eye drops from microbial contamination, moisture and air. Container materials should not be shed or leached into solution, neither should any of the eye drop formulation be sorbed (adsorbed and absorbed) by the container. If the product is to be sterilized in the final container, all parts of the container must withstand the sterilization process used.

Containers may be made of glass or plastic and may be single- or multiple-dose containers. The latter should not contain more than 10 mL. Both single-dose and multiple-dose packs must have tamper-evident closures and packaging.

Single-dose containers

The 'Minims' range manufactured by Smith & Nephew Pharmaceuticals Ltd is the most widely used type of single-dose eye drop container in the UK. It consists of an injection-moulded polypropylene container which is sealed at its base and has a nozzle sealed with a screw cap. This container is sterilized by autoclaving in an outer heat-sealed pouch with peel-off paper backing.

Plastic bottles

Most commercially prepared eye drops are supplied in plastic dropper bottles similar to the illustration in Figure 39.2. Bottles are made of polyethylene or polypropylene and are sterilized by ionizing radiation prior to filling under aseptic conditions with the previously sterilized preparation.

Glass bottles

Most extemporaneously prepared eye drops are supplied in 10 mL amber partially ribbed glass bottles.

The components of the eye dropper bottle are illustrated in Figure 39.3.

It is important to know the glass composition of the bottle. Bottles can be made of either neutral glass or soda glass which has had the internal surfaces treated during manufacture to reduce the release of alkali when in contact with aqueous solutions. The former bottles can be autoclaved more than once but the latter can only be autoclaved once.

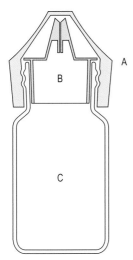

Figure 39.2 • Plastic eye drop bottle. (A) Rigid plastic cap; (B) polythene friction plug containing baffle that produces uniform drops; (C) polythene bottle.

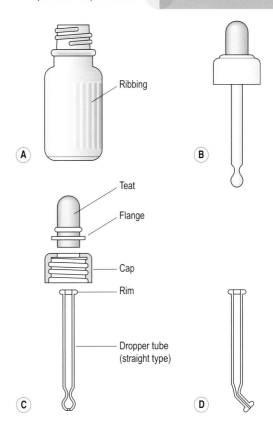

Figure 39.3 • Eye dropper bottle to BS 1679; Part 5 (1974): (A) bottle; (B) assembled closure; (C) components of closure; (D) dropper tube (angled type). (Reproduced by permission of the British Standards Institution (complete copies can be obtained from BSI at Linford Wood, Milton Keynes, MK14 6LE).)

Likewise it is necessary to know whether the teat is made of good-quality natural or synthetic rubber. The former will withstand autoclaving at 115°C for 30 minutes but will not withstand the high temperatures of dry-heat sterilization. The latter teats, made from silicone rubber, will withstand dry-heat sterilization and are suitable for use with oily eye drops. Silicone rubber is permeable to water vapour and this was not realized initially. Aqueous suspensions in bottles with silicone rubber teats sometimes became solid cakes! For this reason aqueous eye drops in bottles having silicone rubber teats are given a limited shelf life of 3 months. This can be lengthened by supplying the sterile eye drops in an eye drop bottle sealed with an ordinary screw cap together with a separately wrapped and sterilized silicone rubber dropper unit. The dropper is carefully substituted for the cap when the eye drops are about to be used.

Teats and caps are used once only. All components are thoroughly washed with filtered distilled or de-ionized water, dried and stored in a clean area until required.

Rubber teats sorb preservatives and antioxidants during autoclaving and storage. It is necessary that individual studies are undertaken during formulation to help counteract preservative and antioxidant loss.

Preparation of eye drops

Extemporaneous preparation of eye drops involves the following:

- Preparation of the solution
- Clarification
- Filling and sterilization.

Preparation of the solution

The aqueous eye drop vehicle containing any necessary preservative, antioxidant, stabilizer, tonicity modifier, viscolizer or buffer should be prepared first. Then the active ingredient is added and the vehicle made up to volume.

Clarification

The BP has stringent requirements for the absence of particulate matter in eye drop solutions. Sintered glass filters or membrane filters of 0.45–1.2 μm pore sizes are suitable. The clarified solution is either filled directly into the final containers which are sealed prior to heat sterilization or temporarily filled into a

Table 39.1 Labelling requirements for eye drop and eye ointment containers at the time of dispensing. (Based on Department of Health guidance HSC(IS)122 1975 revised by the Royal Pharmaceutical Society of Great Britain 2001)

Requirement	Include on label
State route of administration	'For use in the eye only'
Fully identify the product	The name and concentration of the active ingredient(s)
Statement on preservation	Confirm presence or absence of preservative
Directions for use	e.g. 'Add one drop to each eye morning and evening'
State an 'in use' expiry date	Day, month, year
Storage requirements	'Store in a cool place' or 'Protect from light'
Identify patient	Patient's name
Date of dispensing	Day, month, year

Note: When the stability of the final preparation requires it, eye drops may be provided in two containers as a dry powder and an aqueous vehicle. The labels should state 'Powder for eye drops' on one container and the directions for the preparation of the eye drops on the other package or container.

suitable container prior to filtration sterilization. Clarified vehicle is used to prepare eye drop suspensions which are filled into final containers and sealed prior to sterilization.

Sterilization

This can take the form of:

- Autoclaving at 115°C for 30 minutes or 121°C for 15 minutes
- Filtration through a membrane filter having a 0.22 μm pore size into sterile containers using strict aseptic technique. Filling should take place under Grade A laminar airflow conditions (see Ch. 29)
- Dry-heat sterilization at 160°C for 2 hours is employed for non-aqueous preparations such as liquid paraffin eye drops. Silicone rubber teats must be used.

Immediately following sterilization, the eye drop containers must be covered with a readily breakable seal, such as a viskring, to distinguish between opened and unopened containers.

Labelling of containers

Labelling requirements are summarized in Table 39.1 and Box 39.3.

Box 39.3

Additional labelling requirements for use in specific locations

All locations

- Name and concentration of any microbial present

Hospital: wards

- Patient's name. The eye to be treated. Date of opening bottle and/or date to discard (7 days later)

Hospital: operating theatres

- Single dose for once only use. Marked with indication of active ingredient and concentration. No preservative. Outer package fully labelled

Hospital: clinics

- Single dose or multi dose used once only

Domiciliary

- 'Avoid contamination of contents during use'. 'Discard 28 days after opening'. 'Keep out of the reach of children'. Note: If both eyes are to be treated and the patient has an open infection and/or medical opinion dictates, a separate bottle is supplied for each eye and labelled accordingly

Instillation of eye drops

- Wash hands.
- Tilt head back and with one hand gently pull down lower eyelid to form a pouch between the eye and the eyelid.
- Hold dropper bottle (or separate eye dropper containing eye drops) above the eye and drop a single drop into the preformed pouch. Do not touch the dropper on the eye or eyelid. (Using a well illuminated mirror will help.) Administration aids, such as Opticare by Cameron-Graham Limited, are available to assist the self-administration of eye drops contained in plastic eye dropper bottles.
- Release lower lid. Try not to blink more than usual as this removes the medicine from the eye.
- Replace the dropper in the bottle or the cap on the bottle.

Patients who have not used eye drops before need an explanation of how to instil the drops satisfactorily.

Formulation of eye lotions

As stated in the introduction to this chapter, the purpose of eye lotions is to assist in the cleaning of the external surfaces of the eye. This might be to help remove a non-impacted foreign body or to clean away conjunctival discharge. Eye lotions may also be used to impregnate eye dressings. Eye lotions intended for use in surgical or first-aid procedures should not contain antimicrobial preservatives and should be supplied in single-use containers. In keeping with their simple requirements these preparations should have simple formulations and the most common eye lotion consists of sterile normal saline. This preparation typifies the requirements of an eye lotion which are:

- Sterile and usually containing no preservative
- Isotonic with lachrymal fluid
- Neutral pH
- Large volume but not greater than 200 mL
- Non-irritant to ocular tissue.

Labels

These should include:

- Title identifying the product and concentration of contents
- 'Sterile until opened'

- 'Not to be taken'
- 'Use once and discard the remaining solution'
- Expiry date.

Preserved eye lotion would need the additional labelling:

- 'Avoid contamination of contents during use'
- 'Discard remaining solutions not more than 4 weeks after first opening'.

The lotions should be supplied in coloured fluted bottles and sealed to exclude microorganisms.

Powders for the preparation of eye drops and powders for the preparation of eye lotions

These powders are supplied in a dry, sterile form for dissolving or suspending in an appropriate vehicle at the time of use to provide a solution or suspension which complies with the requirements for eye drops or eye lotions as appropriate. The powders may contain suitable excipients to aid dissolution or dispersion, to adjust the tonicity and to improve stability. Unless an exception has been authorized, eye drops in the form of a suspension must pass the same particle size limit test as that applied to the size of particles in eye ointments (see below). In addition single-dose powders for eye drops and eye lotions should either comply with the test for the uniformity of dosage of the *European Pharmacopoeia* (EP), or where appropriate, with the tests for uniformity of content and /or uniformity of mass.

Formulation of eye ointments

Eye ointments are popular and duplicate many of the therapeutic options offered by eye drops. Ointments have the disadvantage of temporarily interfering with vision, but have the advantage over liquids of providing greater total drug bioavailability. However, ointments take a longer time to reach peak absorption.

Eye ointments must be sterile and may contain suitable antimicrobial preservatives, antioxidants and stabilizers. The *United States Pharmacopoeia* (USP 25) requires these ointments to contain one of the following antimicrobials: chlorobutanol, the parabens or the organic mercurials. In addition such ointments should be free from particulate matter that could be harmful to the tissues of the eye. The EP and BP (2007) have limits for the particle size of incorporated solids. Each 10 µg of active solid should have no particles >90 µm, not more than 2 particles >50 µm and not more than 20 >25 µm.

The basic components of an eye ointment are given below:

Liquid paraffin	1 part
Wool fat	1 part (to facilitate incorporation of water)
Yellow soft paraffin	8 parts

Hard paraffin may be substituted as necessary to maintain an appropriate consistency in hot climates.

Containers for eye ointments

Eye ointments should be supplied in small sterilized collapsible tubes made of metal or a suitable plastic. The tube should not contain more than 10 g of preparation and must be fitted or provided with a nozzle of a suitable shape to facilitate application to the eye and surrounds without allowing contamination of the contents. The tubes must be suitably sealed to prevent microbial contamination.

Preparation of eye ointments

Eye ointments are normally prepared using aseptic techniques to incorporate the finely powdered active ingredient or a sterilized concentrated solution of the medicament into the sterile eye ointment basis. Immediately after preparation, the eye ointment is filled into the sterile containers which are then sealed so as to exclude microorganisms. The screw cap should be covered with a readily breakable seal.

All apparatus used in the preparation of eye ointments must be scrupulously clean and sterile. Certain commercial eye ointments may be sterilized in their final containers using ionizing radiation.

Preparation of eye ointment basis

The paraffins and the wool fat are heated together and filtered, while molten, through a coarse filter paper in a heated funnel into a container which can withstand dry-heat sterilization temperatures. The container is closed to exclude microorganisms and together with contents is maintained at 160°C for 2 hours.

Ophthalmic inserts

These are sterile solid or semi-solid preparations for insertion in the conjunctival sac. They contain a reservoir of active material which is slowly released from a matrix or through a rate-controlling membrane over a known time period. Ophthalmic inserts each have their own sterile container which is labelled to state the total quantity of active substance per insert and, where applicable, its rate of release. The EP requires that in the manufacturing of ophthalmic inserts an appropriate product dissolution behaviour is demonstrated.

Monitoring of eye preparations for adverse effects

Pharmacists should be available to counsel patients on the use of their eye medication and advise them about any adverse effects they may experience while using their medicines. Failing to use eye medication appropriately may also have serious consequences. It is important that the pharmacist is able to support the patient in using their medicine correctly. The pharmacist should also be alert to notice any signs/symptoms of adverse effects, that the patient may be experiencing resulting from medication, in order to give appropriate and timely advice. Table 39.2 indicates the signs/symptoms of adverse effects which may occur with eye preparations used in the treatment of primary open angle glaucoma. In addition to adverse effects associated with the eye it should be noted that undesirable systemic effects can also occur with eye medication. Such systemic effects have been reported for certain potent ophthalmic medicines. This is due to excess solution draining from the eye surface through two small channels, the lachrymal canaliculi, into the lachrymal sac and on via the nasolachrymal duct into the gastrointestinal tract. Consequently it is necessary to seek to avoid the instilling of excess eye drops.

Patients who are using an eye drop preparation for a chronic condition may become sensitive to the preservative in the formulation. This may happen with contact lens products also. Changing to a formulation having the same active ingredient but having a different preservative should solve the problem.

Contact lenses and their solutions

Principles of the formulation, purpose and use of contact lenses and their solutions are given. No attempt is

Table 39.2 Signs/symptoms of adverse effects which may occur with treatment for primary open angle glaucoma

| Drugs used | General signs/symptoms of adverse effects | |
Dose frequency as solutions/suspensions	Objective signs	Subjective signs
Beta-blockers	Blood pressure – hypotension	Difficulties in breathing, dry eyes
Timolol 2 × daily	Heart rate – slowed	Itchy and watery eyes
Timolol gel 1 × daily		Pain after instillation
Betaxolol 2 × daily		Blurring of vision
Carteolol 2 × daily		Palpitations
Levobunolol 1 or 2 × daily		Headaches, dizziness, anxiety
Metipranolol 2 × daily		
Parasympathomimetics (Miotics)	Heart rate – rarely affected	Variable blurring of vision
Pilocarpine 4 × daily		Reduction in night vision
Ocusert-Pilo* weekly		Transient headache
A slow-release gel formulation* 24 hourly		Ocular and periorbital pain
		Twitching eyelids
		Sweating, gastrointestinal upsets – rare
Sympathomimetics	Heart rate – quickened	Smarting and redness of eye
	Blood pressure – hypertension	Itchy, watery eyes
Adrenaline (epinephrine) 2 × daily	Conjunctival deposits of oxidized adrenaline[†]	Nasal obstruction
		Dilated pupil, could precipitate acute
Guanethidine 2 × daily	Conjunctival fibrosis on prolonged guanethidine use[†]	glaucoma - dangerous
Dipivefrine* 2 × daily		Headache, blurring vision

* These formulations can reduce adverse effects.
[†] These are specific effects.

made to describe in detail any of the numerous commercial contact lens solutions that are available.

The ready accessibility of the eye and its external structures not only facilitates the use of topical medicines in the conjunctival sac and on the anterior surface of the eye but also facilitates the fitting and wearing of lenses on the precorneal film and on the surface of the eye. Optometrists prescribe and fit contact lenses and monitor their use. Pharmacists should refer patients having persistent problems with wearing their lenses to their optometrist.

Popularity, problems, risks

The popularity of contact lenses results from their cosmetic appeal, optical advantages and their usefulness in sporting activities. Many prefer extended-wear soft lenses to daily-wear soft and hard lenses because of their relative convenience.

The problems that occur with the wearing of contact lenses result from inadequate education of the wearer about lens care. Extended-wear lenses in particular have been marketed in a manner which maximizes the volume of sales at the expense of adequate consumer education. That is, the marketing of lenses has overemphasized the convenient and carefree aspects of overnight lenses to the extent of trivializing the wearing of contact lenses. This has often resulted in poor patient compliance with suggested regimes of lens wear and care. It is estimated that more than 50% of those who wear contact lenses care for them unhygienically.

The risks associated with the wearing of contact lenses include recurrent corneal abrasions, corneal scarring and corneal vascularization. However, the most dreaded complication is microbial ulcerative keratitis or corneal ulcer, caused by microbial invasion of the cornea. Left untreated this can lead to loss of vision. Fortunately the natural defences of the cornea are very effective and the normal cornea resists microbial infection as long as the surface epithelium is intact.

It has been shown that the risk of corneal ulcers is 9–15 times greater for extended-wear lenses worn overnight than for daily-wear soft lenses worn only during the day. The risk increases with the number of consecutive days that lenses are worn without removal.

A serious, but fairly rare, complication that can arise from using non-sterile water in the care of lenses is infection with the free-living opportunistic pathogen *Acanthamoeba*. This is found in most soil and water habitats. *Acanthamoeba* keratitis is hard to diagnose and to treat and can lead to serious loss of vision. *Acanthamoeba* infection has also resulted from wearing soft lenses while bathing in a Jacuzzi; consequently this practice is contraindicated.

The aim of formulators and providers of contact lens systems must be to supply the safest possible system with known and acceptable risks; that is, both convenience and safety must be the aim.

Relevant properties of the eye

Anatomy and physiology

Figure 39.1 indicates the structures of the eye which are particularly relevant to the use of topical medications, contact lenses and contact lens products. First, it is important to note that the cornea, the lens and the humour compartments are avascular and that this property facilitates the transmission of light and vision. Second, exchange of nutrients and waste products in these situations takes place almost entirely by diffusion processes through the aqueous humour, through the lens and cornea and through the lachrymal fluid. Contact lenses reduce the diffusion of oxygen to the cornea and thus can affect corneal metabolism.

Secretions

The secretions of the eye have an important role and influence on the wearing of contact lenses. Tears perform the important functions of lubricating, hydrating, cleaning and disinfecting the anterior surface of the eye. The latter function is performed by the enzyme lysozyme (1,4-N-acetylglycosaminidase) which catalyses the hydrolysis of 1,4-glycosidic linkages between N-acetyl muramic acid and N-acetyl-glucosamine in the peptidoglycan layer of the bacterial cell wall. The peptidoglycan layer of Gram-positive cells is accessible to the action of lysozyme.

Lachrymal fluid

The fluid forming the precorneal film is produced by differing groups of glands. It contains mucus (Henle and Manz), water (Krause and Wolfring) and oil (Meibomian, Moll and Zeis). These fluids are stratified in three distinct layers. The surface-active mucoid layer spreads on the corneal surface and associates with the intermediate aqueous layer externally. The aqueous layer is surfaced with an oily layer which lubricates and protects the mucous membranes of the internal lid surfaces.

Tear electrolyte content

This is broadly similar to that of serum except that the potassium ion is approximately four to six times greater (24 mEq/L compared with 4–6 mEq/L in serum). The protein content of tears is mainly albumin and globulin and is approximately a tenth of that in serum (0.7% compared with 7%).

Tear production

Tears are produced in response to four distinct types of stimuli: emotional via psychological factors, sensory via external irritants, continuous via automatic nervous control and systemic via chemicals in the bloodstream affecting the nerves innervating the lachrymal glands.

Tear pH

This is slightly alkaline at 7.2. Tears have sufficient buffering capacity to adjust rapidly the pH of small volumes of weakly buffered solutions to pH 7.2.

Eyelids

These perform a protecting and a cleaning function. The outer margins of the eyelids close slightly before the inner margins and sweep the fluids across the eye towards the lachrymal duct at the inner angle of the eye and from where it can pass via the lachrymal sac into the gastrointestinal tract. Systemic absorption of excess eye medicament may take place through this mechanism. Conversely, by gentle pressure with the tip of a finger, the lachrymal duct may be closed temporarily and eye medicament maintained in contact with the eye surface for a longer period.

Bacterial flora

There is a common misconception that lachrymal fluid is sterile. It has been known since 1908 that staphylococci and diphtheroids can be found regularly in normal conjunctiva. Gram-negative enteric bacilli have also been isolated from the conjunctivas and lids of about 5% of people. This shows that care is necessary when wearing contact lenses to avoid abrading the corneal epithelium.

Contact lenses

Sir John Herschel used a refractive glass shell in 1823 to protect the cornea from a diseased lid. Dr Eugen Fick, a Swiss physician, first used the term 'contact lens' in 1887. Fick's blown glass lenses were intended to correct defective vision. In 1948 Tuohy introduced the hydrophobic hard plastic corneal lens and in 1962 soft pliable lenses were introduced as the result of work in Prague University. These lenses have been very popular. Gas-permeable hard lenses have also been introduced which allow oxygen perfusion to the cornea. These lenses are more comfortable than the original hard lenses. The first extended-wear lenses were introduced in 1981.

The aim in making contact lenses is to produce lenses which will:

- Correct the patient's vision
- Maintain their position on the eye
- Allow respiration of the cornea
- Permit free flow of tears round or through the lens
- Not release toxic substances
- Not introduce microbial contamination
- Be wearable throughout the day
- Be easy to handle and economical to use.

Hard lenses

Methacrylic acid is esterified to produce the basic monomer methyl methacrylate which is polymerized using benzoyl peroxide as catalyst to produce polymethylmethacrylate (PMMA). This is popularly called 'Perspex' and has optical properties similar to spectacle crown glass. PMMA has hydrophobic properties conferred by the large proportion of methyl groups compared to hydrophilic carboxy ester groups. This means that lachrymal fluid does not readily wet lenses made of this material. Therefore the lenses need to be wetted before mounting on the precorneal

film to reduce or eliminate patient discomfort. Hence the need for a wetting solution to facilitate wear and the need for a storage, hydrating, decontaminating solution to facilitate care of the lenses when not being worn. The original hard lens composition had some major disadvantages for the wearer. Free passage of oxygen and carbon dioxide to and from the corneal epithelium could not take place. Corneal oedema and distortion were a common result. Thus modern lenses have been designed to be gas permeable. These lenses are physiologically more user-friendly and have greater wearer acceptance.

The original gas-permeable lenses consisted of cellulose acetate butyrate (CAB) which was readily wettable and proved quite acceptable. More recently lenses based on silicone and fluorine have been produced which have greater gas permeability. Silicone methacrylate copolymers are very popular. The silicone composition controls the permeability properties and the PMMA composition controls the degree of rigidity. Similarly fluorosilicone methacrylate copolymers which have very high oxygen permeability properties and good wetting properties are proving to be popular. These gas-permeable lenses are cared for using hard lens solutions. These lenses are less subject than soft lenses to deposits of lipids, protein and other substances from the lachrymal fluid. They also have better optical qualities and are generally easier to care for.

Soft lenses

The hydroxyethyl ester of polymethacrylic acid (poly-HEMA) is prepared. The large number of polar hydroxyl groups confers hydrophilic properties to the polymer. Poly-HEMA is flexible and can absorb about 47% of its own weight of water. Thus lenses of this material are comfortable and easy to wear but more difficult to care for than hard lenses. A particular problem is uptake of antibacterial preservatives and subsequent release and irritancy during wear. Although a wetting solution is not needed, cleaning, storing, hydrating and decontaminating functions are required of solutions.

Copolymers of poly-HEMA with vinylpyrrolidine (VP) are also produced which can absorb up to 80% by weight of water depending on the HEMA/VP ratio. The higher water content lenses have the advantage of greater gas permeability and comfort than the poly-HEMA lenses which may occasionally cause corneal oedema. However, they are more fragile and difficult to care for than poly-HEMA, have a greater tendency to attract deposits, more solution problems and less precise optical properties.

Disposable lenses

It is argued that lens design, life span and manufacturing problems can be overcome by the introduction of disposable lenses. Disposable lenses may be discarded after 1 month, 1 week or even 1 day. The latter would obviate the need for the use of solutions and theoretically increase the safety and acceptability of lens wear. However, the original intention of these lenses was for extended wear without removal. It has already been pointed out that the additional risks that are associated with extended wear makes this unattractive and even a dangerous practice. These lenses would seem to offer the greatest advantage to those people who wear lenses on an irregular basis for social and sporting activities and for those children who may need soft lenses.

Hard lens solutions

A 'wetting solution' and a 'soaking/storing/decontaminating solution' are required for the wear and routine care of hard lenses. The first is suitable for placing in the eye but the second must not have contact with the eye.

Wetting solution

Purpose

- Achieves rapid wetting by the lachrymal fluid and thus promotes comfort
- Facilitates insertion of lens
- Provides cushioning and lubrication
- Enables cleaning after removal
- Must be non-irritant during daily use.

Formulation

- Wetting and viscolizing agents – polyvinyl alcohol and hypromellose
- Viscosity 15–20 mPas for comfort
- pH 6.8
- Tonicity 0.9–1.1% sodium chloride

- Antimicrobials – benzalkonium chloride 0.004% plus disodium edetate 0.1%.

Storing solutions

Purpose

- Achieves cleaning and microbial inactivation
- Hydrating.

Formulation

- Surface-active agent not inactivating antimicrobials
- pH 7.4
- Antimicrobials – benzalkonium chloride 0.01% plus disodium edetate 0.1%.

Soft lens solutions

Cleaning solutions

Purpose

- To remove deposits such as lipoprotein adhering to the lens after wear.

Formulation

- Viscolizing surface-active agent such as hypromellose to enable suitable gentle friction with fingertips
- Antibacterial – fast-acting benzalkonium chloride 0.004% may be used if contact time is only 20–30 seconds.

Storing solutions

Purpose

- Hydrating
- Cleaning
- Inactivation of microbial contamination.

Formulation

- Isotonic $\equiv$ 0.9% w/v sodium chloride
- Antibacterial.

Hydrogen peroxide – was introduced into commercially available care systems in 1984. Hydrogen peroxide is a powerful oxidizer and this is the source of its antimicrobial activity. It has good activity against *Acanthamoeba*.

$$2H_2O_2 > 2H_2O + O_2 + Energy$$

Decomposition is more rapid at alkaline than acid pH and many substances catalyse the reaction. These properties are utilized in the formulation of storage, disinfecting and cleaning solutions. For example, a solution containing 3% hydrogen peroxide at acid pH is used to disinfect lenses over a period of 6 hours. This is then followed by suitable inactivation with sodium pyruvate, platinum or the enzyme catalase, to facilitate subsequent safe wearing of the lenses. The procedure is referred to as the two-step system because a separate neutralization step follows the disinfecting step. One-step systems have also been developed for greater patient convenience. The inactivating substance is incorporated with the 3% hydrogen peroxide and the lenses in the disinfecting solution. This system needs to be calibrated to slowly neutralize hydrogen peroxide, but to allow it to have antimicrobial activity over a 6 hour period to ensure effectiveness against *Acanthamoeba* cysts. Some commercial systems may neutralize the effect of the hydrogen peroxide over a period of 30 minutes or so, which is too rapid to guarantee effectiveness. Such systems should be reformulated.

Polyquad – a polyquaternium compound has recently been introduced in soft lens solutions because it is not sorbed (neither adsorbed nor absorbed) by lenses and it has low toxicity to corneal and ocular tissues.

(Thermal disinfection is an alternative disinfection process and the American FDA stipulates heating the lenses in a suitable solution in a lens case at a minimum of 80°C for 10 minutes. Heating reduces the life of the lens and it is also inconvenient in some situations.)

Enzyme protein digest

Purpose

- Occasional cleaning procedure followed by suitable washing and cleansing before wear. Frequency will vary with the individual and his/her state of health. Influenza or hay fever, for example, will increase the need.

Formulation

- Proteolytic enzyme, such as papain, as a solution tablet to produce a suitable solution when dissolved in a stated volume of sterile aqueous vehicle.

Lipid digest or combined protein and lipid digest systems are also available.

All-purpose solutions

The all-purpose solutions initially represented a compromise for hard lens wearers finding it difficult to comply with a two-solution regimen. Single-solution lens care systems are now widely available for use with soft lenses which incorporate an enzyme cleaner combined with a disinfection solution. For example, the serine protease subtilisin A, obtained from the bacterium *Bacillus subtilis*, is used in the presence of hydrogen peroxide to remove protein contamination from contact lenses. Certain all-purpose lens solutions incorporate polyhexamide (polyhexamethylene biguanide) 0.00006–0.0004% as the antimicrobial agent. It is reported to be active against a wide range of bacteria and against *Acanthamoeba*.

All-purpose solutions for soft lenses have become very popular.

Containers

Contact lens solutions are usually packed in plastic containers. It is imperative that the low concentrations of antimicrobials present in these products are not reduced to ineffective levels due to sorption effects with the plastic.

Contact lens storage cases are also of importance to the contact lens wearer. It is important that these containers are kept in a hygienic condition by keeping them scrupulously clean and using the disinfecting/storage solutions strictly in accordance with the manufacturers' instructions. Storage cases should be changed periodically.

Advice to patients

General considerations

Contact lens wearers presenting at the pharmacy with a persistent red eye indicating an infection should not be recommended antibacterial eye drops. They should be referred to an ophthalmologist. This is to guard against the possibility that the person has an infection with *Acanthamoeba*. Such an infection would be more difficult to diagnose after partial treatment.

Disease states leading to a dry eye syndrome such as Sjögren's syndrome, which is mostly confined to menopausal women having osteoarthritis, will also adversely affect the ability of a person to wear contact lenses.

Hard lenses and to a lesser extent soft lenses interrupt the oxygen supply to the cornea and with prolonged wear produce increasing hypoxia. After approximately 16 hours of wear this corneal hypoxia results in a dip in the corneal glycogen level with resultant oedema. Irritation, itchiness, photophobia and blurred vision can result. The patient should be advised not to over-wear the lenses and they may also be recommended to instil sterile sodium chloride 2% w/v every 3–4 hours, after the lenses have been removed, until the oedema has resolved. They should be warned that the hypertonic drops may cause temporary stinging on instillation.

Adverse effects of medicines

Pharmacists should be aware that many medicines taken systemically can also cause problems for wearers of contact lenses and be prepared to offer appropriate counselling.

Certain medicines can affect the eye surface and lachrymal fluid production and thereby influence the comfort of contact lens wear. Medication having anticholinergic properties such as sedative antihistamines, chlorphenamine, antispasmodics, hyoscine, tricyclic antidepressants and neuroleptics can all reduce lachrymal fluid production. Diuretics will also reduce tear volume and topical timolol can cause transitory dry eyes. The consequent lack of lubrication may cause lens discomfort and increased lens deposits.

Oral contraceptives may cause corneal oedema, decreased aqueous and increased mucus and protein production and thus lead to lens intolerance. Pregnancy may also be associated with increased lens awareness and discomfort possibly associated with reduced tear flow and changes in corneal thickness and the curvature of the eye. Clomifene and primidone have also been reported to cause lid and corneal oedema.

Cholinergic drugs and also ephedrine and reserpine will increase tear volume. Aspirin produces low con-

centrations of salicylic acid in the lachrymal fluid. This can be absorbed by soft lenses and subsequently cause irritation. Isotretinoin may cause conjunctival inflammation and consequently cause discomfort to contact lens wearers.

Discolouration, via the lachrymal fluid, particularly with soft lenses, may occur with the administration of certain medicines such as labetalol, nitrofurantoin, phenothiazines, phenolphthalein, rifampicin, sulfasalazine and tetracyclines. Rifampicin for example will stain the lenses and tears orange.

Lenses must be removed before diagnostic dyes such as fluorescein are instilled. In fact it is a general rule that patients should be counselled not to place any ophthalmic preparation on to the eyelids or surface of the eye while contact lenses are in place. Certain eye drops may be instilled while hard lenses are being worn. Sterile 'Comfort drops' may be instilled while lenses are being worn to help maintain the hydration and lubrication of the eye surfaces and lenses when required. Numerous commercial solutions are available. The basic requirements are that the drops should be isotonic, have good wetting properties and be slightly viscous.

Concurrent use of cosmetics

Soft lenses should always be inserted before applying eye makeup but rigid gas-permeable lenses may be put on after. All lenses should be put on before applying nail polish, hand creams, perfumes or using nail polish remover. Aerosol products should be used with caution so that spray does not get between the lens and the eye. All eye makeup should be water based and powders should be avoided. Mascara (not waterproof) should only be applied to the tips of the eyelashes.

The pharmacist should be aware of the various situations mentioned above when offering advice and discussing customers'/patients' questions.

KEY POINTS

- Ophthalmic preparations must be sterile
- Eye drops may be solutions, suspensions or emulsions and contain:
  Active ingredient
  Liquid vehicle free from particulate matter; particle size limits for suspensions
  Antimicrobial preservative
  Adjuvants: tonicity, viscosity, buffering, antioxidants, chelating, dispersing, emulsifying

- Eye drops are contained in a glass or plastic bottle
- Eye lotions are:
  Isotonic
  Neutral pH
  Large volume but not greater than 200 mL
  Non-irritant
  Contained in a fluted, coloured bottle

- Eye ointments contain:
  Semi-solid base
  Active ingredient
  Antimicrobial preservative
  Adjuvants: antioxidants, stabilizers
- Eye ointments are:
  Free from harmful particulate matter; particle size limits
  Contained in a metal or plastic tube
- Ophthalmic inserts:
  Contain a reservoir of active material
  Incorporate a slow-release mechanism

- Properties of the eye affecting formulation of products include:
  Anatomy and physiology
  Secretions
  Lids
  Bacterial flora
- Contact lenses may be:
  Hard lenses including gas permeable
  Soft lenses including disposable
- Contact lens solutions may be:
  Hard lenses – (i) wetting and cleaning; (ii) storing and disinfecting; or (iii) all purpose
  Soft lenses – (i) cleaning; (ii) storing and disinfecting, or (iii) all purpose
- Enzyme cleaning agents are required for all lenses
- Pharmacists should be able to counsel patients on:
  Possible adverse effects of eye medication
  Common problems encountered by lens wearers
  Adverse effects of concurrent medications
  Concurrent use of cosmetics

Specialized services

Graham J. Sewell

STUDY POINTS

- Pharmacy aseptic compounding services and the range of medicines prepared in them
- Equipment and procedures used in centralized cytotoxic reconstitution services
- Occupational health risks of cytotoxic drugs and the effective management of these risks
- Benefits of centralized, pharmacy-operated aseptic compounding services
- Scope and operation of a centralized intravenous additive service (CIVAS)
- Influence of infusion stability on efficacy, patient safety and service provision

Introduction

This chapter describes the specialized services provided by hospital pharmacy departments in the provision of various aseptic dosage forms. These services may include some, or all, of the following elements: cytotoxic or chemotherapy reconstitution services, centralized intravenous additive ser-vices (CIVAS), radiopharmacy services, 'high-tech' home-care services and also the provision of aseptically prepared medicines for clinical trials. In each case, the service involves the provision of aseptically-prepared medicines which are often, but not always, tailored to the specific needs of individual patients. This chapter introduces the scope, practice and pharmaceutical challenges of aseptic compounding services. Parenteral nutrition solutions, which are also compounded aseptically, are considered separately in Chapter 41 and radiopharmaceuticals in Chapter 42.

Cancer chemotherapy

The management of malignant disease is usually based on one or more of the following treatment modes, used singly or in combination: chemotherapy, radiotherapy and surgery. Of these treatment modalities, only chemotherapy is a truly systemic therapy. It has the potential to destroy tumour cells in distant metastasis or in tumour tissue that has infiltrated normal physiological structures and is inaccessible to surgery or radiation therapy without significant damage of healthy tissues. Chemotherapy may be administered with curative intent, but in most adult tumours the intent is normally palliative, with the aim of reducing or controlling symptoms and of prolonging useful life of the patient.

Classification of drugs used in cancer chemotherapy

Traditionally, medicines used in the treatment of malignant disease are cytotoxic in nature, simply meaning that these agents are toxic to cells. This cytotoxic effect is not selective to abnormal cancer cells, and therefore cytotoxic drugs cause severe damage to healthy tissues. Cytotoxic medicines act by interfering with normal cell division preventing DNA and RNA replication. This is often achieved by cross-linking DNA base pairs or by inactivating key enzyme systems or cell-division structures. The mechanisms of action involved and the relative toxicities of cytotoxic medications differ from one agent to another. Most cytotoxic drugs are active only against cells in the replication stages of the cell cycle (cycle-specific) and some are active only in certain phases of the cell cycle, such as S-phase or M-phase (phase-specific). A narrow therapeutic window, severe toxicity and a range of adverse effects characterize all cytotoxic drugs. Healthcare workers involved in handling and administration of cytotoxics must have an understanding of cytotoxic agents and the rationale behind their use in the treatment of cancer.

Cytotoxic agents used routinely in the treatment of cancer can be divided into five main groups. Classification is based on mechanisms of action.

Alkylating agents

These agents form covalent bonds, usually with adjacent DNA bases, either on the same strand of DNA or on opposite strands. Alkylators can also bind to other large molecules such as proteins. Multiple mechanisms of action result from this, including damage to cell membranes, depletion of amino acids and inactivation of enzymes. DNA replication is prevented which arrests cell division. Examples of alkylating agents include: chlormethine (mustine) hydrochloride, cyclophosphamide, ifosfamide, melphalan, chlorambucil, thiotepa, hexamethylmelamine and busulfan.

Antimetabolites

To allow normal cell division, cells must accumulate reserves of protein and nucleic acids. This requires the presence of certain essential metabolites to form the building blocks for the production of larger molecules. The antimetabolite drugs used in chemotherapy have a similar structure to some of these essential metabolites and can take their place in the nuclear material of the cells as a 'false substrate' which then inhibits biological activity. This breakdown in synthesis of essential metabolites and cell components means that cell division will not take place. Also, some antimetabolites have a higher affinity for key enzymes involved in the biosynthesis of nucleic acids than the natural substrate. This 'locks' the key enzyme into a stable complex and effectively inactivates it. An example of this is the inhibition of thymidylate synthetase by 5-fluorouracil. Antimetabolite drugs include methotrexate, 5-fluorouracil, cytosine arabinoside, 6-mercaptopurine and 6-tioguanine.

Vinca alkaloids

These are derived from natural products and the main mode of action is to bind to an intracellular protein,

tubulin, which is involved in the process of cell mitosis. This stops cell division at the second phase of mitosis (metaphase), thus preventing cell reproduction. Cytotoxic agents in this group include vincristine, vinblastine and vindesine.

Antimitotic antibiotics

This is a group of agents historically used in the treatment of infections, which were then found to have an inhibitory effect on dividing tumour cells. Examples of these agents include daunorubicin, doxorubicin and epirubicin. These drugs are associated with multiple mechanisms of action, including intercalation of DNA, enzyme inhibition and free-radical formation which results in damage to the cell nucleus.

Miscellaneous agents

Members of this group do not readily fit into the other above-mentioned categories. However, these agents invariably interfere with DNA biosynthesis and cell replication to exert a cytotoxic effect. The miscellaneous group includes procarbazine and dacarbazine, and the platinum drugs, cisplatin, carboplatin and oxaliplatin, all of which exhibit alkylating activity, and others such as irinotecan and etoposide which act on different topoisomerase enzymes which enable DNA to unwind to facilitate replication. The taxane cytotoxic drugs, which include docetaxel and paclitaxel, act by a different mechanism on the microtubular apparatus of the cell. In summary, the miscellaneous group includes agents with diverse chemical structures and mechanisms of action, some of which are derived from natural products.

Targeted therapies

The recent introduction of the targeted therapies, also known as 'biologicals', has dramatically improved the therapeutic outcomes for many different types of cancer. The targeted therapies are mainly monoclonal antibodies which are directed against specific receptors on the surface of cancer cells. Trastuzumab (Herceptin), for example, is directed against the epidermal growth factor receptor. By inhibiting the stimulation of this receptor, intracellular signalling cascades that promote cell proliferation are blocked. Trastuzumab has been found to significantly improve the treatment of certain types of breast cancer when combined with conventional (cytotoxic) chemotherapy. Other examples of targeted therapies include bevacizumab and rituximab which are used for the treatment of colorectal cancer and certain lymphomas, respectively.

Although the targeted therapies are more specific than conventional chemotherapy agents, toxicity is still a major issue, with the risk of side-effects from conventional agents (e.g. cardiotoxicity caused by doxorubicin) being augmented by the targeted therapy. The targeted therapies are not considered to be cytotoxic agents, although there is some evidence that these drugs can cause indirect cytotoxic effects.

Dosage forms used in chemotherapy

The majority of chemotherapy doses are administered as injections or infusions. The parenteral route offers the advantages of assured bioavailability, careful control over the rate of drug administration and the sequence of administration for regimens based on two or more drugs, and also the ability to stop drug administration immediately in the event of severe, acute adverse effects. However, the parenteral route is invasive, uncomfortable and inconvenient for the patient, and may be associated with complications such as infection, extravasation and thromboembolism. The majority of chemotherapy injections or infusions are given in the hospital setting, usually at specialized outpatient clinics, where nursing and medical support is readily available.

Parenteral cytotoxics are available as sealed vials containing freeze-dried powders or sterile, concentrated solutions. These presentations are designed to provide an adequate shelf life (usually >2 years) for the manufacturer and the user. The freeze-dried powders require reconstitution with an appropriate diluent. The reconstituted solution or the infusion concentrate may then require further dilution before being filled into syringes, infusion bags or infusion devices for administration to patients. The process of taking chemotherapy doses, as provided by the manufacturer, and preparing the required dose in a ready to use form for administration to the patient is often simply termed 'reconstitution', although in practice, it is much more than that.

Parenteral cytotoxics can be administered via the following routes:

- By a syringe as a bolus or slow-bolus injection, usually into a cannula

- By slow bolus injection into the side arm of an infusion
- By addition of a cytotoxic agent directly into an infusion fluid which is then administered over a predetermined infusion period.

Syringe drivers and ambulatory infusion devices can be filled with cytotoxic medicines for use in the community by patients receiving home chemotherapy.

Care must be taken when checking prescriptions and administering chemotherapy that the route of administration has not been transposed. The vinca alkaloids (e.g. vincristine), for example, must never be injected by the intrathecal route, and when this has occurred as a result of an error, the results have always been fatal.

The focus of this chapter is mainly on the provision of parenteral cytotoxic medication for hospital and home patients. However, it should be noted that cytotoxic medicines are available in a range of oral dosage forms including tablets, capsules and suspensions. Recent advances in drug development have overcome some of the bioavailability issues associated with oral chemotherapy and have provided very effective treatments by the oral route. Capecitabine, for example, is a pro-drug of 5-fluorouracil which is selectively activated in the liver and in tumour tissue. A discussion of oral chemotherapy is beyond the scope of this text, and the reader is referred to the British Oncology Pharmacy Association's 'Position statement on care of patients receiving oral anticancer drugs' and the Society of Hospital Pharmacists of Australia's 'Standards of practice for the provision of oral chemotherapy for the treatment of cancer' for more information on this increasingly important area (see Appendix 5).

Dose and schedule of chemotherapy

An explanation is given in Chapter 26 of how to calculate doses on the basis of the patient's body surface area (BSA). The use of BSA is designed to reduce inter-patient variability in responding to chemotherapy, although the scientific validity of this approach is now being challenged. In the case of carboplatin, the dose is calculated according to the patient's renal function and a pre-defined pharmacokinetic parameter (area under the plasma concentration–time curve or AUC). Clinical pharmacists specialized in oncology and haematology are routinely expected to validate chemotherapy protocols and prescribing systems, as well as calculating the doses required. In some parts of the UK, appropriately qualified pharmacists prescribe chemotherapy as supplementary prescribers (see Ch. 17).

Cytotoxic agents can be used individually or in combination. Many oncology centres use a combination of medicines in nationally recognized, evidence-based protocols. These are usually denoted by the initial letters of each medicine used in the regimen, e.g. FEC which stands for 5-fluorouracil, epirubicin and cyclophosphamide in combination. Combinations of cytotoxic agents can increase toxicity, but providing they have a differing spectrum of toxicity, drug combinations may enable the administration of a higher dose-intensity. The risk of emergence of resistant tumour cells is also (at least theoretically) reduced. Further information about chemotherapy regimens can be found in the malignant disorders chapter of *Clinical Pharmacy and Therapeutics* (Walker & Whittlesea 2007).

Occupational exposure risks

For many years there have been concerns regarding the handling of cytotoxic agents by healthcare workers who are involved in the preparation and administration of these medicines. Cytotoxic drug exposure has been associated with various acute toxicities including headache, rash, nausea and dizziness. However, the more serious risks of occupational exposure are related to the potential mutagenic, carcinogenic and teratogenic effects of cytotoxic drugs. The International Agency for Research on Cancer (IARC) classifies 11 cytotoxic drugs and two drug combinations as known human carcinogens, 12 drugs as probable human carcinogens and a further 11 drugs as possible human carcinogens. The United States National Institute of Occupational Health and Safety (NIOSH) issued an alert in 2004 which identified 51 drugs as potential risks to human reproduction. Routes of cytotoxic exposure include ingestion, inhalation, inadvertent inoculation (needle-stick injury) and skin contact. The latter is thought to be the most significant risk for occupational exposure.

The severity of these potential health risks requires that cytotoxic drugs are handled and used in controlled, contained environments by staff provided with adequate training and personal protective equipment (e.g. gloves, gowns, eye protection). To control these risks, and also to reduce the risk of medication errors, cytotoxic agents are prepared under strict aseptic conditions in designated areas within a hospital pharmacy (centralized service) or in dedicated pharmacy aseptic units attached to chemotherapy clinics. In the UK, this requirement is set out and enforced by the Health and Safety Executive.

Pharmacy staff preparing cytotoxic agents must be fully trained in the necessary aseptic and safe handling techniques and must be fully aware of the potential health risks and the precautions that are required when handling cytotoxic drugs. Nursing staff must also be taught strict handling and administration techniques to ensure that they do not expose themselves or patients and carers to any unnecessary risks. At one time, it was thought necessary for annual health checks and full blood counts to be carried out on all staff involved in the preparation and administration of cytotoxic drugs. Current opinion suggests that such checks are of little value, and that resources should instead be invested in the development and validation of safe procedures, staff training, competency assessment, containment facilities (isolators) and protective equipment. Procedures also need to be put in place for emergency situations, such as a cytotoxic spillage.

Published guidelines include the following areas of safe practice:

- Personnel handling cytotoxics, including training and competency
- Facilities and containment systems used for preparation
- Techniques and precautions
- Dealing with spillage
- Disposal of cytotoxic drugs and cytotoxic waste
- Labelling, packaging and distribution
- Administration of cytotoxics drugs.

Useful guidelines on cytotoxic handling include *The Cytotoxics Handbook* (Allwood et al 2002), The Management and Awareness of Risks of Cytotoxic Handling (MARCH) at www.marchguidelines.com and the International Society of Oncology Pharmacy Practitioners (ISOPP) guidelines on safe handling at www.isopp.org.

Provision of a pharmacy-based chemotherapy preparation service

The provision of chemotherapy preparation (reconstitution) services requires that aseptic manipulation of pharmaceuticals is combined with protection of the operator and environment from cytotoxic exposure.

Simultaneous protection of both the pharmaceutical product and the staff involved in its preparation is technically demanding and requires carefully developed systems and procedures together with extensive validation. The principles of the guidelines on cytotoxic handling (above) must be integrated with the principles of good pharmaceutical manufacturing practice. The establishment of a chemotherapy preparation service is not a trivial undertaking and a detailed business case defining the scope and need for the service is fundamental to achieve the support of hospital managers. This should include costings for facilities and equipment, maintenance costs, staff, consumables and drugs costs, together with funding for training and validation of staff. An outline capacity plan should ensure that the service is capable of meeting current and future demand; for example, the service should be able to meet the rising demand for targeted therapies.

The management of chemotherapy preparation services presents numerous challenges; balancing the requirement for stringent safety and quality assurance with the need to provide a timely and responsive service. The demand for chemotherapy, and hence the workload, can fluctuate dramatically. This adds to the difficulty in providing a service that is cost-effective, although new initiatives such as dose-banding (see later in the chapter) have helped in this respect.

Despite the challenges outlined above, it is important that pharmacy staff 'own' chemotherapy preparation services and take a clear lead. In the UK National Patient Safety Agency (NPSA) Alert 20 on injectable medicines, it is clear that application of the risk assessment guidelines places all cytotoxic drugs, and most chemotherapy drugs, in the high-risk category. It is therefore essential that these medicines are prepared by specialized hospital pharmacy aseptic units or, alternatively, by appropriate commercial compounding providers. Pharmacy staff offer a unique combination of skills and expertise, including the practice of aseptic technique, a wide clinical knowledge of cancer chemotherapy, familiarity with formulation and drug stability issues, the application of good manufacturing practice (GMP), quality assurance (QA) and quality control (QC) to aseptic preparation and considerable experience in working with standard operating procedures (SOPs), batch documentation and checking procedures. These are key attributes that help to ensure the provision of safe, effective chemotherapy and contribute towards minimizing the risks of occupational exposure to drugs used in the treatment of cancer.

Training required for staff preparing cytotoxics

All personnel involved in preparing and handling of cytotoxics require training and competency assessment in the appropriate techniques. This should include training for pharmacists, pre-registration graduates and all technical staff and pharmacy assistants working in this field. On a practical level, all staff must be aware of the following over and above standard aseptic technique and the application of GMP to aseptic preparation:

- Procedures required on receipt of a prescription for chemotherapy (electronic or paper), including prescription checking or 'screening'
- Completion of worksheets or batch documents, and assembly of the required materials for chemotherapy preparation
- Changing procedures required prior to working in a clean room environment
- General operation of containment workstations (Class II safety cabinets and isolators) and techniques for the safe handling and manipulation of cytotoxic drugs
- Cleaning and disposal procedures prior to and following aseptic procedures
- Safe storage and transportation of chemotherapy
- Background information on commonly used chemotherapy drugs and protocols
- Local policies and procedures for the operation of pharmacy aseptic services, relevant health and safety legislation and national and/or international guidelines on cytotoxic handling.

Validation of operator techniques

Prior to commencing work on reconstitution of cytotoxics, an operator's competence in this field must be assessed. This is achieved by validating operator techniques. The operator is asked to carry out broth transfer simulations where solutions of sterile broth are transferred from one vial or container to another. The aim of the simulation is to replicate the aseptic transfer techniques which would routinely be used when preparing sterile cytotoxic products. All work is carried out under strictly controlled aseptic conditions. The broth-filled vials can then be incubated for an appropriate time (7–14 days) and examined for microbiological growth. This procedure can be used in conjunction with observing the operator at work to determine operator competence in aseptic transfer techniques (see also Ch. 29).

Each operator undergoing training is required to undertake a predetermined number of broth transfer simulations. Operators must achieve negative results (no growth after incubation) on each occasion before they are deemed capable of preparing cytotoxic agents. The number of broth simulations undertaken can vary from one hospital to another but typically each operator and each process would be re-validated at least every 3 months. Training procedures should be reviewed on a regular basis and retraining and refresher courses made available to all staff. Operators routinely incorporate environmental monitoring tests such as settle plates and finger-dab plates into the production schedule as part of the QA process. A member of staff with environmental monitoring results outside of predefined action levels should be retrained and revalidated before resuming aseptic preparation work. Expert guidance on the validation and monitoring of aseptic compounding has been published in *The Quality Assurance of Aseptic Services* by the NHS Quality Control Committee (Beaney 2006).

Certain handling problems can be encountered when dealing with cytotoxic agents. The formation of an aerosol on removing a needle from a vial containing a cytotoxic agent can result from pressure differences between the inside of the vial and the syringe. This is known as 'aerosolization' and can be prevented by inserting a venting needle into the vial or using a specialized reconstitution device to allow air pressures to equilibrate during addition or withdrawal of solutions. Operator technique in the safe handling of

cytotoxic drugs can be assessed by simulating aseptic transfer processes using a sterile solution containing a fluorescent dye such as quinine hydrochloride. Any splashes or spillage on the work area or equipment, indicative of poor technique, can be visualized using a portable ultraviolet (UV) lamp. Further details on this type of operator competency assessment can be found in *The Cytotoxics Handbook* (Allwood et al 2002). As with assessment of aseptic technique, safe handling should be evaluated using a combination of simulation and expert observation.

Documentation required for cytotoxics

On receipt of a prescription for a cytotoxic agent a number of procedures must be undertaken. Figure 40.1 shows the areas of work in which a pharmacist may have involvement.

When the prescription is received, it is checked by an experienced oncology pharmacist to ensure the accuracy of patient details and dosage calculations and that the presentation or dose form is suitable. The prescription must be validated against an approved chemotherapy protocol, where the drugs, doses, dose intervals and routes of administration are clearly defined. Many chemotherapy regimens are administered in 'cycles', with 2–3 week intervals between them. It is essential that patients receive the correct number of cycles of treatment at the correct intervals. Drug monographs and the manufacturer's Summary of Product Characteristics can be consulted to check drug-specific details including, for example, shelf life of the reconstituted product and the recommended diluents.

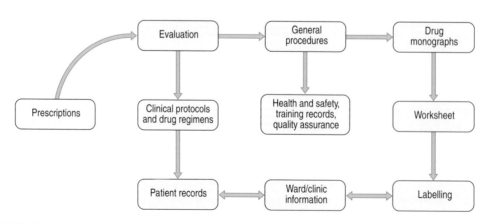

Figure 40.1 • Documentation required for cytotoxic services. (From Allwood et al 1997, reproduced with permission.)

Information from the prescription is transferred to a worksheet or batch document and details of medicine(s) required, diluent and volume for reconstitution are recorded together with the number of drug vials required. Details of batch numbers and expiry date for each component used, all dose and dilution calculations, preparation methods, container(s) to be used, time and date of preparation, and expiry of the final product are also required. Additionally, a sample label is attached to the worksheet. Most chemotherapy preparation units use preprinted worksheets for each chemotherapy protocol, with a pharmacist-approved master document from which copies are made. Alternatively, some units use a computer-based system which contains a database of all approved chemotherapy protocols. Examples of such systems in the UK include Oncology Patient Management Audit System (OPMAS) and Chemocare. These systems produce batch documents and labels, and although computer-generated documents are probably less prone to error, it is essential that all computer systems are fully validated before use.

Labels for cytotoxic medicines are conventionally printed on a yellow background and include the term 'cytotoxic', although many units prefer black print on a white background for clarity. Labels should include the following information:

- Patient's name, hospital number and ward or clinic name
- Drug name, total quantity and final volume of infusion
- Vehicle in which the drug is prepared (e.g. 0.9% sodium chloride)
- Batch number, expiry date and storage conditions required
- Hospital pharmacy name and address
- Route of administration and infusion rate.

When the worksheet is complete, the materials required for the reconstitution procedure are collected together in a marshalling area (adjacent to the clean room) and placed in a suitable plastic tray. The documents and components selected are then subjected to an initial check before transfer to the designated clean room. After preparation has been completed, the finished product(s) and used or part-used vials are returned in the tray, together with batch documents, for labelling, inspection and release. Some cytotoxic agents require protection from light and are sealed in opaque plastic overwraps which will also require labelling. The pharmacist responsible for the release of the prepared medicines will check all details on the worksheets and will reconcile the number of drug vials used in the preparation. If all of these details are in order, the pharmacist will sign the worksheet or batch documents to signify approval, and the medicines are delivered to the clinic, ward or patient, as appropriate. All batch documents must be retained, and many hospitals in the UK are expected to hold these for up to 13 years after the date of preparation.

Cytotoxic preparation areas

In the UK, and in many parts of Europe, pharmaceutical isolators are used for cytotoxic preparation. In addition to providing aseptic conditions for preparation of the product, isolators are designed to protect the operator and the clean room environment from cytotoxic contamination. To achieve this, many isolators operate under negative pressure with respect to the clean room, and the exhaust air is externally ducted via a high-efficiency particulate air (HEPA) filter. All isolators should be located in a classified clean room, although the grade of the clean room environment required is dependent upon the isolator transfer system.

It is generally accepted that isolators offer greater operator protection than open-fronted Class II safety cabinets, although there is little published evidence to support this view. The main disadvantages of isolators include limited access for equipment and difficulties in cleaning and removing cytotoxic residues. Gas sterilizable isolators enable sterilization of the outer surface of vials and components used in the preparation process. Gases such as vapourized hydrogen peroxide are pumped into the isolator to sterilize the inside of the isolator and the outer surface of components in situ, prior to manipulation. This increases assurance that the aseptic environment is maintained, but the validation of gas-sterilization cycles can be complex.

For a more detailed discussion of aseptic preparation facilities, the reader is referred to Chapter 29.

Techniques and precautions

When handling cytotoxics, it is vital that the appropriate protective clothing is worn. Operators using clean room facilities must wear appropriate clean room clothing, with the addition of chemotherapy gowns or armlets for extra protection. These garments are non-shedding and have an absorbent surface and impermeable backing. This design reduces the risk of splashing of solutions on contact with the gown, and also protects the operator from skin contact by cytotoxic drugs. Normally full clean room suits are worn beneath the chemotherapy gown so it is important to ensure that the clean room temperature is carefully controlled. Gloves designed specifically for cytotoxic handling are available and these are normally fabricated from a nitrile material. Gloves should also be worn for handling cytotoxic drug vials outside the clean rooms as these can be contaminated with cytotoxic residues on the outer surface. For operators working in an isolator workstation, the use of a face mask is considered optional from the operator protection viewpoint, but, in accordance with good aseptic practice, face masks should always be used to cover facial hair.

Product segregation is crucial in all aseptic work to avoid any risk of product mix up. In the case of cytotoxic chemotherapy, any such error could be lethal to the patient. For this reason, only one product, or one batch of product, is permitted within the isolator or Class II workstation at any one time.

Reconstitution procedures

When carrying out reconstitution procedures, certain precautions must be taken:

- Vials and outer packs of consumables should be sprayed with sterile 70% alcohol and wiped with a sterile swab before being introduced into the clean room and the process repeated before introducing these materials into the isolator or Class II cabinet workstation. Rubber stoppers on vials should be swabbed with a sterile swab prior to removal of liquid.
- Transfer of liquids to and from vials requires the insertion of a venting needle with hydrophobic filter into the vial or the use of a vented reconstitution device. These devices, which are described below, ensure pressure equalization and reduce the risk of aerosol generation.
- Luer lock syringes with wide-bore needles should be used for all procedures to allow free flow in the fluid pathway and to avoid the risk of syringes and needles becoming disconnected during fluid transfer.
- To ensure that no further additions are made to cytotoxic infusions outside the pharmacy preparation area, all completed products in syringe form should be sealed with a blind hub before removal from the cytotoxic cabinet (Fig. 40.2). An additive plug or cap must be placed on each minibag once additions are complete.

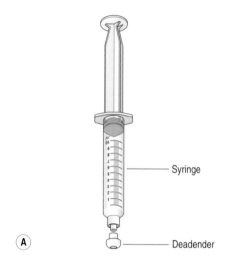

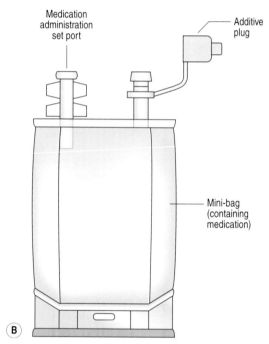

Figure 40.2 • (A) Syringe with deadender or blind hub in position. (B) Minibag with additive plug.

The vials that contain cytotoxic agents are effectively a closed system which contains either a powder requiring reconstitution or a drug concentrate requiring withdrawal from the vial into a syringe. In each case, equalization of pressure within the vial is required to allow withdrawal from it. This can readily be achieved by inserting a sterile 0.2 mm hydrophobic filter venting needle into the vial to facilitate liquid transfer. Ordinary needles with no hydrophobic filter must not be used for venting due to the risk of leakage of cytotoxic solution from the needle. Alternatively, reconstitution devices are available to help with the reconstitution process. Some of these devices consist of a small plastic spike with an integral hydrophobic filter. These devices are useful for rapid transfer of solutions, but the large needle bore can produce large holes in the rubber bung of cytotoxic vials, thus increasing the risk of leakage. The CytoSafe needle is a commonly used example of this type of product. This device consists of a needle which is vented to allow equilibrium of pressure between the vial and the syringe. It is useful for reconstitution of large vials or when more than one vial is required for a dose (Fig. 40.3). However, care must be taken when withdrawing or adding liquid to a vial as the filter may become blocked.

More recently, advanced 'closed systems' using needle-free technologies have been designed for cytotoxic handling. These devices virtually eliminate the risks of cytotoxic aerosol formation and operator needle-stick injuries. An example of this type of device is the Tevadaptor (Fig. 40.4). The Tevadaptor system comprises a vial adaptor to access the drug

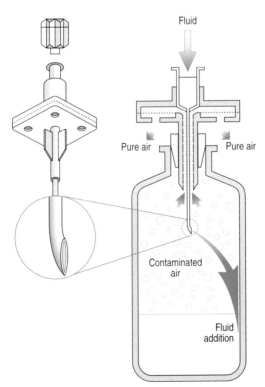

Figure 40.3 • (A) CytoSafe needle and (B) reconstitution set-up. (Courtesy of Baxa Corporation.)

vial, and a syringe adaptor which fits securely onto a luer lock syringe and enables needle-free docking with the vial adaptor. These components allow the closed-system, needle-free addition of diluents to the drug vial for cytotoxic reconstitution, and also the withdrawal of liquids from drug vials into syringes. The spike port adaptor and the connecting set enable a syringe adaptor to dock with an intravenous (IV) bag for addition of additives to the infusion. The two sets provide for connection to the giving set by either a spike (spike port adaptor) or via a luer fitting (connecting set). Alternatively, the luer lock adaptor can be used to access infusion bags fitted with luer additive ports using the syringe adaptor.

The Tevadaptor and other closed reconstitution systems have been shown in studies to be effective in reducing cytotoxic contamination in the work area, and also on products leaving the isolator. The use of these devices will, inevitably, increase costs of the compounding process.

Cleaning the work area

Cytotoxic workstations, particularly isolators, can be difficult to clean. This can result in a build-up of cytotoxic contamination within the isolator with the potential to increase the risk of contamination of both the operator and the outer surfaces of preparations leaving the isolator. The amount of contamination in isolators can be reduced by good technique and by conducting the aseptic manipulation work on a chemotherapy preparation mat. These are sterile mats with an absorbent surface and an impermeable backing which will cover a large proportion of the isolator or Class II cabinet work surface. Any minor spillage is contained on the mat, which is disposable and normally replaced after each day or each work session.

When cleaning isolators or Class II workstations, it is important to recognize that most cytotoxic drugs are water soluble. For this reason, either sterile water or a sterile aqueous-based detergent solution should be used as the first cleaning agent, together with sterile absorbent wipes. This clean should then be followed with a spray and wipe of 70% alcohol to sanitize the surfaces and maintain the aseptic environment.

Effective cleaning is also essential to reduce the risk of cross-contamination of drugs being prepared in the isolator. There is documented evidence of product contamination by the previous infusion prepared in the isolator, and for this reason, the effectiveness of

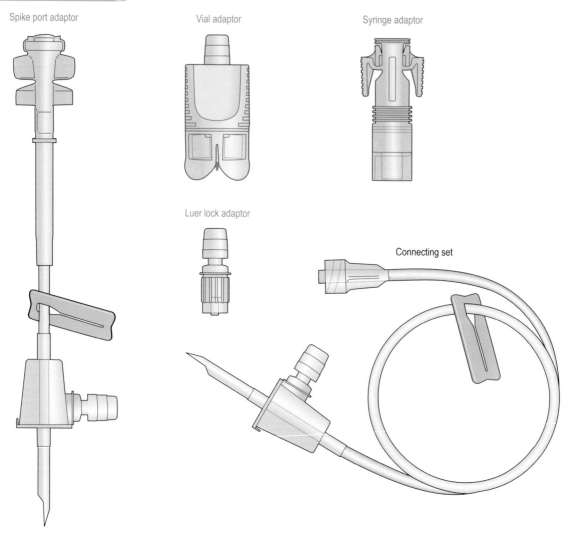

Spike port adaptor

Vial adaptor

Syringe adaptor

Luer lock adaptor

Connecting set

Figure 40.4 • Tevadaptor closed cytotoxic reconstitution and fluid transfer system. (Courtesy of Teva Hospitals.)

cleaning procedures should be validated. This can be done using simulations with fluorescent dyes replacing the cytotoxic drug, and using a UV lamp after the cleaning process to visualize any remaining fluorescent residues. However, a more robust validation would include deliberate contamination by three or four 'marker drugs' from different chemical classes, where wipe samples are analysed after cleaning to detect any low levels of drug residues that persist.

Dealing with cytotoxic spillage

During reconstitution or manipulation, operators must be aware of the procedures required for dealing with a cytotoxic spillage. In the event of a spillage, the problem should be dealt with immediately to prevent the spread of contamination. A written policy on dealing with spillages should be prepared and the operator should be fully competent in the implementation of this. Most policies are based on a spillage kit which contains all the required materials to deal with a spill. These include an absorbent cloth to wipe up liquid spillage and booms to contain a large volume spillage. Spillage involving a powder should be wiped up using a damp cloth to ensure that inhalation of powder particulates does not occur. Contaminated cloths should be disposed of in a cytotoxic hazardous waste bag or cytotoxics sharps bin. All surface areas contaminated by the spillage should be washed with copious amounts of water (sterile water is available in the spillage kit). Cytotoxic spillage kits should be available in pharmacy preparation units, on chemotherapy wards and clinics and in vehicles used to transport cytotoxic medicines.

If the spillage has come in contact with the skin, the contaminated area should be washed thoroughly with soap and water. Contact with eyes should be dealt with by irrigation with a sodium chloride eyewash, the incident reported and medical help sought. In the event of a needle-stick injury involving direct contact with a cytotoxic agent, the puncture wound should be encouraged to bleed and the area should again be thoroughly washed. All accidents involving spillage or needle-stick injury should be reported.

Disposal of cytotoxic waste

Cytotoxic waste materials are regarded as 'hazardous waste' and should be placed in a purple coloured plastic bag, sealed and labelled with a cytotoxic warning label ready for disposal by incineration. Sharp objects including needles, syringes, ampoules and vials should be placed in a sharps bin which is made of rigid plastic and does not allow leakage of cytotoxic waste. When the sharps bin is full, it should be sealed with 'cytotoxic' warning tape and disposed of by incineration. Operators should never put their hands or fingers into a sharps bin, and sharps bins should not be over-filled.

Nursing staff have the task of handling excreta of patients who have received cytotoxic medicines. The potential risks involved will vary depending on the cytotoxic medicine used, dosage given, route of administration and the type of elimination profile. Reports suggest that excreta should be assumed to be potentially hazardous for at least 48 hours after cytotoxic administration is complete. Ward staff should be made fully aware of the patients who pose this risk and should always take the necessary handling precautions, for example wearing chemotherapy gowns and gloves. Patients receiving chemotherapy in the outpatient clinic should have the use of a designated toilet to minimize the spread of contamination. For patients receiving home chemotherapy, family members should be warned about the potential hazards and advised to exercise extreme caution when handling excreta from the patient. The *Cytotoxics Handbook* (Allwood et al 2002) contains useful information on the persistence of cytotoxic drugs in patient excreta.

Packaging of cytotoxic infusions

As a minimum, cytotoxic infusions in syringes or infusion bags should be packaged in a labelled, hermetically sealed overwrap. This has two functions: containment of any leak from the infusion and protection of portering and nursing staff from any cytotoxic residues on the surface of infusion bags and syringes. Ideally (and essentially for transport over long distances), the infusions, in sealed overwraps, should be transported to wards and clinics in a rigid, closed plastic box to provide further protection from any mechanical trauma.

Management of the chemotherapy workload

It is evident from the above text that chemotherapy preparation is very labour-intensive. In recent years, there has been a clear tendency to move from inpatient treatment of cancer patients on hospital wards to chemotherapy outpatient clinics. The operation of outpatient clinics can place significant workload pressures on pharmacy chemotherapy units, partly because several patients often arrive for treatment at the same time, and also because blood test results and other patient-specific data are required before the oncologist is able to confirm the chemotherapy dose and allow treatment to proceed. This often results in several prescriptions arriving in pharmacy at the same time and, consequently, severe delays before some patients receive their chemotherapy on the outpatient clinic. Such delays are not only distressing for patients and chemotherapy nurses waiting to administer treatments, but can also result in treatments over-running normal working hours which can limit the availability of specialist oncology staff to deal with any treatment complications that patients may experience.

Various strategies have been employed to manage these problems. In many centres, it is possible to organize patients' GPs to take blood samples 2 days before the patient is due to visit the outpatient clinic for treatment. Blood counts are then available to the oncologist before the patient arrives at the clinic for treatment. This enables prescriptions to be 'pre-written' so that pharmacy can prepare batch documents and tray-up consumables on the day before treatment, and the go-ahead for preparation can be authorized very early on the day of treatment. Pre-preparing treatments in anticipation of blood results is not recommended, because if treatment does not proceed, or if a dose reduction is required, significant costs are incurred from drug wastage.

More recently, many oncology centres have adopted the approach of 'dose-banding'. Individual patient doses are calculated in the normal way, but the dose is then fitted to predefined dose ranges or 'bands'. If for a given drug the predefined bands were 100–110 mg, 110–120 mg, 120–130 mg, etc. then, for example, a calculated dose of 113 mg would be fitted to the middle band of 110–120 mg. The dose provided to the patient is standardized for each band, normally at the mid-point of the band. So in this example, the standard dose provided would be 115 mg. The key point about dose-banding is that these standard doses are provided with a limited range of standard pre-filled syringes or infusion bags, either singly or in combination. In practice, five or six standard pre-fills are needed to provide the required range of standard doses. Depending on the validated shelf life, these standard pre-fills can be batch prepared, and a stock of them can be stored on the outpatient clinic for immediate dispensing when required. In many centres, this approach has reduced both patient waiting times and drug wastage to almost zero. Further advantages of this approach are that the batches of standard pre-filled syringes or bags can be prepared according to planned work schedules and may also be subjected to prospective QC testing prior to release. Not only is the workload planned and controlled, but quality and patient safety can be improved also. Dose-banding has been widely accepted by oncologists in the UK, largely because the maximum variation of the administered dose from the prescribed dose is limited to <5%.

There is no doubt that managing chemotherapy services is a very challenging task. Operating a patient-focused service which meets clinical needs within the confines of limited resources requires innovation, organization and regular communication with medical and nursing colleagues. The service should be carefully monitored and key outcomes such as errors and patient waiting times should be audited on a regular basis. Requests for new work should be handled efficiently, but a capacity plan to define safe workload limits must be in place to ensure that the service does not become overstretched and compromise patient safety.

Administration of cytotoxic medicines

Specialist chemotherapy nurses are usually responsible for administration of chemotherapy on the oncology or haematology ward and in the outpatient clinic. Some highly specialized, high-risk infusions (e.g. intrathecal and intra-arterial) are still administered by medical staff. Cytotoxic infusions are normally infused using electronic pumps, some of which provide a full audit trail of the infusion time, rate and volume delivered. For many drugs, the chemotherapy infusions are vesicant and can severely damage the lining of blood vessels and blood cells. To reduce such damage, these drugs are infused into a central vein (e.g. cephalic and vena cava) where there is a high blood flow to ensure rapid dilution of the drug infusion. Placing a central venous catheter into a patient is not a trivial procedure and is usually carried out in an operating theatre by an experienced anaesthetist. An alternative is the placement of a peripherally inserted central catheter (PICC), which is tunnelled to a central vein via peripheral veins and can be inserted by a trained nurse in the clinic.

A potential complication of chemotherapy administration occurs when the tip of the catheter used for drug administration locates in the tissues instead of the lumen of the vein. This is known as 'extravasation' or 'tissuing' and can cause extremely serious tissue damage which, in extreme cases, can require the amputation of the limb. In the event of extravasation occurring, administration is halted immediately for staff to aspirate infusion from the tissues and carry out locally agreed policies and procedures which involve, for example, the administration of steroids to reduce tissue inflammation. Extravasation kits should be available on hand in the ward or clinic in anticipation of this problem.

Administration of chemotherapy is clearly a complex and potentially dangerous procedure. National Cancer Standards define the qualification and experience of staff engaged in all aspects of cancer treatment, including drug administration. The NPSA 20 Alert on injectable medicines will place the administration of chemotherapy under particular scrutiny, and will further ensure that only experienced and competent staff are permitted to administer these infusions. Specialized and very high-risk administration routes, such as intrathecal chemotherapy, are the subject of specific and detailed guidelines. For example, in the UK, the NHS Executive published *National Guidance on the Safe Administration of Intrathecal Chemotherapy* (HSC 2003/010) in 2003. Pharmacy has a major role in assuring error-free drug administration. Infusions must be presented in the appropriate form and container, and must be clearly labelled so that nursing staff are provided with unambiguous information about the route, method and rate of administration. The involvement of the oncology clinical pharmacist in the development of drug administration procedures is crucial.

Provision of chemotherapy at home

The introduction of effective oral chemotherapy for cancer, such as capecitabine, has enabled increasing numbers of patients to receive treatment at home. It is also possible to provide parenteral chemotherapy in the domiciliary setting, with home chemotherapy programmes. Patients have more involvement in the administration of their medicines, are able to spend more time with their families and avoid the inconvenience of regular hospital treatment. This, in turn, liberates hospital beds to treat other patients.

Chemotherapy infusions can be administered to patients at home or at work using small, portable ambulatory pumps. These range from sophisticated, programmable electronic devices and battery operated syringe drivers to simple, disposable elastomeric pumps which have a fixed rate of infusion. For a more detailed review of ambulatory infusion devices, the reader is referred to Chapter 38 of this publication and to *The Cytotoxics Handbook* (Allwood et al 2002).

The pharmacist responsible for the centralized cytotoxics service must have a good working knowledge of chemotherapy regimens and the appropriate infusion devices available for home chemotherapy. In certain oncology centres, the pharmacist may also become involved in training patients to manage their infusion devices, and in the safe handling and disposal of cytotoxic drugs. This is necessary to ensure the health and safety of patients and their carers in the home-care environment.

The implications for a pharmacy department setting up a home chemotherapy service are wide ranging. Many home chemotherapy doses are supplied for 1 or 2 weeks at a time. Staff will need to be trained and validated in the techniques used for filling the ambulatory infusion devices required for home chemotherapy. Early home chemotherapy regimens were relatively simple, for example 5-fluorouracil continuous infusion for colorectal cancer. However, more complex, multiple agent regimens are now used. In cases where either the therapeutic response or drug clearance is influenced by a circadian rhythm, it is possible to exploit chronotherapy to optimize treatment using electronic infusion pumps programmed to administer different amounts of chemotherapy over a 24-hour period.

The stability of drug infusions in ambulatory devices is a key element in the provision of home chemotherapy services. In addition to prolonged storage under refrigerated conditions, ambulatory infusion devices are worn under the patient's clothing, exposing drug infusions to elevated temperatures (37°C) for extended periods of time. Stability data on cytotoxic infusions are documented in *The Cytotoxics Handbook* (Allwood et al 2002) and *Handbook on Injectable Drugs* (Trissel 2006). In many cases, stability data appropriate to specific combinations of drug infusions and devices can only be found in the scientific literature, or may need to be determined de novo. In this context, the continuation of research on drug stability under clinical conditions is a crucial role for the few hospital pharmacy departments with a research laboratory.

Centralized intravenous additive service (CIVAS)

The Breckenridge Report produced in the UK in 1976 made recommendations that IV infusions should be prepared, where possible, by hospital pharmacies. Although the preparation of IV cytotoxic medicines was taken up soon after this report, the wider provision of an IV additive service did not commence until the 1980s and then only in a limited number of hospitals.

The establishment of the UK national CIVAS group in 1991 gave more hospital pharmacists the initiative and support for the provision of a CIVAS. By 1998 the *CIVAS Handbook* was produced to provide guidelines for hospital pharmacists setting up a CIVAS. Currently a large proportion of hospital pharmacists in the UK and many European countries provide a CIVAS, and this is augmented by a growing number of commercial compounding units. Despite these developments, it is estimated that of all infusions prepared in UK hospitals, less than 40% are prepared in pharmacy CIVAS units.

Scope of a CIVAS

A CIVAS is set up to provide a range of parenteral dosage forms suitable for administration to patients. Medical, nursing and pharmacy staff involved in patient care in this field will decide the range of dosage forms supplied. A CIVA service can provide the following:

- IV antibiotics, antivirals, antifungals and steroids
- Patient-controlled analgesia, and other opioid infusions for postoperative analgesia and palliative care
- Epidural analgesics infusions
- Ambulatory infusion devices for various IV therapies at home
- Electrolyte infusions (that are not commercially available)
- Clinical trial medicines (if licensed).

Often a CIVAS is operated in conjunction with other aseptic compounding services in the pharmacy (e.g. cytotoxic reconstitution and compounding of parenteral nutrition solutions). Given that CIVAS are resourced to provide only a proportion of the IV additive/compounding needs of a hospital, they normally prioritize the services offered according to clinical risk. Accordingly, CIVAS-produced infusions often include antibiotics for neonates and paediatric patients which require extensive dilution to the required doses. Other high-risk infusions such as complex electrolyte mixtures and ambulatory infusions for home use are often prepared by hospital CIVAS units or are sourced from commercial suppliers. Economic factors can also influence which infusions are prepared in CIVAS units. Many IV medicines contain no preservative and are designed for single use only. Preparation of infusions from these medicines on the hospital ward can often result in significant wastage because only the dose required for immediate use can be taken. However, subject to validated infusion stability, it is possible for a CIVAS unit to prepare a batch of infusions for several days' use, or even longer, so reducing or eliminating drug wastage. In the UK, aseptically prepared medicines may only be assigned a shelf-life of >7 days if supported by validated stability data and providing the unit in which the infusions are prepared holds a 'Specials Manufacturing License' issued by the Medicines and Healthcare products Regulatory Agency (MHRA).

It is likely that the recent NPSA Alert 20 on injectable medicines will provide the stimulus for more ward or clinic-prepared infusions to be transferred to pharmacy CIVAS units to reduce the risk of medication errors.

CIVAS dosage forms

Most hospital pharmacies supply IV additives in the form of a pre-filled syringe or a minibag. Minibags are small volume infusion bags containing volumes of 50–250 mL of common infusion diluents such as 0.9% sodium chloride infusion, 5% glucose infusion or water for injection. Nursing staff often prefer CIVAS doses supplied in minibags as they are easier to administer than syringes, although local preference can vary. Reconstitution procedures are usually required as IV doses are normally received from the manufacturer as sterile freeze-dried powders in sealed vials. The freeze-dried presentation enables the manufacturer to assign a realistic shelf life to these medicines, which are often relatively unstable in aqueous solution. These vials are then reconstituted with the appropriate diluent and drawn up into a syringe. The syringe is then sealed with a blind hub, or if a minibag presentation is required, the dose is transferred to an appropriate minibag ready for administration to the patient. In some cases it will be necessary to withdraw a predetermined volume from the minibag to allow the additive volume to be accommodated. In addition to pre-filled syringes and minibags, CIVAS also provide pre-filled ambulatory infusion devices for domiciliary treatments.

Provision of a CIVAS

Traditionally, IV doses were prepared on the ward or clinic by nursing staff or junior doctors who have limited training in aseptic technique and little experience of calculating appropriate doses and the complex manipulations required for preparing IV medicines. Ward facilities for preparing IV medicines are not ideal and increase the risk of the product being contaminated as it is not prepared under aseptic conditions. A CIVAS operated by trained, competency-assessed pharmacy staff using purpose-built aseptic dispensing facilities ensures that IV products are prepared to the highest possible standards. Clear, comprehensive labelling, full documentation and improved control of ward stocks of IV medicines are also possible with a pharmacy CIVAS. These attributes can significantly improve the risk management of infusions used in a wide variety of therapeutic areas.

The issues to be considered when setting up a CIVAS are essentially the same as those discussed previously for establishing centralized cytotoxic reconstitution services, although the health and safety and occupational exposure aspects are less important with CIVAS. A dialogue should be established between representatives from pharmacy, medical staff, nursing staff and hospital administrators. Information should be gathered on the number of IV doses being used, who prepares them and the conditions under which they are prepared. The proportion of this workload that should be transferred to the proposed pharmacy CIVAS unit can be identified through a risk assessment, and the resources necessary to provide this capacity can be determined. It may be helpful to clearly define the service that wards and clinics can expect through the development of service level agreements.

Any consideration of the resources required to set up a CIVAS must consider the capital costs for the aseptic unit and associated equipment (laminar flow hoods, labelling systems), maintenance costs for facilities and equipment, staff costs for both the CIVAS and the associated QA systems, staff training costs and consumable costs. It should also be possible to estimate the proportion of these costs that can be offset by savings from reduced drug wastage. There may also be the possibility of generating income by providing CIVAS to neighbouring hospitals and private clinics, providing there is adequate capacity.

The main goals of providing a CIVAS should include:

- Improved patient safety
- Improved use of hospital resources
- Improved services to patients, particularly with home infusions
- Improved pharmacy control and reduced risk of medication errors.

Although there are compelling reasons for the provision of pharmacy CIVAS in all major hospitals, it is important in presenting a balanced argument to be aware of potential disadvantages to the hospital and healthcare system:

- Increased pharmacy expenditure, including capital expenditure, diverts funds from other healthcare services.
- Pharmacy CIVAS, once established, should be available 24 hours a day, including weekends and public holidays. This will require a major commitment from pharmacy staff and will also need to be fully funded.
- There is a potential risk of de-skilling ward staff in the preparation of drug infusions. This need not be a problem if the CIVAS is reliable and always available.
- Some wards and departments may be difficult to service, e.g. accident and emergency and intensive care, because doses of some drugs may be required urgently, particularly in an emergency situation.
- Expectations of the CIVAS by medical and nursing staff may not always be realistic. For example, prescribers may not feel the need to furnish prescriptions for infusions in a timely manner, which then places great pressure on the CIVAS unit and causes frustration to nursing staff waiting to administer infusions.
- The capacity of the CIVAS is not infinite but there will always be pressures to add new drugs to the service as soon as these enter clinical use.

Many of these problems can be overcome through good communication, both within the pharmacy department and with medical and nursing staff. A service level agreement (SLA) is a useful device for ensuring that all stakeholders know their responsibilities and that the service operates within the confines of the available resources.

Techniques used in CIVAS

The techniques, procedures, documentation systems and validation requirements of CIVAS are essentially the same as those described previously for chemotherapy services. The main difference is that CIVAS medicines tend to be less hazardous so there is a much lower emphasis on occupational exposure control. This means that instead of isolators and Class II cabinets, CIVAS units tend to use conventional horizontal and vertical laminar flow cabinets. However, it should be recognized that some antibiotics (e.g. penicillins) are sensitizing agents, and some hospitals prefer to use isolator technology for both their cytotoxic and CIVA services.

The reduced hazards associated with CIVAS medicines enable the use of pressurized systems in the reconstitution of freeze-dried drugs and in fluid transfer systems. For example, if minibags are used, a reconstitution device can be used to transfer the diluent into the vial, then, after vigorous shaking, back into the bag again. Throughout this procedure the vial and minibag remain attached via the reconstitution

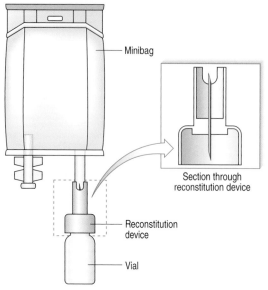

Figure 40.5 ● Reconstitution device used for CIVAS doses. (Courtesy of Baxter Healthcare Ltd.)

device which has a double-ended needle. One end of the needle is placed through the rubber bung of the vial and the other end is connected into the rubber septum of the minibag (Fig. 40.5).

Prior to removal from the laminar airflow cabinet or the isolator cabinet, all prepared syringes are sealed with a blind hub and minibags are sealed with an additive plug or tamper-evident closure. This ensures that no further additions are made to the syringe or minibag outside the pharmacy. All products are labelled and sealed into an outer bag before being transported to the ward.

Quality assurance

All procedures used during preparation of CIVAS doses must be fully validated and documented. Procedures must also be audited and be subject to in-process monitoring. Staff preparing IV products should complete appropriate batch documents and adhere to authorized SOPs and published guidelines. As with the chemotherapy preparation service described previously, batch documents, finished product, used components and records for environmental monitoring and operator validation are all considered as part of the decision-making process for the release of CIVAS medicines for administration to patients. As with any procedure carried out under aseptic conditions, routine environmental monitoring must be

undertaken. This will include the use of settle plates (normally at every work session), finger-dab plates by each operator at the end of each session, and active microbial sampling, air particulate sampling and measurement of air flows from filters at least monthly. Clean room over-pressures should be recorded at least daily, and HEPA filter integrity checks should be carried out at least on an annual basis or in the event of any deviation from defined operating conditions.

Records will be kept for all IV medicines prepared and will include the batch numbers of products used during reconstitution procedures. This ensures that in the event of a product recall or any problems with an IV medicine, a full audit trail documenting all aspects of the process can be reviewed. Records of any errors or complaints should also be maintained, together with the action taken. This information should also be used to inform staff training.

Validation of procedures

Validation of aseptic processes and operator technique will include the use of broth transfer simulations and observation by experienced practitioners. The level of activity and number of staff working in the unit should be taken into account as staff movements are a potential cause of microbiological contamination (see Ch. 29). Validation of processes and operator technique for CIVAS is almost identical to the validations necessary for chemotherapy preparation (see above), with the exception that fluorescent dye simulations are arguably less critical. However, the use of fluorescent dye simulations can still play a valuable role in the validation of cleaning procedures.

Infusion stability and shelf life assignment

The assignment of a shelf life or expiry date to any aseptically prepared medicine is a rigorous, evidence-based process which requires expert interpretation of physical and chemical stability data and a clear understanding of the level of protection afforded to prevent microbiological contamination during the aseptic preparation process.

In the UK, aseptic medicines prepared under Section 10 of the 1968 Medicines Act, which requires pharmacist supervision of the process, are restricted to a maximum shelf life of 7 days, and then only if there is evidence to support this. Even if there is evidence to support a longer shelf life, an expiration of >7 days cannot be assigned to any CIVAS medicines prepared under this system. On the other hand, aseptic medicines made under a manufacturer's 'specials' license issued by the MHRA can be assigned any reasonable shelf life providing this is supported by rigorous evidence on the physical and chemical stability of the infusion, and evidence that the microbiological quality of the product is maintained during both preparation and subsequent storage.

Stability data for CIVAS infusions, including cytotoxic drugs, can be sourced from a number of textbooks including *Handbook on Injectable Drugs* (Trissel 2006), *The Cytotoxics Handbook* (Allwood et al 2002) and the *CIVAS Handbook* (Needle 2007). In many cases, it will be necessary to search the scientific and professional literature for original stability study reports and, on some occasions, the drug manufacturer may be willing to share extended stability data. Whatever the source of information, stability data should always be subjected to critical appraisal before they are used in the assignment of infusion shelf lives.

It is critical that stability studies are carried out under pharmaceutically and clinically relevant conditions. The drug concentration, choice of diluent, container and storage conditions must reflect those used in clinical practice. The method used to assay the drug must be stability indicating, meaning that it will be responsive to any drug degradation and that drug degradation products will not interfere with the accurate determination of the drug itself. This cannot be assumed even for sophisticated and selective analytical methods such as high-pressure liquid chromatography (HPLC). It is vital that validation data support the stability-indicating ability of the assay. In addition to the drug assay, physical stability is assessed by determination of sub-visual particulate matter, visual appearance, pH and the absence of any material or chemicals leaching from the container into the infusion. For more complex biological molecules such as monoclonal antibodies, assessment of stability using simple chemical and physical testing is not adequate. These large molecules are held in secondary and tertiary structures by weak intramolecular hydrogen bonds, and these complex conformations are essential to maintain biological activity. It is important, therefore, to assess the stability of such molecules on the basis of biological activity. In all cases, realistic acceptance limits must be defined for drug degradation.

Typically either 5% or 10% degradation is permitted, depending on the clinical use of the product and the expected toxicity of the degradation product(s).

Normally, aseptically prepared medicines are stored under refrigerated conditions (2–8°C) to inhibit the proliferation of any microbial contaminants. However, the limited physical stability of some infusions under refrigerated conditions requires that room temperature storage is used instead. In some cases, freezing the infusion at −20°C can extend the shelf life of CIVAS prepared infusions. Infusions of the cephalosporin antibiotic ceftazidime are an example in which infusion stability can be increased from 8 days at 2–8°C to 84 days at −20°C. Such infusions must be fully thawed and equilibrated to room temperature before issue to the clinical area.

Assessment of infusion stability is a key responsibility of any pharmacist managing a CIVAS. In the case of infusions which are outsourced from commercial compounding units, it is essential that clear and robust evidence is available to support the assigned shelf life. Care must be exercised when attempting to extrapolate published stability data to infusions with variations in the concentration, diluents or container used. Expert review and a written justification are required to validate a shelf life where there is any variation to the conditions under which the stability data were obtained.

Consideration must also be given to the transportation and storage of aseptically prepared medicines, particularly where infusions are transported over long distances to other hospitals or to patients receiving home infusion treatments. Cold chain transport systems or refrigerated vans must be fully validated to ensure that the stability of infusions is not compromised, and the temperature of refrigerators used for storage of infusions should be monitored at least daily, but preferably by continuous monitoring and data logging (see Ch. 43).

Provision of IV doses for home patients

The potential benefits described previously for home chemotherapy are also applicable to the treatment of other, non-malignant diseases. The range of clinical applications for home infusion therapy is continually expanding; for example pain control (postoperative and terminal care), thalassaemia, infections of the bone, joints and skin, cystic fibrosis (prophylaxis and acute infection flare-up), Parkinson's disease, and non-malignant conditions such as rheumatoid arthritis are treated with cytotoxic drugs. The ambulatory infusion devices used for non-malignant diseases are similar to those described for cancer chemotherapy, with the exception that larger infusion volumes tend to be used and with some drugs, for example antibiotics, the accuracy of the infusion rate is less critical. A number of different options are available for patients receiving home IV therapy (see Ch. 38).

Single-dose bolus injections

These are provided as a pre-filled syringe for bolus administration by either the patient or an outreach nurse. Pre-filled syringes of ceftriaxone, administered once daily for the home treatment of cellulitis, are an example of this type of presentation.

Single-dose infusions

Medicines that need to be given as an infusion at a frequency of one to four times daily are often administered using single-use, disposable elastomeric devices, such as the Baxter Intermate. The drug infusion is filled via a luer lock valve into an elastomeric reservoir which, when expanded, drives the infusion through a flow-restrictor device which may also incorporate a hydrophobic filter to eliminate any air bubbles. These devices require no battery and are available with a wide range of flow rates and infusion volumes. Elastomeric infusors can be used for self-administration by patients who can connect the device to a peripheral or central venous catheter. Examples of home infusions using elastomeric devices include ceftazidime and tobramycin infusions for cystic fibrosis, and desferrioxamine infusion for the treatment of thalassaemia.

Continuous infusions

Prolonged, continuous infusions are required for control of severe pain, where powerful opioid analgesics are infused, often by the subcutaneous route. Continuous infusions, running for 12 hours or more, are also used for other drugs such as the dopamine agonist apomorphine, which is used in the treatment of Parkinson's disease. This type of infusion can be administered with small, portable syringe drivers. These battery-operated infusion devices use a syringe as the infusion reservoir and are ideal for the adminis-

tration of small infusion volumes (<20 mL over 24 hours). More sophisticated electronic infusers work by a peristaltic mechanism and use polyvinyl chloride infusion reservoirs of 50–500 mL volume. These devices are often programmable and are designed to prevent alteration of settings by the patient. However, they are expensive and tend to suffer from a relatively short battery life.

The hospital pharmacy CIVAS has a clear role in providing pre-filled syringes and reservoirs for home infusion patients. Some centres also provide the actual infusion devices and other consumables required by home infusion patients (e.g. sharps bins for disposal of waste, alcohol wipes and sterile gloves). Close liaison between pharmacy, nursing and medical staff is required to ensure home infusions are prescribed and prepared when needed, that the infusion device selected is appropriate to the patient's needs, and that the CIVAS unit can respond to any changes of dose or therapy.

KEY POINTS

- Cancer chemotherapy can include treatment with cytotoxic drugs and biological 'targeted' therapies
- Cytotoxic drugs can be classified as alkylating agents, antimetabolites, anti-tumour antibiotics and miscellaneous drugs
- Cytotoxic agents may be given orally (tablets, capsules or suspensions) or parenterally (slow bolus or IV infusion)
- There are significant occupational exposure risks to healthcare workers who handle cytotoxic drugs
- Compliance with safe handling guidelines, combined with use of protective equipment, containment facilities and validated technique can minimize cytotoxic exposure to healthcare staff and patient's carers
- Use of strict aseptic conditions minimizes the risk of microbiological contamination during preparation
- Detailed standard operating procedures for preparation and administration of chemotherapy must be prepared and implemented
- All personnel involved in provision of a centralized cytotoxic reconstitutions service must be trained and validated in all relevant procedures and techniques
- Transfer of solutions between cytotoxic drug vials and syringes must be carried out using a hydrophobic venting pin or a purpose designed transfer device to avoid the generation of aerosols
- The pharmacy chemotherapy unit has a key role in the provision of home chemotherapy services

- Drug stability is a key issue in assigning infusion shelf lives, particularly those used for home infusion
- Increased use of chemotherapy outpatient or day-case clinics can place significant pressures on the workload of the pharmacy chemotherapy unit
- New strategies such as 'dose-banding' are useful to manage chemotherapy workload
- A CIVAS can provide a wide range of aseptically prepared medicines for hospital and domiciliary use

- Potential benefits of CIVAS include reduced risk of medication errors, improved use of resources, better services to patients and pharmacy control
- Potential difficulties in operating a CIVAS, such as staffing, out-of-hours and emergency provision and unrealistic expectations can be resolved with good communication skills
- Most doses are provided from CIVAS as either pre-filled syringes or minibags
- Home IV therapy may use pre-filled syringes, single-dose infusers, electronic infusers or syringe drivers to administer drug infusions

Parenteral nutrition and dialysis

Lindsay Harper and Liz Lamerton

STUDY POINTS

- Provision of nutritional support for patients
- Indications for total parenteral nutrition (TPN)
- Components and compounding of a TPN/home parenteral nutrition (HPN) formulation
- Addition of medicines to a TPN or HPN bag
- HPN training and potential problems
- Administration of a TPN/HPN formulation
- British Parenteral Nutrition Group and British Association of Parentral and Enteral Nutrition
- Introduction to home care for patients on dialysis
- Haemodialysis (HD), peritoneal dialysis (PD), including continuous ambulatory peritoneal dialysis (CAPD), intermittent peritoneal dialysis (IPD) and automated peritoneal dialysis (APD)
- Dialysis solutions
- Provision of services from a hospital renal unit, including home dialysis

Introduction

Today an increasing number of patients are requesting and being provided with healthcare services at home. Such services include provision of home parenteral nutrition and home dialysis. This chapter will explore the provision of parenteral nutrition and dialysis for patients in hospital and will explain how these services can be transferred to the home-care setting.

Provision of nutritional support

Studies have shown that up to 50% of medical and surgical patients can suffer from nutritional deficiencies. If nutritional support is indicated, enteral feeding is considered as the first option. Patients can receive nutrients orally or via a tube feed, e.g. by nasogastric feeding. This is only possible if the gastrointestinal tract is functional. If this is not the case, parenteral nutrition may be considered. Short-term (e.g. postoperative) intravenous (IV) administration of fluids such as 5% dextrose or saline may be sufficient. This could provide the patient with around 500 calories per day but does not provide any protein, vitamins, minerals or trace elements.

For patients requiring longer-term nutrition, total parenteral nutrition (TPN) may be required. TPN is a method of administering adequate nutrients via the parenteral route. The components of a TPN formulation are added to a sterile infusion bag and administered to the patient via a catheter. Administration can be via a peripheral venflon, a peripherally inserted central catheter (PICC) or a central line. However, TPN fluids are normally highly concentrated mixtures which on a long-term basis could cause damage to peripheral veins. For this reason, peripheral veins are only used for TPN administration lasting up to 4 weeks.

If parenteral nutrition is supplied to patients at home, it is known as home parenteral nutrition (HPN). Patients on HPN administer their nutrition via a central line into a central vein. Commercial pharmaceutical home-care companies most commonly provide the TPN for HPN patients, although some patients may receive the TPN from their local hospital TPN compounding unit.

Parenteral nutrition formulations are prepared under strict aseptic conditions (see Ch. 29) following guidelines published by the Medicines and Healthcare products Regulatory Agency (MHRA) in *Rules and Guidance for Pharmaceutical Manufacturers* (2002) and by the Department of Health in *Aseptic Dispensing for NHS Patients* (Farwell 1995).

HPN is becoming increasingly prevalent, particularly for patients who require long-term parenteral nutrition. Guidelines have been published by the British Association of Parenteral and Enteral Nutrition (BAPEN) and the National Institute for Health and Clinical Excellence (NICE) to ensure that adequate provision is made for patients receiving HPN (Wood 1995). Patients who are suitable candidates for HPN will be initially stabilized on TPN bags while in hospital. They can then undergo appropriate training to enable them to administer their TPN bags at home. If the patient is unable to care for their line, then a carer or nurse would be trained to administer the TPN at home. However, HPN patients will still require to return to the hospital for regular check-ups. This means that pharmacists involved in the care of HPN patients will require a working knowledge of the procedures adopted to provide care for patients in hospital and at home. They may also have to liaise with the patient's GP, the community nurse, primary care trust and other healthcare workers in this field.

This chapter concentrates on the provision of adult TPN in hospital and at home, although neonatal TPN is available.

Indications for TPN

TPN can be required for finite periods of time or can be required for life. Some of the main indications for TPN are:

- Gastrointestinal disease including Crohn's disease, ulcerative colitis, pancreatitis and malabsorption syndrome (e.g. scleroderma patients)
- Major trauma including severe burns, severe septicaemia, intensive care patients and acute renal failure
- Major abdominal surgery; severely malnourished patients may benefit from early peri- and postoperative parenteral nutrition if surgery has resulted in a non-functioning gastrointestinal tract
- Malignancy of the small bowel
- Radiation enteritis when TPN is considered if enteritis is severe after treatment of a primary malignancy

- High-dose chemotherapy, radiotherapy and bone marrow transplantation. Patients are often ill for a limited time (3–6 weeks) and are unable to eat. TPN can be administered during this period to ensure that the patient's nutritional requirements are adequately met.

Several other conditions may require the nutritional support of TPN, e.g. patients in a prolonged coma or AIDS patients.

Assessment of the patient in hospital

TPN aims to provide patients with all their nutritional requirements in one formulation which can then be infused directly into the body via the veins, either central or peripheral. In order to determine exactly what the patient's nutritional requirements are, clinical and biochemical assessments must take place. A clinical patient history is recorded followed by a physical examination to give a clearer picture of the patient's current medical status. The Malnutrition Universal Screening Tool (MUST) is used to identify patients who may benefit from TPN. Patients' body weight, height and body mass index (BMI) can be recorded and comparison made with their ideal body weight which would be available from standard charts. In most hospitals a dietician would review the patient and calculate their nutritional requirements.

Biochemical assessment will be undertaken initially by performing a number of routine tests which can then be repeated as necessary during TPN therapy. Factors investigated will include urea and electrolytes, full blood counts, liver function tests, triglycerides, blood glucose and fluid balance. Trace elements are only required if the patient receives TPN for longer than 28 days. The NICE guidelines for nutrition support contain a section on the monitoring required for TPN patients.

Each hospital has its own particular way of designing a TPN regimen. Most hospitals use a range of standard formulations which are routinely used to treat TPN patients. Standard bags can be altered if the need arises, e.g. intensive care patients may require extra nitrogen in the formulation, renal patients may need an electrolyte-free formulation. In general, additions to the finished TPN bags outside of the pharmacy aseptic unit is not recommended in order to minimize microbial contamination.

More recently pharmaceutical companies have introduced a range of three-in-one ready-to-use multi-chambered TPN bags. These bags have three chambers, which contain amino acid, dextrose and lipid. When a bag of TPN is required, the seal separating the chambers can easily be broken and the three solutions are mixed together in one chamber. Before mixing, these bags have a long expiry date of around 2 years and do not need to be stored in the fridge. Many hospitals have swapped to using these bags as they are cost-effective and reduce the time for manufacture. Trace elements and vitamins need to be added to these bags before use.

Some hospitals tailor regimens to individual patients and carry out a number of calculations to determine baseline requirements for each component. In this way they can build up a formulation by matching up the patient's requirements to commercially available solutions which contain the required components in the correct proportions. During this process, careful consideration is given to the patient's medical condition and the necessary adjustments made. Individualized bags tend to be used in patients on long-term TPN. Patients on HPN will always have bags tailored exactly to their nutritional needs.

The nutrition team

In most hospitals where TPN is supplied there will be a nutrition team to coordinate the delivery of the parenteral nutrition service. This team can include the following:

- Consultant
- Senior registrar/registrar
- Pharmacist
- Clinical psychologist
- Nutrition nurse(s)
- Dietician(s)
- Biochemist(s).

The role of these individuals in provision of patient care can vary from one hospital to another. In general, the consultant is responsible for prescribing the TPN formulation and liaising with the patient's GP to provide care for HPN patients, although with the introduction of non-medical prescribing, this role is increasingly taken over by nurses and pharmacists.

The pharmacist can provide information on aseptic techniques for handling and setting up TPN bags,

formulation requirements, potential complications or stability problems, and storage conditions required. In some hospitals, the pharmacist's role can be extended to include the following:

- Training nursing staff in the techniques required for IV administration of TPN fluids
- Helping with patient training for HPN
- Monitoring of patients in HPN clinics
- Liaising with the staff from the home-care company
- Advising on the patient's drug therapy
- Liaising with the patient's community pharmacist.

The nutrition nurse and dietician will together give advice on a day-to-day basis regarding the nutritional status of the patients and advise on necessary dietary requirements. The nutrition nurse can also be responsible for training patients for HPN.

The biochemist can supply results of daily or weekly analysis of patients' urine and electrolyte levels and alterations can then be made to the TPN formulation if required.

The nutrition team can meet on a weekly basis to discuss the requirements of patients currently receiving TPN both in hospital and at home.

Commercial companies supplying home-care services have a nutrition nurse who provides medical care, support and advice (on a 24-hour basis if required), a patient coordinator who deals with the ordering of HPN bags and ancillaries, and a designated delivery person who will supply the necessary equipment and HPN bags to the patient's home.

In the rare circumstances that the HPN is supplied by the hospital pharmacy, patients can be provided with the support of a small group of people, some of whom may be part of the nutrition team. This group usually includes the nutrition nurse, the hospital pharmacist and the patient's GP.

Components of a TPN formulation

TPN formulations can contain the following components:

- Water
- Protein source – measured in grams of nitrogen
- Energy source – carbohydrate and fat
- Electrolytes
- Trace elements
- Vitamins and minerals.

Baseline water requirements

Water accounts for over 50% of the body weight. To prevent patients becoming dehydrated, daily water losses and gains must be carefully considered. Water can be lost through urine and faeces and through 'insensible losses' – i.e. through the skin and lungs. Patients with burns and gastrointestinal losses will require increased volume. Patients with renal and cardiac failure should be given reduced volumes.

Several methods are available for estimating daily fluid requirements, but most take into consideration body weight and measured urine output, and an allowance is made for insensible losses. The average adult requires between 1500 and 4000 mL of fluid per day. A TPN regimen will require to provide this volume of fluid on a daily basis.

Protein source

Protein requirements vary from one patient to another and are highly dependent on the metabolic status of the patient. Undernourished patients requiring parenteral nutrition are generally said to have a negative nitrogen balance. This means that the amount of nitrogen excreted in urine and faeces is greater than the nitrogen administered.

Lack of nitrogen in the body can result in poor wound healing and interference with body defence mechanisms. To overcome this problem, a utilizable source of nitrogen must be administered to the patient. This is achieved by administering amino acid

---

Example 41.1

A postoperative surgical patient requires 0.2 g/kg/24 h of nitrogen. The patient weighs 47 kg.
Nitrogen requirements per day = 0.2 × 47 kg = 9.4 g nitrogen.
This requirement can then be matched up to commercially available solutions. Each gram of amino acid nitrogen is equivalent to 6.25 g of protein, e.g. Vamin 9 contains 9.4 g of nitrogen per litre. This is equivalent to 60 g of protein and will provide the patient with the required daily nitrogen intake. However, care must also be taken when selecting an amino acid solution for inclusion in a TPN formulation, as most commercially available solutions are hypertonic in nature and have a pH between 5 and 7.4. The pH of the amino acid solution may have an effect on the overall stability of the formulation and must be considered carefully.

---

solutions in a TPN formulation. These solutions act as a source of nitrogen and are said to be the building blocks for the formation of proteins in the body. Nitrogen requirements can be estimated from a 24-hour urine collection. This is done by analysing the total amount of urea excreted and by considering the individual patient's body weight and clinical 'type'.

Energy sources

Carbohydrates and fats are chosen to provide optimal energy sources for TPN patients. The relative proportions of each will be dependent on the clinical requirements of the patient and formulation considerations. The carbohydrate of choice is normally dextrose and is available in solution with concentrations ranging from 5% to 70% weight in volume (w/v). Like amino acid solutions, dextrose solutions are hypertonic and have a low pH (3–5). If high concentrations of dextrose are added to the TPN bags, they must only be given centrally.

The fat component in a TPN formulation is administered in the form of an oil-in-water emulsion. Fat emulsions are isotonic with plasma, have neutral pH and provide a high calorie source in a low volume. As a result, they are often used in combination with dextrose to provide the necessary calorie content, thereby avoiding the potential problems encountered with excessive dextrose administration.

Fat emulsions provide the patient with essential fatty acids and also act as a vehicle for fat-soluble vitamins which are required in the TPN formulation. Fat is not required in every TPN formulation, but fat deficiency can occur in patients who do not receive fat components for periods longer than 1 month. Depending on individual requirements, patients on long-term TPN may require fat added to their TPN bag daily, on alternative days or two or three times weekly.

Commercially available preparations are based on soya bean oils and are composed of varying combinations of long and medium chain triglycerides. Newer fat solutions have been developed incorporating olive oil and fish oils which are claimed to protect patients on long-term parenteral nutrition from complications. Larger and longer trials are required to prove these claims. The energy content of commercially available solutions for both carbohydrates and fats is expressed in kcal/litre, e.g. Intralipid 10% provides 550 kcal/500 mL; Dextrose 5% provides 210 kcal/500 mL.

Table 41.1 Role of electrolytes used in TPN formulations. (From Walker & Edwards 2003, reproduced by permission.)

Electrolyte	Principal function	Daily intravenous requirement	Symptoms of deficiency	Symptoms of excess	Common sources
Sodium	Main extracellular cation Regulation of water balance Neuromuscular contractility	1–2 mmol/kg	Weakness, lethargy, confusion, convulsions, appetite, nausea and vomiting	Lethargy, coma, convulsions, muscle rigidity, thirst	Sodium chloride Sodium acetate Sodium phosphate
Potassium	Main intracellular cation Regulation of acid–base balance Neuromuscular contractility	1–2 mmol/kg	Muscle weakness, ileus, arrhythmias, alkalosis	Muscle weakness, paraesthesia, bradycardia, nausea and vomiting	Potassium chloride Potassium phosphate
Magnesium	Cofactor for enzyme systems Neuromuscular contractility	0.1–0.2 mmol/kg	Lethargy, cramps, tetany, paraesthesia, arrhythmias, excitability, hypokalaemia, hypocalcaemia	Decreased muscular activity, lethargy, depression	Magnesium sulphate Magnesium chloride
Calcium	Mineralization: bones + teeth Neuromuscular contractility	0.1–0.15 mmol/kg	Paraesthesia, tetany, fitting, confusion, arrhythmias	Nausea, anorexia, lethargy, muscle weakness, confusion	Calcium gluconate Calcium chloride
Phosphate	Main intracellular anion Acid–base balance Energy	0.5–0.7 mmol/kg	Weakness, tingling	Non-specific effects on calcium balance	Phosphate salts of sodium and potassium, hydrogen
Chloride	Main extracellular anion Acid–base balance	1–2 mmol/kg	Alkalosis	Acidosis	Chloride salts of above cations

Electrolytes

The main electrolytes of clinical significance in a TPN formulation include sodium, potassium, magnesium, calcium, phosphate and chloride. The requirement for electrolytes can be met in the form of injectable solutions of varying percentage content. Electrolyte content of each is expressed in terms of mmol/L. The individual role of each electrolyte in a TPN formulation is given in Table 41.1.

Trace elements

Trace elements act as metabolic cofactors and are said to be essential for the proper functioning of several enzyme systems in the body. Despite being termed essential, they are only required in very small quantities, expressed in micromoles. The main trace elements required in a TPN formulation are zinc, copper, manganese and chromium. More details on trace element requirements are given in Walker & Edwards (2003).

Vitamins and minerals

Vitamin requirements fall into two categories: fat soluble and water soluble. Four fat-soluble vitamins (vitamins A, D, E and K) and nine water-soluble vitamins (vitamins B_1, B_2, B_3, B_5, B_6, B_{12}, C, folic acid and biotin) are said to be essential. Water-soluble vitamins have an important role in patients at risk of refeeding syndrome, particularly thiamine. The management of refeeding syndrome is discussed in the NICE guidelines on nutrition support.

Vitamins and minerals are normally included in foods taken in orally and must therefore be included in TPN formulations for patients on long-term parenteral nutrition. They are required for several body processes and act as essential coenzymes in carbohydrate metabolism and amino acid and DNA synthesis. Commercially available solutions include Multibionta®, Parentovite®, Solivito N® and Vitlipid N Adult®. The NICE guidelines published in 2006 recommend that patients must receive vitamins and trace elements daily in their TPN bags.

Compounding of TPN and HPN formulations

Compounding can take place within a hospital pharmacy using aseptic dispensing facilities within a clean room or within a designated compounding unit in a commercial pharmaceutical company.

Preparation and training

For patients in hospital, the consultant or non-medical prescriber will prescribe a suitable TPN regimen. On receipt of the prescription, the pharmacist checks the suitability and compatibility of the formulation, the required volume of each component is calculated and details are transferred to a worksheet. Patient details can be entered into a computer and labels generated for the worksheet and the final product. In the preparation area, items required for the compounding process can be collected together in an appropriate tray ready for transfer to the clean room facility. Batch numbers and expiry dates for each product used are recorded on the worksheet. The pharmacist checks all details, including calculations, before the compounding procedure begins.

Compounding of a TPN formulation is carried out under strict aseptic conditions (in a Grade A environment) using a laminar airflow (LAF) cabinet within a clean room facility. Chapter 29 gives details regarding clean room facilities, gowning-up procedures for entry to clean rooms and working procedures for using LAF cabinets. Standard operating procedures (SOPs) should be available for all staff carrying out aseptic dispensing procedures. Operators will undergo appropriate training including validation of operator techniques by broth fill tests (see Ch. 29) prior to commencing work in the field.

TPN/HPN bags

The components of a TPN formulation are sterile and are prepared under sterile conditions as the formulation is eventually infused directly into the bloodstream of the patient. It is therefore essential that the bags used to hold the TPN formulation are also sterile. In the past, only polyvinyl chloride (PVC) bags were used for TPN formulations. However, because of the problems of leaching of plasticizers from PVC bags containing a fat component, ethylvinyl acetate (EVA) bags (which contain no plasticizers) are now recommended. However, EVA bags have been shown to be permeable to oxygen; hence multilayer EVA bags are now available for formulations requiring prolonged storage. These bags are made of layers of plastic with an inert inner layer made of EVA. This arrangement reduces oxygen permeation to a minimum.

Bags are usually supplied with a premounted sterile filling set attached. The filling set consists of a number of hollow plastic tubes (up to six) with a plastic spike attached to the end of each. The spikes are used to pierce the rubber septum of the bottles and bags of amino acids, glucose and fat emulsion to enable filling of the components into the TPN bag. Clamps fitted with air vents are attached to each filling tube to clamp off the source bottles and bags when they are empty. Filling sets are used for compounding purposes only and are disconnected and replaced with a sterile hub before being sent out to the patient. Every HPN bag is supplied with a sterile giving set which allows the bag to be infused into the patient.

TPN bags vary in size, ranging from small 250 mL bags used for neonatal TPN up to 4 L bags for adult TPN. Bags used for HPN patients are identical to those used for TPN in hospitals. Figure 41.1 shows a TPN bag with filling set attached.

Addition of components to a TPN bag

Components are added into the TPN bag in a strictly defined procedure. Small-volume additives can be added directly into large-volume fluids (but not directly into the fat component) or directly into the additive port on the bag (depending on manufacturers' recommendations). Amino acid solutions and glucose are added into the bag first, followed by any fat emulsion if required. To prevent precipitation of

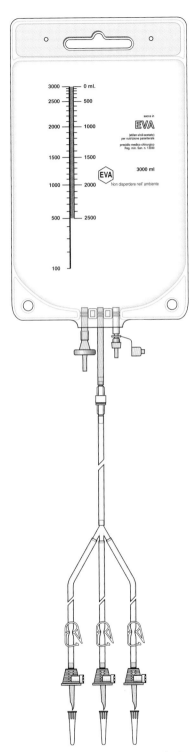

3000
2500
2000
1500
1000
500
100

0 ml.
500
1000
1500
2000
2500

sacca in

EVA

(etilen-vinil-acetato)
per nutrizione parenterale

presidio medico chirurgico
Reg. min. San. n.13030

3000 ml

EVA

Non disperdere nell' ambiente

Figure 41.1 • A TPN bag with filling set attached.

vitamins, they are generally only added immediately before administration.

Filling of the TPN bags can be achieved under gravity. The bag is placed on the floor of the LAF cabinet and the solution components suspended from a retort stand, enabling the solution to flow freely into the bag. If several bags require to be compounded in a limited time period, the bag can be placed in a vacuum chamber to speed up the filling process. Electronic devices, known as compounders, are also available. They are usually under microprocessor control and can be pre-programmed to fill TPN bags with set volumes of individual components. They can be used to achieve rapid filling of a number of TPN bags and are useful devices for compounding neonatal TPN bags where strict control of fluid volumes is required.

When all the components are added, the bag can be clamped off and the filling set removed. A sterile hub replaces the filling set to prevent any further additions being made to the bag outside the sterile production area. The bag is gently shaken to ensure adequate mixing of all components. The TPN bag and compounding materials are transferred back to the preparation area. A visual inspection of the bag is made, including checking of the additive port, for integrity. All necessary documentation is completed and the TPN bag is labelled. Details to be included on the label are shown in Box 41.1.

The TPN bag is then sealed into a dark-coloured outer plastic bag (to protect the formulation from light) and an outer label that is identical to the label on the bag itself is attached.

To maintain stability of the formulated product, it is refrigerated until required. All TPN and HPN formulations must be stored in a designated pharmaceutical grade refrigerator. Cool boxes packed with ice packs can be used for transportation of formulations to the ward or the patient's home.

Box 41.1

Details to be placed on a label of a TPN bag

- Patient name (ward and unit number if hospital patient)
- Components of the bag (expressed in mmol)
- Total volume (mL)
- Energy content (kcal)
- Nitrogen content (g)
- Infusion rate (mL/h)
- Route of administration
- Expiry date and storage conditions

Compounding of HPN formulations by commercial companies

A designated compounding unit is used for preparing HPN formulations. Conditions used will be the same as those used in the hospital sector (aseptic dispensing facilities in a clean room) and the same government regulations apply. If the commercial company does not have its own compounding facilities it may utilize the services of a hospital pharmacy or another industrial pharmaceutical company to compound the HPN bags. The compounding unit must hold a manufacturing licence prior to supplying TPN bags.

Regardless of the compounding arrangements, the commercial company providing the home-care service must be in receipt of a prescription for the HPN formulation prior to compounding. The prescription will be the same formulation which the patient initially had during the stay in hospital.

However, when the health care is transferred to the home-care setting in Scotland, the patient's GP will take on the responsibility for supplying the HPN prescription. In England and Wales the health authority is responsible for providing the HPN prescription. Subsequent prescriptions will then be forwarded to the commercial company in advance of the patient's requirements. The hospital nutrition team will issue the prescriptions for the patients at home. The patient coordinator will deal with orders for sundries and ancillaries such as pumps, dressings, needles, etc.

Potential complications arising during compounding and administration of TPN formulations

The components of a TPN formulation will individually and collectively contribute to the overall stability of the resulting formulation. However, with several hospitals now using standard TPN formulations, many of these problems can be overcome. For hospital pharmacies which have a manufacturing licence, standard bags can be made up in advance of requirements and stored in a refrigerator for periods of 30 days or more. The shelf life given to individual formulations must be based on validated stability studies previously carried out on the formulation. The stability of any regimen will be confirmed before manufacture.

Individual components of the formulation such as vitamins, electrolytes and fat can cause formulation complications. Vitamin stability is very poor, particularly in the presence of light and with extended storage time. Stability is also affected by solution pH, hence the need for careful consideration of the overall formulation.

The requirement for administration of calcium and phosphate in a formulation can lead to precipitation of calcium phosphate. This reaction is said to be affected by factors such as the relative amounts of each component present, solution pH, concentration of amino acid solutions present and the mixing process used. To overcome this type of problem, manufacturers of parenteral nutrition fluids can supply tables which give details of the amount of each component that can be safely combined to ensure stability of the formulation is maintained. These tables are specific to an individual formulation and details cannot be interchanged between formulations.

The presence of fat in a TPN formulation can cause stability problems. As storage time increases, the fat component of the formulation becomes less stable, resulting in a process of 'cracking' where the oil and water phases of the emulsion separate out. If the formulation is administered to the patient in this unstable condition, this can lead to potentially dangerous fat deposits arising in the lungs and other body tissues.

The factors a pharmacist must consider when formulating a TPN bag with a fat component are:

- The order in which components are added to the bag
- The types and amount of electrolytes present and their relative proportions – divalent and trivalent cations reduce stability
- The pH of the resultant mixture – higher pH improves stability
- Conditions arising during storage and administration
- The type of plastic bag used – EVA bags preferred.

Addition of medicines to a TPN or HPN bag

Stability studies have been carried out on a number of medicines to determine their compatibility and stability in a TPN bag. So far, studies have confirmed the suitability of only a limited range of medicines which includes: heparin, insulin, aminophylline, cimetidine, famotidine, ranitidine and certain antibiotics. Reference to manufacturers' literature and compatibility studies will provide current recommendations. Although stability is available on the drugs listed above, the addition of drugs to TPN is not recommended. This is because the drugs may affect the long-term stability of the TPN bag and it will affect the pharmacokinetics of the drugs added to the TPN. Most hospitals in the UK allow no additions to the TPN bags.

Administration of TPN/HPN formulations

For patients requiring TPN for longer than 2 weeks, central venous access is required. During their stay in hospital, patients have a catheter inserted into the subclavian vein under anaesthesia. It has an exit site on the lower chest wall, allowing patients easy access for care of the catheter site.

Catheters can be made of materials such as polyvinyl chloride or silicone. For long-term feeding, a permanent catheter (a Hickman catheter or a portacath) is used. It is held in place by a Dacron cuff (an internal woven plastic used to connect arteries and veins under the skin). Good aseptic techniques are essential to ensure that the catheter site does not become contaminated. Infection around the catheter site can be difficult to treat successfully and may eventually result in removal of the catheter and replacement at another site.

Catheter sites should only be used for administration of TPN fluids and not for blood sampling or administration of other medicines. However, in exceptional circumstances (where venous access is limited) the TPN line may have to be used for these purposes. In some instances, a triple lumen catheter can be used with one line being kept for administration of the TPN bag only. To infuse the TPN formulation into the patient, the catheter is connected via an extension set to a volumetric infusion pump. These devices use positive pressure as the driving force to allow accurate infusion at pre-set rates (see Ch. 40).

Adult TPN formulations can have a volume ranging from about 1500 mL to 4000 mL. The infusion period varies from 24 hours in hospital to around 8–12 hours for home patients (as HPN can often be administered overnight). Infusion rate can be calculated by dividing the total volume of the infusion (mL) by the infusion period (hours) giving a rate of mL/hour. Most pumps now have the ability to be programmed to give an infusion rate which 'steps up' at the beginning and 'steps down' at the end of the infusion period, avoiding potential problems with high concentrations of dextrose in the formulation. They are also fitted with an alarm which will alert the patient if a technical fault arises.

Potential problems for HPN patents

Mechanical problems

Problems of pneumothorax, or air embolism, are more likely to occur in the hospital environment in the early stages of catheter placement and are dealt with before the patient commences on HPN. However, daily connection and disconnection of the catheter hub may result in cracking and possible leakage of the HPN fluid. Repair kits are available, and if used promptly when the problem first arises, catheter replacement may not be necessary.

Internal blockage of the catheter can arise. Patients are taught to flush out the catheter port with heparinized saline to prevent thrombus formation. Blockage of the line arising during administration of the HPN fluid can cause changes in flow rate which are recognized by the pump, and the alarm is activated.

Metabolic problems

Metabolic complications include:
- Problems with electrolyte levels leading to conditions such as hypernatraemia or hyponatraemia
- Problems with glucose levels leading to hyperglycaemia or hypoglycaemia
- Balancing of fluid intake (to ensure adequate hydration is achieved)
- Altered liver enzymes which can be resolved by amending the TPN prescription
- Metabolic bone disease, monitored by regular bone scans.

The majority of the metabolic complications which can affect HPN patients can be overcome by careful monitoring of the patient initially in hospital and with regular check-ups and home visits by the nutrition nurse.

Catheter-related complications

Catheter-related infections can arise as a result of poor management of the catheter exit site. Infection is distinguished by pain, redness and tenderness around the site and rigors when feeding through the line. To minimize such infections, staff in the hospital are trained to use strict aseptic procedures when changing TPN bags and use of the catheter port is restricted to administration of the TPN bag only. HPN patients are taught the same aseptic techniques and are required to carry out these procedures at all times when changing bags at home. Home-care patients are also taught to be aware of their own physical condition and to be alert to any deterioration in their medical condition at the earliest possible time. Patients are asked to contact their nutrition nurse if they experience any signs or symptoms of infection around the catheter site. Many centres will now try and treat the line infection rather than remove the infected line.

Psychological and social problems

Patients receiving TPN in hospital or at home must learn to adapt to the changes occurring in their lifestyle. Some patients have, over a prolonged period of time, suffered from a general deterioration in their health and as a result adapt well to the initiation of parenteral nutrition as it improves their quality of life. Other patients require TPN as a result of major trauma and these patients find the dramatic changes in their lifestyle very difficult to cope with.

While in the hospital receiving treatment, patients have the constant support of medical and nursing staff who can help them to cope with any practical difficulties encountered. The clinical psychologist will review many patients before discharge and coping strategies will be discussed. When patients return to the home-care setting they need continued support to enable them to cope with their HPN therapy on their own. The ability of patients to adapt to HPN is highly dependent on a number of factors:

- Patient's underlying medical condition
- Physical ability and capability of the patient
- Training and counselling prior to leaving hospital
- Home circumstances, particularly support from family members and the patient's GP

- Ability to deal with physical and emotional changes in lifestyle, e.g. dependence on others, potential for mood swings and clinical depression. Disruption to normal sleeping pattern during administration of the HPN bag overnight and loss of 'social' eating can be difficult for many patients, particularly in the initial stages of HPN.

To enable a smooth transition from hospital to home to be achieved, patients require the services of the nutrition nurse and other healthcare workers to teach them the necessary skills required for handling, setting up their HPN bags and disconnecting them once the procedure is complete.

Training for HPN patients

Health care which can be provided at home has a number of advantages. Patients have a better quality of life and can become more independent as their confidence in providing self-care increases. However, motivation and confidence to carry out the required manipulations at home are essential. Thus training in the hospital environment is required to build up the necessary skills and techniques.

When a patient has been selected for home care, a nutrition nurse will begin a training programme with the patient to teach the practical skills required for safe and effective administration of the TPN bag at home. If the patient is unable to care for the line, a carer or district nurse may be trained to administer the TPN. A discharge plan is required for each patient working towards home care. The British Association of Parenteral and Enteral Nutrition (BAPEN), a registered charity formed in 1992, has laid down guidelines for the provision of nutritional care at home. Individual hospitals will develop their own guidelines based on the advice given by BAPEN. The scope of BAPEN includes guidelines on the following matters:

- Details which should be included in a patient discharge plan
- Knowledge and practical skills which must be achieved by patients prior to discharge
- Guidelines for GPs on the provision of HPN
- Advice on how to liaise with patients' GPs to ensure that everyone is aware of their responsibilities
- Information regarding the supplier of the HPN bags and equipment and how this service will be provided

- Details of appropriate people who patients can contact for advice and help with any problems they have.

The length of time required for training can vary depending on the patient's underlying medical condition and personal approach to training. Patients must be taught aseptic techniques and the importance of ensuring that they are carried out correctly. They must demonstrate their skills and competence on several occasions prior to leaving the hospital. Training will take place during the day initially, then, as the patient becomes more confident with the techniques, overnight feeding will be started. This allows the patient to lead as normal a life as possible and allows some patients to return to a working environment. Areas covered during the training period include:

- Aseptic techniques for setting up and disconnecting the HPN bag
- Care of the catheter site
- How to deal with problems of the catheter blocking
- Setting the pump for infusion of the HPN bag
- Dealing with simple mechanical problems with the pump.

Information booklets on HPN and educational videos can be used with patients to reinforce the training received in hospital.

Services provided by home-care companies

Patients receiving home care will require certain practical arrangements to be put in place before HPN can be initiated. Home-care companies who provide services to HPN patients normally provide the following items for patient use: a refrigerator for storing HPN bags; a trolley for patients to set up their HPN bags aseptically; a drip stand and an infusion pump. Patients are required to have adequate storage space to keep any extra components which may be required for HPN administration and easy access to hand washing facilities for use prior to setting up their HPN bag. A home assessment will be completed by the home-care company and a nutrition nurse from the hospital before discharge to ensure the patient's home circumstances are suitable for HPN. Most home-care companies have nurses in their employ to support the patients at home.

Support services provided for HPN patients

Patients will be metabolically stable prior to transfer to the home-care setting, hence frequency of monitoring will be reduced to a minimum. Patients can have monthly check-ups at the hospital initially, reducing to 3-monthly as they adapt to life on HPN. During visits, patients may be seen by the multidisciplinary nutrition team and reviewed by each member of the team. The pharmacist on the team will arrange any changes in the patient's TPN prescription. Routine monitoring can be carried out during these visits, including the following:

- Checking the patient's underlying medical condition
- Reviewing the patient's nutritional status, particularly in relation to their weight
- Routine haematological and biochemical tests
- Checking for any cardiovascular complications
- Reviewing the patient's psychological state.

The nutrition nurse will make home visits if required to check on aseptic techniques and any practical difficulties being encountered by patients and/or their partner or carer.

Patients on HPN can benefit from the support of others undergoing nutrition therapy at home. This is made possible by an organization called 'PINNT' (Patients on Intravenous and Nasogastric Nutrition Therapy). This is a charitable organization which aims to support and bring together people who have similar medical conditions and could benefit from the moral support of others who understand the problems they face. PINNT provides practical help in areas such as provision of portable equipment for people on HPN who wish to go on holiday; help with holiday arrangements including appropriate travel insurance; and general advice on benefits available to HPN patients. A newsletter is produced on a regular basis and close links are kept between PINNT and BAPEN to ensure that patient needs are adequately met.

The British Parenteral Nutrition Group

Pharmacists in the UK can keep up to date with the working of organizations like PINNT and BAPEN by joining the British Parenteral Nutrition Group (BPNG). Currently BPNG has a large membership, most of whom are hospital pharmacists working in the NHS. However, membership also includes dieticians, nutrition nurses, research workers and members of commercial companies who work in the field of TPN and HPN. The BPNG exists to further the practice of TPN through a number of activities including research, contributing to the work of BAPEN and arranging symposia on practical and scientific developments in the field. This group is also one of five constituent groups which make up BAPEN. Hence good communication is achieved between the different sectors of health care who provide care for home and hospital patients receiving nutrition support.

Introduction to kidney disease and dialysis therapy

Like HPN, dialysis at home is now a more regular occurrence. Patients requiring dialysis at home have end-stage renal disease/failure which may have occurred acutely or may be the result of chronic kidney disease.

Chronic kidney disease

Chronic kidney disease (CKD) is relatively common, affecting approximately 1 in 10 people in the general population. The most common causes are hypertension and diabetes, with less common causes such as glomerulonephritis and pyelonephritis. CKD may also be inherited, for example polycystic kidney disease or kidney stones. Some common drug therapy may also lead to kidney disease.

End-stage renal failure (ESRF) is the result of progressive kidney disease which leads to an irreversible and life-threatening loss of function.

Patients with ESRF may be suitable for renal replacement therapy (RRT) or may choose conservative treatment and opt not to have renal replacement therapy at all. There are a number of types of RRT, for example kidney transplantation, haemodialysis or peritoneal dialysis. Unfortunately over 30% of patients are unsuitable for transplantation and for a number of patients a suitable donor may not be found. For these patients, transplantation may not therefore be an option and a chronic RRT is required. For most patients with ESRF who wish to have renal replacement therapy, there are two choices, either long-term haemodialysis (HD) or peritoneal dialysis (PD) therapy, although patients may not be suitable for both

modalities and may change from one to the other at various times according to need.

RRT with dialysis replaces only some of the functions of the kidneys and is an artificial method of filtering toxins and breakdown products from the blood. It does not replicate normal renal function and does not provide any of the metabolic functions of the kidney such as insulin metabolism or the hormonal functions such as erythropoietin production. RRT with HD or PD uses a combination of dialysis therapy to remove unwanted solutes by the process of diffusion and haemofiltration and ultrafiltration to remove water.

Epidemiology

In 2000, over 5000 patients in England and Wales started some form of RRT and the estimated annual rate is 89 per million of the population in the UK. The number of people receiving dialysis varies from 300 to 700 per million of the population.

Dialysis

Dialysis is commenced to treat, or to prevent, life-threatening hyperkalaemia, acidosis or hypervolaemic pulmonary oedema or to treat complications of CKD, for example pericarditis, uraemic neuropathy or seizures.

Haemodialysis

HD is a process where blood is filtered to remove waste products. The patient is connected to a dialysis machine where blood is removed from the patient's body and filtered by passing it over an artificial semipermeable membrane into dialysis fluid. The waste products are retained within the dialysis fluid and the blood returned into the body.

There are a number of different HD machines available and the process varies slightly depending upon the different equipment required, choice of dialysis fluid and the frequency and duration of dialysis session.

To facilitate HD, access to the patient's bloodstream must be established, either using a surgically created arteriovenous fistula where an artery is joined to a vein during a minor surgical operation, a graft, where the join between the artery and vein is made using a synthetic tube, or by inserting a permanent or temporary central vascular catheter into a large vein such as the subclavian, jugular or femoral vein.

HD usually takes 3–4 hours each time and will be required, on average, three times a week for most patients. The blood is removed and passed over a membrane with a large surface area to allow solutes to be exchanged between the blood and dialysis fluid. Dialysis membranes are sterile disposable membranes made of cellulose or polycarbonate materials. Pressure is applied to the blood in the machine to induce an ultrafiltration process and allow removal of excess water in addition to the removal of toxins.

Dialysis fluid is composed of similar constituents to plasma:

- Sodium
- Potassium
- Chloride
- Calcium
- Magnesium
- Glucose
- Bicarbonate, citrate or lactate is added to buffer the solution.

To promote potassium removal from the blood, the dialysate potassium concentration is variable and is usually lower than that in the plasma. To prevent the blood clotting in the dialysis circuit, unfractionated heparin, low molecular weight heparin or prostacyclin may be used.

During the HD process there are a number of potential complications such as low blood pressure, air embolus and blood loss.

HD may be carried out in a variety of settings providing the appropriate equipment and water supply is available. Locations include specialist hospital units at a renal dialysis satellite unit (linked to a specialist unit) or in the patient's own home. The dialysis process follows the same principles in all settings.

Hospital-based haemodialysis

Trained specialist nurses or healthcare assistants usually carry this out. Patients occasionally have direct responsibility for their treatment; however, it is more common for the dialysis to be managed by a team of doctors, nurses and other healthcare professionals. Patients travel to the unit three times a week on a fixed alternate day schedule, though some may have more regular or longer dialysis sessions.

In a satellite unit, patients sometimes play a more active role in their treatment. They are supervised by trained staff but may prepare the dialysis machine or carry out the dialysis process themselves.

Home haemodialysis

Home HD may be suitable for a limited number of patients. At present they represent less than 3% of the dialysis population, although this varies between units from zero to 15% of the dialysis population. The National Institute for Health and Clinical Excellence (TAC 48) recommends that all suitable patients should be offered home HD.

There are a number of advantages to home HD:

- Greater independence for the patient
- Excellent long-term outcome
- Improved blood pressure control
- Lower hospital admission rates
- Fewer limitations on timing of dialysis
- Greater flexibility
- No transport difficulties
- Optimal use of resources.

There are a number of factors that determine a patient's suitability for home HD. For example, patients must be able and motivated to learn and perform dialysis at home and be capable of maintaining and monitoring their own treatment observations. They must be medically stable and be free of complications that make dialysis difficult. Patients also require good functioning vascular access, support from family or carers and suitable space and facilities must be available. Any patients considered suitable for home HD will be assessed, including their home circumstances. They will undergo a comprehensive training programme to develop skills and techniques in addition to developing confidence and self-reliance.

Peritoneal dialysis

In PD, the dialysis fluid is passed directly into the patient's body and, in contrast to HD, no blood removal occurs. The peritoneal membrane which lines the abdominal cavity has a large surface area and a good capillary blood supply. It is this semi-permeable membrane that is used to perform PD and allows excess water and waste products to be removed from the blood.

Dialysis fluid is instilled into the peritoneal cavity through a surgically inserted indwelling catheter which goes through the abdominal wall. The distal end of the catheter has tiny holes in it to allow the dialysis fluid to flow freely into the peritoneal cavity. Fluid is removed from the blood by ultrafiltration down an osmotic pressure gradient. Solutes and toxins cross the peritoneal membrane through diffusion and solvent drag with water.

There are two main methods of PD – continuous ambulatory peritoneal dialysis (CAPD) and automated peritoneal dialysis (APD).

In CAPD, patients generally carry out three or four PD exchanges every 24 hours and this is the most common form of home dialysis. In APD, patients are connected to a machine for 8–12 hours, often overnight. The machine utilizes a pump delivery system which warms the dialysis fluid prior to administration and delivers a carefully programmed volume of dialysis fluid which exchanges throughout the infusion period. The home patient or a carer will set the machine every night by connecting it to the catheter. This method of dialysis has advantages for the patient as it allows freedom from dialysis during the day.

A variety of dialysis fluids is available and each patient will be prescribed a specific tailored regimen of dialysis fluids. The volume will be determined in part by the available abdominal space. For adults, the range is 1 litre to 7 litres.

The composition of the dialysate consists of sodium, calcium, glucose or dextran to increase or decrease osmolality.

The dialysis exchange requires strict aseptic technique and a number of different systems may be employed. The most popular is a disconnect system. Dialysis fluid is warmed to body temperature and both this and a drainage bag are attached to the abdominal catheter. Fluid is drained out from the abdominal catheter into the empty bag and new dialysate is instilled from the warmed bag. The bags are then disconnected and the fluid left in place for 4–8 hours. The dialysate in the abdominal cavity drains in and out under gravity and by capillary blood flow.

The advantages of PD include the following:

- Independence – as the dialysis does not require hospital attendance or complex plumbing or machinery
- Continuous dialysis process is preferable as the haemodynamic fluctuations are minimized
- Blood loss is avoided compared with HD, resulting in less anaemia
- Cost savings in comparison with HD
- Less fluid and dietary restriction.

Disadvantages include:

- Infections of the peritoneum
- Glucose absorption from the dialysate
- Protein loss
- Treatment failure if the peritoneum is damaged.

Community dialysis teams

Community dialysis teams provide support to patients undertaking dialysis at home – both HD and PD. Most teams are multidisciplinary with highly trained medical and nursing staff making decisions regarding the treatment and providing the care and support through regular home visits to monitor patients. The team will usually have strong links with the wider multidisciplinary team which includes dieticians, pharmacists, renal technicians and social workers.

Each member of the renal team will have specific responsibilities:

- The medical and nursing team will be involved with prescribing of dialysis programmes and clinical monitoring
- The dietician advises on nutritional intake and any dietary restrictions required
- The pharmacist provides medicines advice and may have a role in the ordering and supply of dialysis fluids and ancillary products
- The social worker provides advice and practical help for patients
- The renal technician is responsible for the programming, servicing and functioning of dialysis machines.

UK Renal Pharmacy Group (UKRPG)

The UK Renal Pharmacy Group (UKRPG) is affiliated to the British Renal Society and is a specialist interest group for pharmacists and pharmacy technicians working in the field of renal medicine or with an interest in renal pharmacy. The UKRPG uses its clinical pharmacy experience to compile *The Renal Drug Handbook* and *An introduction to Renal Therapeutics*; both publications are excellent reference sources for further reading.

KEY POINTS

- Up to half of medical and surgical patients can have nutritional deficiencies
- TPN/HPN formulations are prepared under strict aseptic conditions
- Before starting TPN, a full assessment of the patient's nutritional needs must be made

- The nutrition team contribute their expertise to provide good patient care by meeting regularly to monitor patient needs
- A TPN formulation may contain water, protein, carbohydrate, fat, electrolytes, trace elements, vitamins and minerals
- Most TPN patients have a negative nitrogen balance and so require amino acids
- Care must be taken when administering dextrose in a TPN/HPN formulation to prevent problems of hyper- or hypoglycaemia
- Strictly defined procedures are followed when adding ingredients to TPN bags during preparation
- Stability of TPN formulations is one of the major issues which must be carefully considered
- Controlling quantities can minimize incompatibilities such as that between calcium and phosphate
- TPN bags containing a fat component become less stable on prolonged storage and could result in fat deposits arising in lungs and capillaries if administered in this unstable condition
- For TPN lasting longer than 4 weeks, a central vein should be used
- A number of problems can arise during TPN/HPN administration. For HPN patients, adequate

- training to deal with problems arising at home is essential
- HPN patients require to make psychological and social adjustments, but can also have an improvement in quality of life
- BAPEN has laid down standards for home nutritional care which are used as the basis for patient training prior to discharge
- Dialysis is used to remove toxic metabolites, correct acid–base balance and avoid fluid overload
- In haemodialysis, the patient's blood is passed over a semi-permeable membrane to allow exchange of small solutes with dialysis fluid
- Peritoneal dialysis uses the peritoneal membrane as the semi-permeable membrane, the dialysis fluid staying in the peritoneal cavity during the exchange
- CAPD has a number of advantages and disadvantages for patients
- HD solutions do not require to be sterile, but PD solutions must be sterile and aseptic technique used in handling
- Home dialysis patients will require training and support

42

Radiopharmacy

David Graham

STUDY POINTS

- Types of radionuclides and the principles of their medical use
- Examples of alpha-emitters, beta$^-$- and beta$^+$- emitters, electron capture and isomeric transitions
- Radionuclide production of beta$^+$-emitters
- Principles of using a molybdenum-technetium generator
- Preparation of ^{99m}Tc radiopharmaceuticals
- Safety in radiopharmacy

Introduction

Elements that emit radiation are known as radionuclides and have a number of applications in medicine. Radiopharmacy in hospital practice is concerned with the manufacture or preparation of radioactive medicines known as radiopharmaceuticals. These have two main applications in medicine:

- As an aid to the diagnosis of disease (diagnostic radiopharmaceuticals)
- In the treatment of disease (therapeutic radiopharmaceuticals).

Diagnostic radiopharmaceuticals may be classified into two types:

- Radiopharmaceuticals used in tracer techniques for measuring physiological parameters (e.g. ^{51}Cr-EDTA for measuring glomerular filtration rate)
- Radiopharmaceuticals for diagnostic imaging (e.g. ^{99m}Tc-methylene diphosphonate (MDP) used in bone scanning).

In diagnostic imaging, gamma-emitting radionuclides are used, since their interaction with tissue is much less than that of particulate emitters and will cause significantly less damage to tissue. Radiopharmaceuticals are administered to the patient, usually by the intravenous (IV) route, and distribute into a particular organ. The radiation is then detected externally using a special scintillation detector known as a gamma-camera. These are used by nuclear medicine departments to image the distribution of the radiopharmaceutical within the patient's body. Using the gamma-camera in conjunction with a computer system it is not only possible to produce static images of an organ, but also to examine how the radiopharmaceutical moves through an organ. These dynamic images describe how the organ is functioning. It is also possible to create images in three dimensions, a process known as single photon emission computerized tomography (SPECT) when used in combination with gamma-emitting radionuclides such as ^{99m}Tc and positron emission tomography (PET) when used in combination with positron-emitting radionuclides such as ^{18}F.

It is important to note that for the safe production of radiopharmaceuticals, the radiopharmacy must be designed to comply with, and procedures must follow, good manufacturing practice and good radiation protection practice. Radiopharmacists working in this field are part of a multidisciplinary team which includes physicians, physicists, radiochemists and technicians from the field of pharmacy as well as nuclear medicine. As part of this team, they not only ensure that the radiopharmaceuticals will give high-quality clinical information, but also that they are safe for both patient and user alike.

Radionuclides used in nuclear medicine

Alpha-emitters

Alpha-decay is the process whereby a nucleus emits a helium nucleus, or alpha-particle. This commonly occurs with heavy nuclei (e.g. ^{226}Ra: $^{226}_{88}$Ra $\rightarrow$ $^{222}_{86}$Rn + alpha).

Because they are heavy and positively charged, alpha-particles travel only short distances in air ($\sim$5 mm) and only micrometer distances in tissues. Their ionizing nature would result in a highly localized radiation dose if taken internally and hence they tend not to be used in radiopharmaceuticals.

Some alpha-emitters (e.g. ^{137}Cs) when encapsulated are used as sealed sources, emitting X-rays or gamma-rays for radiotherapy applications. Here the body is exposed to radiation externally in an attempt to treat malignant tumours.

Beta-emitters

Beta-decay occurs in two ways, one that involves the emission of a negatively charged beta$^-$-particle, or electron, and the other that involves the emission of a positively charged beta$^+$-particle, or positron.

Beta$^-$-emitters

Radionuclides which decay by beta$^-$-decay tend to have nuclei that are neutron rich. They attempt to reach a more stable state by the transformation of a neutron into a proton with the emission of a beta$^-$-particle. (e.g. ^{32}P: $^{32}_{15}$P $\rightarrow$ $^{32}_{16}$S + beta$^-$). Despite beta$^-$-particles having a range in air of up to several meters, their range in tissues is only a few millimetres. Because of this and their highly ionizing nature, beta$^-$-emitters tend to be used in therapeutic radiopharmaceuticals (Table 42.1).

The principle of therapeutic treatment with radionuclides is to target the radionuclide to a specific tissue within the body in an attempt to selectively damage or destroy that tissue. Ideally therapeutic beta$^-$-emitting radionuclides should have energies of 0.5–1.5 MeV and a half-life of several days to provide a prolonged radiobiological effect.

The most widely used example of this is ^{131}I-sodium iodide which is used in the treatment of hyperactive thyroid disease and in certain thyroid tumours. Here the physiological property of thyroid tissue is exploited to target the radionuclide to the site of action. Since thyroid tissue avidly takes up iodine in the normal synthesis of the hormone levothyroxine, radioactive iodine is also taken up and held in the thyroid tissue. Hence the radiation damage is targeted to the thyroid tissue specifically and the normal excretion of any excess iodine results in no significant damage to other organs and tissues.

Beta$^+$-emitters

Radionuclides that emit positrons are becoming more widely used in nuclear medicine. In this transformation, a proton-rich nuclide attempts to achieve stability by converting a proton to a neutron with the emission of a positron (e.g. ^{11}C: $^{11}_{6}$C $\rightarrow$ $^{11}_{5}$S + beta$^+$ + gamma). The positron is very short-lived,

Table 42.1 Examples of radionuclides used in nuclear medicine

Mode of decay	Radionuclide	Radiopharmaceutical	Half-life	Clinical use
Beta$^-$-emitters	^{131}I	Sodium iodide capsules	8 days	Thyrotoxicosis, thyroid carcinomas
	^{89}Sr	Strontium chloride injection	50 days	Palliation of pain from bone metastases
Beta$^+$-emitters	^{15}O	^{15}O$_2$ gas	2.04 min	Brain blood flow imaging
	^{11}C	^{11}C-methionine	20.4 min	Prostate cancer
	^{13}N	^{13}N ammonia	9.97 min	Cardiac perfusion
	^{18}F	Fluorodeoxy-glucose injection	109.8 min	Tumour detection
Electron capture	^{111}In	Indium chloride solution	67 h	Antibody labelling
	^{123}I	Sodium iodide injection	13 h	Thyroid imaging
Isomeric transition	^{99m}Tc	Sodium pertechnetate injection	6 h	See Table 42.2
	^{81m}Kr	Krypton gas	13 s	Lung ventilation imaging

since it interacts with an electron resulting in an an-nihilation reaction and the conversion of both parti-cles into electromagnetic (EM) radiation. This EM radiation is in the form of two gamma-rays, each hav-ing energy of 0.511 MeV, which are emitted at an angle of $180°$ to each other.

When used in conjunction with a specialized gamma-camera with detectors placed $180°$ apart, it is possible to create images in all three dimensions with the position of the radiopharmaceutical being very precisely known. This type of imaging technique is known as positron emission tomography (PET). There are a number of positron emitting radionuclides which are becoming important tools in diagnostic imaging. Currently ^{18}F labelled glucose, known as ^{18}F-fluoro deoxy-glucose (^{18}F-FDG), is the most commonly used PET radiopharmaceutical in hospital practice and as a result the production processes for it will be described in simplified form and used as an example. However, it should be noted there are four main positron emitters used to prepare radio-pharmaceuticals (see Table 42.1). PET imaging with ^{18}F-FDG, in combination with X-ray computerized tomography (CT) is rapidly becoming an important imaging technique in the diagnosis of cancer.

In the manufacture of ^{18}F-FDG there are two main processes required. First there is the production of the radionuclide itself, which is produced in a cyclotron facility. This is followed by the radio-synthesis of the ^{18}F-FDG, which is carried out in an automated appa-ratus, known as a synthesis module. The resulting solution of ^{18}F-FDG has then to be sterilized and may have to be sub-dispensed in some way so as to provide the injection in a ready to administer form. Since the ^{18}F-FDG has been synthesized, it will require analysis and other quality control checks prior to administration to the patient.

Radionuclide production

A cyclotron is a device used to produce radionuclides. It accelerates atomic or subatomic particles in a cir-cular orbit, increasing the energy of the particles until a high-energy beam of particles is created. Once the particles have reached their maximum energy they are extracted using high voltage and allowed to bom-bard target materials. The composition of the target material and the nuclear reactions that take place determine the radionuclides that are produced.

For ^{18}F production, the most common nuclear reaction used is the ^{18}O (p,n) ^{18}F reaction where

protons are produced from hydrogen gas and are accelerated until, at a required energy, a 'beam' of the protons are allowed to bombard a target of ^{18}O-enriched water ($H_2{}^{18}O$). ^{18}O is a naturally occurring isotope of oxygen, but much less abundant than the normal ^{16}O. By forcing a proton into the ^{18}O nucleus the now unstable nucleus ejects a neutron and the result is the production of ^{18}F – a positron-emitting radionuclide.

Radio-synthesis

2-[^{18}F] fluoro-2-deoxy-D glucose (^{18}F-FDG) may be prepared by various chemical pathways, but whatever radio-synthetic route is used it must be rapid to min-imize the radiation risk and be of high yield. An auto-mated apparatus, the synthesis module, is used to synthesize the ^{18}F-FDG to assure production efficien-cy and keep radiation exposure to a minimum. There are now commercially available synthesis modules such as the TRACERlabFx Synthesizer® as shown in Figure 42.1, which are supplied with good manu-facturing practice (GMP) standard raw materials and reagents for use in the module. Using this equipment, the following synthetic pathway is performed:

1. The ^{18}F-fluoride is adsorbed by an anion-exchange resin.
2. The retained ^{18}F-fluoride is eluted using an aqueous potassium carbonate solution.
3. A phase transfer catalyst (Kriptofix 222) dissolved in acetonitrile is then added, to bind the potassium ion and to enhance the nucleophilic reactivity of the ^{18}F-fluoride.
4. After evaporation of the solvents, the ^{18}F-fluoride is allowed to react with the reagent mannose triflate at elevated temperature (1,3,4,6-O-Acetyl-2-O-trifluoromethanesulfonyl-beta-D-mannopyranose). The structure of mannose triflate is similar to that of glucose with a leaving group (triflate) and four acetyl protecting groups to ensure the mannose ring undergoes nucleophilic substitution at the second carbon atom.
5. Hydrolysis under acidic or alkaline conditions also at elevated temperature yields 2-[^{18}F] fluoro-2-deoxy-D glucose (^{18}F-FDG).

Sterilization and sub-dispensing

Sterilization of the ^{18}F-FDG is achieved either by filtration through a 0.2 µm filter, although there are

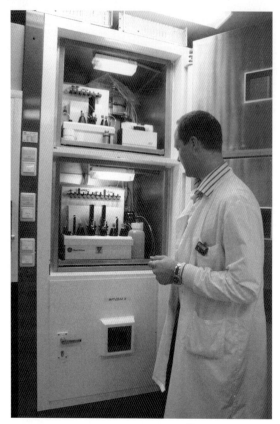

Figure 42.1 • Synthesis module for ^{18}F-FDG production (TRACERlabFx Synthesizer®. (Courtesy of GE Healthcare plc.) Module located in lead-shielded (5.5 cm) specialized fume cupboard known as 'hot cell'.

now automated systems that use high temperature short sterilization cycles (e.g. 10 minute cycle consisting of 4 minutes heat up; 135°C for 3.5 minutes; 2.5 minute cool down). Sub-dispensing or fractionation of the bulk solution into patient doses is then carried out using robotic dispensing systems that perform the aseptic transfers since the radiation hazard is too great for regular manual aseptic transfer. This aseptic manipulation is carried out within a specialized isolator specifically designed for handling PET radiopharmaceuticals.

Quality control

Since the ^{18}F-FDG has been synthesized, it must undergo stringent testing as outlined in the monograph given in the *European Pharmacopoeia*. A detailed description is beyond the scope of this chapter, but in summary the tests will include:

- Identification test
- Determination of pH
- Sterility test
- Determination of bacterial endotoxins
- Determination of chemical purity
- Determination of radionuclide purity
- Determination of radiochemical purity
- Determination of the radioactivity.

Electron capture

Nuclei that are proton rich may, as an alternative to positron emission, capture electrons from the atom's electron orbital. This process results in the transformation of a proton to a neutron within the nucleus. The subsequent rearrangement of the electrons orbiting the nucleus results in a characteristic emission of X-rays or gamma-rays (e.g. ^{123}I: $^{123}_{53}$I + electron → $^{123}_{53}$Te + gamma).

Radionuclides which decay by electron capture are useful in diagnostic imaging since they emit gamma-rays; examples are given in Table 42.1.

Isomeric transition

Some radionuclides exist for measurable periods in excited, or isomeric, states prior to reaching ground state. This form of decay involves the emission of a gamma-ray and is known as isomeric transition. When radionuclides exist in this transitional state, they are known as metastable, which is denoted by the letter 'm' and written thus: ^{99m}Tc.

A simplified decay scheme for ^{99m}Tc-technetium is shown in Figure 42.2 where ^{99m}Tc's parent radionuclide, molybdenum (^{99}Mo), decays by beta$^-$– emission to the ground state ^{99}Tc either directly or indirectly.

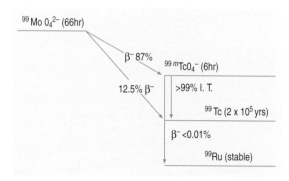

Figure 42.2 • Diagrammatic representation of ^{99}Mo decay.

The indirect route, which is the most common, involves the isomer ^{99m}Tc, which in turn decays from its metastable state to ^{99}Tc by isomeric transition.

Radionuclides which decay by this process are used in diagnostic imaging since they emit gamma-rays (see Table 42.1). It should be noted that ^{99m}Tc is the most widely used radionuclide in hospital radiopharmacy today, making up the radionuclide component of around 90% of the radiopharmaceuticals produced. For these reasons the production processes for ^{99m}Tc-radiopharmaceuticals will be especially emphasized.

Principles of ^{99m}Tc-radiopharmaceutical production

The physical and chemical properties of ^{99m}Tc make it nearly ideal for imaging purposes as outlined below:

- It has a 6-hour half-life ($T_{1/2}$); long enough to allow imaging to take place in the working day, while also being short enough that patients are not radioactive for long periods (in 24 hours, or 4 half-lives, the radioactivity will have decayed by 94%).
- ^{99m}Tc emits gamma-rays of 140 keV energy: ideal for use with the modern gamma-camera.
- There are no particulate emissions that, if present, would add to the patient's radiation dose.
- By purchasing a device known as a ^{99}Mo/^{99m}Tc-generator, ^{99m}Tc can be made readily available to the hospital site in a sterile and pyrogen-free form.
- ^{99m}Tc has versatile coordination chemistry and will allow a large number of ligands to complex with it. By using different ligands in the radiopharmaceutical's formulation, a wide range of radiopharmaceuticals can be prepared in the radiopharmacy, providing for the many different investigations carried out in nuclear medicine departments (Table 42.2).

Table 42.2 Examples of ^{99m}Tc-radiopharmaceuticals

Radiopharmaceutical	Organ or tissue of distribution	Main clinical application
^{99m}Tc-sodium pertechnetate	Thyroid	Imaging the thyroid gland and ectopic tissue
	Salivary gland	Dynamic images of accumulation and drainage to show gland function
	Gastric mucosa	Presence of Meckels diverticulum containing gastric mucosa
^{99m}Tc-methylene diphosphonate (MDP)	Skeleton	Bone metastases from carcinoma of lung, breast and prostrate
^{99m}Tc-macro-aggregates of albumin (MAA)	Lung blood flow	Lung perfusion studies most commonly for the diagnosis of pulmonary embolism
^{99m}Tc-exametazime (HM. PAO)	Brain blood flow	Regional cerebral imaging in stroke and tumours. Diagnosis of Alzheimer's dementia
^{99m}Tc-exametazime (HM. PAO) labelled leucocytes	Infection or inflammation	Identification of abscesses associated with pyrexia of unknown origin. Extent of inflammatory bowel disease
^{99m}Tc-tetrofosmin	Heart	Cardiac perfusion imaging
^{99m}Tc-sestamibi (MIBI)	Heart	Cardiac perfusion imaging
^{99m}Tc-tin colloid	Liver	Location of hepatic tumours, abscesses and cysts. Detection of cirrhosis
^{99m}Tc-mercapto triglycine (MAG 3)	Kidney	Dynamic studies to study kidney function
^{99m}Tc-dimercapto-succinic acid (DMSA)	Kidney	Static imaging showing the kidney structure

The production of ^{99m}Tc – the molybdenum/technetium generator

Radionuclides with long half-lives (e.g. ^{131}I, $T_{1/2}$ = 8 days) can be easily transported from production site to the user hospital. With shorter half-life radionuclides, e.g. ^{99m}Tc, this supply system would be extremely difficult. As a result, a device known as the radionuclide generator is used to provide ^{99m}Tc to the hospital site.

Radionuclide generators work on the principle that they contain a relatively long-lived 'parent' radionuclide that decays to produce a 'daughter' radionuclide. The chemical nature of parent and daughter are different, allowing separation of the daughter from the parent.

The molybdenum/technetium generator consists of ^{99}Mo (long-lived 'parent') absorbed onto an alumina-filled column, the ^{99}Mo being present in the form of molybdate (^{99}MoO$_4^{2-}$). ^{99}Mo decays to its 'daughter' radionuclide ^{99m}Tc, as pertechnetate, ^{99m}TcO$_4^-$ (see Fig. 42.2). The amount of ^{99m}TcO$_4^-$ grows as a result of the decay of ^{99}Mo, until a transient equilibrium is reached. At this point the amount of ^{99m}Tc in the column appears to decay with the half-life of ^{99}Mo (Fig. 42.3).

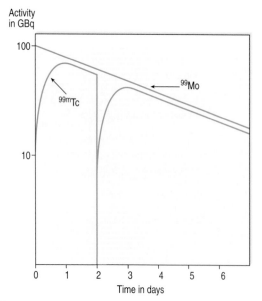

Figure 42.3 • Radioactivity changes with time in a molybdenum/technetium generator column.

By drawing a solution of sodium chloride 0.9% weight in volume (w/v) through the column, ^{99m}Tc is removed from the column in the form of sodium pertechnetate, Na^{99m}TcO$_4$. This process is known as eluting the generator and the resulting solution as the eluate. This process results in the production of a sterile solution of sodium pertechnetate that may now be used to make ^{99m}Tc -radiopharmaceuticals.

^{99}Mo remains on the column where it decays to produce further ^{99m}Tc, the equilibrium being re-established about 23 hours after elution. Elution of the generator is repeated daily to provide the radiopharmacy with a supply of ^{99m}Tc for 7–14 days, beyond which the yield of ^{99m}Tc becomes too small to be useful. Hospital radiopharmacies tend to buy generators on a weekly basis to provide a continuous supply of ^{99m}Tc.

Design of a ^{99m}Tc-generator

The design of a typical generator will be described by reference to the GE Healthcare generator, Drytec (Fig. 42.4). The main components of this generator are:

• A needle connected to the top end of the alumina column by tubing (it is this needle upon which a vial of IV Sodium Chloride Intravenous Infusion BP 0.9% w/v will be placed)
• A sterile alumina column to which is bound ^{99}Mo
• An elution needle which is connected to the bottom end of the alumina column
• Two 0.22 µm filters.

These components are housed within a compact plastic casing. The alumina column is encased in lead to give protection from the radiation.

Operating the generator is fairly straightforward. A vial of Sodium Chloride Intravenous Infusion BP 0.9% w/v, supplied with the generator, is first placed on the left hand needle (see Fig. 42.4). A sterile evacuated vial, also supplied with the generator, is placed in a lead pot designed for the elution process. Then, by placing this on the elution needle, the vacuum draws sterile Sodium Chloride Intravenous Infusion BP 0.9% w/v from the vial through the column and into the evacuated vial. When eluate has been collected, air enters the elution vial after first passing through the column. This dries the column as well as removing excess vacuum in the elution vial. The elution process is now complete and the vial may be removed from the generator.

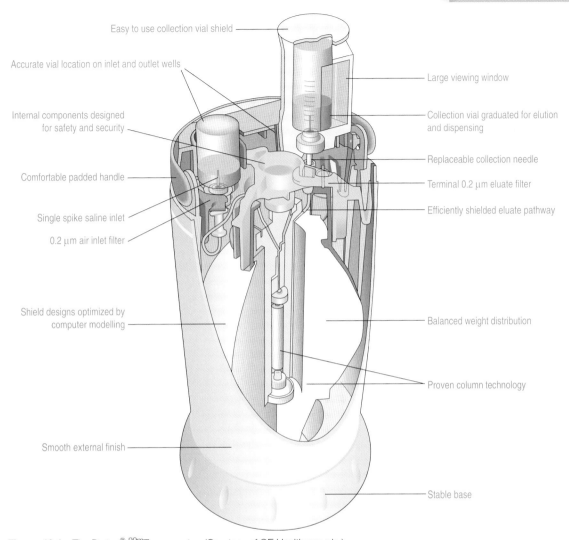

Easy to use collection vial shield

Accurate vial location on inlet and outlet wells

Internal components designed for safety and security

Comfortable padded handle

Single spike saline inlet

0.2 µm air inlet filter

Shield designs optimized by computer modelling

Smooth external finish

Large viewing window

Collection vial graduated for elution and dispensing

Replaceable collection needle

Terminal 0.2 µm eluate filter

Efficiently shielded eluate pathway

Balanced weight distribution

Proven column technology

Stable base

Figure 42.4 • The Drytec® ^{99m}Tc-generator. (Courtesy of GE Healthcare plc.)

The sterility of the eluates is maintained throughout the useful life of the generator by the following means:

- The eluting solution is terminally sterilized Sodium Chloride Intravenous Infusion BP 0.9% w/v
- Air entering the system passes through a 0.22 µm filter
- A terminal eluate 0.22 µm filter is placed between the column and the elution needle
- Between elutions, the needle is protected by a single-use, disposable, sterile needle guard.

The elution of the generator should be carried out in a Grade A environment (see Ch. 29).

Preparation of ^{99m}Tc-radiopharmaceuticals

The daily supply of ^{99m}Tc is provided by the elution of the generator, resulting in a sterile solution of sodium pertechnetate that is subdivided to provide the radioactive component of the radiopharmaceutical. Some nuclear medicine investigations use sodium pertechnetate alone as the radiopharmaceutical (see Table 42.2). In this case, preparation of sodium pertechnetate injection requires only the subdivision from the generator eluate with perhaps some further dilution with Sodium Chloride Intravenous Infusion BP 0.9% w/v.

Other investigations, and these are in the majority, use radiopharmaceuticals that involve the chemical transformation of the sodium pertechnetate into another radiochemical form.

In order to make the preparation of ^{99m}Tc-radiopharmaceuticals as simple as possible, commercially available 'kits' are used to manufacture these radiopharmaceuticals. These kits allow the radiopharmacist, in the hospital environment, to transform the pertechnetate, via complex chemical reactions performed within the vial, into the desired radiopharmaceutical. This is achieved by the simple addition of pertechnetate into the vial followed by shaking to dissolve the contents.

A kit consists of a prepacked set of sterile ingredients designed for the preparation of a specific radiopharmaceutical. Most commonly the ingredients are freeze dried, enclosed within a rubber-capped nitrogen-filled vial. Normally the kit contains sufficient materials to prepare a number of patient doses. In a typical formulation, the following may be found:

- The compound to be complexed to the ^{99m}Tc. These are known as ligands (e.g. methylene diphosphonate)
- Stannous ions (e.g. stannous chloride or fluoride) which are present as a reducing agent. The reduction of ^{99m}TcO$_4^-$ to a lower valance state is required to allow the ligands to form a complex with the ^{99m}Tc
- Other compounds that act as stabilizers, buffers or antioxidants.

Given below is an example of how ^{99m}Tc-radiopharmaceutical production may be performed. The compounding procedures must be carried out within the facilities described in Chapter 29 using aseptic technique and carried out as 'closed' procedures (GMP).

The production method (Fig. 42.5) involves two simple steps:

Step 1. The freeze-dried kit is reconstituted by aseptically transferring the necessary activity of sodium pertechnetate using a sterile syringe and needle. This step may also include a further dilution of the eluate with a suitable diluent. The amount of activity withdrawn for the reconstitution of the kit vial depends on two factors:

- The number of patient doses to be manufactured
- The amount of activity required at injection time for each of the patient doses. The calculation would take into account the decay of ^{99m}Tc.

Manufacturers normally specify a maximum activity that may be added to the vial.

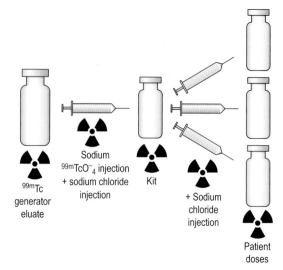

Figure 42.5 • Schematic representation of the preparation of patient doses of radiopharmaceuticals.

Step 2. The reconstituted kit is aseptically subdivided to provide each patient dose with sufficient activity to allow proper imaging after administration. As in Step 1, a diluent may be added to the final dose to give the desired radioactive concentration.

^{99m}Tc-radiopharmaceuticals must be administered on the day of production, for the following reasons:

- *Sterility*. Aseptically prepared pharmaceuticals should ideally be administered within a few hours of production, in accordance with GMP
- *Radioactivity*. ^{99m}Tc has a half-life of only 6 hours
- *Radiochemical stability*. ^{99m}Tc-complexes are generally stable for a period between 4 and 8 hours after production.

Facilities required for the production of radiopharmaceuticals

The majority of radiopharmaceuticals are intended for IV administration; therefore it is of paramount importance that these preparations are sterile. They also contain radionuclides with short half-lives that require their preparation and administration on the same day. Because of the thermal lability of some of these products, it is not possible to use terminal sterilization by autoclaving and hence these injections must be prepared using aseptic techniques. Here highly skilled operators work with sterile ingredients within clean room facilities containing either laminar flow safety cabinets or isolators. The facilities for carrying out such manipulations are more fully described in Chapter 29, but there is specialized equipment as well as design criteria specifically for handling radiopharmaceuticals. A full description of these may be found in Sampson's (1994) *Textbook of Radiopharmacy* (see Appendix 5).

Radiation protection in the radiopharmacy

There are three basic principles to radiation protection:

- *Shielding.* By placing shielding around the radioactive source, the radiation dose rate may be reduced. Materials used as shielding must be appropriate to the type of radiation being emitted by the radionuclide. Plastic, Perspex and metals of low molecular weight such as aluminium are appropriate materials for shielding beta-emitters. For gamma-emitters, high molecular weight metals such as lead and tungsten should be used. The thickness of shielding material necessary for gamma-emitters is dependent on the gamma-ray energy – the greater the energy, the thicker the shield required.
- *Distance.* The radiation dose from a radioactive source is inversely proportional to the square of the distance (i.e. by doubling the distance the radiation dose is quartered).
- *Time.* Minimizing the time spent handling a radioactive source will reduce the radiation dose. It is important for new operators to practice the handling operation prior to working with radioactive materials.

In working practice all three of these principles may be used in isolation or together to reduce the radiation dose to the operator. For example, in the dispensing operation outlined in Figure 42.5, all vials containing radioactive material would be contained in a 3 mm lead pot. This will attenuate ^{99m}Tc's gamma-rays by a factor of approximately 1000. The syringes used to carry out the transfers would be only half full (i.e. 1 mL of radioactive solution would be transferred with a 2 mL syringe) in order to maximize the distance between the operator's fingers and the source,

without compromising the accuracy of the dispensing operation.

The syringes, during the operation, should also be contained within a syringe shield. These are made of materials such as lead, tungsten, lead glass or lead acrylic, the latter two being transparent. Lead and tungsten syringe shields have lead glass/acrylic windows incorporated to allow the operator to see the graduations on the syringe. Alternatively the whole syringe shield may be made of lead glass/acrylic which would have the advantage of giving greater visibility.

Handling the vials outside their lead pots should be carried out using long forceps and not with the fingers. The dispensing process should be carried out over a 'drip tray' that allows easy containment of any accidental spillage. It also should be carried out within a laminar flow safety cabinet or negative pressure isolator that provides operator protection as well as product protection (see Ch. 29).

The staff working in the radiopharmacy will be constantly monitored to assess their radiation exposure and to ensure compliance with safety legislation. Whole-body dose may be monitored with film badges and the radiation dose to the finger pulp with thermo luminescent dosimeters.

KEY POINTS

- Radiopharmaceuticals may be used in therapy or diagnosis, the latter either as tracers or in imaging
- PET CT imaging with ^{18}F-FDG is becoming an important imaging technique in the diagnosis of cancer
- ^{18}F-FDG may be prepared by first producing ^{18}F in a cyclotron, followed by the radio-synthesis of the ^{18}F-FDG, which is carried out in an automated apparatus, known as a synthesis module
- ^{99m}Tc is the most widely used radionuclide
- A molybdenum/technetium generator will provide a daily supply of ^{99m}Tc for 7–14 days, as sodium pertechnetate
- Reacting with a suitable ligand can chemically modify sodium pertechnetate. Different ligands give different bio-distributions, resulting in the wide range of scans that may be performed with ^{99m}Tc
- Radiation protection should be provided for operators using a combination of shielding, distance and time

43

Storage of medicines and waste disposal

David R. Bethell and Judith A. Rees

STUDY POINTS

- Why medicines need to be stored correctly
- Methods of storing medicines
- Methods for procuring (obtaining) stock and the stock supply chain
- Methods for receiving and checking medicines
- Rotation and date checking of stock
- Reasons for storing some medicines in the refrigerator and maintaining records of refrigerator temperatures
- Waste disposal of medicines

Introduction

Medicines, however well formulated, do not keep indefinitely. Some can only be kept for a short time before they have degraded sufficiently to make them unsafe or unsuitable for the patient. Such products are usually referred to as having a short shelf life. Other medicines last longer, sometimes up to several years, but always have a limited, although longer, shelf life. Rhodes (1984) listed six general causes for the degradation of medicines, and hence limited shelf life. These are:

- Loss of drug (due to hydrolysis, oxidation, photolysis, etc.)
- Loss of vehicle (evaporation of water or volatile ingredient)
- Loss of uniformity (such as caking of suspensions or creaming of an emulsion)
- Change in bioavailability (such as ageing of tablets, change in polymorphic form)
- Change in appearance (such as colour change)
- Appearance of toxic or irritant products (as a result of chemical change).

To this list may be added changes which arise from microbiological activity.

All the above causes for the degradation of medicines can be speeded up by poor storage conditions. For example, extremes of temperature, exposure to bright sunlight, moisture, unsuitable packaging and even unsuitable transportation conditions can contribute to degradation and hence shortened shelf lives of medicines. Thus it is important to store medicinal products in the correct conditions at all times. Products that need to be kept cold or in a fridge require to be transported in refrigerated conditions, or if that is not possible, then in insulated containers. Such a transport system is referred to as a cold chain.

Poorly stored medicines may pose a safety hazard to patients – for example, if an incorrect or unavailable amount of drug is provided by a degraded formulation or if a formulation contains toxic degradation products. More information on the degradation of medicines can be found in *Pharmaceutics: The Science of Dosage Form Design* (Aulton 2007).

Pharmacists need to be aware of the potential for the degradation of medicines and the need to store medicines correctly in the pharmacy as well as advising patients about the correct storage of medicines in the home.

Expiry date

The expiry date is the date after which the medicine should not be used. This date is usually determined by accelerated stability testing (see Aulton 2007). The pharmaceutical manufacturer adds the expiry date to the package. In the case of extemporaneously prepared products, the shelf life, and hence the determination of the expiry date, may be found in an appropriate monograph (the *British Pharmacopoeia* or *European Pharmacopoeia* for example), if available. If there is not a monograph for the extemporaneous product, then the pharmacist should label the product with as short an expiry date as possible, bearing in mind the nature of the product. The safety of the patient should remain paramount.

Packaging

Most manufactured medicines will be supplied in purpose designed, elegant containers that will preserve the medicinal product for as long as possible. These containers may specify certain storage conditions, for example store between 2°C and 8°C in a refrigerator, or store in a dry place. Clearly a pharmacist must maintain the packaged medicine at such recommended storage conditions while it is under their control in the pharmacy, and advise the patient on storage conditions when the product is dispensed.

Stock control in the pharmacy

For reasons of economy as well as stability, pharmacists should not keep stocks of medicines on their shelves for long periods of time. The aim is to keep stock at a level which just meets demand. Nowadays, computerized systems of stock control are used in most community and hospital pharmacies. These computerized systems will monitor stock levels and record usage, and in addition, are capable of ordering or suggesting quantities to be ordered, based on past records, or ordering stock as it is used. Uncommon medicines or infrequently used medicines may have to be inputted into the computer system by pharmacy staff. But most everyday ordering decisions are not made by the pharmacist and the pharmacist can concentrate on the stock supply chain. However, the pharmacist should always keep an eye on stock levels and be aware of changes in prescribing, which will directly influence demand. After all, computer systems are only as good as the programming and the information inputted into the computer.

The stock supply chain

The procurement of stock is vital to the well-being of any business, including community and hospital phar-

macy or any other supplier of services. The fundamentals apply whether it is a one man pharmacy, small pharmacy, large multiple pharmacy, hospital dispensary/manufacturing facility or even a robotic supply operation. The stock supply chain can be summed up in four main parts:

- Procurement – this includes ordering/supply and transport by the manufacturer, wholesaler or other sources of medicines
- Receipt of goods, including signing for the stock, safe storage of invoices and reconciliation
- Storage, which includes storage conditions and actual positioning of stock
- Rotation and date checking.

While each section will be looked at in some detail, the whole aim of the process is 'The right product, in the right place, at the right time'. If this aim is followed alongside a robust standard operating procedure (SOP; see Chs 8, 9, 15) then any pharmacy should run in a way that avoids products being out of stock, short dated (near its expiry date) or out of date and, most importantly, the pharmacy should have the right amount of stock that can be afforded.

Procurement

The majority of pharmacies obtain most of their medicines and related products from one or two main wholesalers. These wholesalers are logistics experts and they make their profit by focusing all their efforts on supplying the right amount of product at the right time in the right place in a state that is ready for supply. A 'good' wholesaler makes life easier, not harder, for the pharmacy and generally will provide the following:

- Supply the IT systems that support the dispensing process
- Twice daily delivery, with convenient order and supply times
- Paperwork that allows the simple tracking of the differing types of stock and requirement for signatures, as appropriate
- A large range of stock and more importantly cross-supply with other specialists such as hosiery, appliances and special manufacturers (i.e. units that extemporaneously prepare products to individual prescriptions/requests)
- Payment terms that allow the pharmacy to supply stock at one time and pay for it later

- Reports on products that are out of stock, drug recalls, new products, pack size changes, discontinued medication and many others
- The ability to return stock under certain circumstances. Everyone makes mistakes and the need to occasionally return unused items is vital to cash flow
- Sensible billing and paperwork that allows any level of business to follow their orders and reconcile invoices.

All the main wholesalers do all the above to a greater or lesser extent. The main difference between a well run and a poorly run dispensary is generally the staff training and utilization of systems and not the systems themselves. All the main computer systems will run stock and ordering systems but are dependent on correct information being provided. There must be clear disciplines in place that ensure that the dispensary IT system is up to date at all times. When these disciplines are applied rigidly and in a concise way, the computer system will work to its optimum and time and energy will be saved.

Receipt of goods

It is important that all pharmacy staff including the sales assistant, dispenser, accredited checking technician (ACT), pre-registration student and pharmacist have the same high regard for stock receipt and reconciliation. This is the lifeblood of a business and any amount of IT will not replace staff that are trained to correctly receive goods on delivery and to reconcile the stock. Reconciliation is the process of checking that the stock received is equal to the amount on the invoice or goods delivered documentation. Any pharmacy that does not have a robust checking procedure for the reconciliation of stock will be prone to abuse of that stock, including theft by customers and staff. This will lead to all sorts of potential leakage (loss of stock, usually by theft) and eventually loss of profit and in extreme cases loss of the business. It is absolutely vital that all staff involved in the procurement process are aware of the need for vigilance and security, and one way of doing this is to ensure a member of staff has 'ownership' of this process. There must be a clear and robust SOP for the receipt and reconciliation of stock and this must not be varied. If it is, then a gap in the process will be spotted and leakage will occur. The following is a brief synopsis of the receipt of goods, and

although every pharmacy will be slightly different, the core values will be the same:

- Only authorized staff should sign for goods. This authorization should be commensurate with the type of stock and the risk involved.
- Controlled drugs (CDs) should be checked at the time of receipt and signed for by the pharmacist or delegated staff. Under no circumstances should CD stock be left to check later.
- All 'totals' should be counted – if the driver says there are 10 boxes, then make sure there are 10 before any signature is given.
- When reconciling stock, ensure a tick is made on the invoice for each item received – no one can remember 400 separate lines!
- Where goods are thermo-labile, e.g. insulin, then staff must have a clear understanding of the risks involved with not dealing with these products in good time. Generally all items to be stored in the fridge ('fridge lines') will be identified as such and can be dealt with as a priority.
- Once all received goods are reconciled, any out of stocks, no supplies or shortages must be documented and dealt with straight away. Failure to do so will lead to a lack of urgency and a feeling of, 'well it is only a few tablets'. In some cases those few tablets may be worth a considerable amount of money. Most wholesalers will have special arrangements for problems with CDs and items needing cold storage (cold chain supplies) so extra care must be given to these orders.
- Finally, each day's invoices must be chronologically filed. This process ensures that monthly reconciliation against the monthly bill can be quickly and accurately performed. NB: Invoices for CDs must be kept for a minimum of 2 years (UK law). Most wholesaler systems keep invoices as a data file.

Storage

Once the right goods have been received and reconciled, then it is equally important that they are stored in a way that maximizes their shelf life. All modern medicines are formulated to enhance their stability; however, the general rules of storage are:

- The dispensary temperature should generally be between 16 and 25°C with no direct sunlight onto the packs of medicines.

- Certain medicines will be thermo-labile, that is excess heat or cold will affect them. These will include insulin, many vaccines, some eye drops, new drugs such as Aranesp and many extemporaneously prepared products (specials). It is vital that all dispensary staff are aware of these products and they are stored accordingly (see later).
- In UK law, medicines in a pharmacy may only be stored in the part of the building that is designated as a registered premise. Care must be taken to ensure that medicines are stored in such an appropriate and legal place.
- Medicines must be stored in such a way as to ensure that stock rotation is a routine part of the process. It must be part of the day-to-day procedure that new stock goes to the back of the shelf and old to the front. Concurrent with this is the regular date checking of part of the storage system every week (see later).
- Not to exclude automation, more and more robotic systems are now being utilized in pharmacies. Most of these systems use a 'virtual' storage system where stock is allocated randomly in space but is clearly logged in the computer's memory. While there are undoubted benefits from these systems, they also suffer from lack of correct information and can be adversely affected if non-standard stock lines are used. Nationally it is stated that the level of dispensing supply errors is lower from robotic systems and this is directly related to the way stock is stored and checked. The use of these systems will increase in the future, if they come down in price and size.
- There are some small exceptions but, as a general rule, solid dose stocks should be stored alphabetically. Inhalers, creams and ointments, eye drops and liquids may be stored separately, but alphabetically, and items that require reconstitution with water are generally kept near the sink. CDs must be kept in an approved, lockable cabinet and the key should be under the direct supervision of the pharmacist in charge. Bulk items may be stored outside the dispensary as long as they are on registered premises.

Rotation and date checking

Clinical governance (see Ch. 8) within pharmacy requires that date checking procedures be in place for all pharmacy stock, whether it is in the dispensary, stock room or shop (also see information on the Royal Pharmaceutical Society of Great Britain (RPSGB) website). One of the reasons is to protect the public from date expired medicines. Date expired medicines are likely to be substandard (degraded either chemically, physically or microbiologically) and may pose a safety issue if supplied to the public. Additionally it is professionally unacceptable and potentially illegal.

A SOP should cover rotation and date checking in the pharmacy. Ideally the overall responsibility for these tasks should be delegated to a senior member of staff, with individual staff responsible for certain areas or types of stock. All date checking should be recorded (see Ch. 15). Box 43.1 shows an example of a date checking record.

The general rules for date checking are as follows:

- All incoming stock should be checked to identify short dated expiry dates before being placed in storage or on the shelves.
- All stock should be placed in chronological order of expiry date with shortest dated stock to the front.
- All stock should be date checked every 3 months, that is, four times a year.

Box 43.1

Example of a date checking record chart

Section/area/products	Date checked Initials of checker	Date checked Initials of checker	Date checked Initials of checker
Creams Shelf A	19/7/08 JR	18/10/08 JR	18/1/09 JR
Creams Shelf B	20/7/08 JR	20/10/08 JR	19/1/09 JR

- Short dated stock must have a clear handling system: a good one is a traffic light system, green more than 6 months until expiry date, amber 3–6 months, and red less than 3 months remaining. Where stock is amber, it may be possible to transfer stock to another pharmacy or the wholesalers may be able to facilitate this process. When stock is red, it should be clearly marked short dated. Under no circumstances should this stock enter the dispensing chain when there is less than the treatment cycle remaining.
- All date checking must include lesser used items, items in the fridge, CD cabinet, drawer storage units and other storage areas.
- Date checking should be part of the daily and routine tasks in a pharmacy.
- Under no circumstances must patient-returned medicines be added to the existing stock and storage facilities, since such actions would be both unethical and almost certainly fraudulent. This applies to all returned stock, whether from a patient, nursing/residential home, doctor's bag or nurse's supplies.

It may be possible to incorporate a quantity check at the same time as performing the date check. The benefit of a quantity check is that the position of the IT system can be checked and updated. Every system will corrupt with time and will require a person to update the system with the quantity on the shelf. Ideally a different 100 products a week should be checked and amended where required.

Storage in fridges

Many medicines require storage in a fridge to maintain the stability of the product for a reasonable time period (see examples in Box 43.2). The temperature of the fridge must be kept between the range of +2°C and +8°C. This temperature range should be maintained at all times and, ideally, an emergency power supply should be available in case of a power cut. The emergency power supply should provide power for a minimum of 24 hours.

The fridge cabinet should be sufficiently large to ensure that products are not tightly packed together so that cold air can circulate easily around the products. Airflow should not be obstructed in any way in the fridge.

Box 43.2

List of some medicines requiring storage in a fridge
- Calcitonin injection
- Chloramphenicol eye drops
- Daktacort®
- Fludrocortisone
- Latanoprost
- Proctosedyl® suppositories
- Timodine®
- Xalacom®

As a fridge for storing medicines, it should not be used to store food and drink. Storage of food and drink could result in contamination of medicines.

All fridges for the storage of medicines must be fitted with a maximum–minimum thermometer, either mercury or digital, to enable temperatures to be recorded.

Fridge temperature monitoring

Fridge temperature monitoring is essential to ensure the public receives cold chain supplies of medicines in suitable condition. It is a professional requirement of the RPSGB that daily maximum and minimum temperatures within the fridge are recorded. This ensures correct storage conditions can be demonstrated for clinical governance (see Ch. 8).

Additionally, the fridge should be defrosted at regular intervals to maintain its efficiency. A record should be made of the dates of defrosting, again for clinical governance purposes. Alternative fridge facilities should be found for stock during defrosting procedures.

The following points are important for fridge temperature monitoring processes:
- A member of staff should be delegated to take and record daily maximum and minimum temperatures
- It is important that staff are well trained to know how to use and read the thermometer according to the manufacturer's guidelines
- If a digital thermometer is used, then the probe should be placed in a suitable position
- Staff should be trained so that the reset button is always set after each daily temperature reading in order to obtain a new baseline

Box 43.3

Fridge temperature monitoring chart

Date	Max temp °C	Min temp °C	Action taken	Checked by: Initials	Thermometer reset: Initials
			If outside temp range +2–8°C		
12/8/08	7	3		JR	JR
13/8/08	6	3		JR	JR
14/8/08	9	1	Checked thermometer working. Informed pharmacist	JR	JR

- Staff should be trained to immediately report temperatures outside the appropriate temperature range
- Arrangements should be in place to check a fridge is working correctly
- Arrangements should be in place to replace speedily a non-working fridge
- The pharmacist should review records of temperature readings at least every month.

Box 43.3 shows a typical fridge temperature monitoring chart completed for 3 days, one of which shows an out of temperature range entry.

Waste

As a part of the new pharmacy contract in the UK it was agreed, as part of the essential services provided by all community pharmacies, that patients could return unwanted medicines. This on the face of it was a simple enough agreement and appeared to simply formalize a service that had been provided for years. Unfortunately, owing to a change in the environmental laws in the UK at about the same time, things were not quite as straightforward as planned.

It is vital for the health and safety of us all that medicines are not just dumped into household waste and/or flushed away down the toilet. The pollution of the rivers and lakes is so bad in some areas of the world that fish are changing their sex under the influence of hormonal contraception tablets which have been either disposed of by the patient or have leaked from landfill. The dumping of medicines into landfill is clearly unacceptable in view of the long-term consequences.

As a first step, every pharmacy that handles waste medicine must inform the local environmental health officer (EHO) in writing, or using the appropriate form, that they intend to store such waste.

The exemption for storage is part of the Waste Management Licensing Regulations 1984. The EHO has agreed to allow pharmacies to store waste prior to collection and disposal by an authorized waste carrier. Generally the local primary care trust (PCT) in England will have a contract to collect waste on a regular basis by a third party who is licensed to transport and destroy waste. (NB: A pharmacy must have special registration to transport waste, see later.)

In order to be compliant with the law, it is vital that every pharmacy writes a standard operating procedure for handling of waste and ensures that there are appropriate facilities and tools to do the job properly. As a minimum, this means a dedicated area for storage on the premises, a clear list of questions for the patient returning medicines (see later), a definition of what pharmaceutical waste means (Box 43.4), a special disposal unit for controlled drugs, a clear method for dealing with spills, and a transparent record of what has happened to the waste, that is, a waste transfer note. The authorized waste carrier will always leave a waste transfer note when the waste is collected, and these notes must be stored in a place where they can be checked easily. Also it is important that the pharmacy contractor is clear where the waste is going and what is happening to that waste. It is not enough to hand waste to anyone who asks and then ignore what happens to it.

Another aspect which must be considered is health and safety at work. An employer and employees have a responsibility to work in a way that minimizes risk. Thus the first thing to do when receiving any waste from a patient is to tactfully ask the following questions and act according to the answers:

a. Are you returning only medicines? YES/NO
b. Are you sure there are no sharps or needles in the bag/container? YES/NO
c. Is there anything else that may affect the health and safety of our staff? YES/NO.

Box 43.4

Some definitions of waste from Hazardous Waste Regulations 2005

Hazardous Waste (England and Wales) Regulations 2005
Community pharmacists may only collect waste that is classified as household waste.
Household waste includes:

- Patient's returned medicines
- Waste from a domestic property
- Waste from a caravan
- A residential home providing residential care only (NOT nursing care)
- Waste from a moored vessel used wholly for purposes of living accommodation
- Waste from a home providing nursing care or unwanted/expired stock from a doctor, dentist, vet, midwife or nurse is regarded as industrial waste

Removal of individual tablets or capsules from blister packaging falls within the definition of waste treatment (which is a licensed activity) and should be avoided by pharmacists

If the answer to either a) or b) is NO or the answer to c) is YES then you must reassess the situation, taking care that health and safety regulations are not compromised. For example, if a blood spattered bag containing open needles is offered, then it will be necessary to refuse to accept the bag and contents. Each occasion must be treated on its merits. The majority of patients are considerate individuals.

Generally the law allows sorting of the waste into solids (capsules and tablets), liquids and inhalers. Controlled drugs and hazardous waste should be kept separate and dealt with appropriately. There is a limit imposed on the amount of hazardous waste that may be handled in a year of 200 kg. It is very rare for a pharmacy to exceed this amount but if they do then a separate registration is required. Similarly, any pharmacy that, for business reasons, wished to transport waste, e.g. from a patient's home, must be registered for this and pay a fee. It is not acceptable to pick up medicines from a patient's house and transfer them in a vehicle without the proper registration and documentation. Fines can be hefty.

So as pharmacies have to take part in this valuable waste disposal service, the starting point is registration

followed by writing a robust standard operating procedure which must be the basis of staff training. Any medicines must be stored securely on the registered premises of the pharmacy. An outside shed with no lock is not considered secure and will attract fines and a possible custodial sentence. Controlled drugs and hazardous waste must be treated separately and all spillages must be dealt with promptly and safely.

So is waste a waste of time? Categorically no; if a proper waste medicines management system is in place then there is less likelihood of:

- Hazards to the patient, for example, poisoning and/or overdose
- Hazards to the environment
- Less waste of resources, if pharmacist and GP liaise
- Reduced waste in the local waste system.

These factors alone mean that waste management of medicines is quite correctly an 'essential service' for community pharmacy.

KEY POINTS

- Medicines have a limited shelf life, and expired or poorly stored medicines can pose a threat to patients
- Expiry dates are included on the packaging by manufacturers
- The packaging used by manufacturers may contribute to medicine stability
- Efficient stock control is essential in pharmacies
- The stock supply chain consists of procurement, receipt, storage, rotation with date checking
- Most procurement is now automatic using computer technology
- Reconciliation is an important part of receipt
- Most drugs are stored at 16–25°C, but some require storage in a fridge at 2–8°C
- A fridge must be monitored daily, recording maximum and minimum temperatures
- A standard operating procedure must be in place for date checking
- Pharmacists must register with the environmental health officer if they wish to store returned medicines. This does not include transportation of waste
- Health and safety requires care to ensure that waste is only of medicines and is handled safely
- Staff require training in all these procedures

44

Communication skills – role of the pharmacist in giving advice and information

Judith A. Rees

STUDY POINTS

- The rationale and need for giving information and advice
- Situations suitable for pharmaceutical information and advice
- Assessing the need for giving information and advice
- How to decide on the content and method of giving information and advice
- Aids to information and advice giving

Introduction

It has always been the custom for pharmacists to give information and advice on the use of medicines. As long ago as 1986, the Nuffield Report recognized that there were 'some categories of individuals who certainly will need advice, help and encouragement in the handling of their medicines' and that 'anyone . . . who has to rely on a continuous drug regime, should be a candidate for additional support and help from pharmacies'. These statements highlight the importance placed on the role of the pharmacist in the provision of advice to patients/customers in the Nuffield Report.

Since the Nuffield Report there have been developments in medicines research, production and packaging of medicines, together with changes in society's attitudes towards patient/professional relationships, which have led to advice and information giving becoming an even greater part of the role of the pharmacist.

As a brief explanation of these developments, medicines research has led to the production of new powerful, effective drugs formulated in many specialized dosage forms, such as modified-release formulations, aerosols, patches, nail lacquers, etc. which utilize different absorption routes (e.g. percutaneous, nasal and vaginal) as well as more conventional routes (see Ch. 21). Additionally many medicines are packaged in specialized containers, for example aerosols for rectal use, self-administration parenteral products, metered dose nasal sprays, and often with complicated dosage methods or regimens, e.g. pipettes, times of administration, treatment with multiple drug therapy, such as for tuberculosis. Patients prescribed or purchasing these newer dosage formulations will almost certainly require some information from pharmacists on their method of use and the dosage regimen.

All modern medicines have some side-effects. Some of these side-effects will be relatively insignificant, some inconvenient, while others may be serious and in extreme cases threaten the life of the patient. Clearly it is essential that patients are provided with the knowledge of these side-effects and what to do if they occur. In addition, many medicines interact with other drugs (both over the counter (OTC) and prescribed medicines) and/or with food and drink. Thus, if patients/consumers are to get the best out of their medicines, then they need to know how to correctly use/administer these medicines in as safe a manner as possible, with knowledge about side-effects, interactions, etc. Pharmacists are in an excellent position to provide such advice to patients/consumers. It has been suggested that the advent of providing all medicines in original packs should release time for the pharmacist and thus enable pharmacists to spend more time on patient advice.

Against this background of technological and pharmaceutical advances in the delivery of medicines, attitudes within society have also changed. In recent years there has been a rapid rise in the consumer movement, with consumers questioning and demanding from producers better products, safer products, ecologically friendly products, etc. as well as more information on the products. For example, CFC-free aerosols, including pharmaceutical aerosols, were developed in response to fears of damage to the ozone layer (see Ch. 37). The challenge to the world of global warming due to carbon dioxide emissions will certainly affect the production and packaging of pharmaceuticals.

Alongside and in response to these challenges by consumers, there has been the development of legislation giving consumers more rights and hence more power. Medicines have not been isolated from this consumerism movement and patients and purchasers of medicines have become more demanding in their quest for knowledge about the medicines that they consume. Such patients have also become more questioning about their illness, its treatment and the need for specific medicines, their dosage regimens, alternative medicines, alternative formulations, etc. The introduction of the Internet has produced for consumers a readily available and extensive source of information about medicines, although the quality of some of the information on some websites may be dubious and the ability of the general public to understand the information questionable. However, there are some well recognized factually correct websites (see Ch. 23 for more detail). All the above has led to patients acting as consumers and becoming empowered and much more autonomous, resulting in them wanting more choice in the selection of their medicines/dosage regimens and questioning the justification for the prescribing and use of medicines.

Within the healthcare professions, there has been a move towards the accommodation of the consumer movement and a commitment to patient autonomy and the need for valid patient consent and choice. This has led to the acceptance that the patient has the right to be involved in decisions about their health care. However, in order to make an informed decision the patient needs the information surrounding the issues to make that decision. One of the first documents to accept that patients have the right to choose and the right to be involved in decision making about their medicines was published in 1997. 'From compliance to concordance' (see Ch. 46) outlined the move towards developing patient/professional relationships which represent a negotiation between the patient and the professional and allow the patient to take an active part in decision making about their medicines.

The NHS Plan 2000 in the UK outlined the need for pharmacists to become more involved in helping patients to get the best from their medicines. The aim was for pharmacists to give extra help to patients who have difficulty in using their medicines correctly. The NHS Plan accepts that many patients are receiving less than optimum care because they find their medicines difficult to take or hard to remember when to take, because they do not have anyone to talk to about their medicines, or because they have complicated medication regimens. In 2005, medicine use reviews (MURs) were established as part of the NHS contract for community pharmacists. These are short, face-to-face confidential interviews involving a pharmacist and a patient together reviewing the patient's current medicines. The aim is to help patients find out more about their medicines and to pick up any problems that they are having with the medicines. The pharmacist may advise on finding easier ways to take medicines, different formulations, or the correct method to take the medicine and can sort out any problems, or the problem can be referred to the prescriber. Thus the outcomes may be improved effectiveness of medicines and less unnecessary waste because the patient is more informed about their medicines and has received help from the pharmacist in how to take or use them.

Additionally the NHS Plan aims to 'Give patients the confidence that they are getting good advice when they consult a pharmacist'. In other words, the NHS Plan is advocating a greater role for pharmacists in counselling and advice giving to patients. Furthermore, the NHS Plan emphasizes the need for medicines management services, the aims of which are to prevent, detect and address medicines-related problems to achieve optimum use of medicines. Pharmacists are already providing many of the elements of medicines management informally. However, medicines management implies a coordination and formalization of these elements. The element of relevance to this chapter is the 'provision of support on medicines taking, which includes the identification of an individual's pharmaceutical needs, provision of an opportunity for patients to discuss their medicines and the development of patient–professional partnerships to provide improvements in medicine taking'. Such support could in part be provided in the form of advice giving by pharmacists, when handing out prescription medicines or selling OTC medicines. Other opportunities for such advice giving exist on hospital discharge of patients, during medication reviews and with residential and nursing home staff and residents.

National service frameworks (NSFs) (see also Ch. 48) have been introduced in recent years to define standards for the treatment, health and social services necessary to ensure high-quality care of individuals with specific diseases or conditions, e.g. diabetes, mental health problems, or groups of individuals with special needs, e.g. older people. The use of medicines is a fundamental component of NSF standards. The emphasis is placed on achieving a greater partnership in medicine taking between patients and healthcare professionals, improving choice and addressing information needs. For example, the NSF for older people sets out its aims as ensuring that older people:

- Gain the maximum benefit from their medication to maintain or increase their quality and duration of life
- Do not suffer unnecessarily from illness caused by excessive, inappropriate or inadequate consumption of medicines.

Both these aims encompass the need for pharmacists to advise older people (and their carers) about their medicines. Underlying all the above government documents is an acceptance that individuals need help with using their medicines.

Recently it has been acknowledged that some individuals with chronic conditions are very capable and competent in using their medicines to manage their condition(s). Such individuals have been termed 'expert patients'. At the same time there is an increasing awareness of the importance of self-care and active patient involvement in making decisions about preventing and treating minor and major conditions/illness. Successful self-management programmes for chronic conditions such as arthritis have been developed and have been facilitated by lay individuals with patient experience of the condition. The identification of such 'expert patients' could lead to more user-led self-management programmes. It has been suggested that expert patients could help to 'educate' professionals about the self-management of illness. Healthcare professionals could pass on this 'education' to other patients with chronic conditions via advice giving techniques. However, the self-care of minor ailments will probably require a different approach. Pharmacists will need to facilitate the development of self-care and support the development of competencies by individuals to enable them to use appropriate medicines correctly and effectively. In other words, advice

giving skills will be required by pharmacists to help in the empowerment of patients, so that they will be capable of making informed decisions about self-treatment with medicines for minor ailments.

What is information and advice giving in pharmacy?

Patients and customers have a right to be involved in the decisions about their treatment and their use and choice of medicines. Thus pharmacists require effective communication skills to be able to identify the individual needs of a patient/customer and to determine the type and amount of advice and level of explanation appropriate to provide at that particular time.

The professional standards and guidance which expand the Royal Pharmaceutical Society of Great Britain (RPSGB) Code of Ethics for Pharmacists and Pharmacy Technicians emphasize that when OTC and prescribed products are supplied, then sufficient advice to ensure the safe and effective use of the medicine should be provided. In the case of complementary therapies and medicines, pharmacists and technicians must assist patients in making informed decisions by providing them with necessary and relevant information.

In the UK, the Veterinary Medicines Regulations 2007 make it a legal requirement that any person supplying any veterinary medicine (apart from OTC animal medicines) must:

- Always advise on safe administration
- Advise as necessary on any warnings or contraindications on the label or packaging
- Be satisfied that the person who will use the product is competent to use it safely, and intends to use it for the use for which it is intended.

These conditions seem forward-looking and perhaps one day will apply to human medicines.

The *British National Formulary* (BNF) uses the term 'counselling' rather than advice as a heading in individual monographs to detail the type of advice to be given to a patient. Such advice is above that required on the label of a dispensed product and usually involves unusual/complicated methods or times of administration or the potential interaction with foods. For example, bulk-forming laxatives have the counselling statement 'Preparations that swell in contact with liquid should always be carefully swallowed with water and should not be taken immediately before going to bed'.

While the term counselling is widely used in pharmaceutical literature, the definition of the term is less readily available. The British Association for Counselling (BAC) describes counselling as 'giving clients the opportunity to explore, discover and clarify ways of living more resourcefully and towards greater well-being'. This definition encompasses some aspects of patient counselling, but patient counselling is more about giving information and guidance on medicines to patients and allowing the patient to make informed decisions but with the interests of the patient uppermost. Another description of patient counselling is 'the sympathetic interaction between pharmacists and patients, which may go beyond conveyance of straightforward information about the medicine and how and when to use it'.

The need for information and advice giving

It is generally accepted that some patients have difficulty taking/using their medication and complying with the dosage regimens. Evidence comes from compliance and wastage studies.

It has been estimated that up to 50% of older people do not take their medicines as intended. The scope of this problem can be seen if the facts are considered. It is estimated that 80% of over-75-year-olds in the UK take at least one prescribed medicine and 36% take four or more medicines. Additionally, 50% of patients (not necessarily older people) with hypertension failed to take their medicines correctly and 1 in 10 deaths were attributable to stroke. It has been suggested that advice by pharmacists could lead to better compliance and hence less therapeutic failure and possible death.

The cost of unused medicines returned by patients to pharmacies has been estimated to be in excess of £100 million each year. Many of these unused and hence wasted medicines are because patients do not understand why their medicine(s) has been prescribed or how to take/use them. Hence the introduction of MURs to address these needs (see earlier in the chapter).

Although many medicines are supplied with a patient information leaflet, many patients do not always understand the contents and require further explanation from the pharmacist. Other patients may be scared by the information in the leaflet on, for example, side-effects. Pharmacists are in an ideal situation to provide additional information and advice and/or reassurance when prescription medicines are handed out and when OTC medicines are sold.

The aims of information and advice

There is a lack of evidence that the provision of information alone is sufficient to enable patients to correctly take medicines or to change their existing behaviours and attitudes. Counselling, as the definition from the BAC states, enables clients to explore their beliefs and develop plans for behaviour change. Pharmacists in their patient-advising roles may adapt and make use of the problem-solving model of counselling developed by Egan (1990).

Thus the aims, in addition to the provision of advice, could be to:

- Encourage patients to identify any problems they perceive with medicines and also any solutions to these problems
- Encourage patients to develop their own action plan for taking/using medicines correctly
- Gain an understanding of the patient's perspective
- Respect the patient's beliefs and be non-judgmental of their use (or non-use) of medicines.

Opportunities for giving information and advice

The pharmacist is often the last healthcare professional whom a patient sees before starting drug therapy. It is at this stage that the pharmacist should identify the information and advice needs of the patient. Pharmacists should take a prominent and proactive role, especially since often some patients do not expect it. The opportunities for giving information and advice to patients are many, but the main opportunity is at the end of the dispensing process or the sale of a medicine.

In community pharmacy, information and advice giving should be an integral part of the dispensing of a prescription. No patient should receive a dispensed medicine without the pharmacist making an assessment of the needs of the patient. The availability of prescription medication records and the information contained within will underpin the extent and type of information and advice provided to an individual patient. Some pharmaceutical companies have developed computer-aided systems associated with their products which offer guidelines to pharmacists, when dispensing that product, to assist with information and advice giving. Such computerized systems provide an audit trail and can verify when advising took place.

Another opportunity in community pharmacy for giving advice and information is the provision of prescription only medicines via patient group directions (PGD). All PGDs require that the patient be given advice during the initial assessment of the appropriateness of the medicine for the patient and immediately on supply of the medicine.

The sale of medicines from a community pharmacy is another opportunity. The sale of medicines can be the result of a) a direct request for a named medicine by a customer and b) a request for advice on the treatment of a symptom or minor ailment by a patient. The amount and content of the information and advice given to a patient will vary with the type of initial request, the medicine sold and the patient.

The introduction of self-care programmes for patients with chronic disease or presenting with minor ailments will involve the community pharmacist becoming actively engaged and using their advising skills with patients.

Community pharmacists may provide diagnostic testing and health screening services to the public. In such situations the service specifications to the Code of Ethics requires pharmacists to provide patients with 'any necessary counselling and available information'.

Thus the opportunities for community pharmacists to become involved in patient advice are wide ranging. Other possible areas include:

- During domiciliary visiting
- Visits to care/residential/nursing homes
- Public health (see Ch. 5)
- Dietary advice
- Emergency supply of medicines
- Supply of emergency hormonal contraception
- Special weeks/days, e.g. Asthma Week, Breast Awareness Week, Stop Smoking Day
- Women's and men's health
- Pet medicines.

In some of the above areas it may be necessary to give information and advice to the carer as well as the patient. But remember it is important to maintain patient confidentiality.

Similarly there are many opportunities for hospital pharmacists to counsel patients. Hospital pharmacists, unlike their community counterparts, have the advantage of access to a considerable amount of information about the patient. This information can include details of disease state, current therapy and home circumstances, all of which can be useful in providing information and advice. Patients in hospital often have their medication changed during their stay and so should be made fully aware of any alterations on discharge. Outpatients and inpatients at discharge receiving dispensed medicines will require the same sort of advice and counselling as patients receiving dispensed medicines from community pharmacies. Inpatients may require advice on their medicines during admission and with needs assessment.

Both community and hospital pharmacists may be involved in providing medication to patients in long-term residential homes or prisons. In such situations it may be necessary to give information and advice to both the patient and/or their carers.

How to provide information and advice

Information and advice giving, wherever it occurs, should take place in a thoughtful, structured way. The pharmacist must possess not only a sound knowledge of the drugs and appliances being dispensed or sold, but also excellent communication skills. Pharmacists should be able to provide information and advice in a non-paternalistic way that allows the patient to ask questions in order to understand the information so that they can make decisions about their own treatment and care. Pharmacists must have the ability to explain information clearly and unambiguously and in language the recipient can understand. They must know the right questions and how to ask them and, most importantly, they must know how to listen. For information and advice giving to be successful, it must be a two-way process. Rapport is built up between the pharmacist and the patient and a much more meaningful dialogue can take place.

The Cambridge–Calgary model discussed in Chapter 13 details how to provide explanations to patients. It is important to provide the correct amount and type of information:

- Chunks and checks. The information needs to be given in suitable bite-sized chunks. Observation of patient response should indicate whether the chunks are too small or too large and thus further chunks of information can be adjusted to suit the patient.

- Assess the patient's starting point. How much do they know? This should be assessed early on in the session.
- Ask patients what information would be helpful. For example, a patient may be more concerned about the immediate effects of the drug on their lifestyle rather than the progression of the disease.
- Give explanations at an appropriate time. You should avoid giving advice or information prematurely.

In order to help the patient with recalling and understanding the advice/information that you provide, the pharmacist should:

- Organize the explanation. Try to develop a logical sequences and discrete sections – do not combine information on side-effects with how to administer the medicine.
- Use signposting – in other words, if there are three points to get over, say so, and continue with firstly..., secondly ..., etc.
- Use easily understood and concise language. Avoid using jargon and technical terms where possible and appropriate.
- Use visual methods of explanation. Demonstration models of pharmaceutical packaging can be useful, e.g. aerosols.
- Check patient understanding at regular intervals. Ask the patient to explain to you or to demonstrate the use of a medicine.

The overall communication skills needed for giving advice and information have been discussed in detail in Chapter 13.

What information to include

Each situation and each patient will have different information needs, but as a general summary, no patient who has been given medication should leave a community or hospital pharmacy without knowing:

- How to take or use the medicine
- When to take or use the medicine
- How much to take or use
- How long to continue to take or use
- What to expect, e.g. immediate relief, no effect for several days

- Why the medicine is being taken or used
- What to do if something goes wrong, e.g. if a dose is missed
- How to recognize side-effects and minimize their incidence
- Lifestyle changes which need to be made
- Dietary changes which need to be made.

Who to counsel

Not every patient will require information and advice but it is important that pharmacists can correctly identify those who do. In deciding who to counsel, it is important to consider both the patient and the medication.

Consideration of the medication

The medication can be prescribed or bought. If prescribed, the prescription may contain one or several items. A multiple-item prescription may present more problems to the patient in terms of different drugs, different dosage forms and regimens, etc. and so patients presenting such a prescription may require more counselling than patients presenting single-item prescriptions. Additionally, the individual medicine on any prescription, because of its characteristics, e.g. complex dosage regimen, special delivery methods, novel packaging, etc., may require explanation to ensure the patient has a clear understanding of how to use it.

Other reasons for considering counselling will be if the drug has:

- A narrow therapeutic index. The need for strict adherence to dosing should be emphasized. Drugs such as lithium or theophylline are common examples.
- The potential for interaction with another drug or food. One of the commonest drugs to interact with other drugs is warfarin. Appendix 1 in the BNF lists interactions and Appendix 9 lists any interactions with food.
- The potential to cause side-effects. In these instances the patient should be told not only how to recognize the side-effects, but also how to reduce the incidence or severity of them. See examples in Box 44.1. Many pharmacists are unsure how much information about side-effects should be given to patients. There is concern that the patient may be put off taking the medicine to avoid suffering these

Box 44.1

Some drugs and the type of side-effects that can occur

Some drugs cause side-effects which can be minimized by good management

Drug	Side-effect	Precaution
Chlorpromazine	Photosensitivity	Use sunscreen
NSAIDs	GI disturbances	Take with food
Tamoxifen	Nausea	Take at bedtime
Bisphosphonates	Oesophageal reactions	Stand or sit upright for 30 minutes after taking the tablet

Some drugs have side-effects which require the patient to be warned for their benefit

Drug	Side-effect
CNS drugs	Drowsiness
Co-beneldopa	Colours urine

Some drugs have side-effects that need monitoring

Drug	Side-effect
Penicillamine	Blood and urine tests
Chloroquine	Ocular tests

Some drugs have side-effects that require immediate reporting to the prescriber

Drug	Side-effect
Gold therapy	Sore throat, breathlessness, rashes
Aminosalicylates	Bleeding, bruising

CNS, central nervous system; GI, gastrointestinal; NSAID, non-steroidal anti-inflammatory drug.

unwanted effects. No two situations or patients are alike and it is difficult to make a definite statement about this. However, it has been shown that if patients are informed of commonly occurring side-effects, how to recognize them and how to deal with them, they are less likely to be anxious. Select the side-effects which are most likely to occur and advise on them.

- A recommendation in Appendix 9 of the BNF ('Cautionary and advisory labels') that a cautionary and advisory label should be used. The information on these labels should always be reinforced.

Consideration of the patient

It is part of the pharmacist's role to decide which patients require information and advice. The level and type of information given and how it is given will depend on a variety of factors:

- Is the patient known at the pharmacy and have they been previously identified as having problems with drug therapy?
- What information/advice has the patient previously received?
- What are the patient's comprehension levels?
- What level of support does the patient need or have?
- The age of the patient. In general all patients who are elderly should be offered information and advice. If the prescription is for a child, the parent or guardian should be given advice.
- Is the patient pregnant or breastfeeding? Such patients may require reassurance that the therapy is safe to take. Similarly a breastfeeding mother may require advice on when to take the medication so that it least affects the child.
- Does the patient have physical disabilities? These could include mobility problems, causing problems in opening containers, blindness or deafness. A sight-impaired patient may not benefit from a patient information leaflet, while this may be the best way of providing information for someone who is hearing impaired.

- Does the patient have mental disabilities? These could include states of confusion, anxiety or forgetfulness. Limited intellectual capacity could lead to patients being unable to read labels, etc. or understanding instructions.
- Known poor compliance/concordance.

Other instances which should alert the pharmacist to the need for counselling would be:

- The purchase by a patient of an OTC product which is incompatible with the prescribed medication, for example a patient with hypertension who is taking atenolol and wishes to purchase pseudoephedrine for nasal congestion.
- A patient asking for an item not to be dispensed. This could indicate that the patient is non-compliant with that medication.
- A patient asking to buy an OTC medicine which is to relieve the side-effects of a prescribed medicine. An example of this would be when a patient who is being prescribed NSAIDs asks for an indigestion remedy. This should be investigated. The pharmacist will want to make sure that the stomach problem is not due to inappropriate use of the NSAID.

Stages in the information/advice giving process

If information and advice giving is approached in a structured manner, then time will be used efficiently and there will be a greater likelihood of success. The following stages have been adapted from the guidelines on Counselling and Advice on Medicines and Appliances in Community Pharmacy Practice

produced in 1996 by the Scottish Office Clinical Research and Audit Group:

- Recognizing the need for counselling
- Assessing and prioritizing the needs
- Specifying the assessment methods to be used
- Implementation
- Assessing the success of the process.

Recognizing the need for information and advice

The need for information and advice based on a consideration of the characteristics of the patient and the drug has been discussed earlier. In addition the pharmacist will need to consider the content of the prescription.

Has the medicine been prescribed before for the patient?

This is where a patient medication record (PMR) can be very useful (see Ch. 15). If the PMR cannot provide the answer and the patient is unknown, it is important to find out this information.

Are the instructions clear?

It is the pharmacist's responsibility to make sure that the patient knows what instructions such as 'when necessary' or 'as directed' mean. An open question should be used here, e.g. 'Tell me how you take this medicine'. If the patient does not know, then the necessary information can be provided. In some cases patients may be taking the medication incorrectly. The pharmacist is then in a position to rectify any misconceptions. Checking on imprecise dosage instructions can also pre-empt possible errors, as in Example 44.1.

Example 44.1

A prescription for 60 nitrazepam tablets 5 mg was received. The instructions read 'm.d.u.'.

The prescription was dispensed as written and handed over to the patient without any dialogue taking place. Approximately 2 hours later the patient returned saying that the tablets had a different name and appearance from the ones dispensed previously. On checking with the prescriber, the pharmacist found out that an error in entering the drug details into the surgery computer had

occurred. The patient should have been prescribed Nutrizym 10 capsules. The dose to be taken was 'Two capsules with every meal and one with intervening snacks'. If the pharmacist had asked the patient how he was taking his medication, she would have realized something was wrong. The normal dose for nitrazepam is 'two tablets at bedtime'. Fortunately in this instance no harm was done to the patient, but it illustrates very clearly the importance of the pharmacist's involvement.

Example 44.2

A prescription for colestipol granules, 1 o.d, penicillin tablets 250 mg, 2 q.i.d. and captopril tablets, 25 mg b.d. is received.

Because colestipol interferes with the absorption of drugs, it must be given either 1 hour before or 4–6 hours after other drugs. A considerable amount of organization is needed to get this regimen right. Trying to fit even a single dose of colestipol around the other drug therapy could cause the patient considerable problems.

Is the prescription for drugs which have a complicated or unusual regimen?

In some instances, with a little thought, the pharmacist can simplify matters. Example 44.2 is an illustration.

Assessing and prioritizing the needs

Although all individuals should be considered for information and advice, there will be some for whom little or none is required. For example a customer who asks for an OTC by name and has used it successfully on several previous occasions or an 'expert patient' receiving a dispensed medicine may require minimal information and advice. Giving information and advice is time-consuming and so pharmacists should concentrate their time and efforts on those patients requiring it. This entails assessing the needs of the patient and prioritizing so that efforts are directed at the most needy patients. In addition the pharmacist may have to be selective in what advice is given to a patient. The average number of facts which can be retained at any one time by most individuals is three. Example 44.3 illustrates this point.

Information/advice advice on cautionary labels should always include the reason why the precaution should be taken. Obviously, in this instance, to go into a detailed explanation for each caution could take a considerable amount of time. The large amount of information required might confuse the patient and the whole process becomes self-defeating. In instances like this the most important points should be selected for emphasis. Any other points may have to be left for another time. If only two points could be selected for this prescription, they would differ for different patients. In a patient who never drinks alcohol but is known to have a sensitive GI tract, the alcohol warning is less important than the warning about food intake and swallowing whole.

Specifying assessment methods

It cannot be assumed that because the information and advice has been given, that the patient understands or is able to adhere to that advice. It is

Example 44.3

A prescription for metronidazole tablets is received. Metronidazole tablets have five additional cautionary labels which should be added to the instructions. These are:

'*Avoid alcoholic drink*'. This is because, when combined with alcohol, a disulfiram-like reaction occurs and the patient may suffer nausea and vomiting. Patients who are not aware of this interaction may think, incorrectly, that the drug does not agree with them and stop taking it.

'*Take at regular intervals. Complete the prescribed course unless otherwise directed*'. Because of the antimicrobial effect of metronidazole, blood levels must be maintained and therapy must be continued for a minimum time period to prevent bacterial resistance developing.

'*Take with or after food*'. Metronidazole can cause GI irritation and the presence of food in the stomach will reduce the likelihood of this.

'*To be swallowed whole, not chewed*'. Metronidazole tablets are film coated which gives a degree of protection to the GI tract. If the preparation is chewed the coating will be destroyed, the drug will come into contact with the stomach lining and GI irritation will occur.

'*Take with plenty of water*'.
The film coating on the tablets may become sticky and if not taken with a reasonable draught of water can stick in the oesophagus. The drug will be released and could cause irritation to this least protected area of the GI tract.

therefore important that, before embarking on any information advice giving process, the pharmacist has an idea how the success of the process can be measured.

This assessment could consist of checking that the patient can read the label, use an inhaler device or open a container with a child-resistant cap. Checking on understanding may require follow-up, such as an enquiry the next time the patient visits the pharmacy, to ensure that no problems have occurred and the response to the therapy is as expected.

Implementation

The appearance of the pharmacy is an important factor. The environment should have a professional appearance and it should be apparent that information and advice are offered as a professional service. The service can be advertised in practice leaflets and within the pharmacy. Trying to give patients advice about their medication in a busy pharmacy can be difficult. Most pharmacies have a room or a special area set aside. This is essential for conducting MURs. Constant interruptions and customers milling around nearby are a major distraction and are barriers to good communication.

Time, or rather the lack of it, is a major barrier to good information and advice giving. Patients should be given an indication of why you wish to speak to them and you should always check that they have the time to listen. A patient who is worried about missing a bus or concerned about the car-parking fee is unlikely to give their undivided attention.

How the pharmacist appears is also of importance. An organized, calm person is more likely to inspire confidence in the patient than a pharmacist who appears distracted, harassed and unsure of him- or herself.

Over the last decade or so, through the National Pharmaceutical Association's 'Ask Your Pharmacist' campaign, the public has been made more aware of the pharmacist's role in the provision of healthcare advice. It is important that patients are made aware that pharmacies are sources of information about drug therapy and that information is available. If patients expect to be given information about their drug therapy then they will become more receptive to it.

If the patient is unknown to the pharmacist, it is important at the beginning of the conversation to try to gauge not just the amount of information that is needed but also the patient's level of comprehension. The type of language used is very important, particularly guarding against being patronizing by oversimplification. However, the use of medical terminology must be considered carefully.

The information/advice giving process must not be a monologue by the pharmacist, giving a long list of information points. There should be ample opportunity for the patient to ask questions. The pharmacist should introduce aids to comprehension if this is felt necessary, e.g. an explanatory leaflet or diagram, a placebo device.

Assessing the success of the process

Having given the information, it is then of major importance to check if the process has been successful. What does the patient understand? Can he use his device? Does he have any problems? The ideal, where possible, is to assess compliance/concordance through follow-up.

During the information and advice giving process the pharmacist should be checking if the patient is understanding the information imparted. Watching the patient's body language and maintaining eye contact can give useful clues as to whether the message is being understood and whether compliance/concordance is likely.

Aids to information and advice giving

Patient information leaflets, warning cards and placebo devices are all useful aids when giving advice to patients. Most products are now provided with information leaflets. These should be used where appropriate and important points highlighted. Placebo devices can be used to demonstrate a particular technique and also to check a patient's ability to use a device. The National Pharmacy Association is a useful source of information leaflets and warning cards. Leaflets on how to use ear drops, eye drops, eye ointment, pessaries, suppositories, a nebulizer, malaria tablets and head louse lotions are available. These, along with warning cards for anticoagulant therapy, lithium, monoamine oxidase inhibitors and steroids should be available in all pharmacies, hospitals and any other areas where counselling patients on drug therapy takes place. Whether commercially produced or prepared by individual pharmacists, ensure that the quality of any information leaflet is of the highest standard and is comprehensible to the patient.

Some examples

In the following examples, details of a prescription and some biographical details of the patient are given. Various information and advice points are identified and information which could be given to the patient detailed. These examples illustrate the wide variety of issues which have to be dealt with by pharmacists. They are not intended to be comprehensive, as different situations and different patients will produce a variety of problems and issues.

Example 44.4

Mrs Oak, a lady of about 70 years, presents a prescription for diclofenac sodium 25 mg tablets. She has lived alone since the death of her husband, 2 years ago. When she is signing the back of her prescription she has difficulty holding the pen and complains that her hands and fingers are rather sore and stiff and hopes that the prescription will help. This is the first time she has had these tablets.

Recognize the need for counselling

Mrs Oak has never been prescribed the tablets before, therefore basic information about the drug name and dose timings needs to be given.

NSAIDs can cause GI irritation if not taken with or after food. The warning label which indicates this will need to be reinforced.

Mrs Oak appears to have problems with her hands. Will she be able to open a bottle with a child-resistant cap (CRC)? She lives alone so does not have anyone to help her.

She has not been to the doctor previously for a prescription for her hands but has she been buying anything OTC to try to alleviate the pain? Many of the OTC products available for relief of arthritic pain contain diclofenac or other NSAIDs.

Mrs Oak will need to be advised to swallow the tablets whole and not to chew them. Will she be able to swallow them whole? Other formulations of diclofenac are available and may need to be considered for this patient.

There are a variety of issues here which will need to be checked.

Assessing and prioritizing the information and advice needs

Compliance problems

It is important to ensure that Mrs Oak can open the container and that she will have no difficulty swallowing the tablets.

Side-effects

It is vitally important to alert Mrs Oak to the fact that the tablets may irritate her stomach and how she can avoid this.

OTC purchases

To avoid any duplication of drug therapy it is very important to find out if Mrs Oak is taking any OTC medicines, what they are, and make sure they are not going to cause any problems.

Timing of doses and duration of treatment

Mrs Oak should be told that the tablets are not simply painkillers, to be taken infrequently. NSAIDs should give pain relief within 1 week and successful anti-inflammatory action should be seen within 3 weeks. To achieve these benefits, the drug must be taken at regular intervals. This should be explained to Mrs Oak.

There is obviously a considerable amount of information which needs to be given to Mrs Oak. However, none of it is too complex so it should be possible to deal with all of it.

A simple demonstration with a CRC will identify if she needs a container with a plain cap fitted. Showing her the tablets will also provide a clue as to whether she will be able to swallow them. Patients with swallowing difficulties can rarely conceal a look of horror when presented with tablets they know they cannot cope with. If swallowing is identified as a problem, she can be reassured that alternative therapy is available in liquid or granular form. It may then be necessary to contact the prescriber to alert him to this.

Any potential OTC problems can be dealt with by simple questioning.

It is preferable to give the patient all the drug details, if possible. However, if it is felt this will be counterproductive, dosing in relation to food is one that should have high priority.

Mrs Oak should be invited to let you know how she is getting on with her tablets and to contact you if she has any queries.

Example 44.5

You receive the following prescription:

Pulmicort LS® inhaler
Mitte 1
Sig. 2 puffs m. et n.
Bricanyl Turbohaler®
Mitte 1
Sig. Use m.d.u.

The patient, Mr Yee, is a patient of long standing. He has been on the steroid inhaler for several months and was also prescribed terbutaline as a metered-dose inhaler. He seemed to be well controlled and did not need to use his bronchodilator very frequently. He tells you that recently he has had one or two frightening wheezing attacks where his ability to inhale was severely impaired. For that reason, the doctor has given him a new type of inhaler.

The need for information and advice

Mr Yee has not had the Turbohaler® before. The different method of use will need to be explained. Because of the lack of propellant, some patients are not aware they have inhaled the drug when using this device.

He will need to be told that the Turbohaler® is the same drug as his terbutaline metered-dose inhaler and that he must not use them both.

The maximum dose of one puff four times daily will need to be reinforced, as this is different from the metered-dose inhaler dose.

During the counselling session it is probably worth checking Mr Yee's inhaler technique. The deterioration in his condition may be caused by insufficient steroid being inhaled. This could lead to ineffective prophylaxis.

Although asthmatic patients are normally on long-term treatment, it is dangerous to assume that they have good inhaler technique or are knowledgeable about their drug therapy. There should be regular checking of how devices are used and how frequently they are inhaled. Further information on this is found in Chapter 37.

Example 44.6

The following prescription is received:

Atenolol tablets 50 mg
Hypromellose eye drops
Trimethoprim tablets 200 mg

You notice from your PMR that, other than the atenolol tablets, which had previously been prescribed as the proprietary brand Tenormin®, the other two items are new to the patient. A considerable number of issues need to be dealt with here.

An explanation needs to be given that, although the appearance and name have changed, atenolol and Tenormin® are the same drug. If the patient has any left at home, they should be finished and the generic then started. Unfortunately, cases are reported of patients who end up taking double doses of drugs owing to a generic being prescribed in place of the branded preparation.

Information about shelf life and storage of the eye drops should be given, i.e. the eye drops must be discarded 4 weeks after being opened and should preferably be stored in a fridge.

Compliance with eye drops should be checked and the need for a compliance aid ascertained.

The trimethoprim is for the treatment of a urinary tract infection. Advice on the duration of the therapy must be given. An indication of when an improvement in the condition can be expected should be given. If no decrease in the severity of the symptoms is seen within 48 hours, it is possible that the organism is resistant to the antibiotic and alternative therapy may be needed. Basic advice on maintaining fluid intake should be given as an adjunct to drug therapy.

Conclusion

Develop the habit of thinking about medicines from the patient's point of view. What do patients need to know? What are their concerns about taking the medicine? What can be done to help patients resolve their concerns? Identifying information and advice giving points from the information at your disposal is fundamental to good pharmacy practice. It is important to remember, however, that asking questions and listening carefully to the information provided by patients is critical to the success of the process. Approximately 16% of hospital admissions are directly due to adverse drug reactions. How many of these could have been avoided if the patient had received appropriate information and advice from the pharmacist?

KEY POINTS

- Advice/information giving is an important part of the role of the pharmacist and there are many opportunities for counselling
- It is for the benefit of patients and purchasers of medicines
- Its importance is recognized in many official documents
- It must be structured and deal with the key information in an easily understood form
- The prescription is a useful guide to possible information and advice needs of the patient
- The extent to which patients should be told about side-effects will vary from one patient to another

- Information and advice should be used to reinforce adherence, potential for interactions and warning labels
- Some groups can be identified as requiring special information and advice – the elderly, those where there have been previous problems and parents of children
- It may be necessary to limit the amount of information given to avoid confusion and to meet patients' needs
- Checking is important in ensuring patient understanding
- A busy setting is a barrier to effective communication
- Patients are becoming more aware that pharmacists can give valuable advice
- Information and advice giving is not a lecture – patients must be given the opportunity to ask questions
- There are many aids to help patients with their medicines, including information leaflets, placebos and warning cards

Section Five

Pharmacy services and monitoring the medicine-taking patient

Collection and delivery services

Karen Rice

STUDY POINTS

- Prescription collection services
- Prescription delivery services
- Repeat medication services
- Delivery of medication through Internet pharmacies
- Advertising prescription collection, delivery and repeat medication services
- Handling prescription charges for delivery patients

Introduction

Collection and delivery services have always been undertaken in some form or other in pharmacies. They range from a member of staff 'dropping a prescription off' to a patient's home after the pharmacy has closed to a full blown service which includes ordering the prescription from the patient's surgery and delivering it to their home.

This type of service became more prominent in the late 1980s and now is common to most pharmacies but is not mandatory or funded as an enhanced service.

The service is usually free to patients and has been used as a way of increasing prescription business by improving the service to patients. By offering such services it has brought in a competition element with rival pharmacies for prescriptions. This healthy competition has led to better access to medicines for patients who are housebound or too ill to get to a pharmacy and creates social contact for some hard to reach patients.

Prescription collection services

A prescription collection service involves the collection of a patient's prescription from their doctor's surgery by pharmacy staff, at the request of that patient or their carer.

In order for this to happen there must be an audit trail. To prevent confusion the patient should be asked to give written authorization stating that they are happy for the pharmacy to receive and dispense that patient's prescription (Fig. 45.1).

Usually a patient or their carer orders regular repeat medication by indicating on the repeat medication counterfoil (attached to the last prescription they had dispensed) which items they need. They then hand this into their surgery or ring the request through. Some surgeries have an Internet facility to facilitate this ordering. It usually takes 1–2 days for the request to be translated into a prescription, which can then be picked up from the surgery.

The patient should verbally request collection of this prescription from the surgery by the pharmacy. A written record of this request should be made. This enables production of proof of the request, if necessary, when the prescription is collected from the surgery.

The pharmacy should have a system in place that gives a list of prescriptions requested by patients, which can then be collected at selected times from surgeries. It should indicate the date the prescription was collected from the surgery, the medicines ordered on the prescription and the date the dispensed items were collected by the patient/carer or delivered to the patient's home (Fig. 45.2).

To be retained in the pharmacy
Request for repeat prescription collection and/or delivery service
Please complete this form and hand it in to the pharmacy

Your name: (please print)	
Date of birth:	
Your address:	
Your telephone number:	
Surgery address plus GP name:	
I authorize _____ pharmacy to order ☐ collect ☐ deliver ☐ (please indicate service with a tick) my prescription on my behalf from the surgery above, either in person or by means of electronic transfer. I will inform you should I wish to change this arrangement.	
Signed	
Date	

To be retained in the surgery
Request for repeat prescription collection and/or delivery service
Please complete this form and hand it in to the pharmacy

Your name: (please print)	
Date of birth:	
Your address:	
Your telephone number:	
Surgery address plus GP name:	
I authorize _____ pharmacy to order ☐ collect ☐ deliver ☐ (please indicate service with a tick) my prescription on my behalf from the surgery above, either in person or by means of electronic transfer. I will inform you should I wish to change this arrangement.	
Signed	
Date	

Figure 45.1 ● An example of documentation used for prescription collection services.

Most surgeries expect a written list of patients requesting collection of their prescription by the pharmacy in order to prevent them from going to the wrong pharmacy. Some surgeries may 'direct' a prescription, at the request of the patient, to a specific pharmacy. If this happens, the pharmacy should make sure this patient signs an authorization for future collections. If not, this could lead to disputes with other pharmacies who would usually collect that patient's prescription. If a prescription is received from the surgery that has not been requested by the pharmacy (or patient), they should return it to the surgery.

Patient confidentiality and prescription security should be maintained through all stages of the process.

This collection service is used in conjunction with a prescription delivery service or by patients who find the opening times of the pharmacy more convenient than their surgery opening hours and can then collect their prescription from the pharmacy when the surgery is closed.

Date	Name of patient	Address	GP/ surgery	When is prescription ready to collect?	Collection/ delivery	Date of collection/ delivery

Number of forms/items	Signature of person receiving items	Print name	Reasons for not delivering items	Comments

Figure 45.2 • An example of the records used when delivering prescriptions.

Prescription delivery services

A prescription delivery service is where the patient receives their medication without visiting the pharmacy premises. Some pharmacies restrict this service to the housebound, disabled or elderly only, but most deliver to all patients.

This service is usually in conjunction with the prescription collection service.

If necessary, the pharmacy employs a driver to offer the service. This means the pharmacist does not have direct contact with these patients. In order to overcome the pharmacist's professional responsibility to intervene and give advice on dispensed medicines, the pharmacist must always make sure the patient has the opportunity to speak to them about their medication. This includes advice on how to use their medication safely, effectively and appropriately and to ensure they are not experiencing adverse effects or compliance difficulties. Reviewing patient medication records at regular intervals should highlight when such interventions are needed. A domiciliary medicines use review may be used to facilitate this.

Problems in delivering prescriptions occur when the patient is not at the delivery address. In this case the delivery driver should put some form of written notification through the letterbox to indicate that they have tried to deliver the patient's medication (Fig. 45.3) and make a note on their delivery sheet.

The driver's training should advise how to tackle this type of problem. They should never leave prescriptions with neighbours unless authorized by the patient. They should never put medication through the letterbox or leave it unattended in porches or on a doorstep. This practice can lead to children, unauthorized individuals or an animal taking the medication with possible dire consequences.

The driver should always double-check addresses and make sure they get a signature from the recipient on their delivery sheets (see Fig. 45.2), confirming the name and address at the time of handover. This should prevent delivery to the wrong address.

The driver should always return undelivered stock to the pharmacy.

All medication that has special storage requirements such as fridge items or controlled drugs should have some form of indication on the package to indicate this to the driver and the patient. This may be in

ANOther Pharmacy, address tried to deliver your prescription today (insert date)..............at (insert time).......... but you were out. The medicine will be returned to the pharmacy after (insert time)......... It may be collected from the pharmacy then if there is an immediate need, or it will be delivered tomorrow. If there is an immediate need and you are unable to arrange for collection today, please telephone the pharmacy on (insert telephone number), ...

Figure 45.3 • An example of the notification which may be left if a home delivery fails.

the form of a sticker and should be supplemented by verbal or written advice from the driver.

Deliveries for controlled drugs should have tighter control with regard to who delivers and signs for them when the driver reaches the patient's home. Separate duplicate books may be used to give a receipt to the patient or their representative in line with current controlled drug regulations.

Repeat medication services

A repeat medication service involves the pharmacist ordering repeat medication for the patient directly from a surgery. The pharmacist must always establish with the patient when these requests are being made that they do require all items, and they must look out for issues with concordance or other problems which would indicate referral of the patient back to the prescriber. The pharmacist's aim must always be to help the patient's medicines management and ensure rational and effective use of their medication.

The pharmacist usually keeps the repeat medication counterfoils that are attached to the patient's prescription. The patient contacts the pharmacist when they need to order their medication, usually by telephone. The pharmacist indicates on the prescription counterfoil what is requested and orders the medication from the surgery. They then collect the prescription and, if necessary, deliver the medication to the patient.

Some pharmacists prompt the patient by phoning them when their medication is due to run out. The pharmacist cannot order medication without the patient's consent. Written authorization should be obtained (see Fig. 45.1) from the patient for the service to commence.

Also, the prescriber must be happy for their patient to utilize this service and cooperate with the pharmacy. The prescriber must give informed consent.

There should be clear referral pathways should a patient need to see their doctor or should they need to visit the surgery for a medication review or tests.

The pharmacist must make sure their patient medication records are registered with the Data Protection Commissioner and that a clear audit trail of dispensed medication is available on request.

Since April 2005, pharmacists have been able to dispense patient's medication directly from Repeat master and batch Prescriptions, without the need to order them from the surgery. This service is part of the national pharmacy contract and has clear guidance on

how it should be run. Again, patients must request their medication and the pharmacist must establish the need for the medication.

Delivery of medication through Internet pharmacies

Since April 2005, there has been the ability to apply for an Internet (distant selling) pharmacy contract. These pharmacies have no face-to-face contact with patients so all medication is delivered to the patient, and all prescriptions are posted to the pharmacy (or will be transferred electronically in the future).

As with all pharmacies, online pharmacies must provide the same quality of pharmaceutical care as any other type of pharmacy. This applies to how they handle prescriptions, how they deliver them and how they advise the patient about their medication.

All prescriptions should be valid and legal. The pharmacist must ensure they have checked the prescription's authenticity before dispensing.

When delivering the prescription, the pharmacist has a professional responsibility towards patients. Medicines must be delivered safely and with appropriate instructions. The patient should be able to contact the pharmacist by phone or e-mail with any queries about their medication.

The prescription should not be delivered to the patient's home without the patient's or their representative's consent. This consent should be via the Internet or in writing using a form for authorization. The advice on delivery of the medicines is the same as previously referred to for a prescription delivery service if the pharmacy has a dedicated driver.

If the Internet pharmacy uses a postal delivery system then they are also required to have written consent for this from the patient or their representative. Because it is not recommended that medication be posted through a letterbox, 'special delivery' services, such as recorded delivery or registered post, should be used to guarantee a signature by the recipient and give a verifiable audit trail.

Advertising prescription collection, delivery and repeat medication services

Any publicity for pharmacy services must comply with requirements in the Code of Ethics. Services can be advertised in surgeries via posters and leaflets that are available for self-selection. Surgery staff should not directly promote pharmacies' services as this could be interpreted as endorsing the services of a particular pharmacy and misleading patients. This may be interpreted as prescription direction which could lead to complaints from other pharmacies. Freepost envelopes or freephone numbers are acceptable.

Patients must always have a choice as to where they obtain their pharmacy services.

Handling prescription charges for delivery patients

Currently patients obtaining prescriptions through the NHS either pay or are exempt. When delivering a prescription, this status must be ascertained.

If they pay, they must give the prescription payment to the pharmacy delivery driver who should record this payment being received and take the remittance back to the pharmacy. A receipt should be given to the patient if requested.

If the patient has had their medication posted via an Internet pharmacy, there should be a secure way of paying for the medication.

If the prescription has not been signed and an exemption indicated by the patient, their exemption should be confirmed at the time of dispensing. With age-related exemption this can be verified from the prescription (if it is a computer-generated prescription) and for certified exemption, e.g. medical exemption, a record can be kept on the patient medication record with the expiry date of that exemption certificate. For financial exemptions, the patient should sign the prescription each time. If it is a delivery prescription, the driver should ask the patient or representative to sign the prescription on delivery. If the pharmacy staff sign for a patient exemption, they take responsibility for any fraudulent claims.

The Royal Pharmaceutical Society of Great Britain has produced service specifications and fact sheets for pharmacists which give guidance on these services.

KEY POINTS

- Pharmacists have traditionally offered an ad hoc delivery of medicines
- In a prescription collection service, the pharmacist collects the prescription from the surgery in response to a request from a patient. The medicine is then collected from the pharmacy by the patient
- Prescription delivery services enable the patient to receive their medicine without visiting the pharmacy and are often offered in conjunction with prescription collection services
- Pharmacists must ensure that they offer full services to patients, e.g. counselling and medicines use reviews
- Driver training is essential and must involve procedures for cold chain items and controlled drugs
- Repeat medicine services extend the other services so that the pharmacist initiates the ordering of repeat prescriptions on behalf of the patient
- Since 2005, pharmacists have been able to dispense directly from Repeatable Prescriptions
- Internet pharmacies must offer the same full services to patients and must be able to collect prescription charges or exemption signatures when required
- An audit trail must be created for all aspects of these services

Chapter Forty-Six

Concordance

Marjorie C. Weiss

STUDY POINTS

- What is meant and understood by the term 'concordance'
- How concordance differs from compliance and adherence
- The concordance model and the relationship with patients
- The need for good communication skills in developing a concordant relationship
- Concerns about using a concordance approach with patients

Introduction

'Mrs Jones is being a non-concordant patient (sigh) again'. Or is she? Concordance offers a way forward when we, as pharmacists, notice that patients are not taking their medicines as prescribed. Yet concordance can fundamentally challenge our assumptions about the role of patients in a professional–patient interaction. It states that patients have a legitimate and valuable perspective on taking their medicines and that healthcare professionals should encourage patients, should they wish it, to become involved in decisions about their treatment. For these reasons, concordance is about a consultation process and not an individual patient behaviour. Mrs Jones cannot be non-concordant on her own: it takes at least two, professional and patient, to have a non-concordant (or successfully concordant) encounter. The consultation could have been non-concordant but Mrs Jones, on her own, cannot have been. Mrs Jones can be non-compliant or non-adherent to her medicine but these have a distinctly different meaning from concordance.

What is concordance?

Concordance occurs when 'the patient and the healthcare professional participate as partners to reach an agreement on when, how and why to use medicines, drawing on the expertise of the healthcare professional as well as the experiences, beliefs and wishes of the patient' (Marinker et al 1997). It arose from the recognition that throughout the decades of research investigating interventions to help patients follow prescriptions for medications, there was still a high level of non-adherence. In a review by Haynes et al (2001), interventions that used a combination of approaches in helping patients take their medicines such as providing more convenient care, giving patients more information, providing reminders or offering medicine counselling, did not lead to large improvements in adherence rates. From this synthesis of research findings, there was a call to investigate more innovative approaches to assist patients with taking their medicines. Concordance is one such innovative approach.

This is not to say that terms like adherence and compliance can no longer be used. When referring to the extent to which patients take medicines as prescribed by their doctor or other healthcare professional, the words 'adherence' and 'compliance' are appropriate terms to be used. As a concept distinct from compliance or adherence, concordance may affect adherence although it is mainly concerned with improving the quality of health care through a shared understanding between professional and patient on treatment choices. Yet there are difficulties with words like adherence and compliance which have overtones of the patient being disobedient or 'naughty' in not following the doctor's instructions. Conceptually, terms like compliance and adherence reinforce a paternalistic doctor-knows-best model of health care and implicitly devalue the views and experience of patients as users of medicines. Concordance seeks to redress this balance by acknowledging that patients and customers have a key role in the decision making of whether or not to take their medicine.

The term adherence has been usefully split into those who are intentionally non-adherent and those who are unintentionally non-adherent. Unintentionally non-adherent patients are those who do not take their medicine because of a number of reasons, for example because they are unable to read the label due to poor eyesight, or forgot to take a tablet because a medicine regimen is complex and difficult to remember. Appropriate solutions to unintentional non-adherence are big print labels, improved medicines information, simplified medicine regimens or adherence aids such as a Dosette box. Intentional non-adherence is where concordance can play a role; previous research has suggested that patients make reasoned decisions about whether or not to take their medicines. Patients may alter their medicine-taking behaviour for a number of reasons; for example:

- They have experienced side-effects
- Taking medicines interferes with their daily lives
- They have beliefs about the medicines or illness which conflict with medicine taking
- They are adjusting the medicine dose in response to symptoms.

Concordance has been called a partnership in medicine taking and has three important ingredients: (1) includes an explicit agreement between two people; (2) is based upon respect for each other's beliefs; and (3) gives the patient's view priority although they may choose to have the professional make all the decisions about treatment. This third ingredient recognizes that once the patient leaves the encounter with the healthcare professional, they will ultimately have the casting vote to decide whether or not to take that medicine.

Ethical considerations

The need to involve patients in decisions about their care is enshrined in principle 4 of the Code of Ethics for Pharmacists and Pharmacy Technicians, published by the Royal Pharmaceutical Society of Great Britain. This principle draws upon healthcare professionals' duty to obtain informed consent when initiating new medicines and the ethical principle of respect for patient autonomy, which recognizes that patients should be allowed to have control over their own lives and make decisions that affect their lives. In common with the concordance initiative, this principle advocates working in partnership with patients, to explain the options available and to help patients make informed decisions about different treatment options.

The concordance model

Concordance shares many characteristics with other models and themes currently prevalent in health care, most importantly those of shared decision making and patient-centredness. There is a greater chance of a successfully concordant encounter when each participant knows what the other is thinking. For this reason, concordance shares many characteristics with shared decision making: where both the doctor and patient share information with each other, when both take steps to participate in the decision-making process by expressing treatment preferences and they jointly agree on the treatment to implement. Shared decision making may be considered part of the wider concept of patient-centredness. Patient-centredness has three themes: eliciting the patient's perspectives and understanding them within a psychosocial context; reaching a shared understanding of the patient's problem and treatment; and involving patients, to the extent they wish to be involved, in choices about their care. It is not a coincidence that the concept of concordance arose during the same time period that patient-centred care became dominant in healthcare policy. Concordance can be seen as part of the wider patient-centred political context but one which specifically focuses on medicine-taking behaviour.

Concordance also shares many features with the formative communication teaching guides, the Calgary–Cambridge guides as discussed in Chapter 13. Although designed as a formative aid in teaching medical students communication skills, the Calgary–Cambridge guides have a consultation structure which is readily adaptable to the pharmacy setting. These guides assume a chronology to the consultation with distinct sections on initiating the consultation, gathering information, providing structure to the consultation, building a relationship, explanation and planning and closing the consultation. The Calgary–Cambridge guide has been adapted to reflect two common pharmacy consultation situations of (1) handing out a new prescription and (2) issuing a repeat prescription, as shown in Box 46.1. Sample phrases or 'catchphrases' useful in conducting a concordant consultation in pharmacy are shown in Box 46.2.

The Medicines Partnership at NPC Plus has developed a competency framework for shared decision making with patients, describing the skills and behaviours professionals need to reach a shared agreement about treatment. In this document, shared decision making and concordance are used synonymously, highlighting the common approach underpinning these concepts. These eight competencies are shown in Box 46.3.

 Box 46.1

A concordance model for pharmacy: Involving patients in decisions about their medicines

New prescriptions	Repeat prescriptions

Reinforces prescriber's instructions and provides other important information

- Prioritizes key information: how to take the medicine, what it does, what it is for and important side-effects
- Gives information in manageable chunks so as not to overload patient

Explores patient's ideas, concerns and expectations

- Explores the patient's view on the possibility of having to take a medicine
- Explores previous experience with medicines
- Explores patient concerns about taking the medicine(s)

Explores patient's ideas, concerns and expectations

- Explores previous experience with using the medicine
- Explores patient concerns about taking the medicine(s)

Develops rapport

- Accepts legitimacy of patient's views
- Picks up on patient verbal and non-verbal cues
- Facilitates patient's responses

Develops rapport

- Accepts legitimacy of patient's views
- Picks up on patient verbal and non-verbal cues
- Facilitates patient's responses

Provides additional information

- Discusses the pros and cons of taking and not taking the medicine
- Finds out if the patient wants any other information
- Avoids jargon
- Checks patient understanding

Provides additional information

- Finds out if the patient wants any other information
- Gives information in manageable chunks
- Avoids jargon
- Checks patient understanding

Deciding with the patient

- Discusses other options or issues of importance to the patient
- Negotiates mutually acceptable plan
- 'Safety nets' so patient knows where to go if they experience problems or have further questions and how to follow-up

Deciding with the patient

- Discusses other options or issues of importance to the patient
- Negotiates mutually acceptable plan
- 'Safety nets' so patient knows where to go if they experience problems or have further questions and how to follow-up

Catchphrases useful in involving patients in decisions about their medicines: giving out medicines in a pharmacy

Eliciting the patient's view

- 'How do you feel about starting on a new medication?'
- 'Do you feel you will be able to take this medicine as suggested by your doctor?'
- 'What do you think about taking this medicine on a regular basis?'
- 'How have you been getting on with your medicines?' (repeats)
- 'What makes you think that [particular problem] might be due to the medicine?'

Eliciting patient concerns

- 'Do you have any concerns about starting this medication?'
- 'How can I help you with this medicine?'
- 'Is there anything else you would like to know about?'
- 'Is there anything in particular that worries you?'
- 'Have you had any bad experiences with this kind of thing in the past?'
- 'Could you tell me a bit more about that?'

Giving patients the amount of information they want

- 'Can I give you some more information about that?'
- 'What do you know about it?'
- 'Would you like to know more?'
- 'What do you want to know about it?'
- 'Are there some more questions I can answer for you?'
- 'Would you like to go away and read this and think about it a bit more?'

Deciding with the patient

- 'You're quite right to worry about that kind of thing – it can happen with some medicines. How would you feel about giving this one a go for a month or so and see how you get on?'
- 'How do the good and bad effects of taking this medicine weigh up for you?'

The evidence for concordance

Already presented has been the Haynes Cochrane review regarding the use of interventions to help patients take their medicines: that current methods of improving adherence are complex and not very effective. Much of the information available about concordance relates to the doctor–patient consultation. As shown in Box 46.1, the concordant approach can be readily adapted to the pharmacy situation after a prescribing decision has been made. Examples are handing out new or repeat prescriptions, in repeat dispensing or in conducting a medicines use review. Yet pharmacists also have a role before treatment decisions about medicines are made: when giving over the counter advice or as pharmacist independent prescribers. The next sections will look at evidence drawing upon a predominantly medical literature and may appear to be relevant only in the latter situation, i.e. before prescribing decisions are made. However, the evidence has resonance for the range of pharmacy consultations, both before and after treatment decisions have been made. These are grouped under the headings of: eliciting the patient's view; developing rapport with the patient; providing information; and the therapeutic alliance.

Eliciting the patient's view

Previous research tells us that patients have beliefs about their medicines and illness, and that these beliefs can affect their medicine-taking behaviour. For example, individual patients will vary in their confidence in the medicine to help them. They may have doubts about a medicine and 'test' whether the medicine is having an effect by stopping it on occasions. Patients may believe that they will become 'immune' or addicted to a medicine if they take it long term. These beliefs can occur even when we know these medicines are not associated with a true pharmacological dependence. Many people consider prescribed or over the counter medicines, particularly in comparison with herbal or homoeopathic products, to be unnatural, artificial and potentially harmful to their bodies. They might see themselves as being 'anti-drugs' people where doing without a medicine is the preferred course of action, only resorting to medicine taking when it is absolutely necessary. Evidence also suggests that patients make complex judgments about their medicines, weighing up the benefits and drawbacks of taking a medicine within

Box 46.3

Competency framework for shared decision making with patients: summary. (After Clyne et al 2007 with the permission of NPC Plus)

Building a partnership

Listening

Listens actively to patients

Communicating

Helps the patient to interpret information in a way that is meaningful to them

Managing a shared consultation

Context

With the patient, defines and agrees the purpose of the consultation

Knowledge

Has up-to-date knowledge of area of practice and wider health services

Sharing a decision

Understanding

Recognizes that the patient is an individual

Exploring

Discusses illness and treatment options, including no treatment

Deciding

Decides with the patient the best management strategy

Monitoring

Agrees with the patient what happens next

---

their individual patient experience. All of these patient beliefs have their own rationality when viewed from the patient's perspective of taking medicines within the context of their everyday life.

Research on doctor–patient consultations suggests that these beliefs are important because, if not elicited, they can lead to misunderstandings in consultations when prescribing decisions are made. Misunderstandings in consultations can be caused by non-disclosure of information from either the doctor or the patient, disagreement about causes of side-effects or failure of communication about a decision reached by the doctor. Misunderstandings arise when patients do not play an active role in the consultation by stating their views and beliefs about the medicine or illness under discussion. The consequence of consultation misunderstandings can be non-adherence to prescribed medication. While research has primarily focused on doctor–patient consultations, it can be hypothesized that eliciting the patient's views and beliefs on their medicine and medicine-taking behaviour is equally important in pharmacist–patient or pharmacist–customer interactions as well. The Database of Individual Patients' Experiences of Illness and Health (DIPEx) is a website which gives videoclips of

patients' experiences. It may be useful when professionals want to gain insight into what it is like from a patient's perspective to experience a particular illness or face a specific health-related decision (see Appendix 5).

Developing rapport with the patient

Concordance is focused on a consultation process and, as such, is primarily concerned with professional–patient communication. Although we all tend to think of ourselves as good communicators, to participate in a concordant consultation is actually very difficult. If it seems easy, you are probably not doing it right! All of the 'generic' communication skills such as active listening, avoiding jargon, giving information 'in chunks' or a little bit at a time, using open questions, appropriate body language, encouraging the patient to ask questions, treating the patient as an equal and being non-judgmental are important. Other skills, such as presenting information in a way the patient is able to understand, without being patronizing, are essential. Both people in the consultation need to explore each other's viewpoint and confirm that they understand where the other person is coming from. While a patient may spontaneously volunteer their personal beliefs or views, if they do not, it is down to the skill of the professional to elicit the patient's view and ensure that the patient feels comfortable enough to discuss this information.

Empathy plays a key part in concordance. Empathy is distinct from sympathy. Empathy involves fully understanding an individual's emotions, while sympathy is simultaneously being affected by another's emotions. In interactions with patients, empathy allows for recognition and acknowledgement of the patient perspective. Professionals display their acceptance of the legitimacy of the patient's view by communicating their understanding of the patient's situation. Included within this are expressions of concern, a general willingness to help and an acknowledgement of the efforts the patient may have made thus far in terms of trying to manage their medicines and illness. It requires the professional to be able to deal sensitively with potentially embarrassing or unpleasant issues.

In a concordant consultation it can be useful to overtly draw attention to the structure of the interaction and signpost when a different issue or change of subject will take place. This includes providing information in a logical sequence but may also consist of statements such as 'I would now like to move on to discussing potential options, is that okay with you?' or 'There are three ways in which this medicine can help you. Firstly, ...' or 'I'd now just like to summarize some of the things we've discussed'. Summarizing information at various points in the interaction, asking if the patient has any questions as well as 'safety netting' – identifying appropriate follow-up or what to do if something changes or further questions arise – are important.

Providing information

Studies over the years have consistently shown that patients want information about their medicines. When patients are asked what they would like to know, they frequently respond that they want to know about side-effects, what the medication does, any lifestyle changes they might need to undertake and how to take the medication. Surveys support the view that, while most patients have considerable confidence in their medicines, 30% also have concerns, particularly with regard to side-effects. Patients want

to know information even when the information contains bad news or in terms of side-effects, no matter how rare. This may be impractical during a typically brief pharmacy encounter. Should the patient wish to have information beyond the more frequent and serious side-effects, this information can be provided in a written format. Nonetheless, it is not unusual for patients, when asked retrospectively about whether they would have liked more information about a prescribed medicine, to state that they would have liked more.

Information should be provided in a manner which takes account of what the patient may already know and what, and how much, information they would like to receive. Patients should be offered information on treatment options, to including non-pharmacological options or the choice to have no treatment. Addressing the 'no treatment' option is important, even when there is only one drug of choice or when the doctor has already prescribed the medicine. If the patient has reservations or concerns about a medicine that were not resolved before the medicine was prescribed, the patient will simply walk out of the pharmacy and not take it. This is the pharmacist's opportunity to provide information on both the benefits and risks of taking and not taking a medicine, which may influence the patient's decision-making process long after they have left the pharmacy. Throughout this process, it is important for both pharmacist and patient to communicate their thoughts, perceived dilemmas or uncertainties in treatment options, ideas and reactions to new pieces of information. Only through this process can a mutually agreeable treatment plan be devised.

Verbal information can be supported with written information, the most familiar written format being the patient information leaflet (PIL). European Union legislation requires a comprehensive medicines information leaflet to be provided in every medicines pack. There is strict guidance on the information to be included in this leaflet and, most recently, requirements on the readability of these leaflets. PILs often do not increase patient knowledge, nor do patients value them. This may, however, change as it is now recommended that the wording in PILs be tested with patients. Findings from studies have indicated that patients would like information to be tailored to their particular illness and circumstances, to help with decision making before prescribing occurs, and for it to contain a balance of benefit and harm information.

PILs are not the only way of communicating information. As well as verbal communication and information from PILs, other written information can include condition- or medicine-specific information guides, or use can be made of video, DVD or other interactive media. Information can also be presented in the form of a decision aid. Decision aids are patient decision support tools which facilitate evidence-based patient choice. They normally have a number of informational elements. They provide information on available treatment options, consider the patient's values for benefits versus harm, and facilitate the patient's participation in treatment decisions. Like other educational materials they can be provided as booklets, DVDs, videos or as interactive media. A systematic review of decision aids by O'Connor et al (2003) has shown that they can increase patient knowledge, improve the proportion of patients with realistic perceptions of benefits and harms, reduce the proportion of patients who are undecided after counselling and decrease the proportion of patients who are passive in decision making. There is a library of decision aids at the Ottawa Health Research Institute's website covering a broad range of clinical conditions and health issues (see Appendix 5). On this website library, each decision aid is rated using a series of internationally agreed quality criteria. Many of these decision aids are American but can be adapted to the UK setting. Online initiatives such as NPCi through the National Prescribing Centre will also make available Web-based patient decision aids from late 2007 to support an evidence-based patient choice approach.

A major issue for all types of written, computer-based, audio, video and interactive information is the quality of information available (see Ch. 23). Much of the information available is poor, particularly with regard to providing accurate and adequately detailed clinical information to assist patients in decision making. Other issues exist, such as ensuring topics of relevance to patients are included and that uncertainties in treatment need to be clearly communicated. A number of tools have been developed to assess the quality of health information such as the DISCERN tool and the International Patient Decision Aids Standards (IPDAS) instrument. The tools use a range of criteria to judge the issue information, such as:

- Information accuracy, comprehensiveness and reliability
- Clarity of aims and target audience
- The comprehensibility and balance of information
- References to sources
- How up to date it is

- Support for shared decision making
- Transparency of authorship and sponsorship (if any).

Pharmacists are not the only people who need to be able to judge the quality of health information. Patients are active information seekers and, although their most common source of health information is the doctor, other sources such as the Internet are increasingly playing a part. The pharmacist is in an excellent position to act as the patient's 'Internet guide': to provide advice on accessing and understanding Web resources, to direct them to high-quality Internet sites and to discuss with them any information affecting their decision to take, or not take, a medicine. This will show the pharmacist as a resource for accessing and discussing medicines information to which patients will be likely to return in the future.

Communicating risk

A key aspect of sharing information with patients is the ability to communicate risk: to provide information on the effectiveness of a medicine or the likelihood of a side-effect occurring. Pharmacists often use words such as 'rarely' or 'commonly' to indicate to patients how frequent a particular side-effect is likely to be experienced. In an effort to standardize the interpretation of these words, the European Union (EU) has issued a guideline banding the level of risk into five groups from 'very common' to 'very rare' (Box 46.4). However, even this approach may not ensure consistency. Evidence suggests that the general public has a tendency to reliably overestimate the risk associated with these words in comparison with the risk frequency intended by the EU. Healthcare professionals also consistently overestimate the risk level associated with these words, although not to the same

Box 46.4

EU recommended verbal descriptors and their frequency range

Verbal descriptor	EU assigned frequency level
Very common	>10%
Common	1–10%
Uncommon	0.1–1%
Rare	0.01–0.1%
Very rare	<0.01%

magnitude that the lay public does. The use of these verbal descriptors can lead to people perceiving there is a greater risk to their health than there actually is, suggesting that they need to be used in combination with actual numbers in order to effectively communicate the intended risk level.

Expressing risks as natural frequencies (e.g. 3 out of 10 people will experience dizziness with this medicine) facilitates greater understanding of risk than presenting it as a probability statement (e.g. there is a 30% chance of dizziness with this medicine). As well as textual (or verbal) and numerical presentations of risk, other visual forms can be used such as bar charts, icons (showing how many people in 100 are affected), pie charts, tables or survival curves. Graphical information may result in greater accuracy in determining the relative quantitative difference between risks, although icons have been found to be quite helpful to decision making. Further research is needed on patient preferences and the benefits of alternative risk formats. It is also possible that different people may prefer different formats to aid their individual understanding of risk information. Verbal, textual, visual, graphical and numerical formats may all have a place and the key to communicating risk is a flexible approach. A greater desire for involvement in decision making is associated with a preference for more complex risk information so the need for alternative risk formats, and flexibility in approach, is essential.

A number of factors have been shown to improve people's understanding of risk information. Including both verbal or text information and numerical or graphical information on risks can aid understanding. Presentation of information which is both positive and negative provides a more balanced view of the benefits and risks of taking a particular medicine. Taking account of the starting or baseline risk levels can also improve the accuracy of people's judgments about, for example, the benefit associated with introducing a new medication (e.g. reduction in stroke risk). This allows people to anchor their perception at their starting level of risk and extrapolate more accurately to the potential decrease in stroke risk with starting a new medication.

Finally, whether a risk is presented as an absolute risk reduction or relative risk reduction can also influence people's perception of risk. Absolute risk reduction is the difference in risk between a control group and a treatment group. Relative risk reduction is the event rate in the treatment group divided by the event rate in the control group subtracted from one. For example, if a new hypertensive drug decreases the risk of stroke from 0.004% to 0.003%, the relative risk reduction is 25% although the absolute risk reduction is only 0.001%. Relative risk reduction sounds much more impressive and is more persuasive. Absolute risk reduction is the preferred method for conveying accurate risk information and should be used on its own or in combination with the relative risk reduction.

The therapeutic alliance

What are the benefits of a therapeutic alliance with patients? Once pharmacists have engaged with patients in a pharmacy consultation and a plan of action regarding medicines has been mutually agreed, what are the benefits of this process? Reviews have shown that good adherence to medication is associated with a decreased mortality. This includes adherence to placebo or beneficial drug therapy suggesting that there is a 'healthy adherer effect', where adherence to drug therapy may be a proxy for overall healthy behaviours. The question then becomes, does concordance improve adherence or affect other health outcomes? With concordance embracing a range of competences around the professional and patient sharing beliefs, preferences and information in a collaborative consultation process, the evidence for concordance affecting adherence depends upon how concordance has been defined. Patients rarely voice their concerns about medicines, unless encouraged to do so, and the issue of whether or not patients are taking their medicines is not always discussed in a consultation. Many of the elements perceived to be necessary for concordance (such as establishing whether or not both the professional and patient express their points of view, whether the professional respects the patient's perspective on their illness and medicine use, or whether both work together towards shared decisions) appear not to be taking place in practice, or only taking place to a limited extent. For these reasons, finding evidence that concordance improves adherence or other health outcomes is difficult.

There is evidence on specific aspects of communication which are relevant for concordance. When patients are given information about treatment options and coached to ask questions about their condition, they are more involved in the consultation and have better health outcomes. Improvement in health outcomes can, for example, include decreased blood pressure or blood sugar levels, an improved subjective evaluation of overall health or increased functionality in terms of activities of daily living. When professionals share treatment decision making with patients and focus on the patient as a person and not merely a disease state, patient satisfaction is likely to be increased. Effective communication involving activities such as encouraging the patient to ask questions, providing information and support and sharing the decision-making process has been shown, across a range of research studies, to improve emotional health, resolve symptoms, improve function and reduce pain.

Concerns about concordance

Concerns about concordance centre on four issues:

- Time. That a concordant consultation will take too long
- Anxiety. That providing information to patients makes them anxious and they will either experience the side-effects that have been described to them and/or stop taking their medication
- People do not want to participate in decisions about their medicines
- Concordance will lead to unreasonable patient demands for expensive medicines and healthcare.

Time is a concern for all healthcare professionals. Approaches such as concordance which have the potential to increase consultation times are an issue in any busy pharmacy setting. Research suggests that using a concordant approach with patients may take longer initially, but as professionals gain experience and proficiency in this approach, consultation times will decrease. There is also some evidence that if professionals do not pick up on patient clues, defined as direct or indirect comments made by patients about personal aspects of their lives or emotions, then consultations will be longer. It seems that if a patient has issues or ideas which they hint about during a consultation, it is best to address these issues openly. If not, the patient may feel obliged to continue seeking opportunities throughout the interaction to allude to these issues and this may ultimately prolong the consultation further.

It is also now possible to separate the provision of information about options from the consultation process. This has been facilitated through the use of decision aids and other interactive media. Patients can access the information outside of the consultation and have time to think about their options, discuss them with relevant others, make a list of questions to ask the healthcare professional and then participate as an informed patient in the consultation with their healthcare professional. This may be the best solution to deal with issues of time, i.e. de-couple the provision of information about options from the constraints on consultation length. Decision aids do not replace a consultation with a healthcare professional but may enhance informed discussion by giving patients the time to think about the issues of importance to them, having taken account of the clinical information in the decision aid.

There is a concern that telling patients about the side-effects of their medicines can lead to them experiencing these side-effects. This comes from the idea that humans are suggestible; that telling people about a side-effect makes them experience it. The research on whether forewarning of side-effects affects people's adherence can be conflicting. Yet the weight of research evidence indicates that provision of information about side-effects does not increase anxiety nor does it affect a patient's adherence. What does seem clear is that how this information is presented can affect adherence. So presenting information on both positive and negative effects of treatment, in a manner understandable (without being patronizing) to lay people, that links into lay theories of illness and treatment (see Ch. 3) and which promotes informed choice can avoid the potential negative consequences of information overload or 'information anxiety'.

Patients do not always want to be involved in decisions about what treatment is best for them. It is well known that there are a proportion of patients that want the doctor (most commonly) to decide what treatment is right for them. However, up to two-thirds of patients either want to decide for themselves after the doctor has explained the options to them or want to do so in partnership with a healthcare professional. While older people are less likely to want a more active role in decision making than younger, more affluent people, half of those aged over 65 and those in lower social classes want to have a 'say' in decisions about their care. People need to be involved in decision making to the extent that they want to be. The best way to do this is to ask them.

There is a view that if the patient's view takes priority in an interaction between healthcare professional and patient, the patient will simply demand expensive medicines or healthcare services at the expense of those who are less articulate but more in need of health care. Given the current emphasis on the need to ration scarce healthcare resources, this is a potentially valid concern. High-profile cases in the popular press with patients demanding expensive treatments reinforce this concern. Concordance is about both parties expressing their views and if a healthcare professional has reservations about a particular treatment option (e.g. that it is of uncertain benefit or the costs outweigh the benefits), they need to explain this rationale to the patient. A common cause of litigation is poor communication between professionals and patients, such as devaluing or failing to understand the patient's perspective. The alternative is not to inform patients of all options because one option may be particularly expensive. This can lead to patients seeking out this information on their own and raising a legitimate complaint that they were not informed about all options. Unreasonable demands may occur in a consultation but, provided both parties express their views and the rationale behind their views as part of a concordant consultation process, there is unlikely to be a basis for litigation against an individual practitioner. In the end, both parties may need to agree to differ.

Conclusion

Concordance is an opportunity for pharmacists to engage with patients on an equal level to understand their perspective on taking medicines. It argues for openness in the consultation where both professional and patient are able to express their views. Information is exchanged which may be clinical, personal, experiential and potentially worrying. Decisions are based on all types of information which are relevant for subsequent medicine taking. Ultimately it is

hoped that this will make the best use of medicines and, in situations where the patient has decided not to take a medicine, recognizes that an agreement to differ to include the open acknowledgement of the patient's perspective is preferable to the patient going away with concerns or issues which remain unaddressed.

KEY POINTS

- Concordance promotes the view that patients have a legitimate and valuable perspective on taking decisions about their health care
- The concept of concordance arose because of the need for innovative approaches to help patients with their medicines
- Non-adherence may be unintentional or intentional
- The Code of Ethics indicates that pharmacists have a duty to assist patients reach their own decisions
- The concordance model shares features with other models of effective communication
- Eliciting patient views is the first stage in establishing a concordant relationship
- Because concordance is concerned with the consultation, it is essential to have a good patient–pharmacist relationship
- Empathy plays a key role in concordance
- Patients want information and different techniques can be used including the use of decision aids, PILs, the Internet, medicine guides, video and DVDs
- When communicating risk to patients, pharmacists need to ensure that patients have understood the information fully and have received the breadth and depth of information they desire
- The ultimate aim of concordance is to establish a therapeutic alliance between patient and healthcare provider
- There are strategies for reducing concerns about concordance, particularly with respect to the time it involves

47

Monitoring the patient

Alison Littlewood

STUDY POINTS

- The Yellow Card reporting scheme
- The pharmacist's role in adverse drug reaction reporting
- The medicines use review/prescription intervention service

Introduction

Monitoring the patient may conjure up visions of healthcare professionals, including pharmacists, taking samples of blood and other body fluids from the patient, recording measurements, or merely observing them in order to manage a medical condition. While these are important examples of how monitoring may be achieved, there are other schemes that are used specifically in relation to monitoring patients and their medication.

Pharmacovigilance is the science and activities relating to the detection, assessment, understanding and prevention of adverse effects or any other drug-related problem. This has become increasingly important in evaluating medicines and providing checks, controls and warnings to healthcare professionals and patients.

The Yellow Card scheme

The Medicines and Healthcare products Regulatory Agency (MHRA) is the government agency which is responsible for assessing the safety, quality and efficacy of a wide range of materials from medicines and medical devices to blood and therapeutic products that are derived from tissue engineering. The MHRA authorizes and regulates their sale or supply for human use in the UK.

Medicines are controlled as soon as they are first discovered and undergo clinical trials, but it is recognized that only the most common adverse drug reactions (ADRs) will be detected by the time the drug is marketed.

As part of its activities, the MHRA operates post-marketing surveillance and other systems for reporting, investigating and monitoring adverse reactions to medicines and adverse incidents involving medical devices. Included in this remit, the MHRA and the Commission on Human Medicines (CHM) run the UK's national reporting system for ADRs – called the Yellow Card scheme (YCS).

The YCS was introduced in 1964 initially to provide doctors or dentists with a route to report a suspicion that a medicine could have harmed a patient. The YCS gets its name from the colour of the original document used for reporting the ADR. These 'cards' have become increasingly more accessible and can be sourced by a variety of methods (Box 47.1).

The fundamental principles of the scheme have not changed. Proof of a causal link between a medicine or a combination of medicines does not need to be established, so the reports are suspected ADRs.

In the UK, the MHRA collates data on ADRs via the YCS from a wide range of healthcare professionals working in the NHS or from private healthcare providers. These now include doctors, dentists, pharmacists (from 1997), nurses, midwives and health visitors (from 2002) and also HM Coroners. Reports are received directly from them and via pharmaceutical companies. The scheme is voluntary for

Box 47.1

Ways in which the Yellow Card reporting forms can be accessed

Download	pdf copy (http://www.mhra.gov.uk)
Write to	MHRA, CHM Freepost, London, SW8 5BR or CHM's Yellow Card centres
Copies included in	the *British National Formulary* (BNF), the *ABPI Medicines Compendium* the *MIMS Companion*

healthcare professionals but pharmaceutical companies holding marketing authorizations have legal obligations to report ADRs to the MHRA.

In January 2005 a 6 month limited pilot exercise was launched to include direct reporting by patients, followed by a nationwide pilot scheme in October 2006. This has continued with reports being accepted from patients, parents and carers. The Yellow Card report forms for patients are different from those for healthcare professionals. Standard report forms are shown in Figures 47.1 and 47.2.

There have been over 500 000 reports received in the last 40 years. Yellow Card reports are collected on all types of medicines irrespective of legal status. These include:

- Prescription medicines
- Medicines you can buy without a prescription over the counter (OTC)
- Herbal and other complementary remedies.

The Commission and the MHRA continue to monitor intensively products carrying a black triangle symbol (▼) in the BNF. This identifies newly licensed medicines where the drug is a new active substance.

However, additional criteria have also been applied when products have been selected for intensive monitoring, and include:

- A new combination of active substances
- Administration by a new route which is significantly different from existing routes
- A novel drug delivery system
- A significant new indication which:
  - o may alter the established risk/benefit profile of that drug
  - o is likely to result in a significantly different population being exposed to the drug.

Healthcare professionals are asked to report all suspected ADRs for these products as opposed to focusing only on serious reactions for established products.

It has been suggested that the capacity of the scheme to identify ADRs should be strengthened by including other categories such as:

- Off label use of licensed products
- Delayed drug effects
- Products whose legal status has changed.

A product may retain black triangle status until the safety of the drug or product is well established, which is usually following 2 years of post-marketing experience. Over the last few years there have been 250–300 drugs under intensive surveillance (Black Triangle List) each year. A number are removed but are replaced by approximately the same number of new products each year. The list is regularly updated by the MHRA.

There are a number of problems associated with the scheme but the major one has been, and continues to be, under-reporting. Since October 2002 an Internet electronic Yellow Card has been available (http://www.mhra.gov.uk) to enable all reporters to submit ADR reports via the MHRA website in a paperless way.

Healthcare professionals are now encouraged to register with the site and use this method as it avoids reports being delayed or forgotten, as occurred when they had to be posted. In 2005 there was a 70% increase in the number of Internet reports received compared with the same period in the previous year. The online reporting form has been redesigned to improve clarity and usability by incorporating 'drop-down' menus and dictionaries for technical terms. A recently added feature allows a reporter to save a partially completed report at any point so that it can be finished and submitted at a convenient time or later when more information had been received concerning the ADR. This method may be the best way to encourage spontaneous reporting and it is being strongly promoted to all reporters. The MHRA and CHM also have five Yellow Card centres whose role focuses on follow-up of reports in their areas as this has been shown to improve follow-up rates.

Table 47.1 lists the number of Yellow Card reports received from healthcare professionals and patients in the period 1 November 2001 to 31 December 2006. Reporting of ADRs increased by approximately 5% each year compared to the same period of the previous year, but between January and May 2007 there was a 4% decrease compared with the same period in 2006.

Table 47.2 provides details on the specialty of the reporters for reports received during 1 November

In Confidence

YellowCard

MHRA

SUSPECTED ADVERSE DRUG REACTIONS

If you are suspicious that an adverse reaction may be related to a drug or combination of drugs please complete this Yellow Card. For reporting advice please see over. Do not be put off reporting because some details are not known.

PATIENT DETAILS Patient initials: _____ Sex: M / F Weight if known (kg): _____

Age (at time of reaction) _____ Identification number (Your Practice/Hospital Ref.)*: _____

SUSPECTED DRUG(S)

Give brand name of drug and batch number if known:	Route	Dosage	Date started	Date stopped	Prescribed for

SUSPECTED REACTIONS(S)

Please describe the reaction(s) and any treatment given:

Outcome
Recovered ☐
Recovering ☐
Continuing ☐
Other ☐

Date reaction(s) started: _____ Date reaction(s) stopped: _____

Do you consider the reaction to be serious? Yes / No

If *yes*, please indicate why the reaction is considered to be serious (please tick all that apply):

Patient died due to reaction ☐	Involved or prolonged inpatient hospitalisation ☐
Life threatening ☐	Involved persistent or significant disability or incapacity ☐
Congenital abnormality ☐	Medically significant; please give details: _____

OTHER DRUGS (including self-medication & herbal remedies)

Did the patient take any other drugs in the last 3 months prior to the reaction? Yes / No

If *yes*, please give the following information if known:

Drug (brand, if known)	Route	Dosage	Date started	Date stopped	Prescribed for

Additional relevant information e.g. medical history, test results, known allergies, rechallange (if performed), suspect drug interactions. For congenital abnormalities please state all other drugs taken during pregnancy and the last menstrual period.

REPORTER DETAILS

Name and professional address: _____

Post code: _____ Tel no: _____

Speciality: _____

Signature: _____ Date: _____

CLINICIAN (if not the reporter)

Name and professional address: _____

Post code: _____

Tel no: _____ Speciality: _____

If you would like information about other adverse reactions associated with the suspected drug, please tick this box ☐

* This is to enable you to identify the patient in any future correspondence concerning this report

Please attach additional pages if necessary

COMMISSION ON HUMAN MEDICINES (CHM)

Figure 47.1 • Standard Yellow Card report form for reporting suspected adverse drug reactions by healthcare professionals.

Postage will be paid by licensee

Do not affix Postage Stamps if posted in Gt. Britain, Channel Islands, N. Ireland or the Isle of Man

1

BUSINESS REPLY SERVICE
Licence No. SW 2991

MEDICINES AND HEALTHCARE PRODUCTS REGULATORY AGENCY
CHM FREEPOST
LONDON
SW8 5BR

SECOND FOLD HERE

Remember if in Doubt – Report

SUSPECTED ADVERSE DRUG REACTIONS REPORTING ADVICE

New Black Triangle (▼) Drugs – report ALL suspected adverse reactions
(New medicinal drugs can be identified by the presence of a black triangle (▼)
both on the product information for the drug and in the BNF and MIMS)

Other Drugs – only report SERIOUS suspected adverse reactions
For instance those which are:

- Fatal
- Life threatening
- Involves or prolongs inpatient hospitalisation
- Involves persistent or significant disability or incapacity
- Congenital abnormality
- Medically significant (please exercise your judgement)
      Please remember the areas of particular concern – delayed drug effects, the elderly, congenital
      abnormalities, children (including offlabel use of medications) and any herbal remedies
      For more information contact:
- The National Yellow Card Information Service on Freephone 0800-7316789
- The MHRA website http://mhra.gov.uk
- Reporters can send suspected adverse drug reaction reports by electronic Yellow Card, via the MHRA website
- More detailed guidelines are given in the BNF

DO NOT BE PUT OFF REPORTING BECAUSE SOME DETAILS ARE NOT KNOWN

FIRST FOLD HERE

Figure 47.1 • (*Continued*)

Tear along the dotted line

YellowCard®report

Use blue or black ink. Complete all the lines marked with ✳ and give as much other information as you can

Confidential

1 About the suspected side effect

✳ What were the symptoms of the suspected side effect, and how did it happen?   If there isn't enough space here, attach an extra sheet of paper.

_____

_____

_____

_____

How bad was the suspected side effect?   Tick the box that best describes how bad the symptoms were

✳ ☐ Mild ☐ Unpleasant, but did not affect everyday activities ☐ Bad enough to affect everyday activities ☐ Bad enough to see a doctor
☐ Bad enough to be admitted to hospital ☐ Caused very serious illness ☐ Caused death ☐ Other _____

When did the side effect start?

How is the person feeling now? Tick the box that best describes whether the person still has symptoms of the suspected side effect.

✳ ☐ Better (no more symptoms) ☐ Getting better ☐ Still has symptoms ☐ More seriously ill ☐ Died ☐ Other

Can you give any more details?   For example, did the person take or receive any other treatment for the symptoms?
Did they stop taking the medicine as a result of the side effect?

_____

_____

_____

_____

2 About the person who had the suspected side effect

Who had the suspected side effect?

✳ ☐ You ☐ Your child ☐ Someone else

Information about the person   Supply as much information as you can, even if you prefer not to give a name.

First name or initials _____ Family name _____ ☐ Male ☐ Female

✳ Age _____ Weight _____ ☐ kg ☐ stones/pounds   Height _____ ☐ metres ☐ feet/inches

Any other relevant information? For example, does the person have any medical conditions or allergies?

_____

_____

_____

Make sure you have completed all the lines marked ✳   Please turn over →

Figure 47.2 • Standard Yellow Card report form for reporting suspected adverse drug reactions by patients, parents and carers.

3 About the medicine(s) which might have caused the side effect

Give details of the medicine you suspect of causing the side effect.

✱ **Name of the medicine** _____ ☐ prescription   ☐ bought in pharmacy   ☐ bought elsewhere

Dosage (for example, one 250 mg tablet, twice a day)

What was it taken for?

Start date: _____   End date: _____   Did you stop because of side effects?   ☐ Yes ☐ No

If you (or the person you're reporting for) were taking any other medicine at the same time (which might have caused an interaction), give details of it. If you need to give details of more than one other medicine, attach an extra sheet of paper.

Name of other medicine _____ ☐ prescription   ☐ bought in pharmacy   ☐ bought elsewhere

Dosage (for example, one 250 mg tablet, twice a day)

What was it taken for?

Do you think this medicine might also have caused the side effect?   ☐ Yes   ☐ No   ☐ Possibly

Start date: _____   End date: _____   Did you stop because of side effects?   ☐ Yes ☐ No

Have you taken any other medicines or herbal remedies (as well as the above) within the last 3 months?   ☐ Yes ☐ No

4 About your doctor (optional)

Would you like a copy of this report to be sent to your doctor?
☐ Yes ☐ No   **If Yes, give the doctor's name and address.**

If you want us to send a copy of this report to any other healthcare professional, attach a separate sheet with their contact details.

If we need more medical information (such as test results), do we have your permission to contact your doctor directly for it?
☐ Yes ☐ No

Doctor's name

Address

Postcode

5 About you – the person making the report

We need contact details – please supply a full postal address, even if you prefer not to give a phone number or email address.

✱ Title   First name or initials   Family name

✱ Address

✱   Postcode

Telephone number   Email address

Please sign and date this form   I agree that the Medicines and Healthcare products Regulatory Agency (MHRA) can contact me to discuss the suspected side effect, and to ask for more information that might help understanding of the case.

✱ Signed   Date

Please return this form in the envelope provided to: MHRA, CHM FREEPOST, London SW8 5BR   © Crown Copyright 2008

Figure 47.2 • (Continued)

2005 to 31 December 2006 with 2004/05 figures included for comparison. There has been a steady increase in the number of ADR reports from community pharmacists, other healthcare professionals and patients since the scheme was opened to them.

Patient reporting has been supported by the distribution of improved Yellow Cards to all GP surgeries,

Table 47.1 Reports of suspected adverse reactions (*comparing 1 November to 31 December of the next sequential year)

Year*	No. of registered reports during period
2001/02	20 481
2002/03	22 091
2003/04	23 158
2004/05	25 832
2005/06	27 075

community pharmacies and other NHS outlets across the UK. The patient electronic Yellow Card has been updated and can also be accessed through the website.

Since the launch of the pilot scheme and up to August 2007, over 5500 suspected ADR reports have been received from patients. The patient report form uses a different format and less technical terms than those used by healthcare professionals. As a result, patient reports tend to provide more detail on the impact of the ADR on daily life and activities and initial observations indicate that the reports are of an equivalent level of seriousness to those of healthcare professionals. In September 2007 a 2-year research project was commissioned to formally evaluate the patient reporting component of the YCS and investigate the pharmacovigilance impact of these reports. The project is ongoing.

The Adverse Drug Reactions On-Line Information Tracking (ADROIT) system is the MHRA database used to store and monitor all the reports. Information collected through the scheme is an important means of monitoring drug safety in clinical practice and many important early warnings of new ADRs have been identified in addition to increasing the knowledge of known ADRs.

All data are closely scrutinized by the MHRA/CHM to determine whether a potential health threat is emerging and further investigation is required or more immediate action needs to be taken. The outcomes may be that the product licence for the drug is withdrawn by the regulatory authority when the risks are considered to outweigh the benefits. The company may voluntarily suspend or withdraw the product. In several instances, a drug has continued to be available following amendments to the summary of product characteristics (SPC) and patient information leaflet (PIL) indicating restrictions in use, reduction in dosages and special warnings and precautions. Some examples can be seen in Table 47.3. Complete listings of the suspected ADRs reported to the MHRA through the YCS by healthcare professionals and patients are provided in drug analysis prints. Drug analysis prints can be accessed from the MHRA website.

It is recognized that there are a number of problems with spontaneous reporting systems such as this. Under-reporting arises because healthcare professionals or patients do not recognize an ADR if it is unknown or difficult to spot. Conversely, there may

Table 47.2 Specialty of reporter for reports received between 1 November 2005 and 31 December 2006 (2004/05 figures for same period are given in brackets)

Type of reporter	No. during period	Percentage of all reports
Community pharmacist	689 (676)	2.5 (2.6)
General practitioner	4816 (6164)	17.8 (23.9)
Hospital doctor	5463 (6214)	20.2 (24.0)
Hospital pharmacist	3390 (3477)	12.5 (13.5)
Nurse	2327 (3098)	8.6 (12.0)
Other healthcare professionals (including dentists, coroners, optometrists, psychiatrists, neurologists, paediatricians)	6133 (5241)	2.7 (20.3)
Patients	4257 (962)	15.7 (3.7)
Total	27 075 (25 832)	

Table 47.3 Some major safety issues identified through the Yellow Card scheme

Year	Medicine	Adverse reaction	Resulting action
1995	Quinolone antibiotics	Tendonitis, tendon rupture	Improved warnings
1996	Alendronate (Fosamax▼)	Severe oesophageal reactions	Warnings and revised dosing instructions
1998	Isotretinoin (Roaccutane)	Psychiatric reactions	Improved warnings
1998	Sertindole (Serdolect▼)	Sudden cardiac death	Drug withdrawn**
1999	*Aristolochia* in Chinese herbal remedies	Renal failure	*Aristolochia* banned
2000	Cisapride (Prepulsid, Alimix)	Serious cardiovascular reactions	Use of cisapride suspended in the United Kingdom***
2001	Bupropion (Zyban▼)	Seizures	Improved warnings and revised dosing instructions
2003	Kava-kava	Hepatotoxicity	Supply of Kava-kava prohibited in the United Kingdom
2004	Selective serotonin reuptake inhibitors	Suicidal thoughts/behaviour	Special warnings and precautions for use
2004	Rofecoxib (Vioxx▼)	Cardiovascular risk	Drug withdrawn
2006	Co-proxamol	Drug-related suicides	Licence withdrawn
2007	Lumaricoxib (Prexige▼)	Hepatotoxicity	UK licence suspended
2008	Rimonabant (Acomplia▼)	Depression	Special warnings and precautions for use
2008	Exenatide (Byetta▼)	Acute pancreatitis	Improved warnings

*Black Triangle (▼) drug at the time the major safety issue was identified.
** Sertindole was reinstated in 2002 with increased warnings.
*** Cisapride licences have been cancelled.

be a bias to report ADRs that are well publicized. The true incidence of a particular ADR cannot be determined since there is a lack of information on the total number of patients exposed to the drug. The quality of the data reported is variable and some important details may be omitted and the report only indicates that an ADR is suspected, which does not imply causality, and false positives are mixed with true effects. The YCS is also poor at detecting long delayed reactions.

In addition, reporting systems in different countries differ and it becomes difficult to compare reports of ADRs across international boundaries. However, the World Health Organization's regional monitoring centre in Uppsala is making progress in this area and is able to apply techniques to identify 'signals' of ADRs that require further investigations using reports from 78 countries.

Patient reports are not accepted by the majority of countries despite greater patient usage of complementary and alternative medicines which may increase the incidence of ADRs that are not reported by healthcare professionals.

The role of the pharmacist

Pharmacists have an important contribution to make in the prevention, identification, documentation and reporting of ADRs and in strengthening Yellow Card reporting. Currently the proportion of Yellow Cards received from pharmacists remains around 12%, whereas the proportion of patient reports submitted over a similar time period is 13%.

It is important that pharmacists are not reluctant to report suspected ADRs because they are often the healthcare professional most able to identify ADRs and to play an active role in their prevention.

On a daily basis the pharmacist becomes aware of factors that could indicate an ADR is occurring such as:

- Excessive therapeutic effects of medicines
- Abnormal laboratory values
- Medications prescribed or purchased to treat 'side-effects'
- Drugs being discontinued but alternatives with the same indication being prescribed or purchased.

Their role as prescribers means they are more closely involved with the patient and the choice of medication. The expanding range of over the counter (OTC) medicines and the increasing number of medicines whose legal status has changed means that the responsibility of providing guidance to patients on the safe use of medicines frequently falls to the pharmacist. This also means that they should be advising patients to contribute to the YCS by completing forms themselves or encouraging patients to do so.

The future

For the future it is hoped that the information collected by the YCS can be used by researchers to help studies that will advance knowledge in the safe use of medicines. Examples of research applications that have been accepted include acute renal toxicity reported to the YCS and pharmacogenetics of antimicrobial drug-induced liver injury.

The medicines use review (MUR)/prescription intervention service

Background

The community pharmacy contractual framework (CPCF) for England and Wales was introduced in April 2005. The CPCF comprises 'Essential', 'Advanced' and 'Enhanced' service tiers. The medicines use review (MUR)/prescription intervention service is included under advanced services.

Although there are two service titles, in reality there is only one service, but the trigger which initiates provision is different.

The MUR is the first national service in which community pharmacists are remunerated to discuss the patient's medication and support them in getting the most from their medicines. The pharmacist reviews the patient's use, experience and taking of medicines together with identifying side-effects and interactions. They also aim to resolve any issues around poor or ineffective drug use by the patient and in this way carry out patient monitoring by a different process.

Following the first year of implementation, the national evaluation of the CPCF in 2007 indicated that 60% of pharmacies were providing the MUR service and over 80% of those who were not (mainly independents) planned to do so in the future. At the same time, this research suggested that GPs, primary care organizations (PCOs) and patients were unconvinced of the value of MURs. This was disappointing because the MUR was seen as the first opportunity for the pharmacist to demonstrate the added value that their input could make to patient care. In addition the commissioning of the next phase of 'Enhanced' services was thought to be dependent upon the demonstrated success of this service.

The reasons for the negative comments were linked to issues around the initiation of the service in the pharmacy and integration with general practice (Box 47.2). Since then the directions applying to MURs have been amended to incorporate a revised reporting form and GP (or equivalent) notification requirements. Uptake of the service has steadily increased, and the MUR is becoming more firmly established although it is still less than the suggested targets in some areas.

Prescription interventions involve the same review, but are initiated in response to a significant problem with a person's medication, rather than a periodic

Box 47.2

Suggested barriers to initiation and integration of MUR service

- Accreditation – pharmacist conducting MURs must have an MUR certificate
- Accredited pharmacist must have PCO permission to conduct MURs outside of the pharmacy
- Facilities – pharmacy must have a private consultation area where both the pharmacist and patient can sit down
- Poor understanding by GPs, patients and other staff of the service
- Unfriendly paperwork
- Lack of engagement

check. The same premises and pharmacist accreditation requirement apply.

Accreditation

A pharmacy can only provide advanced services if it is satisfactorily providing all the essential services in the CPCF. In order to provide MUR services, certain criteria must be met by both the pharmacy from which the service is taking place and the pharmacist who is providing the service.

Pharmacy criteria

As well as providing essential services, a pharmacy must have a consultation area:

- Where the patient and pharmacist can sit down together
- Where the patient and pharmacist can talk together without being overheard by other visitors to the pharmacy or staff undertaking normal duties
- Which is clearly designated for confidential consultations, distinct from the general public areas of the pharmacy.

If there is no space for a consultation room, pharmacists may conduct an MUR when the pharmacy is closed, making the whole pharmacy the consultation room. A request form has to be submitted to the PCO in order to do this.

Pharmacists' criteria

Pharmacists must successfully undertake a competency assessment to gain accreditation before providing MURs.

Within the new contract negotiations, it was agreed with the Department of Health and the NHS Confederation that any higher education institution (HEI) should be able to provide training and competency assessments for the MUR service. A national competency framework is used as the basis for these assessments. The framework is not designed to be an exhaustive list of competencies that might be required to undertake MUR, but consists of those key elements that can be assessed in a robust and reliable manner.

There are a number of providers who run courses and/or competency assessments. Additionally some academic institutions that provide postgraduate clinical programmes, such as diplomas, have ensured their courses develop and test the skills of students in order to meet the requirements of the MUR competencies.

A list of providers across the UK is available from the Pharmaceutical Services Negotiating Committee (PSNC) website.

A pharmacist registered with a primary care trust in England has to register separately in Wales – and a pharmacist registered with a local health board in Wales has to register separately in England.

A pharmacist must also apply to the PCO for permission to conduct MURs in special circumstances, for example at a patient's own home, at a residential home, at an external clinic or on the phone. A separate request has to be made for each category of patient on each occasion.

Carrying out an MUR

Although it could be considered to be a simple task to carry out an MUR once the criteria for the premises and pharmacist have been satisfied, it still requires a considerable amount of planning and preparation to achieve a satisfactory result.

Patient selection

The first consideration concerns which patients are suitable, as selection must follow specified criteria. The national criteria for MUR other than prescription intervention indicate:

- An MUR can be conducted with patients on multiple medicines and those with long-term conditions
- Regular MURs, initiated by the pharmacist, must only be provided for patients who have been using the pharmacy for the dispensing of prescriptions for at least the previous 3 months
- The next regular MUR can be conducted 12 months after the last MUR.

Local criteria

Most PCOs, working with their community pharmacies, may identify priority groups who would be appropriate for MURs, based on the needs of the local health economy. The most frequently reported groups being patients with respiratory disease (asthma and/or chronic obstructive pulmonary disease) followed by those on multiple medications. Further examples of the range of patient groups that have been selected can be seen in Box 47.3.

Box 47.3

Examples of patient groups suitable for MUR

- Patients with specified conditions, e.g. diabetes, heart failure
- Patients on specific types of drug, e.g. warfarin, benzodiazepines, analgesics
- Patients who have an inhaler (and a spacer device)
- Patients over 75 on four or more medications
- Any patient taking five or more medicines
- Patients recently discharged from hospital (within last 2 months at time of review)
- Patients with known toxicities
- Patients with known compliance issues
- Patients with repeat prescriptions which contain several items for different durations

Many pharmacists have or are looking to have areas of specialized interest and MURs provide them with an excellent opportunity to use this expertise in certain patient groups.

Pharmacists do not only select suitable patients themselves, they may accept referrals for MUR from the local surgery, other healthcare professionals, e.g. district and practice nurses, key workers and social services. In this way one of the perceived positive aspects for the CPCF, to allow the extended role of the community pharmacist to align with local health needs, may be achieved. The pharmacist can accept requests directly from patients for an MUR as long as the national criteria are met.

Prescription intervention

It should be noted that the patient selection criteria do not apply in the case of a 'prescription intervention', where the requirement for a MUR to be undertaken is initiated by the pharmacist identifying a significant problem during the dispensing of regular prescriptions. In particular, the requirement to have provided pharmaceutical services for a minimum of 3 months is removed. In these cases the initiating issue which led to the need for a prescription intervention is discussed with the patient as part of the MUR and communicated to the patient's GP.

Engaging the patient

Since the service was introduced, engaging with patients to invite them to attend for the MUR has proved to be problematic. Patients must consent to an

MUR being carried out. Initially uptake was poor because few patients had heard of the service and awareness of its purpose was low. Surveys had indicated that patients supported the concept of pharmacists helping them to understand what their medicines were for but patients were less inclined to attend an appointment to discuss their medicines. Many did not perceive that an annual MUR was required.

Similarly GPs and other relevant professionals had received little information about the service, availability was not guaranteed from all pharmacies and there were a number of other problems with the paperwork resulting in reluctance to signpost the service to patients.

Since that time steps have been taken locally and nationally to develop and provide support for those offering the MUR service. A leaflet for patients, explaining what the MUR entails, has been produced and is available from the Department of Health publications. An MUR information leaflet for GPs and practice managers is available from the PSNC (see Appendix 5).

Pharmacists have realized that they have to proactively engage patients to emphasize the benefits of the service and arrange appointments. To incorporate MURs into the daily work of the pharmacy without additional pharmacist cover is also difficult. Experience has now shown that the most successful MUR schemes use skill mix with pharmacy staff assisting with planning and preparatory work for the MUR. Pharmacy staff require an understanding of what MURs are about, but once this has been established they can work together to:

- Identify appropriate patients
- Alert the pharmacist when a potential MUR candidate has presented a prescription or is about to receive the dispensed items
- Organize the appointment system when the MUR pharmacist is available
- Complete as much of the MUR form as possible for the pharmacist prior to the interview
- Keep interruptions to a minimum during the interview.

The patient interview

Despite pharmacists having extensive experience in communicating with patients, many have found the MUR interview difficult initially. Eliciting the information required to complete all sections of the form can be time-consuming if the patient is on multiple medications and sufficient preparation has not taken place. With experience, pharmacists have realized that the key areas they need to address are to:

- Look through the patient medication record (PMR) beforehand
- Note any listed medical conditions
- Prepare a structured format for the session including suitable questions
- Have specific PILs available if necessary.

This is in addition to all the general issues of putting the patient at ease, revising the purpose of the interview, active listening and appropriate responses to any comments or questions from the patient. They must also complete any sections on the form with the information they have received during or soon after the MUR.

Completing the form

In December 2007, the new NHS MUR form (version 2) was published by the Department of Health as a result of feedback provided by stakeholders. Specific changes were made to the MUR form; it has been reduced down to two A4 sheets and the key details required by the patient's GP/practice are all present on the first page – the Overview page (see Fig. 47.3). Sections have been moved to the front page and reworded in order to improve ease of use by GPs. The columns and rows for recording of drug name, dosage form, strength and dose have been revised and unnecessary annotation has been avoided by incorporating 'tick' boxes. Clinical codes for MUR have been added to facilitate recording of the MUR on GP systems (information provided by NHS Connecting for Health). An electronic template is now also available.

In addition, guidance has been provided to give new flexibilities to pharmacists in the way the form is used. The patient must always be provided with a copy of the full MUR form, but pharmacists are now required to send the Overview page of the form to the patient's GP within 7 days of conducting the MUR only when there are items that need to be considered by the GP/practice.

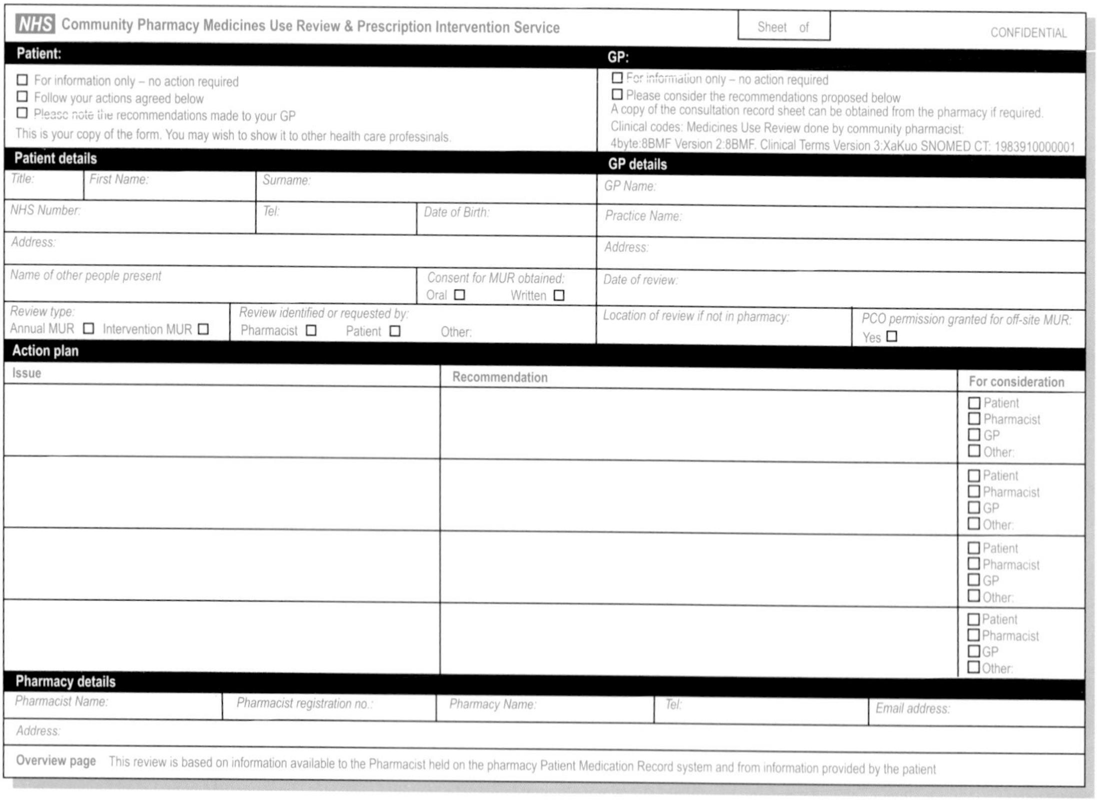

NHS Community Pharmacy Medicines Use Review & Prescription Intervention Service | Sheet of | CONFIDENTIAL

Patient:
☐ For information only – no action required
☐ Follow your actions agreed below
☐ Please note the recommendations made to your GP
This is your copy of the form. You may wish to show it to other health care professinals.

GP:
☐ For information only – no action required
☐ Please consider the recommendations proposed below
A copy of the consultation record sheet can be obtained from the pharmacy if required.
Clinical codes: Medicines Use Review done by community pharmacist:
4byte:8BMF Version 2:8BMF. Clinical Terms Version 3:XaKuo SNOMED CT: 1983910000001

Patient details
Title: | First Name: | Surname:
NHS Number: | Tel: | Date of Birth:
Address:
Name of other people present | Consent for MUR obtained: Oral ☐ Written ☐
Review type: Annual MUR ☐ Intervention MUR ☐ | Review identified or requested by: Pharmacist ☐ Patient ☐ Other:

GP details
GP Name:
Practice Name:
Address:
Date of review:
Location of review if not in pharmacy: | PCO permission granted for off-site MUR: Yes ☐

Action plan

Issue	Recommendation	For consideration
		☐ Patient ☐ Pharmacist ☐ GP ☐ Other:
		☐ Patient ☐ Pharmacist ☐ GP ☐ Other:
		☐ Patient ☐ Pharmacist ☐ GP ☐ Other:
		☐ Patient ☐ Pharmacist ☐ GP ☐ Other:

Pharmacy details
Pharmacist Name: | Pharmacist registration no.: | Pharmacy Name: | Tel: | Email address:
Address:

Overview page This review is based on information available to the Pharmacist held on the pharmacy Patient Medication Record system and from information provided by the patient

Figure 47.3 • NHS form for community pharmacy medicines use review and prescription intervention service.

NHS Community Pharmacy Medicines Use Review & Prescription Intervention Service						Sheet of	CONFIDENTIAL
Title: First name: Surname: NHS Number: Date of birth: Date of review:							

Current medicines (including over the counter & complementary therapies)	Does the patient use the medicine as prescribed?	Does the patient know why they are using the medicine?	More info provided on use of medicine	Is the formulation appropriate?	Are side effects reported by the patient?	General comments relating to advice, side effects and other issues
1 Name/Dosage form/Strength: Dose:	☐ Yes If no, specify:	Yes ☐ No ☐	Yes ☐ No ☐	Yes ☐ No ☐	Yes ☐ No ☐	
2 Name/Dosage form/Strength: Dose:	☐ Yes If no, specify:	Yes ☐ No ☐	Yes ☐ No ☐	Yes ☐ No ☐	Yes ☐ No ☐	
3 Name/Dosage form/Strength: Dose:	☐ Yes If no, specify:	Yes ☐ No ☐	Yes ☐ No ☐	Yes ☐ No ☐	Yes ☐ No ☐	
4 Name/Dosage form/Strength: Dose:	☐ Yes If no, specify:	Yes ☐ No ☐	Yes ☐ No ☐	Yes ☐ No ☐	Yes ☐ No ☐	
5 Name/Dosage form/Strength: Dose:	☐ Yes If no, specify:	Yes ☐ No ☐	Yes ☐ No ☐	Yes ☐ No ☐	Yes ☐ No ☐	
6 Name/Dosage form/Strength: Dose:	☐ Yes If no, specify:	Yes ☐ No ☐	Yes ☐ No ☐	Yes ☐ No ☐	Yes ☐ No ☐	

Consultation record This review is based on information availble to the Pharmacist held on the pharmacy Patient Medication Record system and from information provided by the patient

Figure 47.3 • NHS form for community pharmacy medicines use review and prescription intervention service (*Continued*).

If there are no items to consider, the pharmacist needs only to notify the patient's GP that an MUR has been undertaken within a month of the MUR being conducted.

These changes have made the system more efficient and acceptable to all those involved.

Interactions with GPs

The MUR is the first community pharmacy service where there is a formal requirement for communication between the pharmacist and the GP.

GPs have been slow to accept MURs because of the reasons stated previously. GPs have no authority to prevent pharmacists conducting them for their patients. In order to encourage the roll-out of MURs, pharmacists have produced newsletters and other forms of publicity and written to GPs to ask for practice visits to meet with and explain to them and their staff how the system can be beneficial to the patient. It has been emphasized that there can be significant health gain if MURs are delivered well.

Those practices that have engaged with pharmacists and MURs have generally become enthusiastic supporters.

The future

The potential outcomes from MURs include improved attainment of health goals and quality of life through better use of medicines, reduced wastage and more effective use of resources. It is possible that patients will make fewer visits to the surgery and have reduced unplanned hospital admissions. To some extent these outcomes have been accepted, although a major flaw has been the lack of measurements and monitoring of the quality of the service. In the White Paper on Pharmacy, the government proposed that both of these should be addressed so that the longer term impact of MURs on improved compliance with prescribed medicines can be assessed.

MURs are one of the biggest innovations in community pharmacy in the last few years. They require community pharmacists to undertake functions

545

complementing the work of GPs and other healthcare workers and align them to local health priorities. Improvement in patient knowledge ensures better medicines safety, a more rational approach to the use of medication and better monitoring.

MUR statistics collated for England since April 2005 are available to view on the PSNC website (see Appendix 5).

KEY POINTS

- The MHRA is responsible for assessing safety, quality and efficacy of medicines and medical devices in the UK
- Post-marketing surveillance aims to detect ADRs which did not show during pre-marketing testing
- The YCS was introduced for doctors and dentists in 1964 to report suspected ADRs
- The YCS has been extended to other groups, including pharmacists, and is now being piloted with patients
- The Black Triangle identifies newly licensed drugs, new combinations or new routes for intensive monitoring
- When an ADR is identified, the drug may be voluntarily or compulsorily withdrawn, or it may continue in use with amended SPC or PIL
- Under-reporting appears to be a problem with ADRs
- MUR is an advanced service in the pharmacy contract in England and Wales, but was slow to become established
- For accreditation to carry out MUR, the pharmacy and pharmacist must meet set criteria, the pharmacist applying to the PCO for permission
- There are national criteria for selection of patients for MUR which may be supplemented by local criteria
- Apart from comprehensive preparation, the pharmacist needs to employ effective communication skills
- The MUR form (version 2) has created an overview on page 1 which is to be sent to the GP within 7 days if action is recommended

48

Services for vulnerable patients

Victoria Crabtree

STUDY POINTS

- The problems vulnerable patients experience
- Government policies to care for vulnerable patients
- The pharmacist's role in caring for vulnerable patients
- Drug use in vulnerable patients
- The protection of vulnerable adults and children from exploitation

Vulnerable patients

Vulnerable patients can be described as those in need of care services because of mental ill health, disability, age or illness. They may require protection from harm and exploitation, or may need support to lead healthy and fulfilled lives.

Pharmacists are often involved in the care of vulnerable people. Most commonly these include children and young people, the elderly, drug misusers, people with mental ill health and those who live in care homes.

When developing services for vulnerable people it is important to consider why they are vulnerable. Vulnerable patients tend to experience problems with communication, reduced mental capacity, diminished legal status with regard to treatment or a physical inability to care for themselves.

Communication problems

It is taken for granted that when ill or in need, a person can talk to a healthcare professional to get advice. However, some groups may have problems communicating their needs. Babies and small children cannot talk about how they feel; some who have experienced stroke or head injury can have problems talking; and people suffering with a mental disability may not be able to describe their symptoms or problems. Healthcare professionals may also encounter vulnerable people who are too embarrassed or scared to communicate their needs.

Reduced mental capacity

Children and those with learning difficulties or mental health problems may not have the mental capacity to understand disease and treatment; they rely on parents, carers and healthcare professionals to explain matters on a level that they can understand. When some people are suffering from mental ill health, they may not be able to think clearly enough to understand their disease.

Diminished legal status

When a patient is considered unable to make decisions about disease and treatment they become vulnerable as they rely on others to make decisions for them. In most cases the people involved in the decision-making process have the best interests of the patient at heart. However, occasionally situations occur where patients do not receive the care they require, and they are not in a position to object. Legally a patient should give consent to any treatment given; however, when treating babies and young children, the parent or guardian consents to the treatment on their behalf. As children develop into young adults they acquire more legal rights with regard to consenting to treatment. Decisions can be complex and involve the young person, parents, guardians, the local health authority and courts of law.

Some adults with severe learning difficulties have such reduced mental capacity that they cannot legally consent to treatment; these people are termed 'incapacitated' and the consultant in charge of their care makes decisions about their treatment. Occasionally people suffering from mental ill health have no insight into their illness, and they may not realize they need help. In these situations patients can be 'sectioned' against their will under the Mental Health Act, to ensure they receive appropriate treatment.

Inability to care for themselves

Babies and children rely on adults to feed and care for them. Many vulnerable adults also rely on others for their basic needs. The frail elderly and some with mental or physical disabilities may not have the strength or ability to care for themselves. In these situations people can get support from care services in the community, rely on carers or live in a care home.

Government policies for vulnerable patients

In recent years inequalities and failures in the quality of care that vulnerable groups of people receive from the NHS and social services have been highlighted. High-profile public enquiries such as the Victoria Climbie report and the Bristol enquiry have brought these topics into the public domain. In response, the Department of Health has published a number of national service frameworks (NSFs) and guidance documents that aim to increase the quality of care provided, and protect vulnerable groups from abuse and exploitation.

NSFs set national standards for the care that groups of people should receive, and they also provide strategies and measurable time frames for implementation. The purpose of NSFs is to raise standards and decrease inequalities in care. There are now a number of published NSFs; those relevant to vulnerable patients are:

- NSF for children, young people and maternity services

- NSF for the elderly
- NSF for mental health.

Alongside the NSFs, guidance documents such as 'Working Together to Safeguard Children' and 'The Protection of Vulnerable Adults Scheme' detail how healthcare professionals can work together to protect the vulnerable from harm and exploitation.

Pharmacists and vulnerable patients

There are many services pharmacists provide that contribute to the care of vulnerable people; these services are referred to throughout the NSFs and include:

- Providing health promotion
- Promoting concordance
- Advising on appropriate over the counter (OTC) medicines
- Liaising between primary and secondary care.

Pharmacists also provide enhanced or specialist services to vulnerable patients focusing on the specific care needs of that group. These will be discussed later in the chapter, and services to drug misusers are dealt with in Chapter 49.

Health promotion

All patients benefit from health promotion information (see Ch. 5). However, vulnerable groups may not always receive the information they need. There are a number of health promotion topics that all vulnerable groups benefit from learning about. These include:

- Nutrition
- Physical activity
- Vaccination and immunization
- Smoking cessation
- Drug and alcohol misuse.

Nutrition

A healthy diet is an important component of health and well-being for everyone. When dealing with vulnerable groups of patients it is important to ensure that they receive the correct advice. When considering babies, pharmacists are in an ideal position to promote breastfeeding, give advice on the use of formula milk, and help parents to wean their babies correctly and at an appropriate time. Children have different dietary needs to adults; although children do not require the same volume of food as adults, they may need more energy-releasing foods to support their higher metabolic rate. As children develop in to young adults, pharmacists can advise on what constitutes a healthy diet, promoting the intake of at least five portions of fruit and vegetables a day, with the hope that good eating habits are taken forward into adulthood. Older people may also need advice about healthy diet. Weight loss can have a positive impact on conditions such as hypertension, diabetes and arthritis that develop with age, and ensuring older people eat a diet that provides calcium and vitamin D can help prevent osteoporosis. Some mental health problems, such as bulimia, can present in the pharmacy and pharmacists may be called upon to advise on healthy eating. Care should be taken to refer these patients to specialist services if required.

Many people are confused by health claims related to the use of vitamins, minerals and food supplements. Pharmacists provide a reliable source of information that vulnerable people can turn to. Parents often consult pharmacists for advice about which vitamins are suitable for children. This is an opportunity to discuss what constitutes a healthy diet, and pharmacists can ensure that supplements are used safely. Some people with mental ill health will consult the pharmacist looking for a 'natural' cure and again pharmacists can ensure that any supplements are used safely, but should also be able to signpost people to appropriate help if their symptoms appear severe or worsening. Pharmacists need to be aware of potential interactions between prescribed medicines and dietary supplements, especially in the elderly.

Physical activity

Physical activity provides a vast range of health benefits, and there is no reason why vulnerable groups should not partake. Pharmacists may have to advise on what activities are appropriate and signpost people to relevant services. Physical activity is important to children and young people as it can aid learning and development and prevent weight-related diseases later in life. Physical activity and exercise have been shown to mildly reduce anxiety and depression, thus helping those with mental health problems. Exercise is also of benefit to the elderly, where it has been shown to promote higher bone density, increase muscle strength and flexibility, reduce the risk of stroke and improve memory.

Vaccination and immunization

Immunizations are an essential method of protecting the public and individuals from disease. Pharmacists can ensure that vulnerable groups receive the immunizations they require. Babies and children receive a number of different immunizations, and parents often have concerns about their use. Pharmacists have a role in educating parents about the safety and importance of immunizations, and they can ensure that they are received at the correct age. Some older vulnerable groups of people require immunizations, and again pharmacists have a role informing people of their necessity. For example, it is recommended that all people over 65, those living in long-term residential care homes and those that care for elderly or disabled people receive an influenza vaccination.

Smoking cessation

Stopping smoking is the single most important act an individual can do to improve their health. This is particularly important for vulnerable groups where smoking could have a larger impact on their quality of life. When dealing with children and young people, pharmacists have a role in educating about the risks associated with smoking to try and prevent them taking up the habit. However, if they are already smoking then pharmacists are in an ideal position to advise on giving up. Smoking has been linked with mental health problems such as anxiety and depression, so these groups of people may need more support when trying to give up. Smoking contributes to many illnesses experienced later in life such as heart disease, cancer and osteoporosis, therefore older people also need support to help them stop smoking. This may be particularly difficult if it has been a habit for many years. Community pharmacists provide nicotine replacement therapy (NRT) over the counter or via a NHS stop smoking service if appropriate.

Drug and alcohol misuse

Drug and alcohol misuse is often associated with mental ill health, and can exacerbate existing problems. Issues are usually complex, requiring specialist services; however, pharmacists can advise on safe levels of alcohol consumption, and the dangers associated with illegal drug use. Pharmacists providing drug misuse services may be the first to notice deterioration in a patient's mental state, and can signpost the patient to an appropriate source of help, for example Alcoholics Anonymous or other healthcare professionals involved in their care. As children mature in to young adults they may begin to experiment with alcohol, drugs and volatile substances. Pharmacists have a role in controlling the sale of OTC medicines that are subject to abuse and they can advise against risky behaviours.

Promoting concordance

Concordance is the agreement between the patient and healthcare professionals about what actions are best taken (see Ch. 46). Often actions involve the use of medicines, therefore pharmacists have an important role to play. Achieving concordance can sometimes be challenging, especially when dealing with vulnerable groups. However, if a patient is able to become involved in their treatment decisions, the chances of treatment being successful are increased.

There are a number of different reasons why patients do not adhere to the advice of healthcare professionals, and vulnerable groups may need more support than others to ensure concordance is achieved. Non-concordance may be intentional, where the patient makes a decision not to comply, or unintentional, where there are barriers to following advice given.

Some vulnerable groups are particularly at risk of intentionally not adhering to the advice of healthcare professionals; however, there are actions that pharmacists can take to try and achieve concordance.

As children mature into young adults they should take more responsibility for their own health. Teenagers may be too embarrassed to take medicines to school, or they may decide that they do not need to follow advice as they assert their own independence. To overcome these problems healthcare professionals should involve the patient in any decisions about their treatment, and pharmacists can help by explaining disease and treatment options to the young person in a way that they will understand. Practical support can be given, such as providing modified-release preparations to avoid school time dosing, or supplying discrete appliances such as insulin pens rather than needles and syringes.

Achieving concordance with treatment regimens for people with mental ill health can be difficult, due to the nature of the illnesses involved and the treatments available.

Stigma is attached to some mental health problems such as anxiety, depression, schizophrenia and mania, which can prevent people accepting they have a problem, leading to non-concordance to treatment programmes. Pharmacists can help overcome these problems by discussing mental health issues sensitively and explaining the use of treatment options.

Patients suffering with schizophrenia or mania may lose contact with reality and suffer delusions, posing problems with concordance. Patients may not believe they need treatment, or they believe that a treatment could harm them. These situations require specialist expertise and there are complicated issues with regard to patient consent. Pharmacists can help by providing advice on medication options or the method of drug delivery such as the use of depot preparations.

Drugs used to treat mental health problems often have unacceptable side-effects for patients, resulting in patients choosing not to take the medication at all, or reducing the dose themselves. Identifying and informing patients of potential side-effects before treatment commences may overcome some of these problems. Pharmacists can give advice on how to manage side-effects if they are experienced.

Mental health issues are often related to drug misuse problems, if a prescribed medicine interacts with alcohol or illicit drugs then the patient may choose to discontinue the prescribed medicine in favour of the other. Pharmacists may be the first healthcare professional to become aware of this type of non-compliance. They should advise the patient against risky activities, and signpost them to specialist services such as the local drug misuse team.

Some vulnerable groups experience physical barriers to taking medicines. The frail elderly and some disabled patients are particularly at risk of experiencing difficulties, for example eyesight problems mean some patients may not be able to read instructions. By supplying large print or talking labels the pharmacist can easily overcome this. Problems with dexterity mean some elderly people are unable to remove tablets from bottles or blister packs and again pharmacists can help by ensuring they provide medicines in the most convenient package for the patient. Some patients with a disability may not be able to swallow tablets; therefore the pharmacist can suggest other routes of administration. People with learning difficulties may be unable to read instructions or patient information leaflets, therefore they do not understand why or how to take their medicines. Pharmacists should take time in these situations to ensure they understand. Older people and some with mental health problems may experience memory loss and just forget to comply with a medication regimen. Supplying a memory card can easily solve this problem. If memory problems are severe, such as those experienced with dementia, the pharmacist can repackage solid dosage forms into blistered monitored dosage systems.

Advising on over the counter medicines

The NSFs detail the role pharmacists can play when supplying OTC medicines for minor ailments. Parents consult the pharmacist for advice about their children and the elderly are one of the biggest users of community pharmacies. Drug misusers often have regular contact with community pharmacists, and those living in care homes may rely on pharmacist visits to receive information about minor ailments.

The NSF for children and young people states that they should receive timely and quality effective care when they are ill. Many illnesses that children suffer from, such as coughs, colds, viruses and skin rashes, can be treated quickly and effectively by community pharmacists; however, care should be taken to signpost parents to more appropriate services when a child appears to be more seriously ill. Only OTC products designed and licensed for use in children should be supplied, as they will have been tested for safety and efficacy in this age group. These products are often pleasant tasting colourful liquids, or melt in the mouth sweets, and are more appealing to children, but parents may have concerns about sugar content, artificial flavourings and colourants. Information should be available to parents to help them make informed choices when treating their children. As these medicines are appealing to children, pharmacists must advise parents about the safe storage of medicines in the home.

Minor ailment schemes can provide timely and effective care. When delivering a minor ailment scheme the pharmacy provides advice and medicines, where appropriate, to those people who would have otherwise gone to their GP for a prescription. This saves a GP appointment, and the patient gets the medicine free or at a discounted NHS charge.

It has been estimated that four out of five people over 75 take at least one prescribed medicine, therefore older people are one of the main users of pharmacy services. Pharmacies are not only places where older people collect their prescriptions; they are a source of advice, OTC medicines and social contact. With this in mind, care should be taken to check for interactions with OTC medicines, and any OTC sales

or advice should be recorded in the patient medication record where appropriate. It is important to remember that not all OTC products are suitable for the elderly. For example thrush treatments should not be provided to those over 60 as the incidence of thrush in this group is low and symptoms would require investigation. Vulnerable older people are at risk of becoming socially isolated as family and friends move or pass away. The community pharmacy can become a place of social contact, therefore it should be welcoming, with easy access for those with mobility problems, and pharmacists should take time to talk to people. This gives opportunities to signpost vulnerable people to other services that they may need, and it can give the pharmacist great job satisfaction.

Drug misusers have regular contact with community pharmacies, either as part of a drug treatment programme and a needle exchange service or due to dependence on OTC medication (see Ch. 49). When customers are being treated for opiate addiction they may be taking drugs such as methadone or buprenorphine, and will require advice as to which OTC medicines are suitable. Alcohol dependence can be treated with disulfiram, and patients on this drug need to avoid any alcohol-containing OTC remedies. Customers who use a needle exchange service may be using illicit 'street' drugs and it is important to identify the nature of the drugs being used in order to appropriately deal with OTC requests. Dependence on OTC medicines can occur, for example opiate-based painkillers and cough medicines. Pharmacists should be aware of multiple or repeated sales of these products, and refuse their sale if dependence is suspected. These customers should then be signposted to specialist services to obtain help.

When advising on the use of OTC medicines, pharmacists may become aware that a customer is experiencing mental health problems. For example, people requesting St John's wort or sedating antihistamines may be experiencing anxiety or depression. Customers purchasing large quantities of laxatives could be suffering from an eating disorder. Pharmacists have a duty of care to protect the customer from harm; therefore, if a mental health problem is suspected the customer should be referred to their GP.

When vulnerable patients live in care homes it can be difficult for them to access OTC medicines. If a community pharmacist provides an advisory service to care homes as an enhanced pharmacy service, then they can increase access to OTC advice and treatments. When visiting a care home, the pharmacist can talk to the residents to establish their need for

OTC medicines, and then arrange the safe supply. Many care homes keep OTC medicines for residents to use, known as 'homely medicines'; pharmacists can suggest which are most useful to keep and advise on their safe storage. Most residents in care homes have personalized care plans, and the pharmacist can add in suitable OTC treatments.

Liaising between primary and secondary care

The NSFs for vulnerable groups identify that continuity of care is not always achieved between the primary and secondary sectors. The role of the hospital pharmacist is essential for ensuring a smooth transition between hospital, home and community services.

When vulnerable people enter hospital, a detailed medical history needs to be obtained. Pharmacists often take drug histories which contribute to this process, but this can be more challenging when dealing with vulnerable groups. Children may not know what medicines they are taking, and second hand information from the parent or carer may be more reliable. The elderly often take a number of prescribed and OTC medications, therefore a detailed history is required. It has been estimated that up to 17% of hospital admissions in the elderly can be related to adverse drug reactions. When dealing with those with mental ill health, taking a detailed drug history can help identify any medication issues such as non-concordance or ineffective treatment regimens, which could have contributed to the hospital admission.

Upon discharge the pharmacist can help make the transition from secondary to primary care as smooth as possible. Pharmacists should ensure that when children and young people are discharged from hospital they understand when and how to take their medication. Encouraging them to take responsibility themselves aids concordance and eases the burden on the parent or carer. Pharmacists can also give practical support such as liaising with GPs and community pharmacists to ensure a continual supply of medication, arranging dosage regimens compatible with school hours, and arranging adequate supplies if medicines are needed at school.

Older people may find that changes are made to medication regimens while they are in hospital and pharmacists should ensure these changes are understood and any barriers to taking their medicines are removed.

Most people experiencing mental health problems live in the community; however, from time to time patients may stay in secondary care. When planning discharge from hospital, the pharmacist should be involved in developing a care plan ensuring that patients receive only the necessary medicines, in as simple a regimen as possible, to aid concordance. If a patient relies on a carer then they should be fully involved in this process. Practical support such as liaising with GPs to ensure a continual supply of medication, or writing out compliance charts can be helpful.

Drug use in vulnerable patients

The use of drugs can be complicated in vulnerable groups as often more than one drug is required to achieve the desired effect, or unusual dosages may be required. The differences in response and pharmacokinetics of vulnerable groups must be taken into consideration, i.e. drug absorption, distribution, metabolism and excretion.

Absorption

Drug absorption changes throughout life. Neonates and young infants have prolonged gastric emptying, resulting in slower rates of drug absorption. Neonates and the elderly produce less gastric acid, resulting in a higher stomach pH, possibly affecting the absorption of some basic drugs. Older people experience slower intestinal motility, reduced total surface area for absorption and decreased gastric emptying. Although these factors do not usually have a large effect on total drug absorption, they can slow the rate of drug absorption, resulting in a delayed response.

Distribution

Drug distribution is affected by total body water, adipose tissue and protein binding, three factors which change as a person ages. As children mature, their total body water decreases, therefore neonates and infants may need larger doses of water-soluble drugs. Older people experience a decrease in muscle mass and a gain in adipose tissue. This can sometimes cause problems as lipid-soluble drugs are stored in the adipose tissue, increasing the chances of side-effects and toxicity, therefore lower doses of lipid-soluble drugs should be prescribed.

Neonates have low levels of albumin, therefore less protein binding occurs. This means that lower doses of protein binding drugs are required in this age group. A similar situation occurs in the elderly because as people age, the liver produces less albumin, therefore protein binding drugs such as warfarin and phenytoin may need reduced dosages. In neonates, the protein binding situation is further complicated as they have high levels of bilirubin. Bilirubin attaches to albumin, therefore if a protein binding drug displaces bilirubin from albumin then high circulating levels of bilirubin may result, presenting as jaundice.

Metabolism

Neonates, infants and children have a higher metabolic rate than adults, sometimes resulting in the need for more frequent dosing, or higher doses of drugs on a mg/kg basis. However, care should be taken in neonates as their liver enzyme systems may not be fully mature, and so much lower doses would be required. The elderly experience reduced blood perfusion of the liver, resulting in the slower metabolism of some drugs; lower doses of these would therefore be required.

Excretion

Renal function does not mature until a baby is 6–8 months old and therefore drugs may accumulate and reduced doses should be given to neonates and infants. The elderly may also require reduced dosages of some drugs as renal filtration becomes slower with age, increasing the chances of drug toxicity occurring.

Pharmaceutical services to children and young people

There are a number of services that pharmacists provide to children and young people. Specialist paediatric pharmacists provide prescribing advice in secondary care, and pharmacists may become involved in advising on sexual health and child protection.

Prescribing advice for vulnerable children

Children suffer from a different range of illnesses to adults, and their bodies react differently to disease

states. Ideally drugs used in children will have undergone clinical trials in that age group for the condition that is being treated. However, most drugs are only tested on adults for safety and efficacy, and are therefore unlicensed for use in children. When prescribing decisions are made, pharmacists can provide their expertise by evaluating current clinical evidence. Pharmacists should recommend using a licensed product where possible, or evaluate the safest and most effective unlicensed products available. Parents and carers may be alarmed at the use of unlicensed products, especially if they read an inappropriate patient information leaflet. Explaining the use of the unlicensed medicines to the parent or carer and involving the whole family in any treatment decisions can overcome this. If a drug has not been tested in children, then calculating the dosage can be difficult and the age and weight of the child should be considered. If a high-risk medicine is being used, such as those with a narrow therapeutic range, then the weight of the child and the dose in mg/kg should be stated on all prescriptions to ensure safety. When dosages are being calculated, especially for off-licence medicines, errors may occur and pharmacists have a role in training other healthcare professionals in performing pharmaceutical calculations to ensure correct doses are always given.

Sexual health advice for young people

Pharmacists are often the first healthcare professional that a young person may encounter for advice on contraception and sexual health. Pharmacists sell condoms, provide emergency contraception, signpost people to family planning clinics, provide *Chlamydia* screening and treatment programmes, and provide health promotion about sexually transmitted infections. Emergency hormonal contraception (EHC) can be sold to young people over the age of 16 where appropriate, and some pharmacists supply EHC to under-16-year-olds using a patient group direction.

It can sometimes be difficult for pharmacists to know whether a young person has the intellectual competence to make their own treatment decisions. In the 1980s the Gillick court case raised questions about whether a young person under 16 could receive advice about contraception without the parents' consent. From this court case, the Frazer guidelines were developed to help healthcare professionals make decisions about whether to treat or advise young people without their parents knowing. To provide treatment or advice to an under-16-year-old, the healthcare professional must be satisfied that:

- The young person understands any advice given
- The young person could not be persuaded to inform their parents or agree for the healthcare professional to do so on their behalf
- The young person is likely to start or continue sexual behaviour whether contraceptive treatment is given or not
- Mental or physical health is likely to suffer if contraceptive advice or treatment is not offered
- It is in the best interest of the young person to offer contraceptive services without parental consent.

More recently the Sexual Health Act 2003 states that children under the age of 13 are unable to consent to sexual activity, therefore if a young person under this age requests advice on sexual matters, specialist advice must be sought and it may be appropriate to contact the police. Contacting a third party such as the police can be a difficult decision to make as a pharmacist should respect a patient's confidentiality. Pharmacists must encourage the young person to seek further help if required, or try to get the young person's consent for the pharmacist to contact a specialist service on their behalf.

Child protection services

Children and young people are considered vulnerable as they may not be able to protect themselves from people who harm or exploit them. Pharmacists may become involved in child protection if they have concerns about the welfare of a child and wish to report them. Pharmacists may be asked to provide information on a child or young person to the police or social services, or pharmacists may be involved in a child protection plan.

All healthcare professionals have a duty to safeguard and support the welfare of children. If a pharmacist suspects that a child or young person is being abused they have a legal duty to act upon their suspicions. Abuse can be physical, emotional, sexual or due to neglect. A pharmacist may suspect physical abuse if a child's injuries could not be accounted for by an explanation provided by the parent or carer, or a pharmacist may notice that a child or young person often presents in the pharmacy with injuries. Emotional abuse is more difficult to identify; however, pharmacists may have concerns if a child or young person

became withdrawn or showed signs of self-harm. Pharmacists may encounter children or young people who are suffering from sexual abuse when they are supplying EHC, or the young person may describe sexual activities that are inappropriate for their age. Signs of neglect include failure to provide adequate shelter, food or clothing, which may become apparent to a pharmacist.

If a pharmacist suspects any form of abuse then they must follow the local child protection procedures. Child protection procedures are overseen by the local primary care organization which designates a child protection officer, usually a doctor or a nurse, to coordinate child protection. It is not recommended that pharmacists investigate any suspicions of abuse themselves, but they should record their concerns and any actions taken.

Pharmacists may be asked to give information to social services if a child protection investigation occurs. It is important for pharmacists to cooperate with the police and social services as all agencies involved in child protection should work together if abuse is suspected.

Pharmacists may be directly involved in a child protection plan. These are plans written by social services to help protect a child from harm. For example, a pharmacist may provide drug misuse services to the parent of an at-risk child. Social services may ask the pharmacist for feedback on whether the parent is accessing the drug misuse service.

In situations such as these, conflicts of confidentiality may arise. However, if disclosure is necessary for the protection of children or to prevent serious injury to a person's health, then information should be shared.

Pharmaceutical services to older people

By 2025, one-quarter of the British population will be over the age of 60. Many older people lead active and independent lives late into old age; however, some older people will become frail and increasingly rely on the NHS and social services.

As people age their bodies undergo a number of changes. This increases the number and range of diseases that older people suffer from and changes their response to drugs that treat disease. Older people may find that as family and friends move or pass away they become more socially isolated and therefore vulnerable.

Pharmacists provide a number of specialist services to help prevent the elderly becoming vulnerable, and to fulfil their needs if they are. These services include medicine management and falls prevention.

Medicine management

The NSF for older people estimates that four out of five people over 75 take at least one prescribed medicine, with 36% taking more than four. Pharmacists have a role in ensuring that older people gain maximum benefit from their medication. Medicines should increase quality and duration of life and not cause harm due to excessive, inappropriate or inadequate use. By providing prescribing advice, medicines use reviews and full medication reviews, pharmacists can ensure that this is achieved.

Prescribing advice

Pharmacists are often employed as prescribing advisors either in GP surgeries or within the primary care organization. The role of a prescribing advisor is to evaluate current evidence in the use of medicines and to cascade good prescribing practices down to prescribers. Some drugs are of particular benefit to older people and can increase their quality and duration of life. Prescribing advisors ensure that these drugs are made available to patients. For example, pharmacists can promote the use of statins and anti-thrombotics to help reduce the incidence of stroke. As the clinical evidence for drugs changes, prescribing advisors are in a position to reduce the use of drugs that are of doubtful therapeutic value. In the past phenothiazine antipsychotic drugs have been used for dizziness due to postural hypotension, and benzodiazepines have been prescribed for insomnia due to depression, both of which were not appropriate uses and prescribing advisors can ensure a reduction in such inappropriate medication use.

Medicines use review

A medicines use review is an advanced pharmacy service in which the pharmacist undertakes a structured concordance-centred discussion about medicine use (see Ch. 47). This usually takes place at the time of dispensing and lasts up to 25 minutes. Medicines use reviews are carried out on patients with multiple medicines, or those with long-term conditions, therefore many older people benefit. It is important to state that medicines use reviews are not full medica-

tion reviews, but aim to increase the patient's understanding of their medicine, identify any problems they have taking their medicines and suggest solutions where possible.

Medication review

More detailed than a medicines use review is a full medication review. This is an in-depth evaluation of all a patient's medication, both prescribed and non-prescribed. Full medication reviews are usually carried out at a GP's surgery and can last up to an hour. GPs have a requirement in their NHS contract to review patients at appropriate times and pharmacists can provide a medication review service for GPs to help achieve this. An appropriate time to carry out a full medication review would be in the following circumstances:

- When older people are prescribed more than four medicines
- After a patient has been discharged from hospital
- When an older person lives in a care home
- Where medicine-related problems have been identified
- In patients over 75
- Following an adverse change in health.

When carrying out a full medication review the pharmacist should first explain the purpose and gain the patient's consent to the review process. Sometimes the medication review is carried out with a patient's carer and consent from the patient should be sought if possible. A list of all medications taken by the patient should be compiled which should include OTC remedies, herbal remedies, illicit substances or those borrowed from family or friends. This comprehensive list should then be compared with the GP's records and any ambiguities corrected. While gathering the information, the patient's understanding of what each medicine is used for can be checked and if the patient is unsure why they are taking a medicine, the pharmacist can explain its purpose. During the review the pharmacist should confirm that the patient knows how and when to take their medication and should check that the patient is not having any practical issues such as ordering medicines, getting the medicine out of the container or reading the instruction label. Side-effects should be discussed with the patient, and suggestions made to help overcome them. The medication review is also an opportunity to ensure all relevant monitoring tests have been carried out.

When the pharmacist has gained a comprehensive picture of a patient's drug use, they should evaluate the appropriateness of each medication. Assessing the appropriateness of medication involves checking that the medication is prescribed for an indication listed in the *British National Formulary*, and identifying any inappropriate drug use or dosages. Any recommendations should then be discussed with the prescriber before appropriate changes are implemented.

Fall prevention services

Falls in older people have serious consequences and often result in a healthy active older person becoming vulnerable. Falling has been shown to be a major cause of accidental death in older people and many patients who suffer a fracture never live independently again. The fear of falling can limit what older people do in their day-to-day lives.

Older people are at an increased risk of falling as their muscle mass is decreased which results in a loss of physical strength and a reduction in mobility. Medicines have been implicated in causing older patients to fall. Hypnotic drugs such as benzodiazepines can cause drowsiness, and antihypertensives may cause hypotension and dizziness. Particular care should be taken when an older person suffers from osteoporosis as these patients are much more likely to suffer fractures and consequent deterioration in quality of life. The NSF for older people states that if older people can be prevented from falling, they may live longer, healthier lives, not become vulnerable and therefore ease pressures on the NHS. Many pharmacists have undertaken specialist training to become fall prevention pharmacists. The fall prevention pharmacist reviews a patient's medication, and suggests strategies to withdraw drugs that can predispose a person to falls. They also advise on how to avoid OTC medicines that increase the risk, such as sedating antihistamines or laxatives. Overuse of laxatives can cause dehydration which can result in hypotension.

Fall prevention pharmacists also advise on the prevention of osteoporosis to reduce the risk of fracture. There are some groups of patients that are particularly at risk from osteoporosis and these include those:

- Who are taking long courses of corticosteroids
- Who have had a hysterectomy, premature menopause or suffer from amenorrhoea
- Who have diseases that increase the risk of osteoporosis (liver/thyroid disease, alcoholism, rheumatoid arthritis)
- With a family history of osteoporosis

- With a low body mass
- Who smoke.

The fall prevention pharmacist can identify those at risk of developing osteoporosis and arrange bone density measurements to be taken. If a patient did have osteoporosis, the pharmacist would ensure that corticosteroids were only used when necessary and that preventative measures such as vitamin D and calcium supplementation or bisphosphonates were made available.

Pharmaceutical services to the mentally ill

Mental ill health is a common problem. At any one time, around one in six people of working age have a mental health condition. The Department of Health has increasingly put an emphasis on caring for those with mental ill health in the community. Medication is a fundamental component in the care of the mentally ill.

Managing medication in those with mental ill health is a specialized area and many pharmacists have undertaken further training to become specialist mental health pharmacists. Specialist mental health pharmacists tend to work in secondary care as part of the multidisciplinary team. Their role is to ensure drug use is clinically effective. This means ensuring that the drug is being used at an optimum dose to achieve symptom relief with minimal side-effects and that drugs are administered in a way that is acceptable to the patient. They are also involved in training other healthcare professionals, contributing to the development of treatment guidelines, and are increasingly becoming supplementary and independent prescribers.

In primary care the pharmacist's role is more limited. Prescribing advisors can ensure that prescribers follow up-to-date treatment guidelines with regard to antidepressants, benzodiazepines and antipsychotics. There are increasing opportunities for pharmacists to become involved with local community mental health teams to promote communication between all parties responsible for care planning, and there are increasing opportunities to provide mental health support services to those in prison.

Pharmaceutical services to care homes

Many vulnerable people choose to live in a care home when they can no longer look after themselves or they cannot be adequately cared for by others in their own home. There are a number of different types of care home in the UK which provide different levels of service. Residential care homes provide meals, accommodation, help with personal care such as dressing and bathing and support through short illnesses. This type of home often accommodates the frail elderly or those convalescing after illness. Nursing care homes have a qualified nurse on the premises 24 hours a day and therefore they are often used by those with more severe illness or a disability that requires frequent nursing care. Specialist care homes are available for those who have specific needs or disabilities such as dementia, where specially trained staff or adapted facilities are required. Pharmacists can provide different levels of service to care homes to help them look after their residents.

Providing medicines, dressings and appliances to care homes

Ideally residents should have complete control of their medication which includes ordering their medicines, choosing a pharmacy to dispense them and taking responsibility for taking them. If residents are able to do this they should be encouraged to and provided with a lockable cupboard to store their medicines in. Many care homes like to have some control over medication and often vulnerable people need help storing and taking their medicines correctly. If a home takes responsibility for the residents' medication then a suitably trained person orders the prescriptions from the residents' prescribers. The home usually has a local agreement with a pharmacy to supply all the medicines, dressings and appliances for the residents in the home. Although this reduces the residents' choice, it is much more convenient for the care home staff.

Pharmacists can supply medicines in the manufacturer's original containers or they can put medicines into monitored dosage systems (MDSs). MDSs are a method of repackaging solid dosage forms into individualized blister packs and this is done to help residents or carers in the taking of the medicines. MDSs are time-consuming to prepare; however, they do reduce administration errors as carers and residents can clearly see when to take the medication. Not all solid dosage forms can be repackaged into MDSs. Drugs may deteriorate quickly if not in their original container, and before putting medication into an MDS, the manufacturers should always be consulted.

The way in which the residents receive their medicines depends on the needs of the residents and care home. The care home staff can simply give the resident the manufacturer's container and leave the resident to take the medication themselves or the care home staff can observe the administration. This may be more necessary in care homes for the mentally ill or if a resident is particularly forgetful. If a home chooses to observe administration, then this is often carried out at meal times. This can cause problems if a drug is affected by food and may require the pharmacist to give suitable directions to care home staff when required.

It is important that adequate records of drug administration are kept, especially in homes with large numbers of staff, frequent shift changes and large numbers of residents. Medication administration record (MAR) charts are official records of the medicines that a resident is taking and should be completed every time a drug is administered. MAR charts are provided with the MDS and are kept up to date to reflect any medication changes.

It is good practice for each resident to have an individual care plan which contains details of prescribed medication.

Even if residents look after their own medicines, there is a requirement to consider the storage of medicines in the care home. Steps must be taken to ensure that medicines are kept securely and appropriate storage conditions are considered. Two main types of storage are used – either medicine cupboards or trolleys. Ideally a cupboard should be specially designed and lockable and the person in charge of the home keeps the key. Medicine trolleys should be stored in a room not normally accessible to residents and fastened to a fixed object when not in use. The storage conditions for medicines must be considered, especially controlled drugs (CDs) which must be kept in a CD cupboard. Some items may need to be stored in a refrigerator. The refrigerator ideally would only be used for medicines, but a mixed use refrigerator can be used as long as medicines are kept separately. The refrigerator must be lockable. The temperature inside cupboards should be checked and trolleys should not be kept near radiators.

Pharmacists need to ensure safe disposal of unwanted medicines (see Ch. 43). If a pharmacy supplies a care home, they are responsible for collection and destruction of unwanted medicines. If a resident dies, medicines should be kept for at least a week in case the coroner requests them. In no circumstances should unwanted medicines be kept by a home for use by other residents.

Clinical pharmacy advisory services

Pharmacy advisory services help homes reach the standards set by their regulator. The National Care Standards Commission for England, Care Standards Inspectorate for Wales, or the Scottish Commission for the Regulation of Care regulate care homes. Pharmacists receive payment for these services under the NHS contract.

When providing advisory services, the pharmacist makes an initial visit to the home, and then further annual visits to give advice. These visits entail checking that good practices are followed regarding the supply, administration, storage and destruction of medicines. The pharmacist should be aware of the regulatory body requirements and any advice given to the care home should be recorded. Pharmacists should use these opportunities to talk to the residents. These opportunities can be used to give advice about their medicines. Home visits are a good opportunity to carry out full medication reviews with the residents. Any suggestions for changes in treatment could then be fed back to the prescriber or incorporated into the resident's personal care plan. Pharmacists can use these opportunities to help the home develop safe policies and procedures for drug handling and help train the staff to adopt safe practices, for example helping homes develop protocols for dealing with medication errors. Some pharmacists provide training courses for care workers up to NVQ level, for which extra payment can be claimed from the primary care organization.

While visiting a care home the pharmacist may encounter a scenario where they suspect the residents are at risk of abuse from the care home workers. If a pharmacist becomes concerned that a vulnerable adult may be being harmed, they have a duty to act upon their concerns. Pharmacists should not discuss their concerns with the care home staff, but contact the resident's GP and social services for advice. Pharmacists have a duty to protect a person's confidentiality, therefore consent should be sought from the resident. However, if their health or mental capacity renders them incapable of consent or disclosure is necessary to avoid harm then relevant information can be shared.

KEY POINTS

- There are many reasons patients can be vulnerable, including age, communication problems, reduced mental capacity and legal status and an inability to care for themselves
- It is government policy, through national service frameworks, to support such patients
- The main areas in which pharmacists are involved is with health promotion, promoting concordance, advising on OTC medicines, physical activity, vaccination, smoking cessation and substance misuse
- Patients with mental ill health can present particular difficulties
- People requesting advice on OTC medicines may indicate other problems which require attention
- Patients entering or leaving hospital present an opportunity for pharmacists to ensure medicines are handled correctly
- Pharmacokinetics may be different with some vulnerable patients
- Children and young people may benefit from pharmacist support in a number of ways such as dosage, sexual health and through child protection services
- Medicine management is a particular concern, especially in care settings and with physically and mentally handicapped patients
- Medicines use reviews and medication reviews are valuable pharmaceutical inputs to care
- Some pharmacists have qualified in fall prevention
- Pharmacists will need to provide a wide range of services to care homes

49

Substance use and misuse

Jenny Scott

STUDY POINTS

- List the main psychoactive substances that are taken for non-medicinal purposes
- List the range of professional interventions used in the field of substance misuse and state their aims
- Explain the role of the pharmacist in substance misuse
- State the aim of pharmaceutical interventions and describe their operation
- Explain key factors to consider when providing pharmaceutical care to people with drug misuse problems

Introduction

This chapter begins with some background information before it summarizes current thinking on drug misuse and drug dependence. It then looks at treatment provision in the UK and the range of interventions used, focusing on the practical provision of the two main pharmaceutical interventions – needle exchange and substitute pharmacotherapy provision.

Terminology

Terminology used in the field of drug misuse can be confusing, even for those who work in the area. There are political and philosophical differences behind the use of various terms, a discussion of which is outside the scope of this work. However, it is important to be aware that a variety of terms essentially refer to the same things.

'Drug use' in the context of this chapter is the term commonly used to refer to the consumption of psychoactive substances without medical or healthcare instruction. The term 'drug misuse' refers to drug use that is problematical and incurs a significant risk of harm. These two terms are often used interchangeably. 'Drug abuse' essentially refers to the same thing but its use is less common in recent publications. 'Substance' is sometimes used in place of 'drug' to include non-medicinal chemicals such as solvents, alcohol and nicotine.

'Dependence' or 'addiction' refers to the compulsion to continue administration of psychoactive substance(s) in order to avoid physical and/or psychological withdrawal effects. Drug dependence is defined by the World Health Organization (WHO) as:

> a cluster of psychological, behavioural and cognitive phenomena of variable intensity, in which the use of a psychoactive drug (or drugs) takes on a high priority. The necessary descriptive characteristics are preoccupation with a desire to obtain and take the drug and persistent drug seeking behaviour.
>
> (World Health Organization 1993)

Dependence can be classified in more detail, as found in the *Oxford Textbook of Psychiatry*.

'Drug user' is commonly used to refer to someone who participates in drug/substance use. The term 'drug misuser' refers to someone undertaking drug use in such a way that it is problematical and presents a significant risk of harm. Again the two terms tend to be used interchangeably. Terms such as 'drug addict' and 'drug abuser' are less used in recent literature.

Historical note

Historical works on psychoactive drug consumption make interesting reading and help us to understand how current drug policy came to be formulated. They indicate that psychoactive drug use is not a new phenomenon in society – psychoactive drug use has been recorded as part of some societies more than 7000 years ago. More information is given by Berridge & Edwards (1998).

Substances that are used and their effects

Table 49.1 lists some commonly used psychoactive substances in western societies and summarizes their effects. (Nicotine is included for completeness, but the role of the pharmacist in smoking cessation is covered in Ch. 5.) The unwanted and harmful effects of some drugs relate to prolonged and excessive use, whereas others occur with single doses of smaller amounts. The method of administration also influences the extent of the risks, e.g. injecting opiates presents greater health risks than taking them by vaporization ('chasing the dragon'). Table 49.1 is presented as a guide, but it is not comprehensive. The books *Drugs of Abuse* (Wills 2005) and *Living with Drugs* (Gossop 2007) and the DrugScope website (http://www.drugscope.org.uk/) provide extensive information and the common street names of various drugs. DrugScope is a UK charity that provides information on drugs and support mainly for policy makers and service providers.

Why do people use psychoactive drugs?

Benefits

The question of why people use psychoactive drugs is a multifaceted question to which there is no simple answer. As a crude summary, people who use psychoactive drugs do so because they expect to experience a benefit in some way. They may be aware of risks too, but these are weighed up against the perceived benefits and the decision to take the drug prevails. The extent of the benefits and risks will of course vary depending on the drug, the circumstances and how it is used.

The expected or perceived benefits may include the attainment of pleasurable feelings (e.g. relaxation), increased social interaction (e.g. reduced inhibitions), alteration of the person's psychological condition to a more desirable state (e.g. escapism), physical change (e.g. anabolic steroids taken by bodybuilders) or avoidance of withdrawal symptoms in someone who is dependent on a drug. The reasons for use may change over time with the same user; for example opiate use may be commenced to escape from reality but then continued to avoid the withdrawal effects.

Choice of drug used

The decision to use a drug may be influenced by many things, including:

- Availability and opportunity to try
- Legal status of the drug
- Perceived desired effects
- Perceived risks
- Specifically the desirability of the effects versus the risks as weighed up and assessed by the individual concerned
- Acceptability of the drug and/or method of administration to the individual, the individual's peer group and their wider society.

Risks

The risks from various drugs are not equivalent. Their incidence and nature vary with the drug and how it is used, the individual concerned and the circumstances. Examples of such variables include the drug substance, the presence of impurities, the dose, the frequency of use, the route of administration, the legal status of the drug, related social and financial circumstances, the personality of the individual drug user and the interaction between drug use and lifestyle.

Weighing up benefits vs risks

If the benefits from drug use are experienced before the harm, or to a greater perceived extent than the harm, positive endorsement of drug taking occurs. Following positive endorsement, drug use may, but does not necessarily, continue.

Table 49.1 Some common psychoactive drugs used/misused and selected information on their effects

Common name	Active/main psychoactive component	Most common method(s) of administration	Effect on central nervous system	Examples of desired effects (e.g. reasons for taking)	Examples of unwanted effects/ harm from use
Acid/LSD	Lysergic acid diethylamine	Orally dissolved on the tongue	Hallucinogenic	Altered sensory perceptions e.g. visual hallucinations, time distortion, detachment from reality	Panic attacks, frightening altered perceptions, dysphoria, delusions, psychosis, tachycardia. After-effects include 'flashbacks'
Alcohol	Ethanol	Orally in drinks e.g. wines, spirits, beers, etc.	CNS depressant	Relaxation, disinhibition, promotes social interaction	Aggressive mood, diuresis, dehydration, hypoglycaemia, sedation, vomiting, depression, anxiety, liver cirrhosis, acute hepatitis, gastric cancer
Caffeine	Caffeine	Orally in drinks e.g. tea, coffee, and some soft drinks	CNS stimulation	Increased alertness, combats fatigue, promotes stamina	Diuresis, insomnia, restlessness, anxiety, poor concentration, tremor, headaches
Cannabis	Delta-9-tetrahydrocannabinol (THC) plus other cannabinoids	Hashish (resin) or marijuana (dried flower heads and leaves), both of which are smoked often with tobacco in hand-rolled cigarettes	CNS depressant	Relaxation, enhances mood, disinhibition, sociability	Anxiety, panic reactions, sedation, tachycardia, coughing, lung disorders, loss of motivation
Ecstasy	3,4-methylenedioxy-methamfetamine (MDMA)	Oral ingestion in tablet form often in association with	CNS stimulation, hallucinogenic	Physical and mental stimulation, confidence, sociability, happy, elevated mood, increased energy	Sweating, tachycardia, headache, dry mouth, rhabdomyolysis, hyperpyrexia, hyponatremia, renal

Continued over

561

Table 49.1 *(Continued)*

Common name	Active/main psychoactive component	Most common method(s) of administration	Effect on central nervous system	Examples of desired effects (e.g. reasons for taking)	Examples of unwanted effects/ harm from use
	(other similar amfetamine derivatives also used)	attendance at dance music event			failure. After-effects include depression, insomnia, anxiety, lethargy
Heroin	Diamorphine	Inhalation of vapour produced when heated on tin foil, intravenous injection	CNS depressant	Intense pleasure including euphoria, warmth, relaxation, detachment from emotional distress	Initially nausea and vomiting, constipation, drowsiness, confusion, dry mouth, sweating, in overdose – respiratory depression, pulmonary oedema, hypoxia, arrhythmias
Tobacco	Nicotine	Cigarette smoking, chewing tobacco	CNS stimulation	Social activity, mood elevation, increases concentration, promotes relaxation,	Various cancers, cardiac disease, chronic obstructive airways disease, cough, halitosis
Cocaine	Cocaine hydrochloride (cocaine powder), cocaine base ('crack')	Nasal administration though snorting, injecting, smoking (free base)	CNS stimulation	Euphoria, alertness, increased confidence, excitement, physical stimulation. Intense exhilaration (injection and crack)	Cardiac toxicity, tachycardia, palpitations, hypertension, chest pain, sweating, tremor, mental and anxiety, psychosis. After-effects include dysphoria, depression, fatigue, intense craving
Speed	Amfetamine	Nasal administration through snorting, orally, intravenous injecting	CNS stimulation	Physical and mental stimulation, confidence, increased energy	Sweating, tachycardia, hypertension, anxiety, paranoia and psychosis. After-effects include fatigue and depression

Control and dependence

A lack of specific types of neurological control is sometimes given as the reason why some people develop addictions to specific psychoactive drug(s) whereas others do not. Published studies can be criticized as the models of behaviour are largely shown in animals not humans, making the assumption that the two findings are directly transferable. Nevertheless, neurological processes manifest positive and negative reinforcement of drug seeking and taking behaviours, with genetic variations influencing these.

The level of control a drug user has over his use will influence the balance between the benefits and harms experienced. With controlled use, harms can be prevented or contained, e.g. the quantity of alcohol consumed may be controlled to avoid unwanted effects. In uncontrolled use, harms can escalate. Uncontrolled use is a characteristic of drug dependence.

When a person loses control over his drug consumption, or rather drug consumption controls the person, this may be described as dependence. Drug dependence can present a significant amount of risk and harm to the individual and to society. There is a clear association between drug dependence and social deprivation. In areas where social deprivation is high there tends to be a greater incidence of drug problems. However, drug problems are not exclusive to deprived areas and can be found in most parts of the UK, in both urban and rural environments. Please remember at this stage that drug use and drug dependence do not refer to the same thing.

Withdrawal

When a person stops using a substance they are dependent on they often experience withdrawal. Withdrawal can be described in two forms:

Physical withdrawal effects

These are physical signs and symptoms experienced when the drug is removed. Examples include seizures in alcohol withdrawal, stomach cramps and severe influenza-type symptoms experienced in opiate withdrawal, palpitations and anxiety in cocaine withdrawal, insomnia in nicotine withdrawal. Physical withdrawal effects can be quite severe and tend to be of shorter duration than psychological withdrawal effects. For example the acute physical withdrawal stage from heroin lasts usually no more than 7 days.

Psychological withdrawal effects

These are psychological disturbances experienced when a drug is removed. These cannot be so easily observed or measured in the way that many physical withdrawal effects usually can, but they must not be underestimated. Psychological withdrawal includes intense craving, intense emotional experiences such as unmasking of grief, inability to cope, altered mood and depression, which may be prolonged and severe. It tends to be of long duration and contributes markedly to relapse back to drug use. For example, cravings may be induced by situations, paraphernalia or locations many years after last consumption.

The harms relating to psychoactive drug use and dependence

The risks and harms that drug use and dependence can present to the individual and society vary with the drug taken, the individual and the circumstances in which the drugs are taken. It is not possible to list all possible consequences from drug use/misuse in this chapter, but these are dealt with in the 'Key references and further reading' section (Appendix 5). The risks are categorized below.

Health problems

These affect the individual drug user and include physical and psychological health problems, which can be large and complex. As well as being caused by the individual substances concerned, health problems may relate to the method of administration. For example, injecting drug use is associated with damage to the circulatory system. Blood-borne virus infection (e.g. with HIV, hepatitis B and hepatitis C) is associated with the sharing of injecting equipment. Pharmacists are largely involved in preventing or reducing the harm from drug dependence, benefiting both the individual and society. Hence the role of the pharmacist in drug dependence is about contributing towards individual and public health and safety.

Social problems

The social problems that relate to drug dependence must not be underestimated. It is often these that drive people to seek treatment. Social problems may include poverty (e.g. social deprivation, exclusion or failure in education, inability to obtain or sustain employment, spending of income on drugs), damage to family relationships, difficulties forming relationships, exclusion from society and homelessness.

Drug-related crime

Drug-related crime includes not only the criminal activities committed against the Misuse of Drugs Act (see below) for which the individual is punished, but also crime that impacts on communities and society at large. The latter may relate to the acquisition of drugs or the effects of drugs, e.g. burglary to obtain money to buy drugs, robbery, violence associated with drunkenness, drunk/drug driving. Drug-related crime is of concern to society and is one of the reasons why treatment of drug problems and drug dependence is a key public health issue. Additionally there is evidence that treatment of drug dependence contributes towards a very marked reduction in drug-related crime. Hence treatment benefits not only the individual in terms of improved health but also society by making communities safer.

Drug users are often at greater risk than non-drug users of being victims of crime, e.g. violence associated with debt to drug dealers, prostitution, robbery and mugging if homeless or intoxicated.

Legislation

Misuse of Drugs Act

The Misuse of Drugs Act 1971 classifies drugs into Class A, Class B and Class C. The purpose of this legislation is to define the penalties imposed for the illegal undertaking of various activities, e.g. possession, supply, import, export. These are summarized in Table 49.2. For more information see: http://www.release.org.uk/. This classification system is different from the Misuse of Drugs Regulations that largely govern dispensing and other activities of the pharmacist. For guidance on dispensing of controlled drugs, see the Royal Pharmaceutical Society of Great Britain (RPSGB) website (http://www.rpsgb.org.uk) or the very comprehensive National Prescribing Centre guidance issued in February 2007: http://www.npc.co.uk/controlled_drugs/cdpublications.htm.

Road Traffic Act

This 1988 act makes it illegal to be in charge of a motor vehicle if 'unfit to drive through drink or drugs'. This includes both illicit substances and prescribed medicines. Drivers are required by law to notify the Driving and Vehicle Licensing Agency (DVLA) if there is any reason that the safety of their driving may be impaired, e.g. disability, the misuse of drugs, the need for medicines that impair reactions or cause sedation. The responsibility for notification lies with the patient, not healthcare professionals (see the

Table 49.2 Classification of some commonly misused substances according to the Misuse of Drugs Act 1971

Class	Drugs	Maximum penalties
A	Cocaine including crack cocaine, diamorphine (heroin), dipipanone, ecstasy, LSD, methadone, morphine, opium, pethidine	Seven years imprisonment and/or unlimited fine for possession. Life imprisonment and/or fine for supply*
B[†]	Most amphetamines[§], cannabis[‡], codeine, dihydrocodeine, methylphenidate	Five years imprisonment and/or fine for possession Fourteen years imprisonment and a fine for supply
C	Benzodiazepines, anabolic steroids and growth hormones	Two years imprisonment and/or fine for possession Fourteen years imprisonment and/or fine for supply

* The term 'supply' includes drug trafficking and unauthorized production.
[†] If Class B drugs are prepared for injection they become Class A.
[§] Unless prepared for injection when amfetamines become class A.
[‡] Pure cannabinoids are Class A drugs.

publication *At a Glance Guide to Medical Aspects of Fitness to Drive* (DVLA 2008), which is also available online: http://www.dvla.gov.uk/medical/ataglance. aspx.)

The management of drug use and dependence

This chapter focuses on problematic drug use and specifically on drug dependence. The reason for this is that pharmacists are primarily involved with the treatment of dependence rather than interventions aimed at recreational and non-problematic drug use. Drug dependence must, however, be kept in perspective as not everyone who tries drugs or uses drugs will become dependent on them. The prevalence of drug dependence on a population basis is relatively small compared to national statistics that estimate numbers of people who have ever tried drugs. However, the extent of harm from drug dependence can be large and affect not only the individual but their families and communities, hence the need for effective strategies to support people in changing their drug use is great.

A range of strategies is used to prevent, limit the extent of and address the problems associated with drug use and dependence. These will be summarized in order to illustrate the contribution made by pharmacists. Figure 49.1 illustrates the range of strategies used in preventing, reducing and controlling drug use and dependence and managing the adverse consequences. These will be briefly reviewed.

Primary prevention

Primary prevention is concerned with preventing people from starting to use drugs. Target groups include vulnerable groups such as school children, looked after children and young people who have left education. It includes warning of the harm that can result from drug use and dependence using health promotion and education campaigns. Primary prevention also includes legislation, as the illegal nature of many drugs may prevent some people from using them. It is difficult to evaluate the impact of primary prevention activities as so many factors may influence the person's decision to use or not to use drugs. Reliable research in this area can also be difficult to undertake. This does not mean that primary prevention activities should not be used. They are very important for informing children and young people about drugs and their effects. Such activities should not be scaremongering but need to be factually accurate to give young people an informed knowledge base about drugs which reflects what they may see within society.

Secondary prevention

Secondary prevention is aimed at people who use drugs by discouraging further use. Examples of secondary prevention are giving advice to prevent problems such as overheating and dehydration to ecstasy users, discouraging heroin smokers from progressing to injecting, and warning on the risks and guiding on the use of CNS depressant drugs (such as heroin and methadone) by stimulant users (such as ecstasy and amfetamine) when depressant drugs are used to assist with the 'come down' following CNS stimulation.

Drug education

Drug education is a tool used in primary and secondary prevention campaigns and includes leaflets, booklets, videos and posters. People who are dependent on drugs may also benefit from drug education as they may not be fully informed on the drugs they use or may consider using, e.g. long-term risks and overdose prevention. Drug education is also a key part of harm reduction, giving people information to assist them in minimizing risks from drug taking, e.g. safer injecting information. Drug education may be provided by a range of people, e.g. teachers, youth workers, health promotion workers, medical and nursing staff and

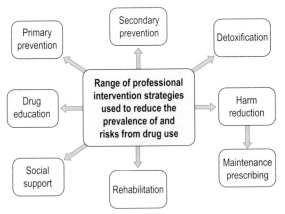

Figure 49.1 • The range of professional intervention strategies used to reduce or manage drug use and dependence.

police officers and should always be appropriate for the target group. For example, advice given to dependent heroin smokers would differ from that aiming to prevent heroin use in school children. Pharmacists may be asked to provide talks and should only deliver such talks if they feel competent to do so and capable of answering questions. Before such talks are given it is advisable to get advice and information from a credible source such as publications by drug charities and health promotion units. Seeking the support of the local drugs service may also be prudent. Inaccurate advice can be harmful and discredited.

Social support

Social support refers loosely to non-medical/pharmacological interventions that can be made. These may include practical advice and assistance (e.g. seeking housing, benefits advice, provision of hostel accommodation) and use of psychological tools such as motivational interviewing. Motivational interviewing aims to assist people in examining their drug use and the impact it has on their lives and those of others to move people towards a psychological state where they are motivated to change their behaviour and attempt to change their drug use. There are many psychological tools that are used by clinical psychologists and counsellors in the treatment and support of people with drug problems. Pharmacists should be aware of the need for a holistic approach to care, using not only pharmacological therapies where appropriate, but non-drug treatments too. Some pharmacists with a special interest (PwSI) who have specialized in drug misuse have developed skills in motivational interviewing and other psychological support tools.

Detoxification

Detoxification refers to the provision of treatment to help someone who is dependent on a drug to stop using it. Examples include the use of diazepam at gradually reducing doses in benzodiazepine dependence and the use of nicotine replacement therapy. The aim of detoxification is for the person to become abstinent from the drug on which they are dependent.

Rehabilitation

Rehabilitation may include a detoxification process followed by a period of social support and intensive psychotherapy to facilitate sustained change. Alternatively, it may comprise the social support and intensive psychotherapy phase only, with successful detoxification being a requirement for entry on the programme. Rehabilitation is usually provided within a 'therapeutic community' – participants live in the environment where treatment is given, often for several months. Often people who enter rehabilitation programmes have serious, complex and chronic drug dependency problems and may previously have experienced community-based treatment. The outcomes from various drug rehabilitation programmes were studied as part of the National Treatment Outcomes Research Study (NTORS), undertaken in the UK. Improvements were seen in drug use, physical health, psychological health and involvement in crime. At 4–5 year follow-up, 47% of people who had previously been dependent on opiates were abstinent, with reductions in frequency of opiate use seen in a significant number of the remainder (Gossop et al 2001).

Harm reduction

Harm reduction is a generic term to describe the range of interventions used to reduce the adverse consequences of drug dependence experienced by both individual drug users and society. Strategies prioritize goals in treatment, recognizing that, whereas abstinence from drug use may be the end goal, in some cases and for some drugs it is not always immediately achievable. Instead the risks and harm to the individual and others are reduced, by a process of prioritization which the individual is involved in defining.

Examples of harm reduction interventions include the provision of sterile injecting equipment and information to drug injectors to prevent the sharing of injecting equipment (to prevent the transmission of viruses such as HIV, hepatitis B and C). Minimizing the prevalence of such diseases also protects the non-injecting community.

Harm reduction also includes the provision of substitute therapies with the aim of reducing illicit drug use and reducing drug-related crime, hence benefiting communities. This is often done by providing substitute therapy, either at an adequate maintenance dose or as a detoxification agent. Pharmacists are frequently involved in the provision of harm reduction services (see later).

Service providers

Drug and alcohol services in the UK can be broadly grouped according to their different sources of funding. The three main groups are described below.

Statutory sector

The statutory sector comprises NHS and local authority services and includes prevention interventions, harm reduction services and abstinence-directed care. A large amount of NHS drug treatment is provided in GP surgeries, either by GPs alone or in partnership with GP liaison workers from specialist drugs services, who advise the GP on prescribing and offer patient counselling and support. Community drug teams (CDTs) are attached to NHS trusts, often led by psychiatrists. CDTs may provide primary care drug treatment, either through GP liaison work or with their own doctors running special clinics, similar to outpatient clinics. CDT services are typically provided by doctors and psychiatric nurses but some employ pharmacists to advise on or undertake prescribing and manage on-site dispensing. Statutory sector needle exchanges also exist, often staffed by specialist nurses.

NHS services also include secondary care, where treatment such as inpatient detoxification from alcohol and other drugs is provided, typically over a short time period such as 2 weeks.

Voluntary sector

Voluntary services are particularly prevalent in the substance misuse field because they developed quickly in response to the threat of HIV in the mid-1980s. The voluntary sector services receive funding from a range of sources (e.g. NHS, criminal justice money, local authorities, grants and donations) and are usually registered charities, with paid workers and/or volunteers operating under a management committee structure. Workers may come from a range of backgrounds, e.g. nursing, social work and community work. Some projects employ current or ex drug users. Services may include:

- Support and/or counselling
- Information and advice including harm reduction information
- Needle exchange
- Preparation for rehabilitation or inpatient detoxification and aftercare
- Client advocacy
- Complementary therapies
- Support to and liaison with GPs
- Specialist services such as women-only sessions
- Outreach and detached street-based work
- Prescribing services
- Input into multidisciplinary groups funded by the statutory service such as pregnancy clinics for drug-using women.

Other voluntary sector services offer spiritual and practical support, e.g. hostel accommodation and self-help groups. The voluntary sector also may represent drug users' views in advocacy, policy and service planning (e.g. The Alliance, see http://www.m-alliance.org.uk).

Private sector

The private sector includes ultra-rapid detoxification units, inpatient detoxification clinics, private primary care doctors and residential rehabilitation providers, private psychotherapists and alternative therapy providers. Funding for some of these treatments may come through the statutory sector but they are most often paid for by the patients or their families. Some pharmacists work in private sector treatment facilities advising on prescribing and dispensing. Private services offer a wide range of choice to patients but access is obviously limited by ability to pay. Ultra-rapid detoxification is not recommended for safety reasons.

Pharmaceutical care

This section focuses on pharmaceutical care of drug users, specifically looking at aspects of good pharmacy practice. The reader is referred for more detail to the National Treatment Agency publication *Best Practice Guidance for Commissioners and Providers of Pharmaceutical Services for Drug Users* (February 2006), available online at: http://www.rpsgb.org/pdfs/pharm servdrugusersguid.pdf.

The role of the pharmacist in drug dependence

Community pharmacists

Community pharmacists are ideally placed to contribute to the care of drug users. In addition to the health gains for the patient, there are several advantages for drug users, the community and pharmacists from providing care:

- Extended opening hours: most pharmacies are open at least part of the weekend and some evenings, when specialist drugs services may be closed.
- Accessibility: pharmacies tend to be based within communities, making them near to need. No appointment is needed so people can access care with little prior planning and at their convenience, which can encourage use.
- Expert advice: pharmacies give access to a trained healthcare practitioner and free advice. Advice may be sought by needle exchange users, people receiving substitute therapies or their families. Alternatively the pharmacist may give advice proactively when an opportunity arises (see Ch. 44).
- Discretion: pharmacies provide a confidential service. Service users tend to see pharmacies as separate from the 'healthcare system' and are encouraged to use them because no personal data are requested.
- Network of service: through widespread provision of services by many pharmacies, the workload can be shared and a network of good practice developed. Joint training with other pharmacists and GPs can develop professional relationships.
- Job satisfaction: the pharmacist may be the only healthcare professional with whom some drug users have regular contact. Over time and with an approachable, non-judgmental service a strong therapeutic relationship can develop between the pharmacist and the service user. The pharmacist may then be approached for advice or be in a position to offer risk-reduction information. Trust in the pharmacist can allow the pharmacist to encourage the person to access drugs services. Over time improvements in health can often be seen in people receiving substitute therapies, bringing job satisfaction.

The two most common services provided by community pharmacists to prevent and reduce harm are needle exchange and dispensing services. These are discussed later. For more detailed information on community pharmacy and drug misuse, the reader is referred to Sheridan & Strang (2002).

Hospital pharmacists

Hospitals should have guidelines for the admission and discharge of drug users to ensure that any on-going prescribing is continued. There should also be policies and specialist support available to ensure treatment can be initiated if a need is identified. This is especially important for cases when people are admitted to general medical or surgical wards for matters not relating to their drug use. The teams on these wards may not be familiar with substance misuse prescribing. Hospital pharmacists may contribute to the formulation of such guidelines. Issues to include are:

- Admissions: how to ensure the safe and prompt continuation of substitute prescribing when someone comes into secondary care from the community, with attention paid to acute and out of hours admissions. Methadone is a controlled drug, unlikely to be kept routinely on wards, so the pharmacy department must establish procedures to supply methadone out of hours.
- Discharge: how to ensure safe continuation of substitute prescribing on discharge without a break in care or doubling up of prescribing. Contact with GPs and community drug teams is vital. Liaison with the patient's nominated community pharmacist is also important to ensure sufficient supplies and to communicate any changes made to treatment while in hospital.
- Initiation of substitute therapy. For example, if a heroin-dependent person is admitted to a ward unplanned via accident and emergency, it will be necessary to control withdrawal symptoms that onset quickly (typically within 4–6 hours). If this is not done, the person will be in severe discomfort, extremely anxious and very reluctant to remain on the ward. As a result, their care may be severely compromised.
- Appropriate referral: there are opportunities for identification of drug users not in contact with service providers especially by accident and emergency staff. Knowledge of local service providers and opening hours, including needle exchanges, is important, and written details should be available on wards. Development of formal rapid access/referral systems should be undertaken in partnership with community-based services. At present some specialist services have waiting lists for care. Guidance on identifying patients at particular risk and rapid referral

from hospital to primary care services is recommended.

Hospital pharmacists also play a key role in advising on co-prescribing for people on substitute therapies such as methadone. Many drug interactions can occur and changes in doses may be necessary if methadone is co-administered with enzyme-inhibiting or enzyme-inducing drugs. Treatments for epilepsy and HIV/AIDS in particular must be carefully considered. Clinical issues of co-prescribing cannot be covered here; instead reference to appropriate texts on drug interactions is advised (e.g. Stockley 2005).

Specialist pharmacists (PwSI)

There are pharmacists who specialize in drug dependency, many of whom come under the umbrella term of 'pharmacist with a special interest' (PwSI). Some provide services from community pharmacies whereas others may be based in GP surgeries or specialist drugs services. They may be prescribers, or provide support to clinical colleagues, e.g. by advising on prescribing or providing drug information. They may also oversee dispensing and liaise with (other) community pharmacists. Others undertake strategic roles such as coordinating local pharmacy needle exchange services or overseeing the pharmacy contribution to shared care (see below).

Needle and syringe exchange

Background

Needle and syringe exchange (NSE) began in the UK in the mid-1980s in response to the threat from HIV. Prior to this, availability of clean injecting equipment was limited due to the belief that this would prevent people injecting. There was grave concern in the mid-1980s regarding the threat to public health that HIV presented and fears of an epidemic unless something was done to reduce its spread. Large health education campaigns were aimed at those at high risk, e.g. gay men, people having casual unprotected heterosexual sex and injecting drug users. In order to enable injecting drug users to follow the advice not to share needles and syringes, NSE programmes were started in many countries. These programmes were studied in several research projects which found that NSE programmes were effective in reducing the transmission of HIV without causing an increase in injecting drug use. A comparative study of 12 cities was conducted by Stimson et al for the World Health Organization (WHO); this is described in the text *Drug Injecting and HIV Infection* (Stimson et al 1998). An excellent summary article was published by MacDonald and colleagues (2003). Ksobiech (2003) published a meta-analysis of 47 studies looking at needle exchange outcomes and concluded that blood-borne virus transmission was significantly reduced by NSE availability.

In the early 1990s hepatitis C (HCV) was identified. This blood-borne virus appears to be highly transmissible among injectors and there is as yet no vaccine, although recent research is promising. It has been shown to be spread through the sharing of injecting paraphernalia, including needles and syringes, but also probably other items used in the preparation of illicit injections, for example the spoon or metal container in which the drug is mixed with water, the makeshift filter used to remove insoluble materials and adulterants and potentially items such as swabs used to clean injecting sites. Recently an odds ratio of 2.44:1 (95% CI, 1.44-4.12) has been calculated predicting the risk of contracting HCV through paraphernalia sharing when never having shared needles and syringes (Mathei et al 2006). It is important that NSE is widely available in order to limit the spread of blood-borne viruses. Community pharmacies contribute to the network of needle exchanges. They increase coverage, especially for those reluctant to access specialist agencies, at times when agencies are closed (such as weekends) and in areas where no such agencies exist. Privacy may be limited in community pharmacies, so there may be limits to the extent of dialogue and examination that can take place. Additionally drug users may not perceive the pharmacist to be knowledgeable about drug misuse so pharmacists need to be proactive in demonstrating their competence.

Practical issues in NSE provision

Training

Before any pharmacist begins to provide any new service it is important that they are adequately trained and competent to provide the service. NSE is no exception. Therefore pharmacists and their staff should undertake training on issues relating to needle exchange. Specialist agencies may be able to offer training for pharmacists and their staff.

Hepatitis B vaccination

Although pharmacists and their staff do not handle loose needles during the needle exchange process, it is a wise health and safety precaution for all staff to be vaccinated against hepatitis B (HBV). There are no vaccines for hepatitis C or HIV. Community pharmacists should discuss HBV vaccination for staff with NSE scheme coordinators or the local public health consultant.

Needle exchange procedure

NSE involves supplying clean, sterile injecting equipment in exchange for used equipment, which is returned in a sealed sharps container. As well as supplying equipment, NSE services should provide advice and check injecting sites, with referral to medical services when problems such as abscesses are identified.

Needle exchange schemes are usually coordinated within the health locality, so local policies may exist and support and guidance should be available to pharmacists. Failing this, policies and procedures for needle exchange need to be put in place in order to minimize risk. Guidance from the National Institute for Health and Clinical Excellence (NICE 2009), National Pharmaceutical Association, National Treatment Agency, public health departments and needle exchange agencies can assist. Adequate storage facilities are essential. Used equipment returned to the pharmacy in a bin should be placed in a larger bin by the client, stored in a separate area from clean equipment and away from medicines. These bins are sealed when full and collected for incineration by clinical waste disposal companies.

To maximize the public health benefits, injecting drug users need to be able to use a clean set of equipment for each injection and every set of equipment supplied should be returned for incineration. In order to try to meet this aim, adequate amounts of injecting equipment should be supplied, bearing in mind that some crack cocaine injectors may be injecting very frequently (e.g. 15 times per day or more). Also the number of needles and syringes supplied does not necessarily equate with the number of injections the person themself takes, as needles can be damaged or broken during access attempts or distributed to peers. The number of needles and syringes that can be supplied in any one visit may be dictated locally by scheme coordinators. It is wise to discuss supply quantities with local needle exchange agencies to ensure continuity in service provision. Capping of numbers of sets of equipment allowed is not advocated and dilutes harm reduction effectiveness. In Scotland the Lord Advocate's Guidance dictates the number of sets that can be supplied. A sharps bin should be supplied with every exchange. Bins range from pocket size to large clinical waste tubs. The return of equipment should be strongly encouraged and local campaigns to promote returns participated in. Written advice on safe disposal accompanied by verbal emphasis is important. However, if a person requests needle exchange but has no used equipment to return, it is advocated that supply of clean needles and syringes is made, as the health risks of not supplying are great. Pharmacy staff should not open disposal bins to count the number of sets returned. Instead estimates of returned numbers should be made based on the number of returns reported by the service user and the size and estimated fullness of the returned disposal bin.

Record keeping and audit

Records need to be kept in order to audit the pharmacy NSE service. In order to encourage use, pharmacy NSE should be provided on an anonymous basis (no names recorded). Attractions of pharmacy-based NSE are the anonymity and low threshold access. Too many obstacles will discourage use. In some schemes, pharmacies issue cards which give the service user an identification number or code. This can be used to record service usage but it also allows discreet service provision, as the person only needs to show the card to indicate that they require needle exchange. This can be helpful in a crowded pharmacy. The advantage of having a record for each service user is that it can quickly be seen if someone returns used equipment or not. Those who do not can be targeted with information and firm requests to return equipment. The disadvantage is that in a busy pharmacy this system can be too time-consuming. Additionally some people do not want to carry a card that identifies them as an injector. As a basic requirement, the daily number of sets of injecting equipment supplied and the approximate number returned should be recorded and data compiled for weekly or monthly audit purposes. Data should be returned to the scheme coordinator where one exists. Pharmacies with poor return rates should seek the advice of specialist drugs agencies and the scheme coordinator on strategies to increase return rates and be proactive in encouraging returns. In some areas, including Leeds, novel ideas such as client completed 'order forms' have been successful in minimizing the pharmacy burden of paperwork but providing auditable records of supplies.

Risk management

A written procedure for needle exchange should be in place and followed. Body fluid spillage kits should be kept in all pharmacies as a matter of routine, irrespective of whether the pharmacy is part of an NSE scheme, and staff should be trained in their use. In the event of an incident (e.g. a patient bleeds or vomits on the floor), the kit should be used. It should be noted that use of the kit is dictated by the situation and not the perceived risk presented by the patient, i.e. use of the kit does not depend on whether the patient is a known injector or not.

Chain mail gloves should be kept in needle exchange pharmacies for use in the event of loose used injecting equipment requiring disposal. However, this is only a precaution, as the needle exchange scheme procedure should be such that it minimizes the risk of such events. If any such events occur they should be documented as part of the pharmacy's critical incident scheme. Procedures should then be reviewed to see if anything could be done to avoid such an incident in the future.

Links with specialist services

Pharmacy NSE providers should have links with local drugs agencies and know what services they provide. Often younger and newer injectors use pharmacy needle exchanges because of the low threshold and discretion. These people may also not want to stop injecting and consider agencies to be for people with drug 'problems' or people who want to stop using. Women may also prefer the anonymity of using pharmacy services. Female drug users are often extremely stigmatized, especially if they are also mothers. The pharmacist may be the only healthcare professional these service users have contact with. Knowledge of other local services means that the pharmacist can advise when a need is identified or an opportunity arises. The pharmacy should consider itself a gateway to specialist services. Some specialist agencies may be able to supply pharmacists with targeted written information for drug injectors, such as safer injecting leaflets, and with free condoms to reduce sexually transmitted diseases. Safer injecting leaflets should

not be available for self-selection but should be targeted at injectors. The pharmacist needs to ensure they are competent to provide advice and allow a rapport with the client to develop over time. This in turn will facilitate the provision of information, advice and signposting when the time is right.

Use of pharmacotherapies in drug dependence

The term pharmacotherapy in this context refers to any drug treatment used to assist in the management of drug dependence or symptoms of withdrawal. Substitute therapy refers to drug treatment that replaces an illegal drug with a legal one of the same or similar pharmacological class. For example methadone is a substitute for opiates such as heroin. Non-substitute drugs may also be used to control withdrawal symptoms (e.g. lofexidine to manage opiate withdrawal) and to manage symptoms secondary to withdrawal (e.g. loperamide to manage diarrhoea associated with opiate withdrawal).

Role of pharmacotherapy

Pharmacotherapy can be mistaken both by patients and by professionals as an all-encompassing solution. However, it is one of several tools used in the care of drug dependence. Alone it cannot stop someone using drugs but it can facilitate change in motivated people by providing what many describe as 'breathing space'. For example substitute therapy can prevent withdrawal symptoms thus giving the person a chance to sever links with illicit drug suppliers. Substitute therapy also removes the need to commit crime to obtain money for drugs. Pharmacotherapy therefore has benefits for both the individual and society. Substitute therapy, from a risk-reduction point of view, is also preferable to illicit drugs because the quality and dose of the product is assured.

There is an ever increasing evidence base of literature to support the provision of pharmacotherapy in drug dependence. In particular most literature focuses on methadone and high-dose buprenorphine. Evidence shows maintenance doses of treatment alone improve patient physical health and mental health outcomes, reduce drug-related deaths and improve social functioning. However, outcomes can be enhanced with appropriate 'wrap around' services providing support and counselling, where the person freely is willing to take part. Coercion into such services or psychotherapy is not advocated.

The psychoactive and non-psychoactive effects of substitute therapies are not usually the same as the illicit drugs they replace and an awareness of this in the patient at the start of treatment is important. For example, methadone is used as a long-acting substitute in opiate dependence. When taken orally it does not produce euphoria and it can cause lethargy and a feeling of 'heaviness' not associated with heroin use.

All who receive pharmacotherapy, especially in the early stages of treatment, may not achieve complete abstinence from illicit drug use. It is a common misconception that substitute treatment should be given at a reducing dose leading in a short time period to abstinence from illicit drug use. Whereas in a minority of patients this will produce sustained benefits, for many, rapid detoxification has been shown not to produce long-term abstinence from illicit drugs. Instead a period, often prolonged, of maintenance therapy at an adequate dose may be necessary. This may last for many years.

Methadone

Methadone is used as a substitute drug in opiate dependence. Its long half-life (24–48 hours) makes it suitable for once-daily dosing in the majority of cases, although a few patients prefer to divide the dose. Providing it is given in adequate doses and for a satisfactory length of time, there is substantial evidence to suggest that methadone treatment has several benefits:

- Improved physical health
- Improved psychological health
- Reduced illicit drug consumption
- Reduced incidence and frequency of injecting episodes
- Reduced drug-related crime.

As can be seen, the benefits extend beyond the individual patient into the community. Less injecting will reduce the risks of blood-borne virus transmission. The reductions seen in drug-related crime have been large. These findings have been reported in a range of publications. As a summary, the reader is referred to the NICE technology appraisal of methadone and buprenorphine (January 2007), available online at: http://www.nice.org.uk/TA114. An updated version of the Department of Health publication *Drug Misuse and Dependence, Guidelines on Clinical Management* is now available.

Failure to reduce or prevent illicit drug consumption is associated with maintenance doses of methadone less than 60 mg per day and premature pressure to abstain from methadone (Ward et al 1999). Before detoxification can be considered, treatment may need to be given at maintenance dose level for prolonged periods of time, with some people remaining on maintenance doses indefinitely. Withdrawal of treatment should begin only when the patient is willing to attempt this, as motivation is the key to success. Regular review of patients on maintenance doses and on detoxification schemes is necessary. In detoxification, the speed of dose reduction largely depends on how well the patient is coping. Reductions should be calculated as a percentage of the dose; hence towards the smaller end of the scale, dosing will be reduced by smaller quantities. For some people the small doses can be the hardest to reduce and some people remain on doses of as little as 1 mg and 2 mg per day for several months until they feel capable of stopping treatment completely. Psychological adjustment is very important at this stage, especially if drug use has been used as a coping mechanism. Withdrawal can take several months, even years. If the dose needs to be increased at any point during detoxification, emotional support and reassurance may be necessary as some people can regard such increases as failure.

It is important to discuss with patients potential overdose risks from combining CNS depressants, including alcohol. Healthcare teams need to understand that some illicit drug use may continue, especially at the early stages of treatment. During the initiation of treatment, this can be a time when there is a greater risk of overdose, due to the fact that treatment dosing will not yet be optimized and withdrawal effects are likely, leading to 'on top' illicit drug use. The patient must be advised of this risk and monitored closely. Several information leaflets are available which explain this to patients, e.g. the 'Methadone Briefing' from Exchange Health or the Department of Health-supported *Going Over* DVD. If illicit drug use continues at a similar frequency as it was before substitution therapy was introduced, it is important to review the dose and treatment goals with the patient. Methadone treatment may be suboptimal or the person is not ready to change their drug use. In this case methadone may be compounding the risks and other harm reduction strategies may be more appropriate.

Pharmacists should have a good understanding of the clinical aspects relating to methadone treatment before they begin providing methadone dispensing services. This should be gained as part of a continuous professional development plan if needed.

Safe storage in the home

If take-home doses are dispensed, pharmacists should discuss safe storage of methadone and other drugs in the home with patients, especially those with children. As little as 5 mg of methadone can kill a small child. Parents on methadone prescriptions should store take-home doses in overhead cupboards, which should be locked to prevent access by children. In addition parents should be advised not to consume medicines in front of children to prevent copying behaviours.

Other treatments

Buprenorphine is a partial agonist, used as an opiate substitution therapy instead of methadone. Its use is becoming more widespread as the evidence base develops. As it is a partial agonist, it antagonizes the effects of other opiates if they are used on top. The patient needs clear advice on initiation and counselling on the risks of attempting to overcome the antagonist properties, for example by using large amounts of opiate. This may present an overdose risk. Buprenorphine is used in sublingual tablet form and also has a long half-life, which facilitates daily or even every second day administration, although in practice daily use is usually preferred.

Lofexidine and naltrexone are also used in the management of opiate withdrawal. The former reduces some of the physical withdrawal effects from opiates by acting on the noradrenergic system, while the latter is an opiate antagonist used in relapse prevention. There are also recognized regimens to assist withdrawal for those with stimulant, benzodiazepine and alcohol dependence. When a person is dependent on more than one drug, withdrawal should be done one drug at a time. Further reading regarding these treatments is advised.

Urine screening and responding to symptoms

People receiving treatment for drug dependence may have their urine screened. This is done to check for evidence of compliance with prescribed regimens or to confirm for the consumption of illicit drugs. In some areas urine screen results may be used to make a decision on whether treatment is continued or not. Pharmacists should undertake training in this area of toxicology, as some over the counter and prescribed medicines can interfere with urine screens, giving false results. It is important to have an understanding of what medicines to avoid in people receiving treatment for dependence, so that patients and prescribers can be advised. This is also relevant to athletes subject to urine screens for banned substances.

Pharmaceutical dispensing services

Shared care

Shared care with regard to substance misuse is GPs, pharmacists, drugs services and the patient being in partnership to manage dependence within a formalized, structured scheme. Pharmacists participating in such schemes receive additional remuneration. Examples of schemes in the UK include those in Glasgow and Berkshire (Roberts & Bryson 1999; Walker 2001). Daily dispensing of controlled drugs is often advocated by prescribers, especially at the start of treatment, as it is believed to prevent leakage onto illegal markets. This means that the pharmacist is likely to be the healthcare professional with the most frequent contact with the patient as they see the patient daily, while the prescribing team may see them weekly or fortnightly. Pharmacists can play an important role in monitoring the patient's health.

One of the benefits of shared care is that the workload of providing care is distributed locally. This prevents one or two pharmacies becoming overburdened and allows patients access to care within their communities. Participation of all or the majority of community pharmacies in the area is therefore vital for the scheme to succeed. To date this has not always been the case as some pharmacies have refused to provide services to drug users.

Before joining a shared-care scheme, pharmacists should consider any changes within the pharmacy that may be necessary. These should be discussed with the scheme coordinator who may be able to source financial assistance for such changes. For example is there enough space in the controlled drug cabinet to store dispensed controlled drugs waiting for collection? Consider the layout of the premises. What can be done to ensure an appropriate area is available to allow a respectful service to be provided? Is there a private area for methadone consumption? A private room is not always desired by patients but a discrete area can be very welcome. The Department of Health guidelines on drug misuse and dependence give more detail on the role of the pharmacist in shared care and cover issues such as information sharing and confidentiality.

Supervised consumption

The development of shared-care schemes for the management of drug dependence has led to an increased involvement of pharmacists, especially community pharmacists, in providing care to drug users. Many shared-care schemes require daily dispensing and supervision of consumption of all or most doses of substitute therapy, at least for the first 3–6 months of treatment. Supervised consumption was introduced because of leakage of methadone and other drugs to the illicit market contributing to overdoses in people who had not been prescribed the drugs.

Supervised consumption is a contentious area. Some patients view it as a useful part of treatment whereas others dislike it (Neale 1999). Supervised consumption can cause the patient much embarrassment. In a busy shop it may be very humiliating for a person if a pharmacist presents them with a measure of green liquid to drink or some tablets to take in front of other customers. As it is not 'normal' to take medicines in front of the pharmacist, people can quickly be identified as drug users. Much can be done by the pharmacist to show respect and consideration for someone when they are required to consume their treatment in the pharmacy, e.g. ask if they wish to wait until the shop is free of other customers before their dose is given. Pharmacists should also ask patients whether they wish to use a private area, if one is available. Patients appreciate such respect.

To assist with organization, it is suggested that pharmacists prepare all daily dispensed prescriptions the day before or early in the day required. Doses should be packaged appropriately in individually labelled containers and stored in the controlled drug cupboard, or as legislation dictates, with the prescription attached. When the patient presents for supervised consumption, the pharmacist should recheck the dispensed item. The patient should then be given the substance to be consumed together with a drink of water. The water helps take the taste of the medicine away, rinses the mouth (methadone has a high sugar content and is acidic, which could damage tooth enamel) and helps ensure the dose has been swallowed. Disposable cups should be used. Under no circumstances should patients be expected to share the same cup for water in case this presents a risk of infection transmission. The pharmacist should take the opportunity for discussion with the patient to assess their well-being and offer any advice as the opportunity arises. Over time a good rapport and therapeutic relationship can develop with patients.

The Royal Pharmaceutical Society of Great Britain website on controlled drugs should be consulted for legal updates including recent guidance on instalment prescriptions.

Confidentiality

Communication between healthcare professionals is key in shared care. However, patient confidentiality must be borne in mind. Information should not be shared without consent. The patient should be involved in negotiations about care and treatment changes. When consulation with another service provider about a patient is necessary, this should be discussed with the patient. They should be informed of what the other service provider is to be told and their permission sought. Patient's wishes should only be breached when a severe risk to health or well-being is considered to exist if confidentiality is not broken. All matters relating to the upholding or breaching of confidentiality should be documented.

Contracts

Some shared-care schemes advocate the use of contracts, which clearly state what is expected of the patient and what the patient can expect from the service. Often they dictate standards of behaviour and include clauses requiring the patient to fulfil certain criteria, including restricting the times when patients can collect prescriptions. It is debated whether contracts should be used specifically for patients with drug problems. They imply that it is expected that the person will not behave appropriately and as such stereotypes patients. Contracts are not routinely used within pharmacy health care for other patients and it can be argued that using one for drug users is unfair and discriminatory. Pharmacies should have practice leaflets as a matter of routine which are available to all pharmacy users. These may include a statement that all pharmacy customers have a right to privacy and respect and all pharmacy staff have a right to be treated with courtesy. If individuals present any problems, the pharmacist should deal with these individually. This applies to any customers who cause difficulty within the pharmacy. Pharmacies should have a complaints procedure which can be useful for reviewing response to such incidents.

When pharmacists are asked to use contracts as part of the shared-care scheme, the pharmacist should review the contract before agreeing. Pharmacists should ask themselves whether they, as a patient, would consider it fair to sign such terms. The contract should not imply that it is expected that the person cannot behave or will cause problems.

Restricted collection hours for drug users should also be considered with caution. Pharmacists are required to dispense prescriptions with 'reasonable promptness'. Refusing to dispense a prescription during opening hours because a person has not arrived within a designated collection time may be considered discriminatory and is certainly unfair.

Locums

All standard operating procedures for pharmacy services should be documented and available for locums to use. This includes needle exchange and supervised consumption. It is important that all locums are aware of all the services provided,

including those to drug users, and are briefed on the completion of any necessary documentation such as needle exchange usage.

KEY POINTS

- Pharmacists can make an important contribution to the care and support of people with drug misuse problems
- Treatment of substance misuse benefits not only the patient but the community as well by reducing blood-borne virus transmission and drug-related crime
- Pharmacists should seek adequate continuous professional development to increase their competence in providing services to drug users. This should include clinical and therapeutic knowledge of treatment in this area as well as service provision skills
- Pharmacists should seek to be informed on local specialist services for drug users and have good professional links with such treatment providers
- Pharmacists should treat all pharmacy users with respect. This includes not discriminating on the basis of a person's disease state or drug dependence
- Local pharmacy scheme coordinators can be of great benefit in supporting pharmacists who provide services to drug users

Appendices

Medical abbreviations

Megan R. Thomas

Introduction

Abbreviations are widely used throughout all areas of life. While some abbreviations are so well known as to be accepted as part of everyday conversation, other abbreviations are very specific to a particular profession or even a specialty within a profession. This can easily lead to confusion, as the meaning of the abbreviation may not be immediately clear to the reader or listener. Indeed some abbreviations have a number of different interpretations and it is important to take them within context. For instance, 'aka' is widely understood to mean 'also known as', but can also stand for above knee amputation. While NPA might immediately suggest the National Pharmaceutical Association to the majority of the readers of this book, found in a set of medical records it is more likely to refer to nasopharyngeal aspirate. Perhaps more confusingly BM can be used for bone marrow, bowel movement, or blood sugar level (in reference to the type of reagent strip used to measure the blood sugar). It would be easy to recommend that abbreviations were never used, but with the sheer volume of information that requires recording and the often linguistically challenging terminology, their use is inevitable. Listed below are some of the more widely used terms adopted by the medical profession in the UK including a separate section on the abbreviations commonly used to document physical examination findings. A useful Web-based resource offers over 200 000 medical, pharmaceutical, biomedical and healthcare acronyms and abbreviations and can be found at http://www.medilexicon.com/. However, it is best, as with all things in life, never to assume.

Common medical abbreviations

AAA Abdominal aortic aneurysm
Ab Antibody, abortion
Abd Abdomen
ABG Arterial blood gas
ABO Blood group classification
ABX Antibiotic
ACTH Adrenocorticotrophic hormone
AD(H)D Attention deficit (hyperactivity) disorder
ADH Antidiuretic hormone
ADL Activities of daily living
ADR Adverse drug reaction
A&E Accident and emergency
AED Antiepileptic drug

AF Anterior fontanelle, atrial fibrillation
AFB Acid fast bacilli
AFL Atrial flutter
AFO Ankle-foot orthosis
AFP Alpha fetoprotein
A/G Albumin/globulin ratio
Ag Antigen
AIDS Acquired immunodeficiency syndrome
aka Also known as
AKA Above knee amputation
ALL Acute lymphocytic leukaemia
ALT Alanine aminotransferase

ALTEs Acute life-threatening episodes
AMA Against medical advice
AML Acute myeloid leukaemia
amnio Amniocentesis
ANA Antinuclear antibody
ANF Antinuclear factor
AOB Alcohol on breath
AP Anteroposterior
A&P Anterior and posterior
APLS Advanced paediatric life support
appt Appointment
AR Aortic regurgitation
A-R Apical-radial pulse

ARDS Adult respiratory distress syndrome

ARF Acute renal failure

AS Aortic stenosis

ASAP As soon as possible

ASCVD Arteriosclerotic cardiovascular disease

ASD Atrial septal defect

ASHD Atherosclerotic heart disease

ASO(T) Antistreptolysin O (titre)

AV Arteriovenous, atrioventricular

A&W Alive and well

AXR Abdominal X-ray

Ba Barium

Bact Bacteriology

BaE Barium enema

BBA Born before arrival

BBB Bundle branch block, blood–brain barrier

BCC Basal cell carcinoma

BCG Bacillus Calmette–Guerin vaccine (against tuberculosis)

BEAM Brain electrical activity mapping

Beta HCG Human chorionic gonadotrophin

BID Brought in dead

bil Bilateral

bili Bilirubin

BKA Below knee amputation

BLS Basic life support

BM Bowel movement, bone marrow, blood sugar

BMR Basal metabolic rate

BNO Bowels not open

BOM Bilateral otitis media

BOR Bowels open regularly

BP Blood pressure

BPD Bipolar disorder, borderline personality disorder, bronchopulmonary dysplasia

BPH Benign prostatic hypertrophy

BPLS Basic paediatric life support

bpm Beats per minute

BS Bowel sounds, breath sounds, blood sugar

BSA Body surface area

BSER Brain stem-evoked response

BTL Bilateral tubal ligation

BUN Blood urea nitrogen

BW Birth weight, body weight

Bx Biopsy

c Cum (with)

C₁ First cervical vertebra, etc.

Ca Calcium

CA,Ca,ca Cancer, carcinoma

CAB(G) Coronary artery bypass (graft)

CAD Coronary artery disease

CAPD Continuous ambulatory peritoneal dialysis

C(A)T Computed (axial) tomography

cath Catheter

CBC Complete blood count

CBG Capillary blood gas

CC Chief complaint

CCF Congestive cardiac failure

CCU Coronary care unit, clean catch urine

CDs Controlled drugs

CDH Congenital diaphragmatic hernia, congenital dislocated hips

CF Cystic fibrosis

CHD Congenital heart disease

CHF Congestive heart failure

CIBD Chronic inflammatory bowel disease

CI Chloride

CLL Chronic lymphocytic leukaemia

CMV Cytomegalovirus

CN Cranial nerves

CNS Central nervous system

CO Carbon monoxide, cardiac output

c/o Complains of

COAD Chronic obstructive airway disease

co-arct Coarctation of the aorta

COLD Chronic obstructive lung disease

COPD Chronic obstructive pulmonary disease

CP Chest pain, cerebral palsy

CPAP Continuous positive airways pressure

C(P)K Creatinine (phospho)kinase

CPR Cardiopulmonary resuscitation

CRF Chronic renal failure

CRP C-reactive protein

C&S Culture and sensitivity

CSF Cerebrospinal fluid

C section Caesarean section

CTS Carpal tunnel syndrome

CVA Cerebrovascular accident, costovertebral angle

CVP Central venous pressure

CVS Cardiovascular system, chorionic villus sampling

Cx Cervix, cervical

CXR Chest X-ray

D(x) Diagnosis

D&C Dilatation and curettage

DH Drug history

DIC Disseminated intravascular coagulation

diff Differential blood count

DIP Distal interphalangeal joint

DKA Diabetic ketoacidosis

DM Diabetes mellitus

DNA Did not attend (outpatient)

DNR Do not resuscitate

DOA Dead on arrival

DOB Date of birth

DOE Dyspnoea on exertion

DPL Diagnostic peritoneal lavage

DPT Diptheria, pertussis, tetanus vaccine

DSA Digital subtraction angiography

DTR Deep tendon reflexes

DTs Delirium tremens

DU Duodenal ulcer

D&V Diarrhoea and vomiting

DVT Deep vein thrombosis

D/W Discussed with

DXT Deep X-ray treatment

ECF Extracellular fluid

ECG Electrocardiogram

ECMO Extracorporeal membrane oxygenation

ECT Electroconvulsive therapy

EDD Expected date of delivery (baby)

EEG Electroencephalogram

ELBW Extremely low birth weight

EMG Electromyogram

EMU Early morning urine

ENT Ear, nose and throat

EOM Extraocular muscles

Ep Epilepsy

ERCP Endoscopic retrograde cholangiopancreatography

ERG Electroretinogram

ESM Ejection systolic murmur

ESR Erythrocyte sedimentation rate

ET Endotracheal

ETA Expected time of arrival

EUA Examination under anaesthetic

exc Excision

FB Finger breadths, foreign body

FBC Full blood count

FBS Fasting blood sugar

FDPs Fibrin degradation products

FEV₁ Forced expiratory volume (in 1 second)

FFA Free fatty acids

FFP Fresh frozen plasma

FH Family history

FISH Fluorescent in situ hybridization

FOB Faecal occult blood, foot of the bed

Frax Fragile X syndrome

FROM Full range of movement

FSH Follicle stimulating hormone

FTNVD Full-term normal vaginal delivery

FTT Failure to thrive

FU Follow-up

FUO Fever of unknown origin

FVC Forced vital capacity

Fx Fracture

GA General anaesthetic

GCS Glasgow coma scale

GFR Glomerular filtration rate

GI(T) Gastrointestinal (tract)

GN Glomerulonephritis

G6PD Glucose-6-phosphate dehydrogenase

G&S Group and save

GSW Gun shot wound

GTN Glyceryl trinitrate

GTT Glucose tolerance test

GU Genitourinary, gastric ulcer

GYN, gyn Gynaecology

Hb, Hgb Haemoglobin

HC Head circumference

Hct Haematocrit

HCVD Hypertensive cardiovascular disease

HDL High density lipoprotein

HDN Haemolytic disease of the newborn

HDU High-dependency unit

Hep Hepatitis

HFO High-frequency oscillation

HH Hiatus hernia

HI Haemaglutination inhibition, head injury

HIE Hypoxic ischaemic encephalopathy

HIV Human immunodeficiency virus

HL Hodgkin's lymphoma

HLA Human leukocyte antigen

HMD Hyaline membrane disease

HO History of

HOCM Hypertrophic obstructive cardiomyopathy

H&P History and physical

HPI History of presenting illness

HR Heart rate

HRT Hormone replacement therapy

HSM Hepatosplenomegaly

HSP Henoch–Schönlein purpura, hereditary spastic paraparesis

HT Hypertension

ht Height

HUS Haemolytic uraemic syndrome

HVS High vaginal swab

Hx History

IA Intra-arterial

IABP Intra-aortic balloon pump

IBS Irritable bowel syndrome

ICF Intracellular fluid

ICM Infracostal margin

ICP Intracranial pressure

ICS Intercostal space

ICU Intensive care unit

ID Intradermal, initial dose

I&D Incision and drainage

IDD Insulin-dependent diabetic

IDM Infant of a diabetic mother

Ig Immunoglobulin

IHD Ischaemic heart disease

IHSS Idiopathic hypertrophic subaortic stenosis

IM Intramuscular

imp Impression

IMV Intermittent mandatory ventilation

inf Inferior

inj Injury, injection

INR International normalized ratio (prothrombin time)

I&O Intake and output

IO Intraosseous

IOP Intraoccular pressure

IP Intraperitoneal, inpatient

IPPV Intermittent positive pressure ventilation

IRDS Idiopathic respiratory distress syndrome

IVC Inferior vena cava

ISQ No change (in status quo)

ITP Idiopathic thrombocytopenic purpura

ITU Intensive therapy unit

IUD Intrauterine device, intrauterine death

IUGR Intrauterine growth retardation

IV, iv Intravenous

IVH Intraventricular haemorrhage

IVP Intravenous pyelogram

IVU Intravenous urography

Ix Investigations

J Jaundice

JRA Juvenile rheumatoid arthritis

jt Joint

JVP Jugular venous pulse

K Potassium

KO Keep open

KO'd Knocked out

KUB Kidneys, ureters, bladder

L₁ First lumbar vertebra, etc.

LA Local anaesthetic, left atrium

Lab Laboratory

labs Results of tests

lac Laceration

LAD Left anterior descending (coronary artery), left axis deviation

lat Lateral

LBBB Left bundle branch block

LBW Low birth weight

LD Lethal dose

LDH Lactate dehydrogenase

LDL Low density lipoprotein

LE Lupus erythematosus

LFTs Liver function tests

LH Luteinizing hormone

LIH Left inguinal hernia

LMN Lower motor neurone

LMP Last menstrual period

LN Lymph node

LOC Loss of consciousness

LP Light perception, lumbar puncture

LSCS Lower segment caesarean section

LSE Left sternal edge

Lt Left

LUQ Left upper quadrant

LV Left ventricle

LVF Left ventricular failure

LVH Left ventricular hypertrophy

LVOT Left ventricular outflow tract

LWBS Left without being seen

MAOIs Monoamine oxidase inhibitors

MAP Mean arterial pressure

MCH Mean corpuscular haemoglobin

MCHC Mean corpuscular haemoglobin concentration

MCT Medium chain triglyceride

MCU Micturating cystourethrogram

MCV Mean corpuscular volume

mets Metastasis

Mg Magnesium

MI Mitral incompetence or insufficiency, myocardial infarction

MMR Mumps, measles, rubella vaccine

MR Mitral regurgitation

MRI Magnetic resonance imaging

MRSA Meticillin-resistant *Staphylococcus aureus*

MS Mitral stenosis, morphine sulphate, multiple sclerosis

MSU Midstream urine

MVA Motor vehicle accident

N Normal

Na Sodium

NAD Nothing abnormal detected, no active disease, no acute distress

NAI Non-accidental injury

NBI No bony injury

NBM Nil by mouth

NCPAP Nasal continuous positive airways pressure

Neb Nebulizer

NEC Narcotizing enterocolitis

Neuro Neurology

NF Neurofibromatosis

NFR Not for resuscitation

NG New growth

NG(T) Nasogastric (tube)

NHL Non-Hodgkin's lymphoma

NICU Neonatal intensive care unit

NIDDM Non-insulin-dependent diabetes mellitus

NKA No known allergies

NMR Nuclear magnetic resonance

NPA Nasopharyngeal aspirate

NPN Non-protein nitrogen

NPO Nothing orally

NSR Normal sinus rhythm, no sign of recurrence

NTD Neural tube defect

N&V Nausea and vomiting

NWB Non-weight-bearing

O Oedema

O/A On admission

OA Osteoarthritis

Obs-Gyn Obstetrics and gynaecology

OD Overdose, right eye

OGD Oesophagogastroduodenoscopy

OOB Out of bed

op Operation

OP Outpatient

OPA Outpatient appointment

OPD Outpatient department

open + shut Inoperable case

OPV Oral polio vaccine

OR Operating room

ortho Orthopaedics

OS Left eye

O$_2$ sat Oxygen concentration

OT Occupational therapy

OTC Over the counter (medicine)

OU Both eyes

P Pulse

PA Posteroanterior, pulmonary artery

PaCo$_2$ Partial pressure of carbon dioxide in arterial blood

Paeds Paediatrics

PaO$_2$ Partial pressure of oxygen in arterial blood

Pap Papanicolaou smear

path Pathology

PBI Protein bound iodine

PC Presenting complaint

PCA Patient-controlled analgesia

PCO$_2$ Partial pressure of carbon dioxide

PCR Polymerase chain reaction

PCV Packed cell volume

PD Peritoneal dialysis

PDA Persistent ductus arteriosus

PE Physical examination, pulmonary embolus

PEEP Positive end expiratory pressure

PEFR Peak expiratory flow rate

PERRLA Pupils equal, round, react to light and accommodation

PET Positron emission tomography

PF(R) Peak flow (rate)

PFO Persistent foramen ovale

PFT Pulmonary function tests

PG Prostaglandin

PH Past history

PHT Pulmonary hypertension

PID Pelvic inflammatory disease, prolapsed intervertebral disc

PIP Proximal interphalangeal joint

PKU Phenylketonuria

Plt Platelets

PM Post mortem

PMD Post micturition dribbling

PMH Past medical history

PMS Premenstrual syndrome

PND Paroxysmal nocturnal dyspnoea

PO Per oral

PO$_2$ Partial pressure of oxygen

POD Postoperative day

post op After operation

PP Private patient

PPD Purified protein derivative (of tuberculin)

PPHN Persistent pulmonary hypertension of the newborn

PR Per rectum, pulmonary regurgitation

pre op Before operation

prep Prepare for surgery

prn As required

PROM Premature rupture of membranes

PS Pulmonary stenosis

PSM Pansystolic murmur

Psych Psychiatry

Pt Patient

PT Physiotherapy, prothrombin time

PTA Prior to admission

PTC Percutaneous transhepatic cholangiogram

PTCA Percutaneous transluminal coronary angioplasty

PTH Parathyroid hormone

PTT Partial thromboplastin time

PUO Pyrexia of unknown origin

PV Per vagina

PVC Premature ventricular contraction

PVD Peripheral vascular disease

PVL Periventricular leukomalacia

PVR Pulmonary vascular resistance

RA Rheumatoid arthritis, right atrium

RAIU Radioactive iodine uptake

RBBB Right bundle branch block

RBC Red blood cell, red blood count

RBS Random blood sugar

RCA Right coronary artery

RCC Red cell count

RDS Respiratory distress syndrome

rehab Rehabilitation

REM Rapid eye movement

RF Renal failure, rheumatic fever, rheumatoid factor

RHD Rheumatic heart disease

Rh neg. (Rh−) Rhesus factor negative
Rh pos. (Rh+) Rhesus factor positive
RLF Retrolental fibroplasia
RLQ Right lower quadrant
RN Registered nurse
R/O Rule out
ROM Range of movement, ruptured membranes
ROP Retinopathy of prematurity
ROS Review of systems
RR Respiratory rate
RS Respiratory system
RSV Respiratory syncytial virus
rt Right
RT Radiotherapy
RTA Road traffic accident
RUQ Right upper quadrant
RV Residual volume, right ventricle
RVH Right ventricular hypertrophy
RVT Renal vein thrombosis
Rx Prescription
s Without
SA Sino-atrial
Sab Spontaneous abortion
SAH Subarachnoid haemorrhage
SB Stillbirth, short of breath
S/B Seen by
SBE Subacute bacterial endocarditis
SBFT Small bowel follow through
SBO Small bowel obstruction
SBS Short bowel syndrome
SC Subcutaneous
SCC Sickle cell crisis, squamous cell carcinoma
SCBU Special care baby unit
SCID Severe combined immunodeficiency
SGA Small for gestational age
SH Social history, serum hepatitis
SIADH Syndrome of inappropriate antidiuretic hormone
SIDS Sudden infant death syndrome
SL Sublingual
SLE Systemic lupus erythematosus
S(A)LT Speech (and) language therapist
SOA Swelling of the ankles
SOB(OE) Short of breath (on exertion)
SOL Space occupying lesion
SOS Swelling of the sacrum
spec Specimen

SPECT Single photon emission computed tomography
SR Sinus rhythm
S&S Signs and symptoms
SSS Sick sinus syndrome
stat Immediately
STD Sexually transmitted disease
STOP Suction termination of pregnancy
SVC Superior vena cava
SVD Spontaneous vaginal delivery
SVT Supraventricular tachycardia
SW Social worker
Sx Symptoms
SXR Skull X-ray
T Temperature
T_1 First thoracic vertebra, etc.
T_3 Tri-idothyronine
T_4 Levothyroxine (thyroxine)
T&A Tonsillectomy and adenoidectomy
Tabs Tablets
TB Tuberculosis
TBA To be arranged, to be administered
TBI Total body involvement
T&C Type and crossmatch
TCI To come in
TED stocking Thromboembolic deterrent stocking
temp Temperature
TFTs Thyroid function tests
TGA Transposition of great arteries
THR Total hip replacement
TIA Transient ischaemic attack
tib and fib Tibula and fibula
TIBC Total iron binding capacity
TKVO To keep vein open
TL Tubal ligation
TLC Tender loving care, total lung capacity
TLE Temporal lobe epilepsy
TMJ Temporomandibular joint
TOF Tetralogy of Fallot, tracheo-oesophageal fistula
TOP Termination of pregnancy
TORCH screen Toxoplasma, rubella, cytomegalovirus, herpes simplex infection screen
TPN Total parenteral nutrition
TPR Temperature, pulse, respirations
TR Tricuspid regurgitation
Trachy Tracheostomy
TS Tricuspid stenosis

TSH Thyroid stimulating hormone
TTAs To take away (discharge medicines)
TTN Transient tachypnoea of the newborn
TTOs To take out (discharge medicines)
TURP Transurethral resection of prostate
TVH Total vaginal hysterectomy
Tx Treatment
UA Uric acid, urinalysis
UAC Umbilical artery catheter
UC Ulcerative colitis, umbilical cord
U&Es Urea and electrolytes
UMN Upper motor neurone
UR(T)I Upper respiratory (tract) infection
U/S Ultrasound
UTA Unable to attend (outpatient appointment)
UTI Urinary tract infection
VA Visual acuity
VD Venereal disease
VDRL Venereal disease research laboratory
VE Vaginal examination
vent Ventilator
VEP Visual evoked potential
VF(ib) Ventricular fibrillation
VF Visual fields
VLBW Very low birth weight
VMA Vanilmandelic acid
VMI Very much improved
VP Venous pressure, ventriculoperitoneal
VPB Ventricular premature beats
VQ scan Ventilation perfusion scan
VS Vital signs
VSD Ventricular septal defect
VT Ventricular tachycardia
VZIG Varicella zoster immune globulin
WBC White blood count
WBS Whole body scan
WC Wheelchair
WNL Within normal limits
WPW Wolff Parkinson White
WR Ward round, Wasserman reaction
wt Weight
X-match Crossmatch
XR X-ray
y.o. Year old

Common abbreviations used to document physical examination findings

AAL Anterior axillary line
AB Apex beat
HO Hernial orifices
HS Heart sounds
ICS Intercostal space
MAL Mid-axillary line
MCL Mid-clavicular line
N/P Not palpable
° Absent
° **JACICyL** No jaundice, anaemia, clubbing, cyanosis or lymphadenopathy
° **LKKS** No liver, kidney, kidney, spleen palpable

O/E On examination
PAL Posterior axillary line
S_1 First heart sound
S_2 Second heart sound
TGR Tenderness, guarding and rebound
VF Vocal fremitus
VR Vocal resonance
∵ Because
↑**BP** High blood pressure
Δ Diagnosis
† Died
ΔΔ Differential diagnosis
Fracture

−**ve** Negative
+**ve** Positive
↔ No change
1° Primary
2° Secondary
∑ Sigmoidoscopy
∴ Therefore
1/7 One day
2/52 2 weeks
3/12 3 months

Appendix Two

Latin terms and abbreviations

Arthur J. Winfield

Introduction

Prescriptions written in the UK should be written in English and the use of Latin is strongly discouraged. However, the use of some Latin terms persists and abbreviations are often used, especially to indicate the frequency of dosing. Abbreviations may have different meanings in different countries. Great care is required to avoid errors arising through misunderstanding.

The following lists include terms which may be encountered in current practice. For more comprehensive lists, see previous editions of this book, Carter (1975) and the *Pharmaceutical Handbook* (Wade 1980).

Dosage forms

Latin name	Abbreviation	English name
Auristillae	aurist.	ear drops
Capsula	caps.	capsule
Cataplasma	cataplasm.	poultice
Collunarium	collun.	nosewash
Collutorium	collut.	mouthwash
Collyrium	collyr.	eye lotion
Cremor	crem.	cream
Guttae	gtt.	drops
Haustus	ht.	draught
Liquor	liq.	solution

Continued over

Lotio	lot.	lotion
Mistura	mist.	mixture
Naristillae	narist.	nose drops
Nebula	neb.	spray solution
Oculentum	oculent.	eye oinment
Pasta	past.	paste
Pigmentum	pig.	paint
Pulvis	pulv.	powder
Pulvis conspersus	pulv. consp.	dusting powder
Trochiscus	troch.	lozenge
Unguentum	ung.	ointment
Vapor	vap.	inhalation
Vitrella	vitrell.	glass capsule (crushable)

Terms used in prescriptions

Latin	Abbreviation	English name
ante cibum	a.c.	before food
ante meridiem	a.m.	before noon
Ana	aa.	of each
Ad	ad	to
ad libitum	ad lib.	as much as desired
Alternus	alt.	alternate
Ante	ante	before
applicandus	applic.	apply
aqua	aq.	water
bis	b.	twice
bis die	b.d.	twice daily
bis in die	b.i.d.	twice daily
calidus	calid.	warm
cibus	cib.	food
compositus	co.	compound
concentratus	conc.	concentrated
cum	c.	with
dies	d.	a day
destillatus	dest.	distilled
dilutus	dil.	diluted
duplex	dup.	double
ex aqua	ex aq.	in water
fiat	ft.	let it be made
fortis	fort.	strong
hora	h.	at the hour of
hora somni	h.s.	at bedtime
inter cibos	i.c.	between meals

Continued over

Latin	Abbreviation	English name
inter	int.	between
mane	m.	in the morning
more dicto	m.d.	as directed
more dicto utendus	m.d.u.	to be used as directed
mitte	mitt.	send
nocte	n.	at night
nocte et mane	n. et m.	night and morning
nocte maneque	n.m.	night and morning
nomen proprium	n.p.	the proper name
nocte	noct.	at night
omnibus alternis horis	o.alt.hor	every other hour
omni die	o.d.	every day
omni mane	o.m.	every morning
omni nocte	o.n.	every night
parti affectae	p.a.	to the affected part
parti affectae applicandus	part. affect.	apply to the affected part
partes aequales	p.aeq.	equal parts
post cibum	p.c.	after food
post meridiem	p.m.	afternoon
partes	pp.	parts
pro re nata	p.r.n.	when required
parti dolente	part. dolent.	to the painful part
quarter die	q.d.	four times daily
quarter die sumendus	q.d.s.	take four times daily
quarter in die	q.i.d.	four times daily
quaque	qq.	every
quaque hora	qq.h.	every hour
quarta quaque hora	q.qq.h.	every fourth hour

	q.q.h	every fourth hour		ter de die	t.d.d.	three times daily
quantum sufficiat	q.s.	sufficient		ter die sumendus	t.d.s.	take three times daily
recipe	R$_x$	take		ter in die	t.i.d.	three times daily
secundum artem	sec. art.	with pharmaceutical skill		Tussis	tuss.	a cough
semisse	ss.	half		tussi urgente	tuss. urg.	when the cough troubles
si opus sit	s.o.s.	if necessary		ut antea	u.a.	as before
signa	sig.	label		ut dictum	ut. dict.	as directed
Statim	stat.	immediately		ut directum	ut. direct.	as directed
sumendus ter	sum. t.	take thrice		Utendus	utend.	to be used

Continued over

Table A2.1 Roman numerals: Roman symbol and corresponding Latin names for the cardinal and ordinal numbers and their adverbs

Arabic number	Roman symbol	Cardinals	Ordinals	Adverbs
1	I	unus	primus, -a, -um	semel (once)
2	II	duo	secundus or alter	bis (twice)
3	III	tres, tria(n.)	tertius	ter (three times)
4	IV	quattuor	quartus	quater (four times)
5	V	quinque	quintus	quinquies
6	VI	sex	sextus	sexies
7	VII	septem	septimus	septies
8	VIII	octo	octavus	octies
9	IX	novem	nonus	novies
10	X	decem	decimus	decies
11	XI	undecim	undecimus	undecies
12	XII	duodecim	duodecimus	duodecies
14	XIV	quattuordecim	quartis decimus	quattuordecies
15	XV	quindecim	quintus decimus	quindecies
20	XX	viginti	vicesimus	vicies
50	L	quinquaginta	quinquagesimus	quinquagies
100	C	centum	centesimus	centies

Appendix Three

3

Systems of weights and measures

Arthur J. Winfield

Introduction

In 1960 the Système International d'Unités (SI system), based on the metric system, was adopted as the standard. Since 1969 all prescriptions in the UK have been dispensed in this system. The older Imperial and Apothecary systems are still found in older books and formularies. This appendix outlines the three systems for weight and volume.

General

When expressing quantity, it is important to avoid the risk of error or misinterpretation. To reduce this it is best to avoid decimal fractions where possible. Thus, it is better to use 50 mg rather than 0.05 g. Where a decimal point is used, it should be preceded by a 0 (zero); thus it should be 0.1 g rather than .1 g.

Units of weight

Metric (SI) system

The basic unit is the kilogram (kg), which is the mass of the International Prototype Kilogram.

Name of unit	Abbreviation	Relationship
Kilogram	kg	
Gram	g	1/1000 (0.001) kg
Milligram	mg	1/1000 (0.001) g
		Continued over

Microgram	µg (or mcg)	1/1000 (0.001) mg
Nanogram	ng	1/1000 (0.001) µg
Picogram	pg	1/1000 (0.001) ng

To avoid confusion between mg, mcg and ng it is advisable not to use these abbreviations in dispensing.

Imperial system

The pound (avoirdupois) (lb) is the basic unit.

Name of unit	Abbreviation	Relationship
Pound	lb	
Ounce	oz	1/16 lb
Grain	gr	1/7000 1b 1/437.5 oz

Apothecary system

The grain is the basic standard and is the same as the Imperial grain (gr).

Name of unit	Abbreviation	Relationship
Grain	gr	
Scruple		20 gr
		Continued over

Name of unit	Abbreviation	Relationship
Drachm		60 gr
Ounce (Apoth.)		480 gr
		8 drachms

Note: The Imperial and Apothecary ounces are not the same weight.

Volume

Metric (SI) system

The basic unit is the litre (L) which is defined as 1 cubic decimetre.

Name of unit	Abbreviation	Relationship
Litre	L	
Millilitre	mL	1/1000 (0.001) L
Microlitre	μL	1/1000 (0.001) mL

Imperial system

The basic unit is the pint (pt).

Name of unit	Abbreviation	Relationship
Pint	pt	
Fluid ounce	fl oz	1/20 pt

Apothecary system

The minim (m) is the basic unit.

Name of unit	Abbreviation	Relationship
Minim	m	
Fluid drachm	fl dr	60 m
Fluid ounce	fl oz	8 fl dr
		480 m

Amount of substance

The basic unit is the mole which is the amount of substance containing as many formula units as there are in 12 g of carbon-12. The formula units may be atoms, molecules, ions, etc.

Name of unit	Abbreviation	Relationship
Mole	mol	
Millimole	mmol	1/1000 (0.001) mol
Micromole	μmol	1/1000 (0.001) mmol

Concentration

Concentration can be expressed as g per L (g per dm^3) or mol per L. In dispensing, the former is normally used for drug concentration. Electrolyte concentration may be expressed as amount of substance (mol per L). In medical records and literature, mol per L is normally used.

Length

The metre (m) is the basic unit.

Name of unit	Abbreviation	Relationship
Metre	m	
Centimetre	cm	1/100 (0.01) m
Millimetre	mm	1/1000 (0.001) m
Micrometre	μm	1/1000 (0.001) mm
Nanometre	nm	1/1000 (0.001) μm

4

Presentation skills

R. Michael E. Richards and Megan R. Thomas

Introduction

Short presentations by students, often known as 'giving a seminar', have become an integral part of most academic courses. Although you may regard it as a bit of an ordeal at first, it does in fact have many benefits. You will gain confidence at putting across your ideas and answering questions. This will be very beneficial for you in interview situations. It is also likely that you will be expected to make presentations all through your future career and so the skills you develop in making presentations as a student will have lifelong benefits. Pharmacy students may expect to present short reviews of academic material or research findings and also present case studies. Case studies are not dealt with specifically in this appendix but many of the skills needed are similar. Basically a good presentation is a form of effective communication between two or more individuals. As such, making a good presentation is something which can be learned. The good news is that every pharmacy student is capable of making a good presentation provided they make adequate preparation. This appendix provides information on the basic skills needed for helping with that preparation. These basic skills are concerned with:

- Preparation
- Visual aids
- Communication
- Delivery.

There is considerable overlap between these areas and this is obvious from a study of Figure A4.1. Nevertheless, for the purpose of this appendix each area will be discussed separately.

Preparation

Subject material

Once the subject for the presentation is known, the initial preparation is to ensure a thorough grasp of the relevant material which will provide the basis of the presentation. This knowledge may be gained as the result of some form of literature survey or as the result of carrying out a research project plus a literature study. The material given here follows the general outline of the 'preparation' section of the spidergram given in Figure A4.1.

The study of the original material, literature or research findings will involve a critical assessment and interpretation of the material in order to assemble the relevant and valid information. Through a process of integration, synthesis and refinement, the body of knowledge thus obtained will be applied to compose the draft outline of the text. Before this is done, however, it would be wise to take a step back and consider the level of knowledge and the expectations of the intended audience. For the undergraduate preparing a presentation for his/her peers, this is fairly straightforward. Should it be a postgraduate or multidisciplinary audience, the situation would need careful consideration. It is very discouraging for an audience to be talked down to by someone assuming that they do not have the most basic knowledge of the subject. On the other hand it is equally discouraging for the presenter to assume knowledge which the audience in general does not possess. It is also important to understand the expectations the audience has of the presentation. Do they wish to have a broad

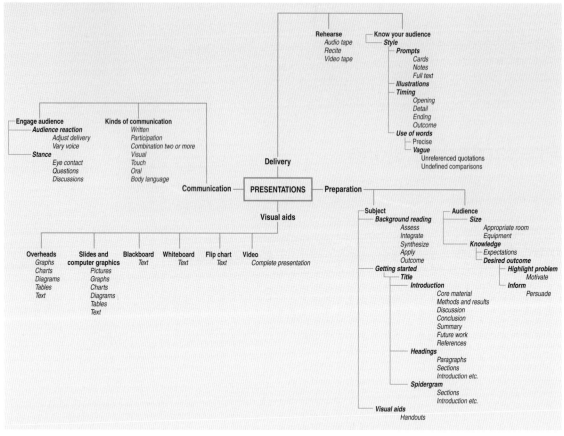

Figure A4.1 • Spidergram of the individual factors and overall picture involved with presentations.

overview of a subject or are they expecting to have considerable detail on part of the subject which is of particular interest to them at that point in time? The other side of this coin is that you may have been given a brief of what you were expected to achieve with the presentation. That is, the purpose it was intended that the presentation would achieve. In the student situation the main purpose of the presentation is likely to be to provide accurate and reliable information on a particular subject. It could also be to highlight a problem. In other situations it could be to motivate, involve, persuade or encourage creativity.

Having assembled the required information on the subject, the level of knowledge and expectations of the audience and the purpose of the presentation, the draft outline of the text can be prepared. There are several ways this may be done. If the presentation is to follow an accepted scientific communication format,

the structure has already been decided for one. It will follow the sequence:

- Title
- Introduction
- Core material (methods and results)
- Discussion, conclusions
- Suggestions for future work
- References.

In order to produce the material in this format it might be convenient to assemble information under headings and subsequently produce paragraphs which are built up into the required sections: 'introduction', etc. On the other hand it may sometimes be helpful to adopt the spidergram approach which was used to note down ideas for this appendix. In this approach, a rectangle is drawn in the middle of a blank sheet of paper. One or two words describing the subject of the presentation are written into this rectangular block. A line is then drawn from each of the corners representing the main points which will form the basis of the presentation. Spider-like legs are then developed consisting of words or phrases which develop outwards from each of the central main points. Some words may be repeated in the different legs. Audience and outcomes, for example, are seen to be present in three of the subject areas. In general, however, the legs represent different aspects of the main subject in the central rectangle.

The first draft would then be revised as many times as necessary to produce a polished text which is clear and as interesting as possible. Decisions would also be made on the relevant visual aids needed to illustrate and support the presentation. A short attractive handout summarizing the main points of the seminar would also be helpful. This would give your aim or objective and act as a guide to your presentation for the audience. It could be in the form of questions which were subsequently answered in your presentation. The handout should not only reinforce the presentation but also be useful for taking away as a record and reminder of the presentation.

Physical facilities

For groups of more then 20 people, it is usual to use a purpose built lecture room for the presentation. These are mostly arranged with an overhead projector in the format indicated in Figure A4.2A. The head-on arrangement centres the audience attention on both the illustrations and the presenter at the same time. A slide projector may also be in the central position of Figure A4.2A but situated further from the screen at the back of the lecture theatre with the controls near to the presenter. For groups of fewer than 20 people, ideally 12–15 people, the bench or table seating arrangement of Figure A4.2B is convenient. This encourages a good degree of interaction and provides a flat surface for note taking and consulting other documents. The half circle arrangement, Figure A4.2C, also allows for easy discussion, but if note taking is required, each seat would need its own small table attached. Other arrangements of these basic configurations are obviously possible. Whichever small group arrangement is chosen, the common requirement is for ease of interaction between presenter and participants and participant and participant.

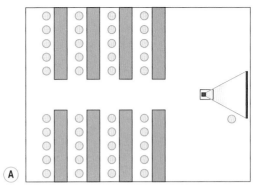

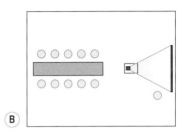

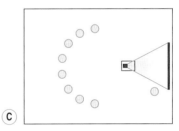

Figure A4.2 • (A) Arrangement for the overhead projector (OHP) with lecture theatre-type seating arrangement. (B) Table seating arrangement for use with small groups and the OHP. (C) Half circle seating arrangement for use with small groups and the OHP.

Visual aids

A presentation is usually improved by the appropriate use of visual aids and these are included in Figure A4.1.

Writing directly

Writing and/or drawing on a blackboard with chalk has been the traditional visual aid used in teaching. It has the advantage of being cheap and widely available. It has now been replaced in the majority of higher education establishments by more effective methods. The whiteboard with coloured felt tipped pens is now more commonly used. Whiteboards are suitable for informal meetings and discussions with groups of up to 20 people. The felt tips need to be kept capped when not in use or the pens rapidly dry out. Care also needs to be taken not to use permanent inks or the board cannot be cleaned without the use of the appropriate solvent.

Flipcharts, again with the use of coloured felt tipped pens, are useful with small groups for presenting and recording textual material. They are especially useful in brainstorming sessions and the sheets can be torn off and displayed like posters around the room. Flipcharts are cheap but can be rather fragile and somewhat difficult to handle. Their final appearance, however, can look somewhat scrappy.

Projection

General points

Whenever visual aids are projected, a number of issues need to be considered:

- Care needs to be taken to ensure that the seating positions allow all present to see the whole screen
- Ensure you are familiar with the equipment and technology you will be using
- Font or letter size needs to be sufficiently big to be read easily, i.e. a minimum of 6–7 mm in height or 24–28 point font
- The number of words should be restricted with a maximum of seven words to a line and seven lines to a slide, or 15–20 words per acetate sheet
- Appropriate spaces between lines are required to aid clarity
- When using graphs, do not use more than five different lines per graph and try to use different colours for each line
- Bar charts should not contain more than six bars or groups of bars
- Pie charts should not contain more than six wedges. One floating wedge may be used to highlight a particular set of information (Fig. A4.3)
- Do not use red and green for data that are to be compared or contrasted – it will cause difficulties for those who are colour blind
- Colour is helpful but should be limited and used consistently throughout the presentation to aid understanding
- Information can be revealed either as a complete acetate or slide at a time or by progressively revealing the information

PSEUDOMONAS AERUGINOSA

Resistant opportunistic pathogen

- Burn wounds
- Immunocompromised
- Cystic fibrosis
- Indwelling catheter
- Corneal abrasions
- Contaminant of non-sterile pharmaceuticals

Figure A4.3 • Sample text for use with an OHP.

- Do not simply read the visual aid information to the audience but use it to focus their attention on the main points of your message.

Overhead projector

The overhead projector (OHP) plus acetate sheets and coloured felt tipped pens have become one of the most popular methods for presenting textual or graphical material. This is because of the great versatility of the OHP for use in a large number of situations and without the need for complete blackout facilities. The OHP should ideally be used with an angled white screen to avoid distorting the picture. Although not ideal, the OHP can be used with a light coloured wall or flat white screen. In fact the versatility of the OHP is such that it is often used in less than ideal circumstances. This also applies to the preparation of the text on the acetate sheets for projection. It is not uncommon to see typewritten pages and tables copied directly onto the acetates. No one but the presenter is then able to read the text. Figure A4.4 gives an indication of what an acetate

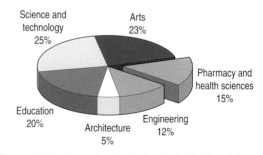

Figure A4.4 • Example of a pie chart – distribution of students by faculty.

should look like. The life of the projector bulb is related to the number of times it is switched on and off, so rather than switch the projector on and off it is better to use blank coloured acetates between the acetates containing information.

Slides

Slides are another very versatile visual aid and can be used with large and small audiences. Producing the slides is more expensive than producing overheads and requires more skill, but good slides can be used repeatedly.

Computer-generated slides

Microsoft PowerPoint is the most frequently used software to produce slides and presentations and has rapidly become a common method which will be expected in more formal situations and conferences. It is extremely versatile and easy to use but the general points above must not be forgotten. The aim is for the audience to focus on the content of your presentation rather than the special effects. In particular, sound effects are best avoided and animation sequences kept simple. Restrict yourself to the use of two fonts, and if you use the design templates in a software package, complimentary fonts will be offered.

In contrast to OHP acetates where a light background with a dark text is recommended, with slides, a dark background with light text is often very effective. It has been shown that for individuals with a visual impairment, a dark blue background with yellow text is easiest to read. A red or orange background should be avoided but a green background is supposed to stimulate interaction and sharing of opinions and therefore could be useful in training and educational settings. Avoid fancy background designs that distract and make the text difficult to read. Underlining is also difficult to read and therefore use bold lettering for emphasis.

It is straightforward to insert pictures, clip art or other graphics and these are best placed off centre to leave room for text and to help lead eyes to the text. Only use art work if it offers a positive contribution. It is also possible to insert video clips but make sure these work on the equipment you are using during your presentation. Indeed it is important to be aware that later versions of software may offer animation sequences and other features that will not run on earlier versions, and special fonts may be changed into the nearest similar fonts with disastrous effects on your slide layout. Not all computer and multimedia projectors are compatible and re-writable CDs are not always readable by older laptops. A USB memory stick is very useful for safe storage of data and is compatible with any current computer equipment. Handouts are easy to generate from a PowerPoint presentation and can be produced in a variety of layouts and formats.

Videos

Video presentations are not usually a suitable means for making small group or specifically academic presentations. To prepare a high-quality video presentation oneself is very difficult. However, it can be a useful training tool, particularly for role play to develop communication skills, with participants' or actors' videos being discussed and analysed.

Communication

This is the subject of Chapters 13 and 44, but in those chapters the emphasis is on one-to-one communication. In this appendix, the emphasis is on the communication skills required for making an effective oral presentation to different groups.

Kinds of communication

Figure A4.1 indicates that there are several kinds of communication such as written, oral, body language, visual, touch, participation and combinations of these. Estimates vary but it is likely that after 3 hours the average person will remember about 70% of a verbal presentation and possibly only 10% after 3 days. A visual presentation improves the retention rate to about 75% after 3 hours and 20% after 3 days. When the presentation consists of a mixture of verbal and visual media, the retention improves to 85% after 3 hours and 66% after 3 days. This shows that it is important for a presenter to ensure that their audience has the opportunity to both hear and see what they are seeking to get across by using appropriate visual aids. Where possible the audience should also be given opportunities to interact with the speaker during the presentation as well as through questions at the end of the presentation. How all three aspects can be included should be considered at the time the text outline is being prepared. It should also be mentioned that it is important to keep the presentation short and simple. This will be referred to again in the section on 'Delivery'.

Another sobering thought about the means we use to communicate is that for most members of the audience, the presenter's body language and the way they speak have a greater influence on their credibility with the audience than the content of what they say. In general a person who speaks fairly slowly in a medium or low tone without frequent extravagant gestures is perceived as a credible person. The stance of the presenter is also important. It is good to be as natural and relaxed as possible. Fixed stances like folding arms, placing hands on hips or clasping hands in front of the body act as a barrier to communication with the listeners. Hands in pockets and fiddling with the contents of pockets can be considered sloppy and distracting. Neither is continuously clicking a ball-point pen an endearing habit. Sitting on the table provided for your notes, etc. may be interpreted as indicating a superior and disrespectful attitude to your audience.

Engage with your audience

Think carefully how you will manage the first half minute of your presentation. This often sets the tone and influences the impact of the whole presentation. The object will be to attract the listeners' attention by using something which you know will be of interest to them. A quote from a well chosen reference relating to your subject could be a good way of attracting attention and easing them into your presentation at the same time. The quote could take the form of a shocking statistic related to the subject of your presentation. This would be especially so if you were going to be able to show that the statistic could be greatly improved. For example – 'Four million of the world's children die needlessly each year from diarrhoea. Oral rehydration fluids are simple to prepare and cheap and could save the majority of those lives. I am going to explain what oral rehydration consists of.'

Eye contact provides a useful link between you and your audience. This should consist of a few seconds of contact with certain sympathetic members of your listeners. The eye contact indicates to you the level of interest and understanding of your audience. It answers the question 'How am I doing?' It enables you to adjust your delivery if necessary, vary your voice, or to even interpose a question, or ask the audience if they have a question.

Questions

A time for questions is usually included after the presentation has been completed but there is no reason why a question should not be asked by the speaker, or invited from the audience, during the course of the presentation. This promotes interaction between speaker and audience and helps to clear up misunderstandings before they result in restlessness among the participants and discussions between themselves. There are potential pitfalls in taking questions, however, and it would be good for the speaker to be aware of some helpful hints in answering questions.

First listen carefully to the whole question. Keep your mind from wandering to thinking about the answer to the question while the questioner is still speaking. Worse still is to second guess the questioner and start answering the question before it has been completed.

Second repeat the question clearly so that all can hear. This helps you to have time to think about the answer to the question. It also helps other people to understand the question, which everyone might not have heard clearly when it was asked initially, and it reassures the questioner that you have understood the question correctly.

Third avoid having a dialogue with one questioner by breaking eye contact with the questioner as you complete your answer. If you do not know the answer to a relevant question then say that you will let them have an answer at some specific time later. Always seek to be calm and polite in answering questions and be relaxed enough to allow the final question time to develop into a discussion, with you as the moderator, if that seems helpful.

Delivery

Timing

This is where the mnemonic KISS is useful. KISS stands for Keep It Short and Simple (less politely expressed, Keep It Short Stupid!). It is good advice and easy to remember. Failing to keep to the allocated time and inadequate preparation are the two main causes for poor presentations. KISS will help you to avoid the first and this appendix should encourage you to avoid the second.

Most presentations will be of a pre-agreed length of time. Knowing how much time is available means that the preparation must be geared to that time. When the first outline draft has been prepared as described in the section on 'Preparation', the delivery will need to be practised and modified until it fits the time available.

Recording the presentation on an audio cassette and listening to the playback is a good way to improve the delivery of the presentation and to tailor it to the allocated time.

Structure

In addition to the time for the presentation being stated, it is quite likely that an indication may be given for the structure of the presentation. For a piece of research, this would follow the headings: title, brief introduction, methods, key results, discussion – placing the work in context, conclusion and summary. This would be followed by an opportunity for the listeners to question the speaker. If the presentation was based on a literature review, it might follow the headings: title, brief introduction – putting the subject in context, presentation of the relevant information, summary of the main points giving the advantages and disadvantages, followed by a time of questions and discussion. Key references for both types of presentation could be given on a handout.

Style

The style of the delivery is important, and for a pharmaceutical topic, the presentation should use precise language with a few apt illustrations probably using an OHP. Vague language and unsubstantiated quotations should be avoided. Prompts as aides-memoire should be used and may take the form of numbered hand-held notes on filing cards or equivalent size pieces of strong paper. These will contain clearly written headings and key phrases. A full text is not really recommended but might be used as a handout. Overheads could contain the same headings and key phrases as the cards.

In addition to a well thought out, interesting, attention grabbing introduction, the delivery should end with a well prepared set of closing remarks. Some people keep saying that they are just about to finish but seem unable to do so. Just stop the presentation after the summary. If there is time for questions, however, and you wish to draw the question time to a close, say 'the next question will be the last question', then after you have answered it, stop.

In general, the content of your presentation will be judged on its accuracy and usefulness and the delivery of your presentation will be judged on its clearness and its interest. Be positive and enjoy yourself.

5

Key references and further reading

Introduction

This section includes guides to further reading and the references used in some chapters. Several books are referred to many times, especially pharmacopoeias and similar books. Others are important textbooks, including the two companion volumes to this book. These have been grouped together in the first section. This is followed by a chapter by chapter listing of other suggested reading to expand on the individual chapters and the references cited within the chapters where appropriate. When using a pharmacopoeia, you must always use the information in the most recent edition. Sometimes the information you require, such as the formula for a particular medicine, may not be in the current edition. You then have to work back until you find the most recent edition in which it occurs.

Frequently used references

Allen LV, Popovich NG, Ansel HC 2004 Ansel's pharmaceutical dosage forms and drug delivery systems, 8th edn. Lippincott, Williams and Wilkins, Philadelphia.

Aulton ME 2007 Aulton's pharmaceutics: the design and manufacture of medicines, 3rd edn. Churchill Livingstone, Edinburgh.

British national formulary (BNF), current edition. British Medical Association and Royal Pharmaceutical Society of Great Britain, London.

Gives technical details on many ingredients

Harman RJ 2002 Patient care in community practice, 2nd edn. Pharmaceutical Press, London.

Lawson DG, Richards RME 1998 Clinical pharmacy and hospital drug management. Hodder Arnold, London.

Marriott JF, Wilson KA, Langley CA et al. 2006 Pharmaceutical compounding

British national formulary (BNF) for children, current edition. British Medical Association, Royal Pharmaceutical Society of Great Britain and Royal College of Paediatrics and Child Health, London.

British pharmaceutical codex 1973 Pharmaceutical Press, London.

British pharmacopoeia, current edition. Stationery Office, London.

Committee of inquiry into pharmacy: a report to the Nuffield Foundation. 1986 Nuffield Foundation, London.

and dispensing. Pharmaceutical Press, London.

Martindale: the complete drug reference, current edition. Pharmaceutical Press, London.

Medicines compendium, current edition. Datapharm Publications, London.

Medicines Control Agency. 2002 Rules and guidance for pharmaceutical

Diluent directories (internal and external), current edition. National Pharmaceutical Association, St Albans.

European pharmacopoeia, current edition and supplements. Maisonneuve, Saint Ruffine, France.

Farwell J. 1995, Aseptic dispensing for NHS patients (the Farwell Report). Stationery Office, London.

Handbook of pharmaceutical excipients, current edition. Pharmaceutical Press, London.

manufacture. Stationery Office, London.

Pharmaceutical codex, 11th edn. 1979, Pharmaceutical Press, London.

Pharmaceutical codex, 12th edn. 1994, Pharmaceutical Press, London.

Royal Pharmaceutical Society of Great Britain Medicines, ethics and practice: a guide for pharmacists, current edition. Royal Pharmaceutical Society of Great Britain, London.

Stephens M 2002 Hospital pharmacy. Pharmaceutical Press, London.

Stone P, Curtis SJ 2002 Pharmacy practice, 3rd edn. Pharmaceutical Press, London.

United States pharmacopoeia, current edition. Mack, Easton, PA.

Wade, E. editor. (1980) *Pharmaceutical handbook*. 19th edn. Pharmaceutical Press, London.

Walker R, Whittlesea C 2007 Clinical pharmacy and therapeutics, 4th edn. Churchill Livingstone, Edinburgh.

Waterfield J 2008 Community pharmacy handbook. Pharmaceutical Press, London.

Part 1: Pharmacy in society

Chapter 1: The role of pharmacy in health care

Bond C 2000 Evidence-based pharmacy. Pharmaceutical Press, London.

Clinical Resources Audit Group1996 Clinical pharmacy in the hospital pharmaceutical service: a framework for practice. Stationery Office, Edinburgh.

Department of Health. 1996 Choice and opportunity. Primary care: the future. Stationery Office, London.

Department of Health. 2001 Response to the report of the public inquiry into children's heart surgery at the Bristol Royal Infirmary, 1984–1995. Stationery Office, London.

Department of Health. 2002 Pharmacy in the future: implementing the NHS plan – a programme for pharmacy in the National Health Service. Stationery Office, London.

Farwell I 2001 The Bristol Royal Infirmary inquiry (the Kennedy Report). Stationery Office, London.

Royal Pharmaceutical Society of Great Britain1996 Pharmacy in a new age: the new horizon. Royal Pharmaceutical Society of Great Britain, London.

Scottish Executive. 2002 The right medicine: a strategy for pharmaceutical care in Scotland. Stationery Office, London.

Weller PJ (Ed.) Pharmacists' directory and yearbook, current edition. Royal Pharmaceutical Society of Great Britain, London.

Chapter 2: Models of pharmacy practice within healthcare systems

Health and Safety Executive 2002 COSHH A brief guide to the regulations. Online. Available: http://www.hse.gov.uk/pubns/indg136.pdf. (accessed 16 October 2008).

Medicines and Healthcare products Regulatory Agency 2006 The supply of unlicensed relevant medicinal products for individual patients. MHRA Guidance Note No. 14. Online. Available: http://www.mhra.gov.uk. (accessed 16 October 2008).

National Patient Safety Agency Community pharmacy reporting to the NRLS. Online. Available: https://www.eforms.npsa.nhs.uk/staffeform/. (accessed 16 October 2008).

Pharmaceutical Services Negotiating Committee Pharmacy contract, essential services, service specifications. Online. Available: http://www.psnc.org.uk/index.php?type=page&pid=106&k=2 (accessed 16 October 2008).

Pharmaceutical Services Negotiating Committee 2006 PSNC briefing on the NHS complaints procedure. Online. Available: http://www.psnc.org.uk/data/files/PharmacyContractandServices/ClinicalGovernance/complaintsprocess/briefingpdf.pdf. (accessed 16 October 2008).

Royal Pharmaceutical Society of Great Britain 2005 Confidentiality audit, December 2005. Online. Available: http://www.rpsgb.org/pdfs/confidentiality.pdf. (accessed 16 October 2008).

Royal Pharmaceutical Society of Great Britain 2006 Guidance on recording interventions. Online. Available: http://www.rpsgb.org.uk/pdfs/recinterventionsguid.pdf. (accessed 16 October 2008).

Stationery Office 1998 The Data Protection Act 1998. Online. Available: http://www.opsi.gov.uk/acts/acts1998/ukpga_19980029_en_1. (accessed 16 October 2008).

Chapters 3 and 4: Socio-behavioural aspects of health, illness, treatment and medicines

Bissell P, Traulsen JM 2005 Sociology and pharmacy practice. Pharmaceutical Practice, London.

FIP (International Pharmaceutical Federation) Standards for quality of pharmacy services. Online. Available: http://www.fip.org.

Florence AT, Taylor KMG, Harding G 2001 Pharmacy practice. Taylor and Francis, London.

Gard P 2000 A behavioural approach to pharmacy practice. Wiley Blackwell, Oxford.

Taylor K, Nettleton S, Harding G. 2003 Sociology for pharmacists, 2nd edn. Taylor and Francis, London.

Lilja J, Larsson S, Hamilton D 1996 Drug communication. How cognitive science can help the health professionals. In: Pharmaceutical Sciences No. 24. Kuopio University Publications, Kuopio, Finland.

Marmot M, Wilkinson RG. 2005 Social determinants of health, 2nd edn. Oxford University Press, Oxford.

Miller DF, Price JH 1998 Dimensions of community health, 5th edn. McGraw-Hill, Boston.

Panton R, Chapman S 1998 Medicines management. Pharmaceutical Press, London.

Quick JD 1997 Management sciences for health: managing drug supply, 2nd edn. Kumarian Press, West Hartford, CT.

Sarafino EP 2005 Health psychology: biopsychosocial interactions, 5th edn. John Wiley, New York.

Smith FJ 2002 Research methods in pharmacy practice. Pharmaceutical Press, London.

Smith MC, Knapp DA 1992 Pharmacy, drugs and medical care, 5th edn. Williams and Wilkins, Baltimore.

Smith MC, Wertheimer AI 2002 Social and behavioural aspects of

pharmaceutical care. Pharmaceutical Products Press, New York.

Taylor KMG, Nettleton S, Harding G 2003 Sociology for pharmacists, 2nd edn. Taylor and Francis, Andover.

Chapter 5: Public health

Acheson D 1998 Independent inquiry into inequalities in health: report. Stationery Office, London.

Dahlgren G, Whitehead M 1991 Policies and strategies to promote social equity in health. Institute of Future Studies, Stockholm.

Department of Health. 2004 Choosing health: making healthy choices easier. Stationery Office, London Online. Available: http://www.dh.gov.uk/en/Publicationsandstatistics/Publications/PublicationsPolicyAndGuidance/DH_4094550.

Department of Health. 2005 Choosing health through pharmacy: a programme for pharmaceutical public health 2005–2015. Stationery Office, London Online. Available: http://www.dh.gov.uk/en/Publicationsandstatistics/Publications/PublicationsPolicyAndGuidance/DH_4107494.

Marmot MG, Shipley MJ, Rose G 1984 Inequalities in death: specific explanations of a general pattern. Lancet I: 1003—1006.

Marmot MG, Davey Smith G et al. 1991 Health inequalities among British civil servants: the Whitehall II study. Lancet 337: 1387—1393.

NHS Health Scotland 2004. Online. Available: http://www.healthscotland.com/topics/index.aspx (accessed 16 October 2008).

Walker R 2000 Pharmaceutical public health: the end of pharmaceutical care? Pharmaceutical Journal 264: 340—341.

Chapter 6: Types of patient charges for medicines and their impact

Cox ER, Henderson RR 2002 Prescription use behaviour among Medicare beneficiaries with capped prescription benefits. Journal of Managed Care Pharmacy 8: 360—364.

Cox ER, Jernigan C, Joel Coons SJ et al. 2001 Medicare beneficiaries' management of capped prescription benefits. Medical Care 39: 296—301.

Lexchin J, Grootendorst P 2004 Effects of prescription drug user fees on drug and health services use and on health status in vulnerable populations: a systematic review of the evidence. International Journal of Health Services 34: 101—122.

Lundberg L, Johannesson M, Isacson DGL et al. 1998 Effects of user charges on the use of prescription medicines in different socio-economic groups. Health Policy 44: 123—134.

Rice T, Matsuoka KY 2004 The impact of cost-sharing on appropriate utilization and health status: a review of the

literature on seniors. Medical Care Research and Review 61: 415—452.

Safran DG, Neuman P, Schoen C et al 2005 Prescription drug coverage and seniors: findings from a 2003 national survey. Health Affairs Web Exclusive W5 (April):152–166.

Schafheutle EI, Hassell K, Noyce PR et al. 2002 Access to medicines: cost as an influence on the views and behaviour of patients. Health and Social Care in the Community 10: 187—195.

Schafheutle EI, Hassell K, Noyce PR 2004 Coping with prescription charges in the UK. International Journal of Pharmacy Practice 12(4) (4): 239—246.

Soumerai SB, Avorn J, Ross-Degnan D et al. 1987 Payment restrictions for prescription drugs under Medicaid: effects on therapy, cost, and equity. New England Journal of Medicine 317: 550—556.

Soumerai SB, McLaughlin TJ, Ross-Degnan D et al. 1994 Effect of limiting Medicaid drug-reimbursement benefits on the use of psychotropic agents and acute mental health services by patients with schizophrenia. New England Journal of Medicine 331: 650—655.

Stuart B, Grana J 1998 Ability to pay and the decision to medicate. Medical Care 36: 202—211.

Tamblyn R, Laprise R, Hanley JA et al. 2001 Adverse events associated with prescription drug cost-sharing among poor and elderly persons. JAMA 285: 421—429.

Weiss MC, Hassell K, Schafheutle EI, Noyce PR 2001 Strategies used by general practitioners to minimise the impact of the prescription charge. European Journal of General Practice 7: 23—26.

Chapter 7: WHO and the essential medicines concept

Quick JD 1997 Management sciences for health: managing drug supply, 2nd edn. Kumarian Press, West Hartford, CT.

World Health Organization. 1999 The world health report: making a difference. World Health Organization, Geneva.

World Health Organization. 2002 WHO's policy perspectives on medicines, The selection of essential

medicines. World Health Organization, Geneva.

World Health Organization 2004a, WHO medicines strategy: countries at the core 2004–2007. Document reference WHO/EDM/2004.5. World Health Organization, Geneva.

World Health Organization. 2004b WHO model formulary 2004. World Health Organization, Geneva.

World Health Organization. 2005 The world health report 2005 – make every

mother and child count. World Health Organization, Geneva.

World Health Organization. 2006a Engaging for health. 11th general programme of work, 2006–2015. A global health agenda. World Health Organization, Geneva.

World Health Organization 2006b, The use of essential medicines. WHO Technical Report Series 933. World Health Organization, Geneva.

World Health Organization 2007a, About WHO. Online. Available: http://www.who.int/about/en/.

World Health Organization 2007b, Constitution of the World Health Organization 1946. Online. Available: http://www.who.int/library/collections/historical/en/index3.html.

World Health Organization 2007c, International Health Regulations enter into force. Online. Available: www.who.int/mediacentre/news/releases/2007/pr31/en/.

World Health Organization 2007d, Essential medicines. Online. Available: http://www.who.int/topics/essential_medicines/en/.

World Health Organization 2007e, WHO model list of essential medicines. 15th list, March 2007. Online. Available: http://www.who.int/medicines/publications/EML15.pdf.

World Health Organization 2007f, Better medicines for children. Sixtieth World Health Assembly. WHA60.20, 23 May 2007.

World Health Organization 2008, Public-private partnerships for health. Online. Available: http://www.who.int/trade/glossary/story077/en/.

Part 2: Governance and good professional pharmaceutical practice

Chapter 8: Clinical governance – an overview

Dean B 2000 What is clinical governance? *Pharmacy in Practice* 10: 182—184.

Department of Health. 1998 A first class service: quality in the new NHS. Stationery Office, London.

Department of Health. 2000 Organisation with a memory. Stationery Office, London.

Department of Health. 2001 Clinical governance in community pharmacy. Stationery Office, London.

NHS Executive and National Prescribing Centre 2000 Competencies for pharmacists working in primary care. Online. Available: http://www.npc.co.uk/publications/CompPharm/competencies.htm.

Royal Pharmaceutical Society of Great Britain 2000, Pharmacy audit support pack. Online. Available: http://www.rpsgb.org/registrationandsupport/audit.

Royal Pharmaceutical Society of Great Britain, 2005, Scottish Executive 2005 Audit to excellence. CD-ROM See details on: http://www.rpsgb.org/registrationandsupport/audit.

Chapter 9: Risk management

Department of Health 2000 An organisation with a memory: a report from an expert working group on learning from adverse events in the NHS. Department of Health, London.

Department of Health. 2004 Building a safer NHS for patients: improving medication safety (a report by the Chief Pharmaceutical Officer). Department of Health, London.

National Patient Safety Agency. 2007b Design for patient safety: a guide to the design of the dispensing environment. National Patient Safety Agency, London.

National Patient Safety Agency. 2007c Healthcare risk assessment made easy. National Patient Safety Agency, London.

National Patient Safety Agency 2008 Exploring incidents – improving safety: a guide to root cause analysis from the NPSA. E-learning programme at: http://www.msnpsa.nhs.uk/rcatoolkit/course/iindex.htm.

Reason J 2000 Human error: models and management. *BMJ* 320: 768—770.

Chapter 10: Continuing professional development and fitness to practise

Royal Pharmaceutical Society of Great Britain website: www.rpsgb.org.uk.

Royal Pharmaceutical Society of Great Britain CPD recording site: www.uptodate.org.uk.

Department of Health. 1998 The new NHS: a first class service. Stationery Office, London.

Department of Health. 2007 Trust, assurance and safety – the regulation of health professionals in the 21st century. HMSO, London.

Pharmacists and Pharmacy Technicians Order 2007, HMSO. London.

Chapter 11: Audit

Healthcare Commission National Clinical Audit 2008 Online. Available: http://www.healthcarecommission.org.uk/serviceproviderinformation/nationalclinicalaudit.cfm (accessed 14 October 2008).

National Institute for Health and Clinical Excellence 2002 Principles for best practice in clinical audit. Radcliffe Medical Press, Oxford. Online. Available: http://www.nice.org.uk/usingguidance/implementationtools/auditadvice/audit_advice.jsp?domedia=1&mid=79613703-19B9-E0B5-D4F14A0429022FC0 (accessed 16 October 2008).

NHS Clinical Governance Support Team 2005 A practical handbook for clinical audit. Online. Available: http://www.cgsupport.nhs.uk/downloads/Practical_Clinical_Audit_Handbook_v1_1.pdf.

Royal Pharmaceutical Society of Great Britain Clinical Audit Unit. Online. Available: http://www.rpsgb.org/registrationandsupport/audit/. (accessed 14 October 2008).

Chapter 12: Ethics
Websites

Ethox Centre Department of Public Health and Primary Health Care, University of Oxford: http://www.ethox.org.uk/. (accessed 14 October 2008).

EthicsWeb.ca: http://www.ethicsweb.ca/ (accessed 14 October 2008).

Kennedy Institute of Ethics Georgetown University: http://bioethics.georgetown.edu/ (accessed 14 October 2008).

Stanford Encyclopaedia of Philosophy: http://plato.stanford.edu/contents.html (accessed 14 October 2008).

Internet Encyclopaedia of Philosophy http://www.iep.utm.edu/ (accessed 14 October 2008).

Textbooks

Beauchamp TL, Childress JF 2001 Principles of biomedical ethics, 5th edn. Oxford University Press, New York.

Gillon R 1999 Philosophical medical ethics. John Wiley, Chichester.

Hawley G 2007 Ethics in clinical practice: an interprofessional approach. Pearson Education, Harlow.

Hill TE, Zweig A 2002 Kant: groundwork for the metaphysics of morals. Oxford University Press, Oxford.

Hope T, Savulescu J, Hendrick J 2008 Medical ethics and law, the core curriculum, 2nd edn. Churchill Livingstone, Edinburgh.

Leathard A, McLaren S 2007 Ethics: contemporary challenges in health and social care. Policy Press, Bristol.

Schwartz L, Preece PE, Hendry RA 2002 Medical ethics: a case-based approach. Saunders, Edinburgh.

Thompson M 2003 An introduction to philosophy and ethics. Hodder Murray, Manchester.

Vardy P, Grosch P 1999 The puzzle of ethics. Fount, London.

Wingfield J, Badcott D 2007 Pharmacy ethics and decision making. Pharmaceutical Press, London.

References

Aggarwal R, Bates I, Davies JG et al. 2002 A study of academic dishonesty among students at two schools of pharmacy. *Pharmaceutical Journal* 269: 529—533.

Belmont Report 1979 Ethical principles and guidelines for the protection of human subjects of research. National Commission for the Protection of Human Subjects of Biomedical and Behavioral Research, April 18 1979. Online. Available: http://ohsr.od.nih.gov/guidelines/belmont.html (accessed 14 October 2008).

Benson A 2006 Pharmacy values and ethics: a qualitative mapping of the perceptions and experiences of UK pharmacy practitioners, in Centre for Public Policy. Department of Education and Professional Studies. King's College London, London.

Benson A, Cribb A, Barber N 2007 Respect for medicines and respect for people: mapping pharmacist practitioners' perceptions and experiences of ethics and values. Royal Pharmaceutical Society of Great Britain, London.

Berwick D, Davidoff F, Hiatt H et al. 2001 Refining and implementing the Tavistock principles for everybody in health care. Commentary: Justice in health care a response to Tavistock. *BMJ* 323: 616—620.

British Medical Association. 1995 Core values of the medical profession in the 21st century – survey report. British Medical Association, London.

Department of Health. 2008 White Paper: Pharmacy in England. Building on Strengths – Delivering the Future. HM Government, London.

Gillon R 1985 Medical oaths, declarations, and codes. *BMJ* 290: 1194—1195.

Hawksworth G 2003 From the president: a personal professional pledge. *Pharmaceutical Journal* 271: 849—850.

Hawksworth G 2004 The president promotes a personal professional pledge for pharmacists. *Pharmaceutical Journal* 272: 684—685.

Hurwitz B, Richardson R 1997 Swearing to care: the resurgence in medical oaths. *BMJ* 315: 1671—1674.

Rennie SC, Crosby JR 2001 Are tomorrow's doctors honest? A questionnaire study exploring the attitudes and reported behaviour of medical students to fraud and plagiarism *BMJ* 322: 274—275.

Rogers R, John D 2006 Paternalism to professional judgement – the history of the code of ethics. *Pharmaceutical Journal* 276: 721—723.

Smith R, Hiatt H, Berwick D. 1999a Shared ethical principles for everybody in health care: a working draft from the Tavistock group. *BMJ* 318(7178)(7178): 248—251.

Smith R, Hiatt H, Berwick D [Tavistock group]1999b A shared statement of ethical principles for those who shape and give health care: a working draft from the Tavistock group. *Annals of Internal Medicine* 130(2)(2): 143—147.

Sritharan K, Russell G, Fritz Z et al. 2001 Medical oaths and declarations. *BMJ* 323: 1440—1441.

Thimbleby CEH 2003 Drug tariff. Do we have to dispense a prescription item at a loss? *Pharmaceutical Journal* 271: 47.

Tonks A 2002 What's a good doctor and how do you make one? *BMJ* 325: 711.

Wingfield J 2007a New emphasis in the code of ethics. *Pharmaceutical Journal* 279: 237—240.

Wingfield J 2007b Consent: the heart of patient respect. *Pharmaceutical Journal* 279: 411—414.

Wingfield J 2007c When confidences should be kept and what constitutes an exception. *Pharmaceutical Journal* 279: 533—536.

Chapter 13: Communication skills for the pharmacist

Argyle M 1983 The psychology of interpersonal behaviour, 4th edn. Penguin, Harmondsworth.

Beardsley RS, Kimberlin CL, Tindall WN 2007 Communication skills in pharmacy practice, 5th edn.

Lippincott Williams and Wilkins, Baltimore.

Burnard P 1997 Effective communication skills for health professionals, 2nd edn. Chapman and Hall, London.

Dickson D, Hargie O, Morrow N 1997 Communication skills training for health professionals, 2nd edn. Chapman and Hall, London.

Kurtz SM, Silverman JD 1996 The Calgary–Cambridge referenced observation guides: an aid to defining the curriculum and organizing the teaching in communication training programmes. *Medical Education* 30 (2)(2): 83—89.

Ley P 1988 Communicating with patients. Croom Helm, London.

Pease B, Pease A 2006 The definitive book of body language. Bantam Books, Atlanta.

US Pharmacopeia Medication counseling behaviour guidelines. Online. Available: www.usp.org.

Part 3: The prescribing process

Chapter 16: Access to medicines and prescribing – introduction

Bradley C 1992 Factors which influence the decision whether or not to prescribe: the dilemma facing general practitioners. *British Journal of General Practice* 42: 454—458.

Denig P, Haaijer-Ruskamp F 1995 Do physicians take cost into account when making prescribing decisions? *Pharmacoeconomics* 8: 282—290.

Department of Health. 1998 A review of the prescribing, supply and administration of drugs – a report of the supply and administrations of medicines under group protocols. HMSO, London.

Department of Health 1999 Review of prescribing, supply and administration of medicines – final report. HMSO, London.

Department of Health 2005 Supplementary prescribing by nurses and pharmacists within the NHS in England: a guide for implementation. HMSO, London.

Department of Health. 2006 Improving patients' access to medicines: a guide to implementing nurse and pharmacist independent prescribing within the NHS in England. HMSO, London.

Haayer F 1982 Rational prescribing and sources of information. *Social Science and Medicine* 16: 2017—2023.

Jones M, Greenfield S, Bradley C 2001 Prescribing new drugs: qualitative study of influences on consultants and general practitioners. *BMJ* 323: 378.

McGettigan P, Golden J, Fryer J et al. 2000 Prescribers prefer people: the sources of information used by doctors for prescribing suggest that the medium is more important than the message. *British Journal of Clinical Pharmacology* 51: 184—189.

Muller C 1972 The overmedicated society: forces in the marketplace for medical care. *Science* 176: 488—492.

Prosser H, Amond S, Walley T 2003 Influences on GPs' decision to prescribe new drugs – the importance of who says what. *Family Practice* 20: 61—68.

Royal Pharmaceutical Society. 2006 Better management of minor ailments: using the pharmacist. Pharmaceutical Press, London.

Stevenson F, Greenfield S, Jones M et al. 1999 GPs' perceptions of patient influence on prescribing. *Family Practice* 16: 255—261.

Chapter 17: The prescribing process and evidence based medicine

Barber N 1995 What constitutes good prescribing? *BMJ* 310: 923—925.

Clinical Knowledge Summaries (formerly PRODIGY). Online. Available: http://cks.library.nhs.uk/ (accessed 14 October 2008).

Department of Health. 2006 Improving patients' access to medicines: a guide to implementing nurse and pharmacist independent prescribing within the NHS in England. HMSO, London.

Eccles M, Freemantle N, Mason J 1998 North of England evidence-based guideline development project. *BMJ* 317: 526—530.

MeReC Bulletin 1995 Evidence based medicine. MeReC Bulletin 6(12):45–48.

National Institute for Health and Clinical Excellence. Online. Available: http://www.nice.org.uk/page.aspx?o=cg (accessed 14 October 2008).

National Prescribing Centre 2006 Maintaining competency in prescribing: an outline framework to help pharmacist prescribers. NPC Plus, Keele.

Chapter 18: Formularies

Cambridgeshire Primary Care Trust Formulary, latest update. Online. Available: http://www.cambsphn.nhs.uk/default.asp?id=149 (accessed 14 October 2008).

Central Services Agency Northern Ireland COMPASS Therapeutic Notes. Online. Available: http://www.centralservicesagency.com/display/compass (accessed 14 October 2008).

Furniss L 2000 Formularies in primary care. *Primary Care Pharmacy* 1(2)(2): 37—39 Online. Available: http://www.pharmj.com/PrimaryCarePharmacy/200003/

medicines/formularies.html (accessed 14 October 2008).

Health Solutions Wales. Online. Available: http://www.hsw.wales.nhs.uk/page.cfm?orgid=166&pid=3997 (accessed 14 October 2008).

Information Services Division (Scotland) Online. Available: http://www.isdscotland.org/isd/1038.html (accessed 14 October 2008).

Lothian Joint Formulary Online. Available: http://www.ljf.scot.nhs.uk/ (accessed 14 October 2008).

National Prescribing Centre 2007 Managing medicines across a health community: making area prescribing committees fit for purpose. Online. Available: http://www.npc.co.uk/apcguide/apc_guide_may_2007_core.pdf. (accessed 14 October 2008).

NHS Tayside Area Prescribing Guide (TAPG) Online. Available: http://www.nhstaysideadtc.scot.nhs.uk/approved/formular/formular.htm.

Pegler S 2007 Whatever the appeal of drug lunches, take STEPS to avoid indigestion!. *Pharmaceutical Journal* 278: 612—614 Online. Available:

http://www.pharmj.com/pdf/ articles/pj_20070526_steps.pdf.

Prescribing Support Unit Items Online. Available at (both accessed 14 October 2008).

Measures of prescribing: http://www.ic. nhs.uk/services/prescribing-support-unit-psu/measures.

Prescribing indicators: http://www.ic.nhs. uk/our-services/prescribing-support-unit/indicators.

Prescription Pricing Division (England). Online. Available: http://www.ppa. org.uk/index.htm.(accessed 14 October 2008).

Twycross R, Wilcock A, Charlesworth S, Dickman A 2002 Palliative care formulary, 2nd edn. Radcliffe Publishing, Oxford.

Chapter 19: Drug evaluation and pharmacoeconomics

Briggs AH, O'Brien BJ 2001 The death of cost-minimization analysis? *Health Economics* 10: 179—184.

Drummond MF, Sculpher MJ, Torrance GW et al. 2005 Methods for the economic evaluation of health care programmes, 3rd edn. Oxford University Press, Oxford.

Elliot R, Payne K 2004 Essentials of economic evaluation in healthcare. Pharmaceutical Press, London.

Heart Protection Study Collaborative Group2005 Cost-effectiveness of simvastatin in people at different levels of vascular disease risk: economic analysis of a randomised trial in 20 536 individuals. *Lancet* 365: 1779—1785.

Hughes DA 2004 Modelling in health economics. In: Walley, T., Haycox, A.,

and Boland, A. editors., *Pharmacoeconomics*. Churchill Livingstone, Edinburgh.

Hughes DA, Vilar FJ, Ward CC et al. 2004 Cost-effectiveness analysis of HLA B*5701 genotyping in preventing abacavir hypersensitivity. *Pharmacogenetics* 14(6)(6): 335—342.

Lowson KV, Drummond MF, Bishop JM 1981 Costing new services: long-term domiciliary oxygen therapy. *Lancet* 1 (8230)(8230): 1146—1149.

Medicines and Healthcare products Regulatory Agency. Online. Available: http://www.mhra.gov.uk/. (accessed 14 October 2008).

National Institute for Health and Clinical Excellence 2004 Guide to the methods of technology appraisal.

Online. Available: http://www.nice. org.uk/. (accessed 14 October 2008).

Prescribing Support Unit Online. Available: http://www.ic.nhs.uk/ services/prescribing-support-unit-psu. (accessed 14 October 2007).

Scottish Intercollegiate Guidelines Network 2008, SIGN Guideline 50. A guideline developer's handbook, revised edn. Online. Available: http:// www.sign.ac.uk/guidelines/fulltext/ 50/index.html. (accessed 14 October 2008).

Scottish Medicines Consortium Online. Available: http://www. scottishmedicines.org.uk/smc/. (accessed 14 October 2008).

Walley T, Haycox A, Boland A 2003 Pharmacoeconomics. Churchill Livingstone, Edinburgh.

Chapter 20: Complementary/alternative medicine

Ang-Lee MK, Moss J, Yuan C-S. 2001 Herbal medicines and perioperative care. *JAMA* 286: 208—216.

Barnes J, Anderson LA, Phillipson JD 2007 Herbal medicines: a guide for healthcare professionals, 3rd edn. Pharmaceutical Press, London.

Commission of the European Communities 2002 2002/0008 Proposal for amending the directive 2001/83/EC as regards traditional herbal medicinal products. European Commission, Brussels.

Department of Health. 2001 Government response to the House of Lords Select Committee on Science and Technology's report on complementary and alternative medicine. Stationery Office, London.

Directive, 2004, 2004/24/EC of the European Parliament and of the Council of 31 March 2004 amending, as regards traditional herbal medicinal products, Directive 2001/83/EC on the Community code relating to medicinal products for human use. Online. Available: http://europa.eu. int/eur-lex/lex/LexUriServ/ LexUriServ.do?

uri=CELEX:32004L0024:EN: HTML. (accessed 14 October 2008).

Eisenberg DM, Davis RB, Ettner SL et al. 1998 Trends in alternative medicine use in the United States, 1990–1997. Results of a national follow-up survey. *JAMA* 280: 1569—1575.

Ernst E, White A 2000 The BBC survey of complementary medicine use in the UK. *Complementary Therapies in Medicine* 8: 32—36.

Gunther S, Patterson RE, Kristal AR et al. 2004 Demographic and health-related correlates of herbal and specialty supplement use. *Journal of the American Dietetic Association* 104: 27—34.

House of Lords Select Committee on Science and Technology 2000 Session 1999–2000, 6th report. Complementary and alternative medicine. Stationery Office, London.

Information Centre Prescriptions. Online. Available: http://www.ic.nhs. uk/statistics-and-data-collections/ primary-care/prescriptions (accessed 14 October 2008).

Kayne S 2002 Complementary therapies for pharmacists. Pharmaceutical Press, London.

MCA (now MHRA) 2002 Safety of herbal medicinal products, July 2002. Online. Available: http://www.mhra. gov.uk/home/groups/es-herbal/ documents/websiteresources/ con009293.pdf (accessed 16 October 2008).

Medicines for Human Use (Marketing Authorisations etc.) Regulations 1994 (SI 1994/3144) Stationery Office, London.

Medicines for Human Use (Marketing Authorisations etc.) Amendment Regulations 2000 (SI 2000/292). Stationery Office, London.

Medicines for Human Use (Marketing Authorisations etc.) Amendment Regulations 2005 (SI 2005/768). Stationery Office, London.

Medicines (Aristolochia and Mu Tong etc.) (Prohibition) Order 2001 (SI 2001/1841). Stationery Office, London.

Mills S, Peacock W 1997 Professional organisation of complementary and alternative medicines in the United

Kingdom 1997. A report to the Department of Health. University of Exeter, Exeter.

Mintel International. 2005 Complementary medicines. market intelligence. Mintel International Ltd, London.

Thomas KJ, Nicholl JP, Coleman P 2001 Use and expenditure on complementary medicine in England: a population based survey. *Complementary Therapies in Medicine* 9: 2—11.

Medicines Control Agency 2001 Traditional ethnic medicines. Public health and compliance with medicines law. Medicines Control Agency, London. Online. Available at http://www.mhra.gov.uk/.

Zollman C, Vickers A 1999 What is complementary medicine? *BMJ* 319: 693—696.

Chapter 22: Prescribing for minor ailments

Blenkinsopp A, Paxton P, Blenkinsopp J 2005 Symptoms in the pharmacy, 5th edn. Blackwell Science, Oxford.

Edwards C, Stillman P 2006 Minor Illness or major disease? The clinical pharmacist in the community, 4th edn. Pharmaceutical Press, London.

Harman RJ, Mason P 2002 Handbook of pharmacy healthcare, 2nd edn. Pharmaceutical Press, London.

Nathan A 2006 Non-prescription medicines, 3rd edn. Pharmaceutical Press, London.

OTC Directory. Treatments for common ailments, current edition [updated annually]. Proprietary Association of Great Britain, London.

Rutter P 2004 Community pharmacy. Churchill Livingstone, Edinburgh.

Rutter P 2005 Symptoms, diagnosis and treatment. Churchill Livingstone, Edinburgh.

Chapter 23: Information retrieval

Anon. 1995 An introduction to assessing medical literature. *MeReC Briefing* 9: 1—8.

Aronson JK 2006 Meyler's side effects of drugs: the international encyclopedia of adverse drug reactions and interactions, 15th edn. Elsevier Science Publishers, Amsterdam.

Brazier H, McCabe G 1998 Making the most of Medline. *Hospital Medicine* 59(10)(10): 756—761.

Covell DG, Uman GC, Manning PR 1985 Information needs in office practice: are they being met? *Annals of Internal Medicine* 103: 596—599.

Ely JW, Osheroff JA, Bell MH et al. 1999 Analysis of questions asked by family doctors regarding patient care. *BMJ* 319: 358—361.

Ely JW, Osheroff JA, Ebell MH et al. 2002 Obstacles to answering doctors' questions about patient care with evidence: qualitative study. *BMJ* 324: 710—713.

Gardner M 1997 Information retrieval for patient care. *BMJ* 314: 950—954.

Greenhalgh T 1997 Assessing the methodological quality of published papers. *BMJ* 315: 305—308.

Hands D, Judd A, Golightly P, Grant E 1999 Drug information and advisory services – past, present and future. *Pharmaceutical Journal* 262: 160—162.

Impicciatore P, Pandolfini C, Casella N et al. 1997 Reliability of health information for the public on the world wide web: systematic survey of advice on managing fever in children at home. *BMJ* 314: 1875—1881.

McKibbon KA, Wilczynski NL, Walker-Dilks CJ 1996 How to search for and find evidence about therapy. *Evidence-Based Medicine* 1(3)(3): 70—72.

Malone P 1998 Drug information technology and Internet resources. *Journal of Pharmacy Practice* 11: 196—218.

Shaughnessy AF, Slawson DC, Bennett JH 1994 Becoming an information master: a guidebook to the medical information jungle. *Journal of Family Practice* 39: 489—499.

Slawson DC, Shaughnessy AF 1997 Obtaining useful information from expert based sources. *BMJ* 314: 947—949.

Slawson DC, Shaughnessy AF, Bennett JH 1994 Becoming a medical information master: feeling good about not knowing everything. *Journal of Family Practice* 39: 505—513.

Smith R 1996 What clinical information do doctors need? *BMJ* 313: 1062—1068.

Baxter K 2007 Stockley's drug interactions, 8th edn. Pharmaceutical Press, London.

Wright SG, LeCroy RL, Kendrach MG 1998 A review of the three types of biomedical literature and the systematic approach to answer a drug information request. *Journal of Pharmacy Practice* 11: 148—162.

Section 4: Dispensing and related pharmaceutical practice activities

Chapter 24: The prescription

Department of Health 1999 Review of prescribing, supply and administration of medicines, final report. Stationery Office, London. Online. Available: http://www.dh.gov.uk/. (accessed 14 October 2008).

Drug tariff, current edition. Stationery Office. Online. Available: http://www.ppa.org.uk/ppa/edt_intro.htm (accessed 16 October 2008).

Editorial. 2001 Consultation on SOPs for dispensing. *Pharmaceutical Journal* 266: 616—619.

National Prescribing Centre. Prescribing analysis terms. Online. Available: http://www.npc.co.uk/publications/prescribingTerms/frames.htm. (accessed 15 October 2008).

National Prescribing Centre 1999 Signposts for prescribing nurses. Prescribing Nurse Bulletin 1(1):1–4.

Review of prescribing supply and administration of medicines 1998 Initial report (Crown review). Department of Health, London.

Review of prescribing supply and administration of medicines 1999

Final report (Crown review).
Department of Health, London.

Chapter 26: Pharmaceutical calculations

Ansel HC, Stoklosa MJ 2007
Pharmaceutical calculations, 12th
edn. Lippincott Williams and
Williams, Baltimore.

Rees JA, Smith I, Smith B 2004
Introduction to pharmaceutical

calculations, 2nd edn. Pharmaceutical
Press, London.

Smith I, Rees JA 2005 Pharmaceutical
calculations workbook.
Pharmaceutical Press, London.

Winfield AJ, Edafiogho IE 2005
Calculations for pharmaceutical
practice. Churchill Livingstone,
Edinburgh.

Chapter 27: Packaging

Dean DA, Evans ER, Hall IH 2000
Pharmaceutical packaging technology.
Taylor and Francis, Andover.

Chapter 28: Labelling

Royal Pharmaceutical Society 1990
Working Party Report. Labelling of

dispensed medicines. Pharmaceutical
Journal 245:128–129.

Chapter 29: Production of sterile products

Beaney AM 2005 Quality assurance of
aseptic preparation service, 4th edn.
Pharmaceutical Press, London.

European Commission 2005 The rules
governing medicinal products in the
European Union, vol 1V: EU

guidelines to good manufacturing
practice for medicinal products for
human and veterinary use. European
Commission, Brussels.

Midcalf B, Phillips M, Neiger JS et al.
2004 Pharmaceutical isolators.
Pharmaceutical Press, London.

Rules and Guidance for Pharmaceutical
Manufacturers and Distributors 2007
Pharmaceutical Press, London.

Chapter 33: External preparations

Williams AC 2003 Transdermal and
topical drug delivery. Pharmaceutical
Press, London.

Chapter 34: Suppositories and pessaries

Allen LV 2007 Suppositories.
Pharmaceutical Press, London.

Chapter 37: Inhaled route

ABPI compendium of patient information
leaflets current edition. Datapharm
Publications, London.

Electronic medicines compendium 2001.
Online. Available: http://emc.
medicines.org.uk. (accessed 15
October 2008).

Murphy A 2006 Asthma in focus.
Pharmaceutical Press, London.

Purewal TS, Grant DJW 2002 Metered
dose inhaler technology. Interpharm
Press, Buffalo Grove, IL.

National Institute for Health and Clinical
Excellence Chronic obstructive
pulmonary disease. Online. Available:
http://guidance.nice.org.uk/cg12.
(accessed 15 October 2008).

National Prescribing Centre 1998
Chlorofluorocarbon (CFC) free
inhalers. MeReC Bulletin 9(5):17–20.

SIGN Guideline No. 101, May 2008
British guideline on the management
of asthma. Online. Available: http://
www.sign.ac.uk/guidelines/fulltext/
101/index.html. (accessed 16
October 2008).

Chapter 38: Parenteral products

Akers MJ, Larrimore DS, Guazzo DM
2002 Parenteral quality control:
sterility, pyrogens, particulate and
package integrity testing, 3rd edn.
Marcel Dekker, New York.

Avis KE, Lieberman HA, Lachman L.
editors. (1992) *Pharmaceutical
dosage forms: parenteral medications*,
vol. 1, 2nd edn. Marcel Dekker,
New York.

British Standards Institute 2004 BS EN
ISO 1135-4:2004. British Standards
Institute, London.

Collentro WV 2008 Pharmaceutical
water: systems design, operation and
validation, 2nd edn. Interpharm Press,
Buffalo Grove, IL.

DeLuca PP, Boylan JC 1992 Formulation
of small volume parenterals. 2nd edn.
In: Avis, K.E., Lieberman, H.A., and
Lachman, L. editors., *Pharmaceutical
dosage forms: parenteral medications*.
Marcel Dekker, New York.

Demorest LJ, Hamilton JG. 1992
Formulation of large volume
parenterals. 2nd edn. In: Avis, K.E.,
Lieberman, H.A., and Lachman, L.

editors., *Pharmaceutical dosage forms:
parenteral medications*. Marcel
Dekker, New York.

Levchuk JW 1992 Parenteral products in
hospital and home care pharmacy
practice. 2nd edn. In: Avis, K.E.,
Lieberman, H.A., and Lachman, L.
editors., *Pharmaceutical dosage forms:
parenteral medications*. Marcel
Dekker, New York.

Turco S 1994 Sterile dosage forms: their
preparation and clinical application,
4th edn. Lippincott Williams and
Williams, Baltimore.

Williams KL 2001 Endotoxins, pyrogens, LAL testing and depyrogenation, 2nd edn. Marcel Dekker, New York.

Chapter 39: Ophthalmic products

Royal Pharmaceutical Society. 2001 Guidance for use of ophthalmic preparations in hospital and care homes. *Pharmaceutical Journal* 267: 307.

Chapter 40: Specialized services

Allwood M, Stanley AP, Wright P. editors. 2002 *The cytotoxics handbook*. 4th edn. Radcliffe Medical Press, Oxford.

Beaney AM (formerly from NHS Quality Control Committee) 2006 The quality assurance of aseptic services, 4th edn. Pharmaceutical Press, London.

British Oncology Pharmacy Association. 2004 Position statement on care of patients receiving oral anticancer drugs. *Pharmaceutical Journal* 272: 423—424.

Department of Health and Social Security, 1976, Breckenridge working party: report of the working party on addition of drugs to intravenous infusion fluids. HC (76)9. HMSO, London.

International Society of Oncology Pharmacy Practitioners (ISOPP) Guidelines on safe handling and other information. Online. Available: www.isopp.org. (accessed 15 October 2008).

Management and Awareness of Risks of Cytotoxic Handling (MARCH) guidelines. Online. Available: www.marchguidelines.com. (accessed 15 October 2008).

Needle RA 1995 Survey of hospital centralised intravenous additive services. *Pharmaceutical Journal* 225: 326—327.

Needle RA 2007 CIVAS handbook. Pharmaceutical Press, London.

Pharmaceutical Society. 1983 Working party report: guidelines for the handling of cytotoxic drugs. *Pharmaceutical Journal* 230: 230—231.

Society of Hospital Pharmacists of Australia. 2007 Standards of practice for the provision of oral chemotherapy for the treatment of cancer. *Journal of Pharmacy Practice and Research* 37: 147—150.

Trissel LA 2006 Handbook on injectable drugs, 14th edn. American Society of Health-System Pharmacists, Bethesda.

Chapter 41: Parenteral nutrition and dialysis

Austin P, Stroud M 2007 Prescribing adult intravenous nutrition. Pharmaceutical Press, London.

Walker R, Edwards C 2003 Clinical pharmacy and therapeutics, 3rd edn. Churchill Livingstone, Edinburgh.

Wood S 1995 Home parenteral nutrition: quality criteria for clinical services and the supply of nutrient fluids and equipment. British Association for Parenteral and Enteral Nutrition, Maidenhead.

Chapter 42: Radiopharmacy

Department of Health Social Security. 1982 Guidance notes for hospitals on the premises and environment required for the preparation of radiopharmaceuticals. HMSO, London.

Sampson CB 1994 Textbook of radiopharmacy: theory and practice, 2nd edn. Gordon and Breach Science Publishers, New York.

Sharp PF, Gemmell HG, Murray AD 2005 Practical nuclear medicine, 3rd edn. Springer-Verlag, London.

Chapter 43: Storage of medicines and waste disposal

Rhodes CT 1984 An overview of kinetics for the evaluation of the stability of pharmaceutical systems. *Drug Development and Industrial Pharmacy* 10(8&9)(8&9): 1163—1174.

Chapter 44: Communication skills – role of pharmacists in giving advice and information

Beardsley RS, Kimberlin CL, Tindall WN 2007 Communication skills in pharmacy practice, 5th edn. Lippincott Williams and Wilkins, Baltimore.

Burnard P 1997 Effective communication skills for health professionals, 2nd edn. Chapman and Hall, London.

Cromarty JA 1996 Counselling and advice on medicines and appliances in community pharmacy practice, Clinical Research and Audit Group. Stationery Office, Edinburgh.

Dickson D, Hargie O, Morrow N. 1997 Communication skills training for health professionals, 2nd edn. Chapman and Hall, London.

Ley P 1988 Communicating with patients. Croom Helm, London.

Tindall WN, Beardsley RS, Kimberlin CL. 2002 Communication skills in pharmacy practice, 4th edn. Lippincott Williams and Wilkins, Baltimore.

US Pharmacopeia Medication Counseling Behaviour Guidelines. Online. Available: www.usp.org.(accessed 15 October 2008).

Part 5: Services to particular groups of patients

Chapter 45: Collection and delivery services

Royal Pharmaceutical Society of Great Britain 2004. 2004 Fitness to practice and legal affairs directorate fact sheet: seven. Prescription collection, home delivery and repeat medication services, November 2004. Royal Pharmaceutical Society of Great Britain, London.

Royal Pharmaceutical Society of Great Britain 2006. 2006 Guidance for Internet pharmacy services, March 2006. Royal Pharmaceutical Society of Great Britain, London.

Royal Pharmaceutical Society of Great Britain. Medicines, ethics and practice – a guide for pharmacists, current edition. Royal Pharmaceutical Society of Great Britain, London.

Chapter 46: Concordance

Berry D 2004 Risk, communication and health psychology. Open University Press, Maidenhead.

Bond C 2004 Concordance: a partnership in medicine taking. Pharmaceutical Press, London.

Britten N, Stevenson FA, Barry CA et al. 2000 Misunderstandings in prescribing decisions in general practice: qualitative study. *BMJ* 320: 484—488.

Charnock D, Shepperd S, Needham G et al. 1999 Discern: an instrument for judging the quality of written consumer health information on treatment choices. *Journal of Health Epidemiology and Community Health* 53: 105—111.

Clyne W, Granby T, Picton C 2007, A competency framework for shared decision-making with patients: achieving concordance for taking medicines, first edn, January 2007. NPC Plus, Keele. Online. Available: http://www.npc.co.uk/med_partnership/resource/our-publications/concordant.html (accessed 15 October 2008).

Coulter A 1997 Partnerships with patients: the pros and cons of shared clinical decision-making. *Journal of Health Services Research and Policy* 2: 112—121.

Coulter A, Ellins J, Swain D et al. 2006 Assessing the quality of information to support people in making decisions about their health and healthcare. Picker Institute, Oxford.

DIPEx Database of individual patient experiences of illness and health. Online. Available: http://www.healthtalkonline.org/ and http://www.

youthhealthtalk.org/. (both accessed 15 October 2008).

Gigerenzer G, Edwards A 2003 Simple tools for understanding risks: from innumeracy to insight. *BMJ* 327: 741—744.

Haynes RB, Montague P, Oliver T et al 2001. Interventions for helping patients to follow prescriptions for medications (Cochrane Review). Cochrane Library, Issue 2. Oxford Update Software, Oxford.

IPDAS Collaboration. International patient decision aid standards (IPDAS). Online. Available: http://ipdas.ohri.ca/ (accessed 15 October 2008).

Kurtz SM, Silverman JD 1996 The Calgary–Cambridge referenced observations guides: an aid to defining the curriculum and organising the teaching in communication training programmes. *Medical Education* 30: 83—89.

Lewin SA, Skea ZC, Entwistle V et al 2001 Interventions for providers to promote a patient-centred approach in clinical consultations. Cochrane Database of Systematic Reviews, Issue 4. article no. CD003267. DOI:10.1002/14651858.

Marinker M, Blenkinsopp A, Bond C et al. 1997 From compliance to concordance: achieving shared goals in medicine taking. A joint report by the Royal Pharmaceutical Society of Great Britain and Merck, Sharpe and Dohme. Royal Pharmaceutical Society, London.

O'Connor AM, Stacey D, Entwistle V et al 2003. Decisions aids for people facing health treatment or screening decisions. Cochrane Database of Systematic Reviews, Issue 1. Article no. CD001431. DOI:10.1002/14651858.

Ottawa Health Research Institute. Patient Decision Aids. Online. Available: http://decisionaid.ohri.ca/index.html. (accessed 15 October 2008).

Raynor DK, Blenkinsopp A, Knapp P et al. 2007 A systematic review of quantitative and qualitative research on the role and effectiveness of written information available to patients about individual medicines. *Health Technology Assessment* 11(5)(5): 1—178.

Simpson SH, Eurich DT, Majumdar SR et al. 2006 A meta-analysis of the association between adherence to drug therapy and mortality. *BMJ* 333: 15 Online. Available: http://bmj.bmjjournals.com/cgi/content/abstract/333/7557/15.

Stevenson FA, Cox K, Britten N et al. 2004 A systematic review of the research on communication between patients and health care professionals about medicines: the consequences for concordance. *Health Expectations* 7: 235—245.

Stewart MA 1995 Effective physician–patient communication and health outcomes: a review. *Canadian Medical Association Journal* 152: 1423—1433.

Weiss MC 2007 The informed patient: friend or foe? *Pharmaceutical Journal* 278: 143—146.

Weiss MC, Britten N 2003 What is concordance? *Pharmaceutical Journal* 271: 493.

Chapter 47 Monitoring the patient

Books

Randall M, Neil KE 2004 Disease management. Pharmaceutical Press, London.

Sexton J, Nickless G, Green C 2006 Pharmaceutical care made easy. Pharmaceutical Press, London.

Websites

MHRA Black Triangle list. Online. Available: http://www.mhra.gov.uk/ Safetyinformation/ Howwemonitorthesafetyofproducts/ Medicines/BlackTriangleproducts/ index.htm (accessed 15 October 2008), 2001.

MHRA Yellow Card Scheme. Online. Available: http://yellowcard.mhra. gov.uk/ (accessed 15 October 2008).

PSNC website for Advanced Services 2001. Online. Available: http://www. psnc.org.uk/pages/advanced_services. html. (accessed 15 October 2008).

PSNC website for MUR forms. Online. Available: http://www.psnc.org.uk/ pages/mur_forms.html. (accessed 15 October 2008).

WHO regional monitoring center. Online. Available: http://www.who-umc.org. (accessed 15 October 2008).

Chapter 48 Services for vulnerable patients

Department of Health 1997, Consultation Paper: Who decides? HMSO, London.

Department of Health. 1999 National service framework for mental health. HMSO, London.

Department of Health. 2001 National service framework for older people. HMSO, London.

Department of Health. 2001 Medicines for older people: implementing medicines-related aspects of the NSF for older people. HMSO, London.

Department of Health. 2003 National service framework for children young people and maternity services. HMSO, London.

Department of Health. 2006 Protection of vulnerable adults scheme. HMSO, London.

Hudson SA 1997 Pharmaceutical care of the elderly. *Pharmaceutical Journal* 259: 686—688.

Livingston S 2003 The older patient. *Pharmaceutical Journal* 270: 862—863.

Livingston S 2003 Effective interventions to support medicine use in older people. *Pharmaceutical Journal* 270: 893—895.

Livingston S 2003 Falls prevention and management. *Pharmaceutical Journal* 271: 49—50.

National Prescribing Centre 2000, Prescribing for children. MeReC Bulletin 11(2):5–8.

National Prescribing Centre 2000, Prescribing for the older person. MeReC Bulletin 11(10):37–40.

Royal Pharmaceutical Society of Great Britain. 2000 Caring for people with mental health problems. *Pharmaceutical Journal* 265: 391—392.

Royal Pharmaceutical Society of Great Britain. 2003 The administration and control of medicine in care homes and children's services. Royal Pharmaceutical Society of Great Britain, London.

Royal Pharmaceutical Society of Great Britain. 2003 Practice guidance

advisory services to care homes. Royal Pharmaceutical Society of Great Britain, London.

Royal Pharmaceutical Society of Great Britain. 2005 Practice guidance for the provision of printed medication administration record charts by community pharmacists for use in health and social care settings. Royal Pharmaceutical Society of Great Britain, London.

Royal Pharmaceutical Society of Great Britain. 2006 Guidance on child protection. Royal Pharmaceutical Society of Great Britain, London.

Royal Pharmaceutical Society of Great Britain. 2007 Guidance on the protection of vulnerable adults. Royal Pharmaceutical Society of Great Britain, London.

United Kingdom Psychiatric Pharmacy Group1995 Community care: pharmaceutical care for people with enduring mental health needs. *Pharmaceutical Journal* 255: 501—503.

Chapter 49: Substance use and misuse

Berridge V, Edwards G 1998 Opium and the people, 2nd edn. Free Association Books, London.

Department of Health 2007 Drug misuse and dependence: guidelines on clinical management. Stationery Office, London. Online. Available: http:// www.nta.nhs.uk/areas/ Clinical_guidance/clinical_guidelines/ docs/clinical_guidelines_2007.pdf (accessed 15 October 2008).

Driver and Vehicle Licensing Agency 2008 At a glance guide to medical aspects of fitness to drive. DVLA, Swansea. Online. Available: http:// www.dvla.gov.uk./medical/ataglance. aspx. (accessed 15 October 2008).

Gelder M, Mayou R, Harrison P. 2006 Misuse of alcohol and drugs. *The shorter Oxford textbook of psychiatry.*

5th edn. Oxford University Press, Oxford.

Gossop M 2007 Living with drugs, 6th edn. Ashgate Publishing, Aldershot.

Gossop M, Marsden J, Stewart D 2001 NTORS (National Treatment Outcome Research Study) after five years: changes in substance use, health and criminal behaviour during the five years after intake. National Addiction Centre (Crown copyright), London. Online. Available: http://www.erpho. org.uk/Download/Public/5367/1/ ntors5yr.pdf. (accessed 15 October 2008).

Ksobiech K 2003 A meta-analysis of needle sharing, lending, and borrowing behaviors of needle exchange program attenders. *AIDS Education and Prevention* 15(3)(3): 257—268.

MacDonald M, Law M, Kaldor J et al. 2003 Effectiveness of needle and syringe programmes for preventing HIV transmission. *International Journal of Drug Policy* 14: 353—357.

Mathei C, Shkedy Z, Denis B et al. 2006 Evidence for a substantial role of sharing of injecting paraphernalia other than syringes/needles to the spread of hepatitis C among injecting drug users. *Journal of Viral Hepatitis* 13(8)(8): 560—570.

Neale J. 1999 Drug users' views of substitute prescribing conditions. *International Journal of Drug Policy* 10: 247—258.

Roberts K, Bryson SM 1999 The contribution of Glasgow pharmacists to the management of drug misuse. *Hospital Pharmacist* 6: 244—248.

Sheridan J, Strang J 2002 Drug misuse and community pharmacy. Taylor and Francis, Andover.

Stimson GV, Des Jarlais DC, Ball A 1998 Drug injecting and HIV infection. Taylor and Francis, London.

Walker M 2001 Shared care of opiate misusers in Berkshire. *Pharmaceutical Journal* 266: 547—552.

Ward J, Hall W, Mattick R 1999 Role of maintenance treatment in opioid dependence. *Lancet* 353: 221—226.

Wills S 2005 Drugs of abuse, 2nd edn. Pharmaceutical Press, London.

World Health Organization 2007 Expert Committee on Drug Dependence. 34th Report. World Health Organization, Geneva.

Appendix A2: Latin terms and abbreviations

Carter S 1975 Dispensing for pharmaceutical students, 13th edn. Pitman Medical, London.

Appendix A4: Presentation skills

Bradbury A 2006 Successful presentation skills, 3rd edn. Kogan Page, London.

Index

NB: Page numbers in **bold** refer to boxes, figures and tables